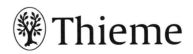

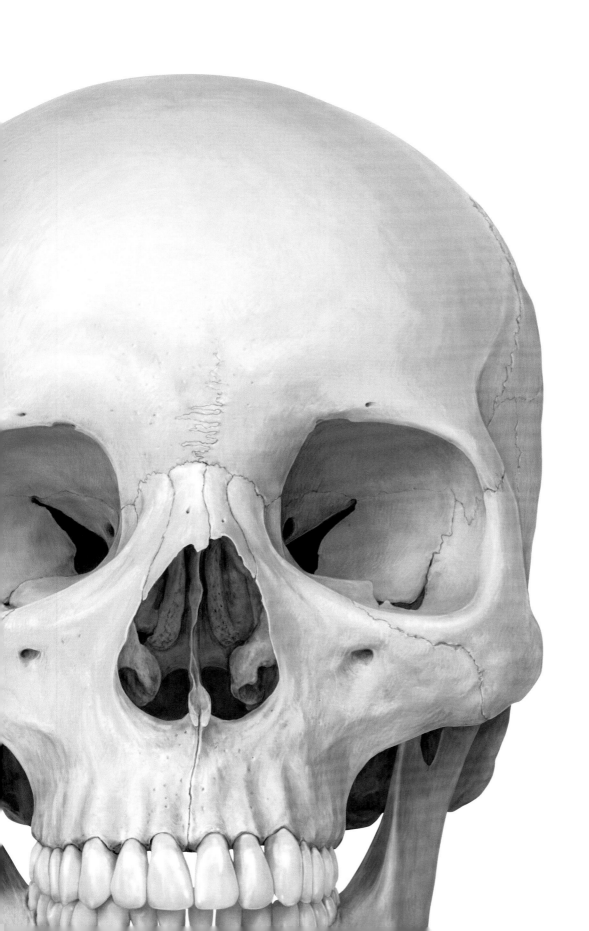

Head
and Neuroanatomy

THIEME
Atlas of Anatomy

Consulting Editors

Lawrence M. Ross, M.D., Ph.D.,
The University of Texas Medical School at Houston

Edward D. Lamperti, Ph.D.,
Boston University School of Medicine

Ethan Taub, M.D.
Neurosurgeon, Zurich

Authors

Michael Schuenke, M.D., Ph.D.,
University of Kiel Medical School

Erik Schulte, M.D.,
University of Mainz Medical School

Udo Schumacher, M.D.,
FRCPath, CBiol, FIBiol, DSc,
Hamburg University Medical Center

In collaboration with Juergen Rude

Illustrations by

Markus Voll

Karl Wesker

1182 Illustrations
72 Tables

Thieme
Stuttgart · New York

Library of Congress Cataloging-in-Publication Data is available from the publisher.

This book is an authorized and revised translation of the German edition published and copyrighted 2006 by Georg Thieme Verlag, Stuttgart, Germany. Title of the German edition: Schuenke et al.: Kopf und Neuroanatomie: Prometheus Lernatlas der Anatomie.

Illustrators
Markus Voll, Fürstenfeldbruck, Germany;
Karl Wesker, Berlin, Germany (homepage: www.karlwesker.de)

Translator
Terry Telger, Fort Worth, Texas, USA

© 2007 Georg Thieme Verlag
Rüdigerstraße 14
D-70469 Stuttgart
Germany
http://www.thieme.de
Thieme New York, 333 Seventh Avenue,
New York, NY 10001, USA
http://www.thieme.com

We wish to thank the leading manufacturer of anatomical teaching aids, 3B Scientific (www.3bscientific.com), for the kind support.

Typesetting by weyhing digital, Ostfildern-Kemnat
Printed in Germany by Appl, Wemding

Softcover
ISBN-10: 1-58890-441-5 (The Americas)
ISBN-13: 978-1-58890-441-6 (The Americas)
ISBN-10: 3-13-142121-5 (Rest of World)
ISBN-13: 978-3-13-142121-0 (Rest of World)

Hardcover
ISBN-10: 1-58890-361-3 (The Americas)
ISBN-13: 978-1-58890-361-7 (The Americas)
ISBN-10: 3-13-142101-0 (Rest of World)
ISBN-13: 978-3-13-142101-2 (Rest of World)

Important note: Medicine is an ever-changing science undergoing continual development. Research and clinical experience are continually expanding our knowledge, in particular our knowledge of proper treatment and drug therapy. Insofar as this book mentions any dosage or application, readers may rest assured that the authors, editors, and publishers have made every effort to ensure that such references are in accordance with **the state of knowledge at the time of production of the book**.

Nevertheless, this does not involve, imply, or express any guarantee or responsibility on the part of the publishers in respect to any dosage instructions and forms of applications stated in the book. **Every user is requested to examine carefully** the manufacturer's leaflets accompanying each drug and to check, if necessary in consultation with a physician or specialist, whether the dosage schedules mentioned therein or the contraindications stated by the manufacturers differ from the statements made in the present book. Such examination is particularly important with drugs that are either rarely used or have been newly released on the market. Every dosage schedule or every form of application used is entirely at the user's own risk and responsibility. The authors and publishers request every user to report to the publishers any discrepancies or inaccuracies noticed. If errors in this work are found after publication, errata will be posted at www.thieme.com on the product description page.

Foreword

Preface

Our enthusiasm for the THIEME Atlas of Anatomy began when each of us, independently, saw preliminary material from this Atlas. We were immediately captivated by the new approach, the conceptual organization, and by the stunning quality and detail of the images of the Atlas. We were delighted when the editors at Thieme offered us the oppertunity to cooperate with them in making this outstanding resource available to our students and colleagues in North America.

As consulting editors we were asked to review, for accuracy, the English edition of the THIEME Atlas of Anatomy. Our work involved a conversion of nomenclature to terms in common usage and some organizational changes to reflect pedagogical approaches in anatomy programs in North America. In all of this, we have tried diligently to remain faithful to the intentions and insights of the original authors.

We would like to thank the team at Thieme Medical Publishers who worked with us. Heartfelt thanks go firtst to Kelly Wright, Developmental Editor, and Cathrin E. Schulz, M.D., Executive Editor, for her assistance and checking and correcting our work and for their constant encouragement and availability. We are also grateful to Bridget Queenan, Developmental Editor, who provided a uniquely thorough, thoughtful, and cooperative approach from the moment she entered the process in the editing of this volume.

We would also like to extend our heartfelt thanks to Stefanie Langner, Production Manager, for preparing this volume with care and speed.

Lawrence M. Ross,
Edward D. Lamperti
Ethan Taub

As it started planning this Atlas, the publisher sought out the opinions and needs of students and lecturers in both the United States and Europe. The goal was to find out what the "ideal" atlas of anatomy should be—ideal for students wanting to learn from the atlas, master the extensive amounts of information while on a busy class schedule, and, in the process, acquire sound, up-to-date knowledge. The result of this work is this Atlas. The THIEME Atlas of Anatomy, unlike most other atlases, is a comprehensive educational tool that combines illustrations with explanatory text and summarizing tables, introducing clinical applications throughout, and presenting anatomical concepts in a step-by-step sequence that allows for the integration of both system-by-system and topographical views.

Since the THIEME Atlas of Anatomy is based on a fresh approach to the underlying subject matter itself, it was necessary to create for it an entirely new set of illustrations—a task that took eight years. Our goal was to provide illustrations that would compellingly demonstrate anatomical relations and concepts, revealing the underlying simplicity of the logic and order of human anatomy without sacrificing detail or aesthetics.

With the THIEME Atlas of Anatomy, it was our intention to create an atlas that would guide students in their initial study of anatomy, stimulate their enthusiasm for this intriguing and vitally important subject, and provide a reliable reference for experienced students and professionals alike.

"If you want to attain the possible, you must attempt the impossible"
(Rabindranath Tagore).

Michael Schünke, Erik Schulte, Udo Schumacher,
Markus Voll, and Karl Wesker

Acknowledgments

First we wish to thank our families. This atlas is dedicated to them.

We also thank Prof. Reinhard Gossrau, M.D., for his critical comments and suggestions. We are grateful to several colleagues who rendered valuable help in proofreading: Mrs. Gabriele Schünke, Jakob Fay, M.D., Ms. Claudia Dücker, Ms. Simin Rassouli, Ms. Heinke Teichmann, and Ms. Sylvia Zilles. We are also grateful to Dr. Julia Jürns-Kuhnke for helping with the figure labels.

We extend special thanks to Stephanie Gay and Bert Sender, who composed the layouts. Their ability to arrange the text and illustrations on facing pages for maximum clarity has contributed greatly to the quality of the Atlas.

We particularly acknowledge the efforts of those who handled this project on the publishing side:

Jürgen Lüthje, M.D., Ph.D., executive editor at Thieme Medical Publishers, has "made the impossible possible." He not only reconciled the wishes of the authors and artists with the demands of reality but also managed to keep a team of five people working together for years on a project whose goal was known to us from the beginning but whose full dimensions we came to appreciate only over time. He is deserving of our most sincere and heartfelt thanks.

Sabine Bartl, developmental editor, became a touchstone for the authors in the best sense of the word. She was able to determine whether a beginning student, and thus one who is not (yet) a professional, could clearly appreciate the logic of the presentation. The authors are indebted to her.

We are grateful to Antje Bühl, who was there from the beginning as project assistant, working "behind the scenes" on numerous tasks such as repeated proofreading and helping to arrange the figure labels.

We owe a great dept of thanks to Martin Spencker, Managing Director of Educational Publications at Thieme, especially to his ability to make quick and unconventional decisions when dealing with problems and uncertainties. His openness to all the concerns of the authors and artists established conditions for a cooperative partnership.

Without exception, our collaboration with the entire staff at Thieme Medical Publishers was consistently pleasant and cordial. Unfortunately we do not have room to list everyone who helped in the publication of this atlas, and we must limit our acknowledgments to a few colleagues who made a particularly notable contribution: Rainer Zepf and Martin Waletzko for support in all technical matters; Susanne Tochtermann-Wenzel and Manfred Lehnert, representing all those who were involved in the production of the book; Almut Leopold for the Index; Marie-Luise Kürschner and her team for creating the cover design; to Birgit Carlsen and Anne Döbler, representing all those who handled marketing, sales, and promotion.

The Authors

Table of Contents

Head

Neuroanatomy

10 Sectional Anatomy of the Brain

11 Autonomic Nervous System

12 Functional Systems

Appendix

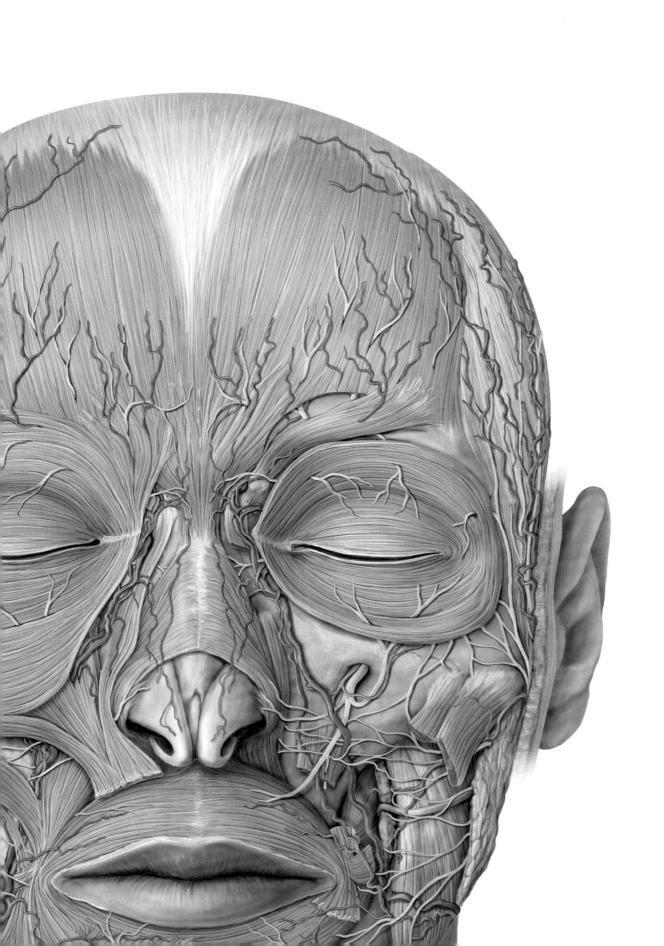

Head

1.1   Skull, Lateral View

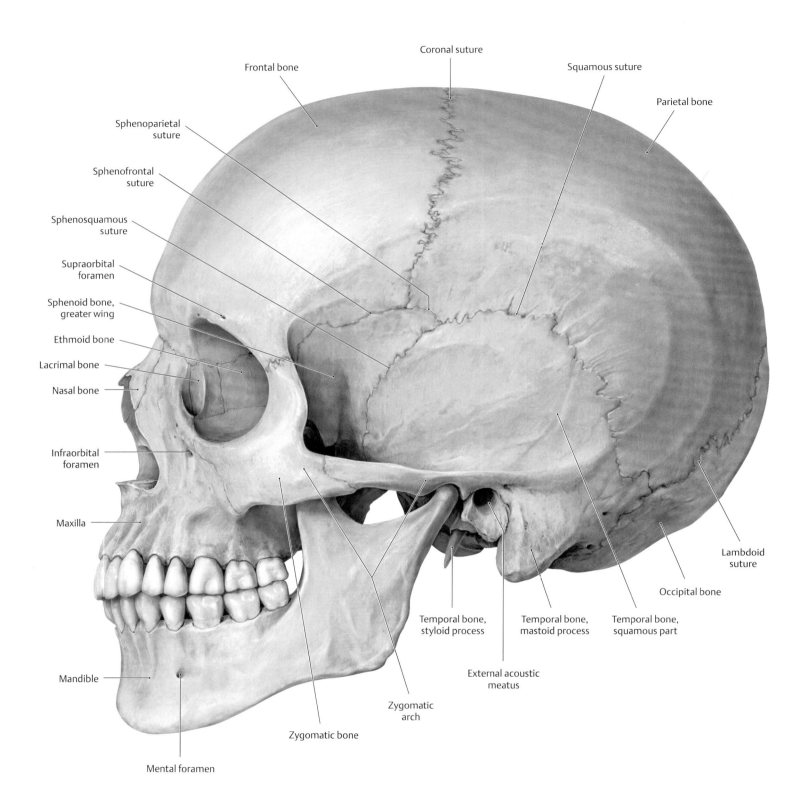

Coronal suture

Frontal bone

Squamous suture

Parietal bone

Sphenoparietal suture

Sphenofrontal suture

Sphenosquamous suture

Supraorbital foramen

Sphenoid bone, greater wing

Ethmoid bone

Lacrimal bone

Nasal bone

Infraorbital foramen

Maxilla

Mandible

Mental foramen

Zygomatic bone

Zygomatic arch

Temporal bone, styloid process

External acoustic meatus

Temporal bone, mastoid process

Temporal bone, squamous part

Occipital bone

Lambdoid suture

A Lateral view of the skull (cranium)

Left lateral view. This view was selected as an introduction to the skull because it displays the greatest number of cranial bones (indicated by different colors in **B**). The individual bones and their salient features as well as the cranial sutures and apertures are described in the units that follow. This unit reviews the principal structures of the lateral aspect of the skull. The chapter as a whole is intended to familiarize the reader with the names of the cranial bones before proceeding to finer anatomical details and the relationships of the bones to one another. The teeth are described in a separate unit (see p. 36 ff).

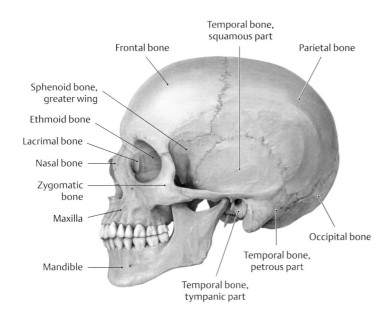

Temporal bone, squamous part

Frontal bone

Parietal bone

Sphenoid bone, greater wing

Ethmoid bone

Lacrimal bone

Nasal bone

Zygomatic bone

Maxilla

Mandible

Occipital bone

Temporal bone, petrous part

Temporal bone, tympanic part

B Lateral view of the cranial bones
Left lateral view. The bones are shown in different colors to demonstrate more clearly their extents and boundaries.

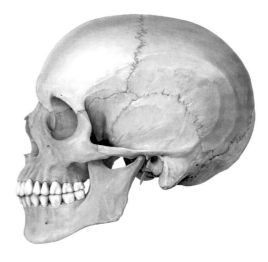

C Bones of the neurocranium (gray) and viscerocranium (orange)
Left lateral view. The skull forms a bony capsule that encloses the brain, sensory organs, and viscera of the head. The greater size of the neurocranium (cranial vault) relative to the viscerocranium (facial skeleton) is a typical primate feature directly correlated with the larger primate brain.

E Bones of the neurocranium and viscerocranium

Neurocranium (gray)	Viscerocranium (orange)
• Frontal bone • Sphenoid bone (excluding the pterygoid process) • Temporal bone (squamous part, petrous part) • Parietal bone • Occipital bone • Ethmoid bone (cribriform plate)	• Nasal bone • Lacrimal bone • Ethmoid bone (excluding the cribriform plate) • Sphenoid bone (pterygoid process) • Maxilla • Zygomatic bone • Temporal bone (tympanic part, styloid process) • Mandible • Vomer • Inferior nasal turbinate • Palatine bone • Hyoid bone (see p. 31)

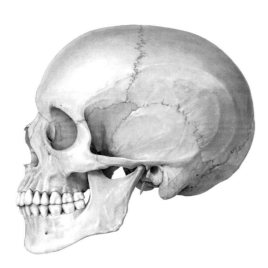

D Ossification of the cranial bones
Left lateral view. The bones of the skull either develop directly from mesenchymal connective tissue (intramembranous ossification, gray) or form indirectly by the ossification of a cartilaginous model (enchondral ossification, blue). Elements derived from intramembranous and endochondral ossification (desmocranium, chondrocranium) may fuse together to form a single bone (e.g., the occipital bone, temporal bone, and sphenoid bone).
The clavicle is the only tubular bone that undergoes membranous ossification. This explains why congenital defects of *intramembranous* ossification affect both the skull and clavicle *(cleidocranial dysostosis).*

F Bones of the desmocranium and chondrocranium

Desmocranium (gray)	Chondrocranium (blue)
• Nasal bone • Lacrimal bone • Maxilla • Mandible • Zygomatic bone • Frontal bone • Parietal bone • Occipital bone (upper part of the squama) • Temporal bone (squamous part, tympanic part) • Palatine bone • Vomer	• Ethmoid bone • Sphenoid bone (excluding the medial plate of the pterygoid process) • Temporal bone (petrous and mastoid parts, styloid process) • Occipital bone (excluding the upper part of the squama) • Inferior nasal turbinate • Hyoid bone (see p. 31)

3

1.2 Skull, Anterior View

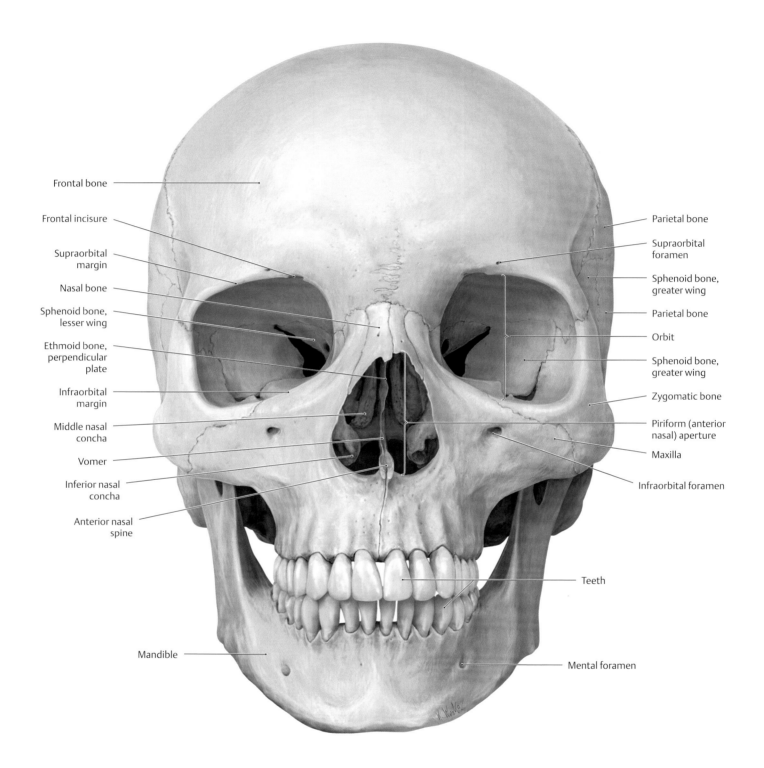

Frontal bone

Frontal incisure

Supraorbital margin

Nasal bone

Sphenoid bone, lesser wing

Ethmoid bone, perpendicular plate

Infraorbital margin

Middle nasal concha

Vomer

Inferior nasal concha

Anterior nasal spine

Mandible

Parietal bone

Supraorbital foramen

Sphenoid bone, greater wing

Parietal bone

Orbit

Sphenoid bone, greater wing

Zygomatic bone

Piriform (anterior nasal) aperture

Maxilla

Infraorbital foramen

Teeth

Mental foramen

A Anterior view of the skull
The boundaries of the facial skeleton (viscerocranium) can be clearly appreciated in this view (the individual bones are shown in **B**). The bony margins of the anterior nasal aperture mark the start of the respiratory tract in the skull. The nasal cavity, like the orbits, contains a sensory organ (the olfactory mucosa). The *paranasal sinuses* are shown schematically in **C**. The anterior view of the skull also displays the three clinically important openings through which sensory nerves pass to supply the face: the supraorbital foramen, infraorbital foramen, and mental foramen (see pp. 77 and 93).

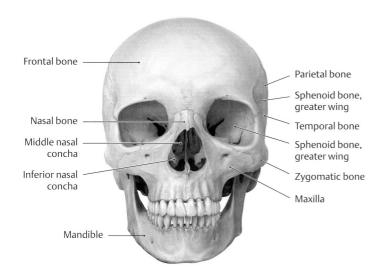

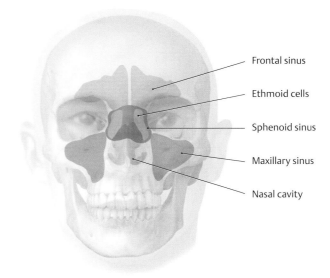

B Cranial bones, anterior view

C Paranasal sinuses: pneumatization lightens the bone

Anterior view. Some of the bones of the facial skeleton are pneumatized, i.e., they contain air-filled cavities that reduce the total weight of the bone. These cavities, called the paranasal sinuses, communicate with the nasal cavity and, like it, are lined by ciliated respiratory epithelium. Inflammations of the paranasal sinuses (sinusitis) and associated complaints are very common. Because some of the pain of sinusitis is projected to the skin overlying the sinuses, it is helpful to know the projections of the sinuses onto the surface of the skull.

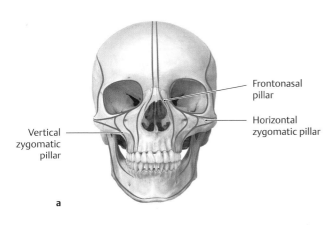

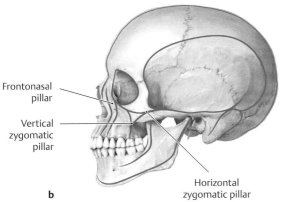

D Principal lines of force (blue) in the facial skeleton

a Anterior view, **b** lateral view. The pneumatized paranasal sinuses (**C**) have a mechanical counterpart in the thickened bony "pillars" of the facial skeleton, which partially bound the sinuses. These pillars develop along the principal lines of force in response to local mechanical stresses (e.g., masticatory pressures). In visual terms, the frame-like construction of the facial skeleton may be likened to that of a frame house: The paranasal sinuses represent the rooms while the pillars (placed along major lines of force) represent the supporting columns.

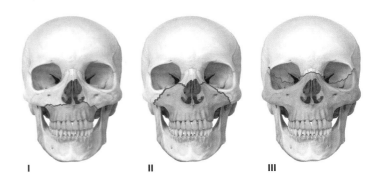

E LeFort classification of midfacial fractures

The frame-like construction of the facial skeleton leads to characteristic patterns of fracture lines in the midfacial region (LeFort I, II, and III).

LeFort I: This fracture line runs across the maxilla and above the hard palate. The maxilla is separated from the upper facial skeleton, disrupting the integrity of the maxillary sinus (*low transverse fracture*).

LeFort II: The fracture line passes across the nasal root, ethmoid bone, maxilla, and zygomatic bone, creating a *pyramid fracture* that disrupts the integrity of the orbit.

LeFort III: The facial skeleton is separated from the base of the skull. The main fracture line passes through the orbits, and the fracture may additionally involve the ethmoid bones, frontal sinuses, sphenoid sinuses, and zygomatic bones.

1.3   Skull, Posterior View and Cranial Sutures

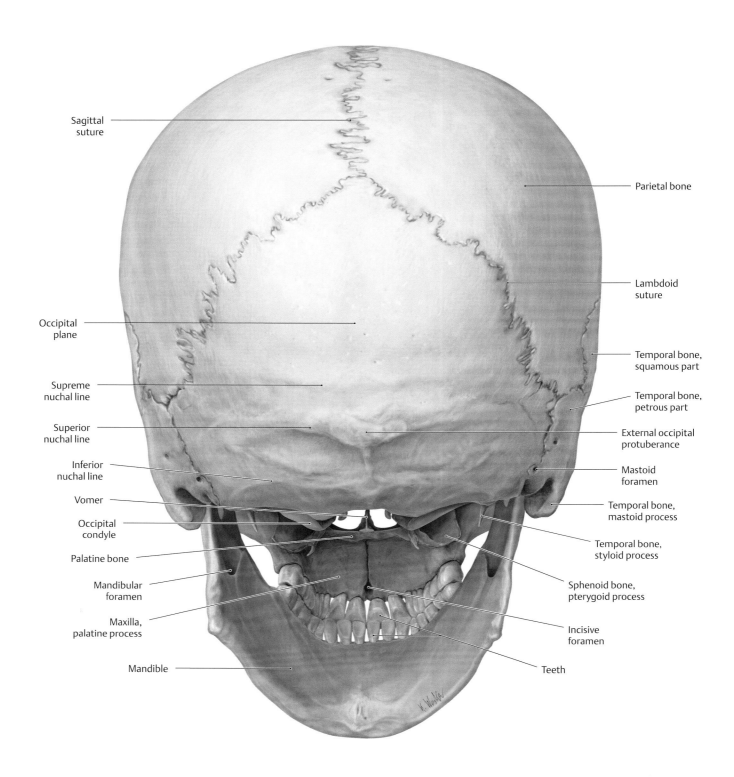

Sagittal suture

Parietal bone

Lambdoid suture

Occipital plane

Temporal bone, squamous part

Supreme nuchal line

Temporal bone, petrous part

Superior nuchal line

External occipital protuberance

Inferior nuchal line

Mastoid foramen

Vomer

Temporal bone, mastoid process

Occipital condyle

Temporal bone, styloid process

Palatine bone

Sphenoid bone, pterygoid process

Mandibular foramen

Maxilla, palatine process

Incisive foramen

Mandible

Teeth

A   Posterior view of the skull
The occipital bone, which is dominant in this view, articulates with the parietal bones, to which it is connected by the lambdoid suture. The cranial sutures are a special type of syndesmosis (= ligamentous attach- ments that ossify with age, see **F**). The outer surface of the occipital bone is contoured by muscular origins and insertions: the inferior, su- perior, and supreme nuchal lines.

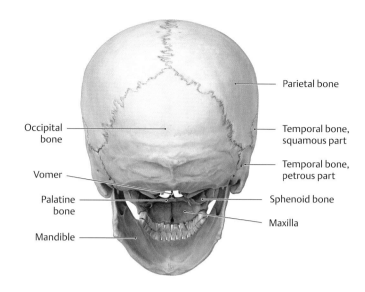

B Posterior view of the cranial bones

Note: The temporal bone consists of two main parts based on its embryonic development: a squamous part and a petrous part (see p. 22). The petrous part of the temporal bone is also referred to as the "petrous bone."

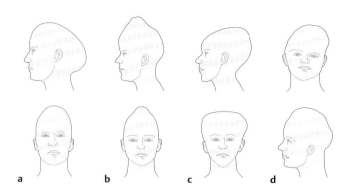

D Cranial deformities due to the premature closure of cranial sutures

The premature closure of a cranial suture (craniosynostosis) may lead to characteristic cranial deformities. The following sutures may close prematurely, resulting in various cranial shapes:

a Sagittal suture: scaphocephaly (long, narrow skull)
b Coronal suture: oxycephaly (pointed skull)
c Frontal suture: trigonocephaly (triangular skull)
d Asymmetrical suture closure, usually involving the coronal suture: plagiocephaly (asymmetrical skull)

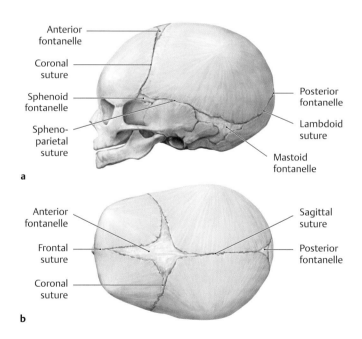

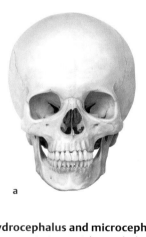
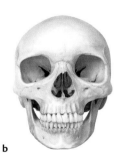

E Hydrocephalus and microcephaly

a Characteristic cranial morphology in *hydrocephalus*. When the brain becomes dilated due to cerebrospinal fluid accumulation *before* the cranial sutures ossify (hydrocephalus, "water on the brain"), the neurocranium will expand while the facial skeleton remains unchanged.
b *Microcephaly* results from premature closure of the cranial sutures. It is characterized by a small neurocranium with relatively large orbits.

C The neonatal skull

a Left lateral view, **b** superior view.

The flat cranial bones must grow as the brain expands, and so the sutures between them must remain open for some time (see **F**). In the neonate, there are areas between the still-growing cranial bones that are not occupied by bone: the fontanelles. They close at different times (the sphenoid fontanelle in about the 6th month of life, the mastoid fontanelle in the 18th month, the anterior fontanelle in the 36th month). The *posterior fontanelle* provides a reference point for describing the position of the fetal head during childbirth, and the *anterior fontanelle* provides a possible access site for drawing a cerebrospinal fluid sample in infants (e.g., in suspected meningitis).

F Age at which the principal sutures ossify

Suture	Age at ossification
Frontal suture	Childhood
Sagittal suture	20–30 years of age
Coronal suture	30–40 years of age
Lambdoid suture	40–50 years of age

1.4 Exterior and Interior of the Calvaria

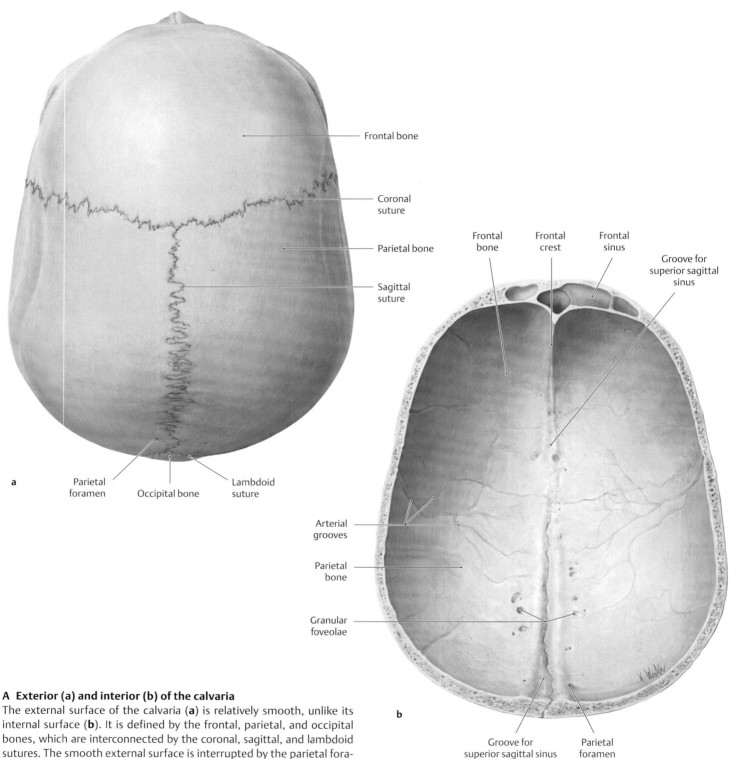

A Exterior (a) and interior (b) of the calvaria

The external surface of the calvaria (**a**) is relatively smooth, unlike its internal surface (**b**). It is defined by the frontal, parietal, and occipital bones, which are interconnected by the coronal, sagittal, and lambdoid sutures. The smooth external surface is interrupted by the parietal foramen, which gives passage to the parietal emissary vein (see **F**). The internal surface of the calvaria also bears a number of pits and grooves:

- The granular foveolae (small pits in the inner surface of the skull caused by saccular protrusions of the arachnoid membrane covering the brain)
- The groove for the superior sagittal sinus (a dural venous sinus of the brain, see **F** and p. 65)

- The arterial grooves (which mark the positions of the arterial vessels of the dura mater, such as the middle meningeal artery which supplies most of the dura mater and overlying bone)
- The frontal crest (which gives attachment to the falx cerebri, a sickle-shaped fold of dura mater between the cerebral hemispheres, see p. 188).

The frontal sinus in the frontal bone is also visible in the interior view.

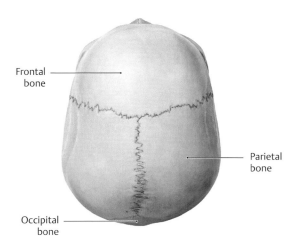

B Exterior of the calvaria viewed from above

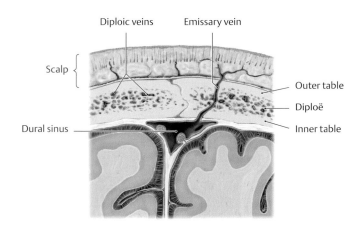

C The scalp and calvaria
Note the three-layered structure of the calvaria, consisting of the outer table, the diploë, and the inner table.
The diploë has a spongy structure and contains red (blood-forming) bone marrow. With a plasmacytoma (malignant transformation of certain white blood cells), many small nests of tumor cells may destroy the surrounding bony trabeculae, and radiographs will demonstrate multiple lucent areas ("punched-out lesions") in the skull. Vessels called *emissary veins* may pass through the calvaria to connect the venous sinuses of the brain with the veins of the scalp (see panels **E** and **F**).

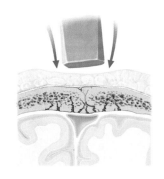

D Sensitivity of the inner table to trauma
The inner table of the calvaria is very sensitive to external trauma and may fracture even when the outer table remains intact (look for corresponding evidence on CT Images).

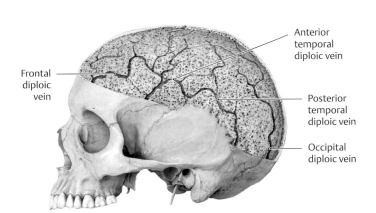

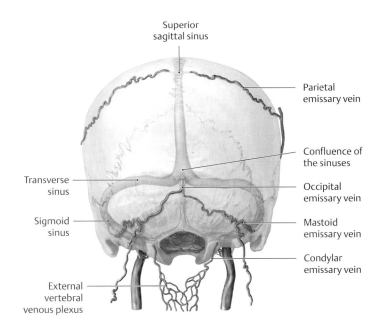

E Diploic veins in the calvaria
The diploic veins are located in the cancellous or spongy tissue of the cranial bones (the diploë) and are visible when the outer table is removed. The diploic veins communicate with the dural venous sinuses and scalp veins by way of the emissary veins, which create a potential route for the spread of infection.

F Emissary veins of the occiput
Emissary veins establish a direct connection between the dural venous sinuses and the extracranial veins. They pass through preformed cranial openings such as the parietal foramen and mastoid foramen. The emissary veins are of clinical interest because they may allow bacteria from the scalp to enter the skull along these veins and infect the dura mater, causing meningitis.

1.5 Base of the Skull, External View

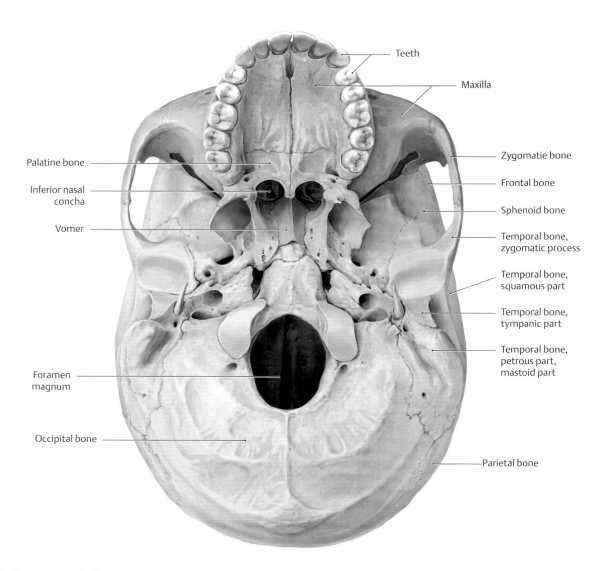

A Bones of the base of the skull
Inferior view. The base of the skull is composed of a mosaic-like assembly of various bones. It is helpful to review the shape and location of these bones before studying further details.

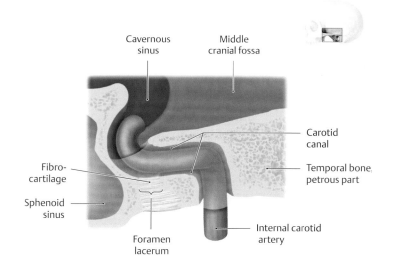

B Relationship of the foramen lacerum to the carotid canal and internal carotid artery
Left lateral view. The foramen lacerum is not a true aperture, being occluded in life by a layer of fibrocartilage; it appears as an opening only in the dried skull. The foramen lacerum is closely related to the carotid canal and to the internal carotid artery that traverses the canal. The greater petrosal nerve and deep petrosal nerve pass through the foramen lacerum (see pp. 81, 85, and 90).

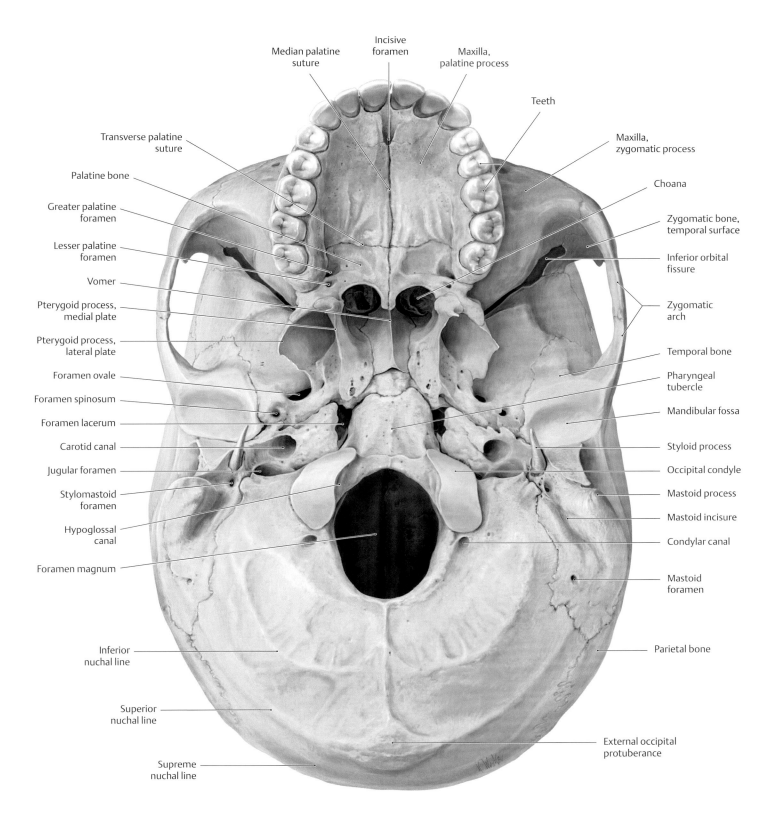

Median palatine
suture

Incisive
foramen

Maxilla,
palatine process

Teeth

Transverse palatine
suture

Maxilla,
zygomatic process

Choana

Palatine bone

Zygomatic bone,
temporal surface

Greater palatine
foramen

Inferior orbital
fissure

Lesser palatine
foramen

Zygomatic
arch

Vomer

Pterygoid process,
medial plate

Temporal bone

Pterygoid process,
lateral plate

Pharyngeal
tubercle

Foramen ovale

Mandibular fossa

Foramen spinosum

Styloid process

Foramen lacerum

Occipital condyle

Carotid canal

Jugular foramen

Mastoid process

Stylomastoid
foramen

Mastoid incisure

Hypoglossal
canal

Condylar canal

Foramen magnum

Mastoid
foramen

Inferior
nuchal line

Parietal bone

Superior
nuchal line

External occipital
protuberance

Supreme
nuchal line

C The basal aspect of the skull

Inferior view. The principal external features of the base of the skull are labeled. Note particularly the openings that transmit nerves and vessels. With abnormalities of bone growth, these openings may remain too small or may become narrowed, compressing the neurovascular structures that pass through them. If the optic canal fails to grow normally, it may compress and damage the optic nerve, resulting in visual field defects. The symptoms associated with these lesions depend on the affected opening. All of the structures depicted here will be considered in more detail in subsequent pages.

1.6 Base of the Skull, Internal View

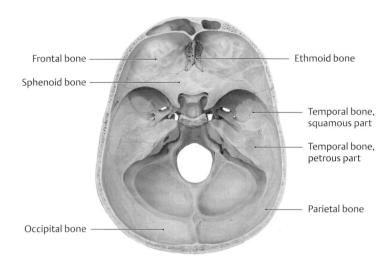

Frontal bone — Ethmoid bone

Sphenoid bone —

— Temporal bone, squamous part

— Temporal bone, petrous part

— Parietal bone

Occipital bone —

A Bones of the base of the skull, internal view
Different colors are used here to highlight the arrangement of bones in the base of the skull as seen from within the cranium.

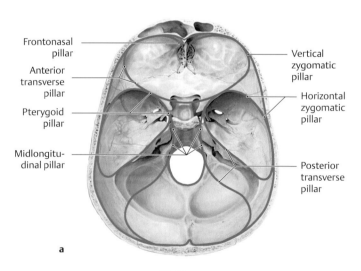

Frontonasal pillar —

Anterior transverse pillar

Pterygoid pillar

Midlongitu-dinal pillar

— Vertical zygomatic pillar

— Horizontal zygomatic pillar

— Posterior transverse pillar

a

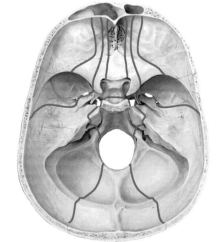

b

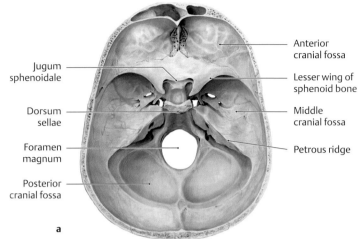

Jugum sphenoidale —

— Anterior cranial fossa

— Lesser wing of sphenoid bone

Dorsum sellae —

— Middle cranial fossa

Foramen magnum —

— Petrous ridge

Posterior cranial fossa —

a

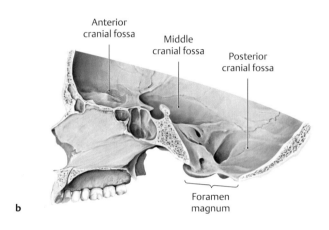

Anterior cranial fossa

Middle cranial fossa

Posterior cranial fossa

Foramen magnum

b

B The cranial fossae
a Interior view, **b** midsagittal section. The interior of the skull base is not flat but is deepened to form three successive fossae: the anterior, middle, and posterior cranial fossae. These depressions become progressively deeper in the frontal-to-occipital direction, forming a terraced arrangement that is displayed most clearly in **b**.
The cranial fossae are bounded by the following structures:

- Anterior to middle: the lesser wings of the sphenoid bone and the jugum sphenoidale.
- Middle to posterior: the superior border (ridge) of the petrous part of the temporal bone and the dorsum sellae.

C Base of the skull: principal lines of force and common fracture lines
a Principal lines of force, **b** common fracture lines (interior views). In response to masticatory pressures and other mechanical stresses, the bones of the skull base are thickened to form "pillars" along the principal lines of force (compare with the force distribution in the anterior view on p. 5). The intervening areas that are not thickened are sites of predilection for bone fractures, resulting in the typical patterns of basal skull fracture lines shown here. An analogous phenomenon of typical fracture lines is found in the midfacial region (see the anterior views of LeFort fractures on p. 5).

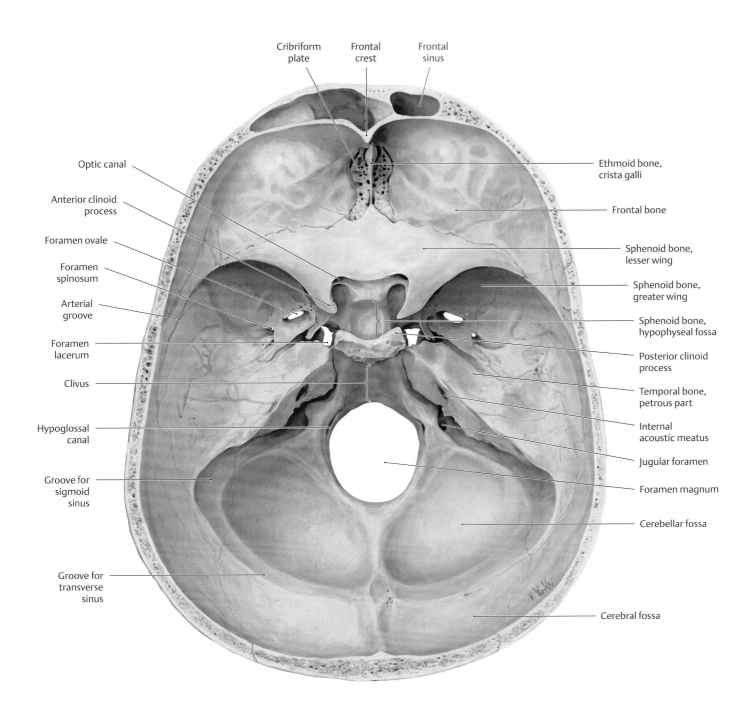

Cribriform plate • Frontal crest • Frontal sinus

Optic canal

Anterior clinoid process

Foramen ovale

Foramen spinosum

Arterial groove

Foramen lacerum

Clivus

Hypoglossal canal

Groove for sigmoid sinus

Groove for transverse sinus

Ethmoid bone, crista galli

Frontal bone

Sphenoid bone, lesser wing

Sphenoid bone, greater wing

Sphenoid bone, hypophyseal fossa

Posterior clinoid process

Temporal bone, petrous part

Internal acoustic meatus

Jugular foramen

Foramen magnum

Cerebellar fossa

Cerebral fossa

D Interior of the base of the skull

It is interesting to compare the openings in the interior of the base of the skull with the openings visible in the external view (see p. 11). These openings do not always coincide because some neurovascular structures change direction when passing through the bone or pursue a relatively long intraosseous course. An example of this is the internal acoustic meatus, through which the facial nerve, among other structures, passes from the interior of the skull into the petrous part of the temporal bone. Most of its fibers then leave the petrous bone through the stylomastoid foramen, which is visible from the external aspect (see pp. 80, 91, and 149 for further details).

In learning the sites where neurovascular structures pass through the base of the skull, it is helpful initially to note whether these sites are located in the anterior, middle, or posterior cranial fossa. The arrangement of the cranial fossae is shown in **B**. The cribriform plate of the ethmoid bone connects the nasal cavity with the anterior cranial fossa and is perforated by numerous foramina for the passage of the olfactory fibers (see p. 116).

Note: Because the bone is so thin in this area, a frontal head injury may easily fracture the cribriform plate and lacerate the dura mater, allowing cerebrospinal fluid to enter the nose. This poses a risk of meningitis, as bacteria from the nonsterile nasal cavity may enter the sterile cerebrospinal fluid.

1.7 Orbit:
Bones and Openings for Neurovascular Structures

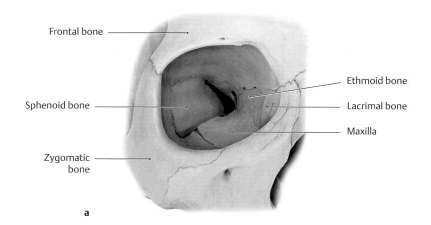

Frontal bone

Ethmoid bone

Sphenoid bone

Lacrimal bone

Maxilla

Zygomatic bone

a

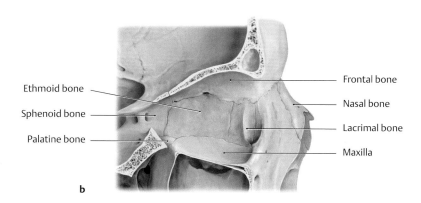

Ethmoid bone

Sphenoid bone

Palatine bone

Frontal bone

Nasal bone

Lacrimal bone

Maxilla

b

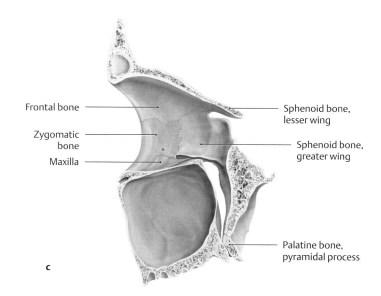

Frontal bone

Sphenoid bone, lesser wing

Zygomatic bone

Maxilla

Sphenoid bone, greater wing

Palatine bone, pyramidal process

c

A Bones of the right orbit

Anterior view (**a**), lateral view (**b**), and medial view (**c**). The lateral orbital wall has been removed in **b**, and the medial orbital wall has been removed in **c**.

The orbit is formed by seven different bones (indicated here by color shading): the frontal bone, zygomatic bone, maxilla, ethmoid bone, sphenoid bone (see **a** and **c**), and also the lacrimal bone and palatine bone, which are visible only in the medial view (see **b**).

The present unit deals with the bony anatomy of the orbits themselves. The relationships of the orbits to each other are described in the next unit.

B Openings in the orbit for neurovascular structures

Note: The supraorbital foramen is an important site in routine clinical examinations because the examiner presses on the supraorbital rim with the thumb to test the sensory function of the supraorbital nerve. The supraorbital nerve is a terminal branch of the first division of the trigeminal nerve (CN V_1, see p. 76). When pain is present in the distribution of the trigeminal nerve, tenderness to pressure may be noted at the supraorbital site.

Opening or passage	Neurovascular structures
Optic canal	• Optic nerve (CN II) • Ophthalmic artery

Superior orbital fissure	• Oculomotor nerve (CN III)
	• Trochlear nerve (CN IV)
	• Ophthalmic nerve (CN V_1)
	  – Lacrimal nerve
	  – Frontal nerve
	  – Nasociliary nerve
	• Abducent nerve (CN VI)
	• Superior ophthalmic vein

Inferior orbital fissure	• Zygomatic nerve (CN V_2) • Inferior ophthalmic vein • Infraorbital artery, vein, and nerve (CN V_2)
Nasolacrimal canal	• Nasolacrimal duct
Infra-orbital canal	• Infraorbital artery, vein, and nerve
Supra-orbital foramen	• Supraorbital artery • Supraorbital nerve (lateral branch)
Frontal incisure	• Supratrochlear artery • Supraorbital nerve (medial branch)
Anterior ethmoidal foramen	• Anterior ethmoidal artery, vein, and nerve
Posterior ethmoidal foramen	• Posterior ethmoidal artery, vein, and nerve

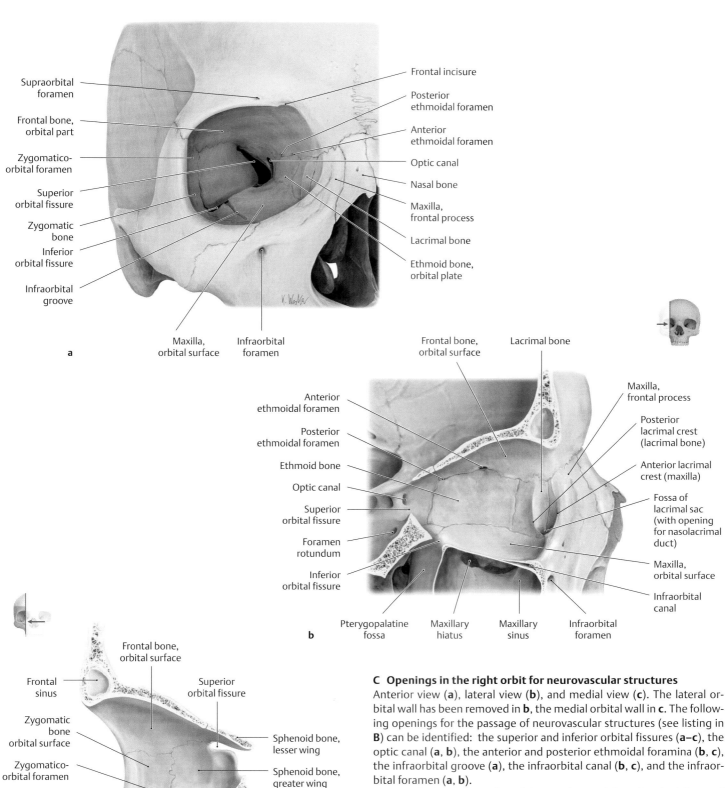

Supraorbital foramen

Frontal bone, orbital part

Zygomatico-orbital foramen

Superior orbital fissure

Zygomatic bone

Inferior orbital fissure

Infraorbital groove

Frontal incisure

Posterior ethmoidal foramen

Anterior ethmoidal foramen

Optic canal

Nasal bone

Maxilla, frontal process

Lacrimal bone

Ethmoid bone, orbital plate

Maxilla, orbital surface

Infraorbital foramen

a

Anterior ethmoidal foramen

Posterior ethmoidal foramen

Ethmoid bone

Optic canal

Superior orbital fissure

Foramen rotundum

Inferior orbital fissure

Frontal bone, orbital surface

Lacrimal bone

Maxilla, frontal process

Posterior lacrimal crest (lacrimal bone)

Anterior lacrimal crest (maxilla)

Fossa of lacrimal sac (with opening for nasolacrimal duct)

Maxilla, orbital surface

Infraorbital canal

Pterygopalatine fossa

Maxillary hiatus

Maxillary sinus

Infraorbital foramen

b

Frontal sinus

Frontal bone, orbital surface

Superior orbital fissure

Zygomatic bone orbital surface

Zygomatico-orbital foramen

Maxilla, orbital surface

Infraorbital canal

Inferior orbital fissure

Sphenoid bone, lesser wing

Sphenoid bone, greater wing

Maxillary sinus

Palatine bone, pyramidal process

c

C Openings in the right orbit for neurovascular structures

Anterior view (**a**), lateral view (**b**), and medial view (**c**). The lateral orbital wall has been removed in **b**, the medial orbital wall in **c**. The following openings for the passage of neurovascular structures (see listing in **B**) can be identified: the superior and inferior orbital fissures (**a–c**), the optic canal (**a**, **b**), the anterior and posterior ethmoidal foramina (**b**, **c**), the infraorbital groove (**a**), the infraorbital canal (**b**, **c**), and the infraorbital foramen (**a**, **b**).

Diagram **b** shows the orifice of the nasolacrimal duct, by which lacrimal fluid is conveyed to the inferior meatus of the nose.

The lateral view (**b**) demonstrates the funnel-like structure of the orbit, which functions like a socket to contain the eyeball and constrain its movements. The inferior orbital fissure opens into the pterygopalatine fossa, which borders on the posterior wall of the maxillary sinus. It contains the pterygopalatine ganglion, an important component of the parasympathetic nervous system (see pp. 81, 101). The upper part of the exposed maxillary sinus bears the ostium (in the maxillary hiatus) by which the sinus opens into the nasal cavity superior to the inferior concha (see pp. 20–21).

1.8 Orbit and Neighboring Structures

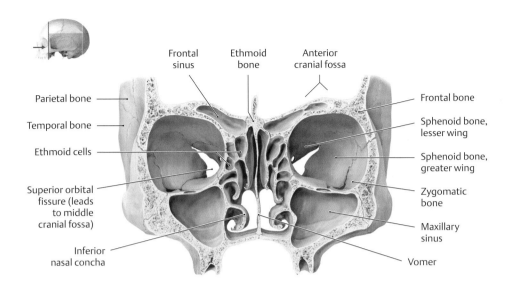

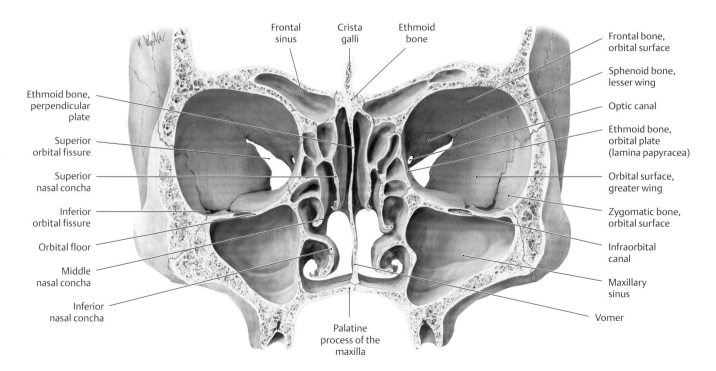

A Bones of the orbits and adjacent cavities

The color-coding here is the same as for the bones of the orbit on pp.14–15. These bones also form portions of the walls of neighboring cavities. The following adjacent structures are visible in the diagram:

- Anterior cranial fossa
- Frontal sinus
- Middle cranial fossa
- Ethmoid cells*
- Maxillary sinus

Disease processes may originate in the orbit and spread to these cavities, or originate in these cavities and spread to the orbit.

*The *Terminologia Anatomica* has dropped the term "ethmoid sinus" in favor of "ethmoid cells."

B Clinically important relationships between the orbits and surrounding structures

Relationship to the orbit	Neighboring structure
Inferior	• Maxillary sinus
Superior	• Frontal sinus • Anterior cranial fossa (contains the frontal lobes of the brain)
Medial	• Ethmoid cells

Deeper structures that have a clinically important relationship to the orbit:

- Sphenoid sinus
- Middle cranial fossa
- Optic chiasm
- Pituitary
- Cavernous sinus
- Pterygopalatine fossa

C Orbits and neighboring structures

Coronal section through both orbits, viewed from the front. The walls separating the orbit from the ethmoid cells (0.3 mm, lamina papyracea) and from the maxillary sinus (0.5 mm, orbital floor) are very thin. Thus, both of these walls are susceptible to fractures and provide routes for the spread of tumors and inflammatory processes into or out of the orbit. The superior orbital fissure communicates with the middle cranial fossa, and so several structures that are not pictured here—the sphenoid sinus, pituitary gland, and optic chiasm—are also closely related to the orbit.

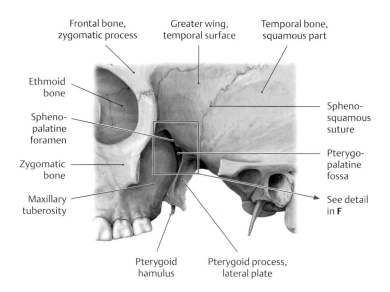

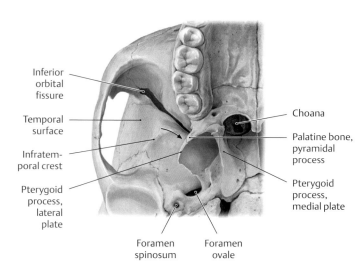

D Close-up view of the left pterygopalatine fossa

Lateral view. The pterygopalatine fossa is a crossroads between the middle cranial fossa, orbit, and nose, being traversed by many nerves and vessels that supply these structures. The pterygopalatine fossa is continuous laterally with the infratemporal fossa. This diagram shows the lateral approach to the pterygopalatine fossa through the infratemporal fossa, which is utilized in surgical operations on tumors in this region (e.g., nasopharyngeal fibroma).

E Structures adjacent to the right pterygopalatine

Inferior view. The arrow indicates the approach to the pterygopalatine fossa from the skull base. The fossa itself (not visible in this view) is lateral to the lateral plate of the pterygoid process of the sphenoid bone.

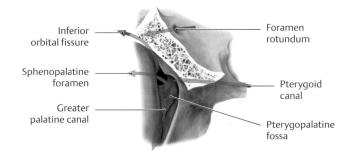

F Connections of the left pterygopalatine fossa with adjacent structures

Detail from **D**. The contents of the pterygopalatine fossa include the pterygopalatine ganglion (see pp. 81, 101), which is an important ganglion in the parasympathetic nervous system.

H Pathways to the pterygopalatine fossa

Pathways	From:	Transmitted structures
Foramen rotundum	Middle cranial fossa	• Maxillary nerve (CN V$_2$)
Pterygoid canal (Vidian canal)	Skull base (inferior surface)	• Greater petrosal nerve (parasympathetic branch of facial nerve) • Deep petrosal nerve (sympathetic fibers from carotid plexus) • Artery of pterygoid canal with accompaning veins • Nerve of pterygoid canal
Greater palatine canal (foramen)	Palate	• Greater palatine nerve • Descending palatine artery • Greater palatine artery
Lesser palatine canals	Palate	• Lesser palatine nerves • Lesser palatine arteries (terminal branches of descending palatine artery)
Sphenopalatine foramen	Nasal cavity	• Sphenopalatine artery (plus accompanying veins) • Lateral and medial superior posterior nasal branches of the nasopalatine nerve (CN V$_2$)
Inferior orbital fissure	Orbit	• Infraorbital nerve • Zygomatic nerve • Orbital branches (of CN V$_2$) • Infraorbital artery (plus accompanying veins) • Inferior ophthalmic vein

G Structures bordering the pterygopalatine fossa

Direction	Bordering structure
Anterior	Maxillary tuberosity
Posterior	Pterygoid process
Medial	Perpendicular plate of the palatine bone
Lateral	Infratemporal fossa (via the pterygomaxillary fissure)
Superior	Greater wing of the sphenoid bone, junction with the inferior orbital fissure
Inferior	Retropharyngeal space

17

1.9 Nose: Nasal Skeleton

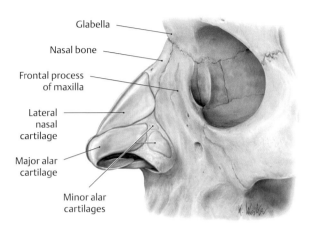

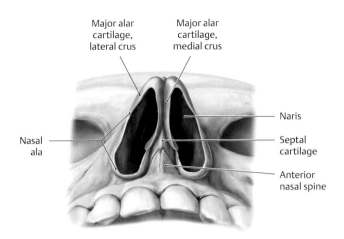

A Skeleton of the external nose

Left lateral view. The skeleton of the nose is composed of bone, cartilage, and connective tissue. Its upper portion is bony and frequently involved in midfacial fractures, while its lower, distal portion is cartilaginous and therefore more elastic and less susceptible to injury. The proximal lower portion of the nostrils (alae) is composed of connective tissue with small embedded pieces of cartilage. The lateral nasal cartilage is a winglike lateral expansion of the cartilaginous nasal septum rather than a separate piece of cartilage.

B Nasal cartilage

Inferior view. Viewed from below, each of the major alar cartilages is seen to consist of a medial and lateral crus. This view also displays the two nares, which open into the nasal cavities. The right and left nasal cavities are separated by the nasal septum, whose inferior cartilaginous portion is just visible in the diagram. The wall structure of a single nasal cavity will be described in this unit, and the relationship of the nasal cavity to the paranasal sinuses will be explored in the next unit.

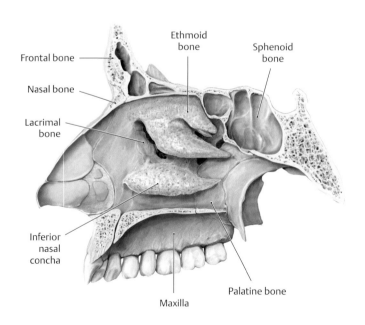

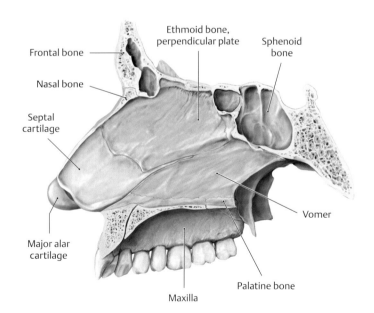

C Bones of the lateral wall of the right nasal cavity

Left lateral view. The lateral wall of the right nasal cavity is formed by six bones: the maxilla, nasal bone, ethmoid bone, inferior nasal concha, palatine bone, and sphenoid bone. Of the nasal concha, only the inferior is a separate bone; the middle and superior conchae are parts of the ethmoid bone.

D Bones of the nasal septum

Parasagittal section. The nasal septum is formed by the following bones: the nasal bone (roof of the septum), ethmoid bone, vomer, sphenoid bone, palatine bone, and maxilla. The latter three contribute only small bony projections to the nasal septum.

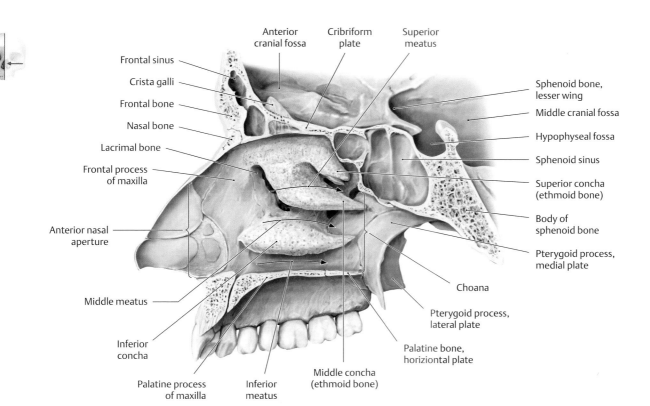

Anterior cranial fossa
Cribriform plate
Superior meatus
Frontal sinus
Crista galli
Frontal bone
Nasal bone
Lacrimal bone
Frontal process of maxilla
Anterior nasal aperture
Middle meatus
Inferior concha
Palatine process of maxilla
Inferior meatus
Middle concha (ethmoid bone)
Palatine bone, horizontal plate
Pterygoid process, lateral plate
Choana
Pterygoid process, medial plate
Body of sphenoid bone
Superior concha (ethmoid bone)
Sphenoid sinus
Hypophyseal fossa
Middle cranial fossa
Sphenoid bone, lesser wing

E Lateral wall of the right nasal cavity
Medial view. Air enters the bony nasal cavity through the anterior nasal aperture and travels through the three nasal passages: the superior me-atus, middle meatus, and inferior meatus. Air leaves the nose through the choanae, entering the nasopharynx. The three nasal passages are separated into meatuses by the inferior, middle, and superior conchae.

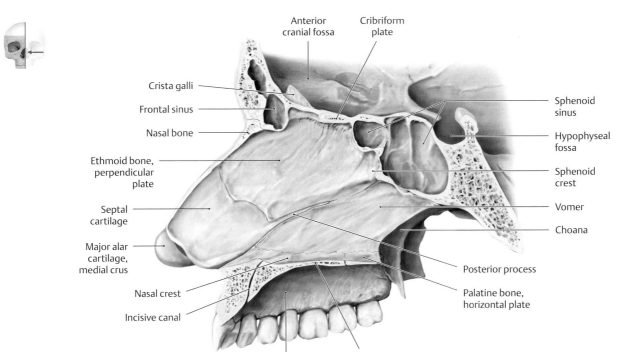

Anterior cranial fossa
Cribriform plate
Crista galli
Frontal sinus
Nasal bone
Ethmoid bone, perpendicular plate
Septal cartilage
Major alar cartilage, medial crus
Nasal crest
Incisive canal
Oral cavity
Palatine process of maxilla
Posterior process
Palatine bone, horizontal plate
Vomer
Choana
Sphenoid crest
Hypophyseal fossa
Sphenoid sinus

F Nasal septum
Parasagittal section viewed from the left side. The left lateral wall of the nasal cavity has been removed with the adjacent bones. The nasal sep-tum consists of an anterior cartilaginous part, the septal cartilage, and a posterior bony part (see **D**). The posterior process of the cartilaginous septum extends deep into the bony septum. Deviations of the nasal sep-tum are common and may involve the cartilaginous part of the septum, the bony part, or both. Cases in which the septal deviation is sufficient to cause obstruction of nasal breathing can be surgically corrected.

1.10 Nose: Paranasal Sinuses

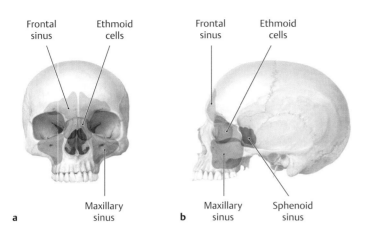

a

b

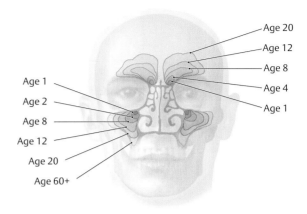

A Projection of the paranasal sinuses onto the skull

a Anterior view, **b** lateral view.

The paranasal sinuses are air-filled cavities that reduce the weight of the skull. Because they are subject to inflammation that may cause pain over the affected sinus (e.g., frontal headache due to frontal sinusitis), knowing the location of the sinuses is helpful in making the correct diagnosis.

B Pneumatization of the maxillary and frontal sinuses

Anterior view. The frontal and maxillary sinuses develop gradually during the course of cranial growth (pneumatization)—unlike the ethmoid sinuses, which are already pneumatized at birth. As a result, sinusitis in children is most likely to involve the ethmoid cells (with risk of orbital penetration: red, swollen eye; see **D**).

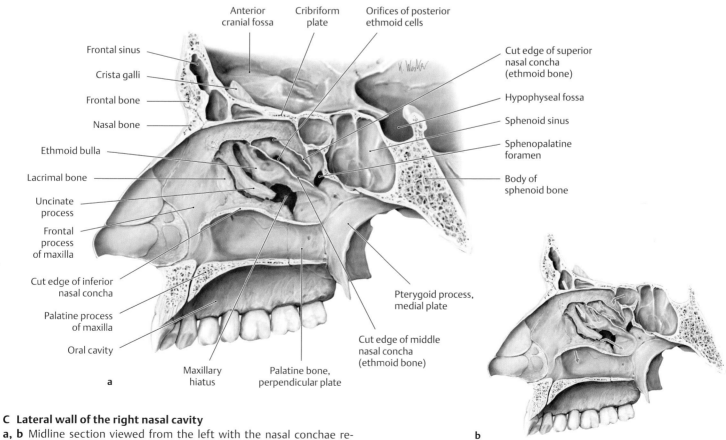

a

b

C Lateral wall of the right nasal cavity

a, b Midline section viewed from the left with the nasal conchae removed to display the openings of the nasolacrimal duct and paranasal sinuses into the nasal cavity (see colored arrows in **b**: red = nasolacrimal duct, yellow = frontal sinus, orange = maxillary sinus, green = anterior and posterior ethmoid cells, blue = sphenoid sinus; drainage routes are described in **F**).

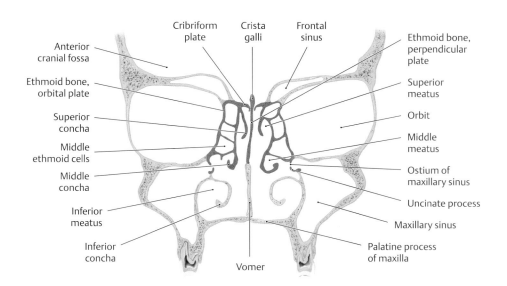

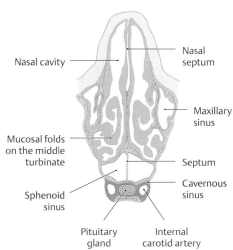

D Bony structure of the paranasal sinuses

Anterior view. The central structure of the *paranasal sinuses* is the ethmoid bone (red). Its cribriform plate forms a portion of the anterior skull base. The frontal and maxillary sinuses are grouped around the ethmoid bone. The inferior, middle and superior meatuses can be identified within the nasal cavity and are bounded by the coordinately-named conchae. The bony ostium of the maxillary sinus opens into the middle meatus, lateral to the middle concha. Below the middle concha and above the maxillary sinus ostium is the ethmoid bulla, which contains the middle ethmoid cells. At its anterior margin is a bony hook, the uncinate process, which bounds the maxillary sinus ostium anteriorly. The middle concha is a useful landmark in surgical procedures on the maxillary sinus and anterior ethmoid. The lateral wall separating the ethmoid bone from the orbit is the paper-thin orbital plate (= lamina papyracea). Inflammatory processes and tumors may penetrate this thin plate in either direction.

E Nasal cavity and paranasal sinuses

Transverse section viewed from above. The mucosal surface anatomy has been left intact to show how narrow the nasal passages are. Even relatively mild swelling of the mucosa may obstruct the nasal cavity, impeding aeration of the paranasal sinuses.

This diagram also shows that the pituitary gland, located behind the sphenoid sinus in the hypophyseal fossa (see **C**), is accessible to transnasal surgical procedures.

F Sites where the nasolacrimal duct and paranasal sinuses open into the nose

Nasal passage	Structures that open into the meatus
Inferior meatus	• Nasolacrimal duct
Middle meatus	• Frontal sinus • Maxillary sinus • Anterior ethmoid cells • Middle ethmoid cells
Superior meatus	• Posterior ethmoid cells
Spheno-ethmoid recess	• Sphenoid sinus

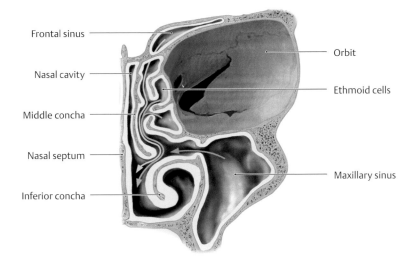

G Ostiomeatal unit on the left side of the nose

Coronal section. When the mucosa (ciliated respiratory epithelium) in the ethmoid cells (green) becomes swollen due to inflammation (sinusitis), it blocks the flow of secretions (see arrows) from the frontal sinus (yellow) and maxillary sinus (orange) in the ostiomeatal unit (red). Because of this blockage, micro-organisms also become trapped in the other sinuses, where they may incite an inflammation. Thus, while the anatomical focus of the disease lies in the ethmoid cells, inflammatory symptoms are also manifested in the frontal and maxillary sinuses. In patients with *chronic sinusitis*, the narrow sites can be surgically widened to establish an effective drainage route, thereby curing the disease.

1.11 Temporal Bone

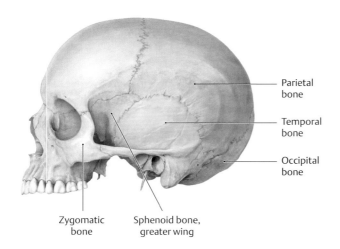

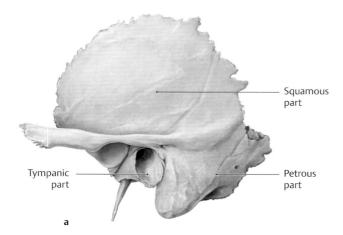

a

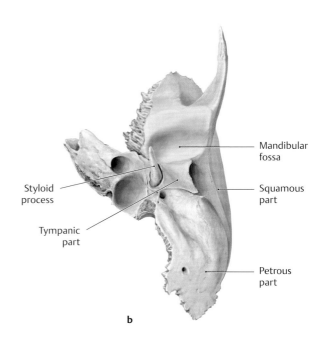

b

A Position of the temporal bone in the skull
Left lateral view. The temporal bone is a major component of the base of the skull. It forms the capsule for the auditory and vestibular apparatus and bears the articular fossa of the temporomandibular joint.

B Ossification centers of the left temporal bone
a Left lateral view, **b** inferior view.
The temporal bone develops from three centers that fuse to form a single bone:

- The squamous part, or temporal squama (light green), bears the articular fossa of the temporomandibular joint (mandibular fossa).

- The petrous part, or petrous bone (pale green), contains the auditory and vestibular apparatus.
- The tympanic part (darker green) forms large portions of the external auditory canal.

Note: The styloid process appears to belong to the tympanic part of the temporal bone because of its location. Developmentally, however, it is part of the petrous bone.

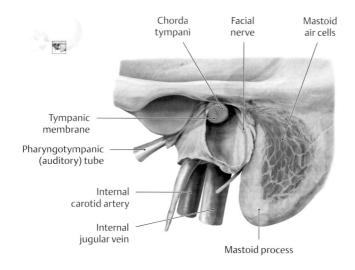

C Projection of clinically important structures onto the left temporal bone
The tympanic membrane is shown translucent in this lateral view. Because the petrous bone contains the middle and inner ear and the tympanic membrane, a knowledge of its anatomy is of key importance in otological surgery. The internal surface of the petrous bone has openings (see **D**) for the passage of the facial nerve, internal carotid artery, and internal jugular vein. A fine nerve, the chorda tympani, passes through the tympanic cavity, and lies medial to the tympanic membrane. The chorda tympani arises from the facial nerve, which is susceptible to injury during surgical procedures (see **C**, p. 79). The mastoid process of the petrous bone forms air-filled chambers, the mastoid cells, that vary greatly in size. Because these chambers communicate with the middle ear, which in turn communicates with the nasopharynx via the pharyngotympanic (auditory) tube (also called Eustachian tube) bacteria in the nasopharynx may pass up the pharyngotympanic tube and gain access to the middle ear. From there they may pass to the mastoid air cells and finally enter the cranial cavity, causing meningitis.

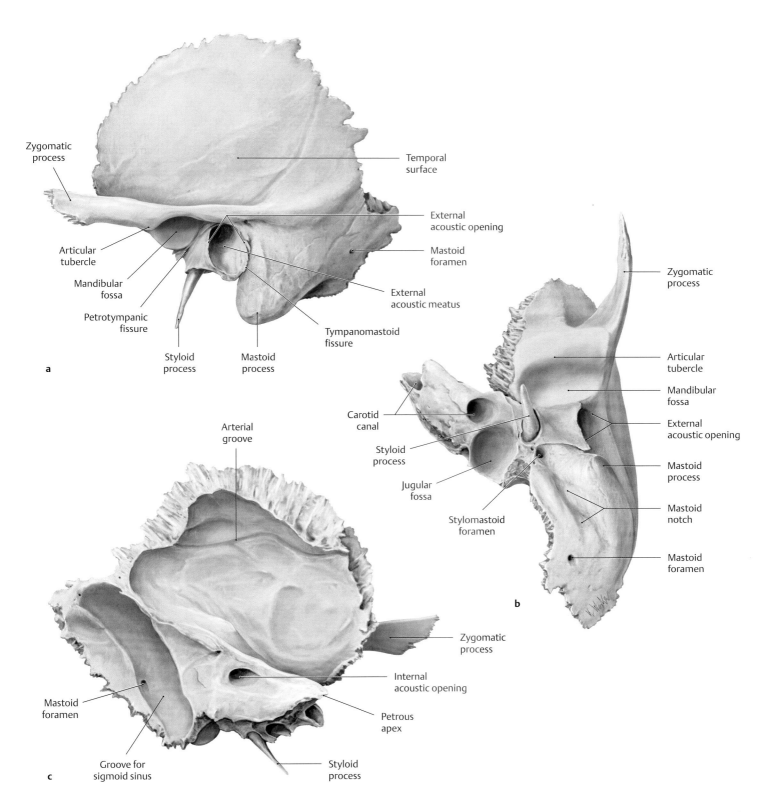

D Left temporal bone

a Lateral view. The principal structures of the temporal bone are labeled in the diagram. An emissary vein (see p. 9) passes through the mastoid foramen (external orifice shown in **a**, internal orifice in **c**), and the chorda tympani passes through the medial part of the petrotympanic fissure (see p. 147). The mastoid process develops gradually in life due to traction from the sternocleidomastoid muscle and is pneumatized from the inside (see **C**).

b Inferior view. The shallow articular fossa of the temporomandibular joint (the mandibular fossa) is clearly seen from the inferior view. The facial nerve emerges from the base of the skull through the stylo-

mastoid foramen. The initial part of the internal jugular vein is adherent to the jugular fossa, and the internal carotid artery passes through the carotid canal to enter the skull.

c Medial view. This view displays the internal orifice of the mastoid foramen and the internal acoustic meatus. The facial nerve and vestibulocochlear nerve are among the structures that pass through the internal meatus to enter the petrous bone. The part of the petrous bone shown here is also called the *petrous pyramid*, whose apex (often called the "petrous apex") lies on the interior of the base of the skull.

1.12 Sphenoid Bone

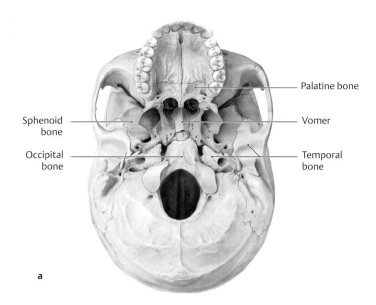

Palatine bone

Sphenoid bone

Vomer

Occipital bone

Temporal bone

a

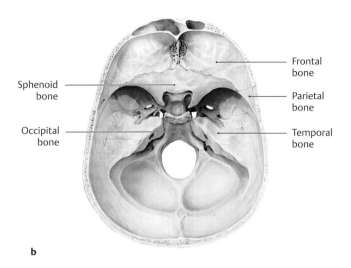

Frontal bone

Sphenoid bone

Parietal bone

Occipital bone

Temporal bone

b

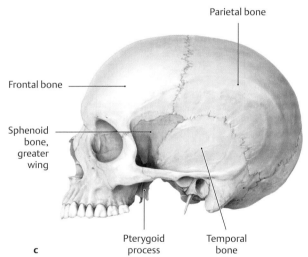

Parietal bone

Frontal bone

Sphenoid bone, greater wing

Pterygoid process

Temporal bone

c

A Position of the sphenoid bone in the skull

The sphenoid bone is the most structurally complex bone in the human body. It must be viewed from various aspects in order to appreciate all its features (see also **B**):

a Base of the skull, external aspect. The sphenoid bone combines with the occipital bone to form the load-bearing midline structure of the skull base.

b Base of the skull, internal aspect. The sphenoid bone forms the boundary between the anterior and middle cranial fossae. The openings for the passage of nerves and vessels are clearly displayed (see details in **B**).

c Lateral view. Portions of the greater wing of the sphenoid bone can be seen above the zygomatic arch, and portions of the pterygoid process can be seen below the zygomatic arch.

Note the bones that border on the sphenoid bone in each view.

B Isolated sphenoid bone

a Inferior view (its position in situ is shown in **A**). This view demonstrates the medial and lateral plates of the pterygoid process. Between them is the pterygoid fossa, which is occupied by the medial pterygoid muscle. The foramen spinosum and foramen rotundum provide pathways through the base of the skull (see also in **c**).

b Anterior view. This view illustrates why the sphenoid bone was originally called the sphecoid bone ("wasp bone") before a transcription error turned it into the sphenoid ("wedge-shaped") bone. The apertures of the sphenoid sinus on each side resemble the eyes of the wasp, and the pterygoid processes of the sphenoid bone form its dangling legs, between which are the pterygoid fossae. This view also displays the superior orbital fissure, which connects the middle cranial fossa with the orbit on each side. The two sphenoid sinuses are separated by an internal septum (see p. 21).

c Superior view. The superior view displays the sella turcica, whose central depression, the hypophyseal fossa, contains the pituitary gland. The foramen spinosum, foramen ovale, and foramen rotundum can be identified posteriorly.

d Posterior view. The superior orbital fissure is seen particularly clearly in this view, while the optic canal is almost completely obscured by the anterior clinoid process. The foramen rotundum is open from the middle cranial fossa to the external base of the skull (the foramen spinosum is not visible in this view; compare with **a**). Because the sphenoid and occipital bones fuse together during puberty ("tribasilar bone"), a suture is no longer present between the two bones. The cancellous trabeculae are exposed and have a porous appearance.

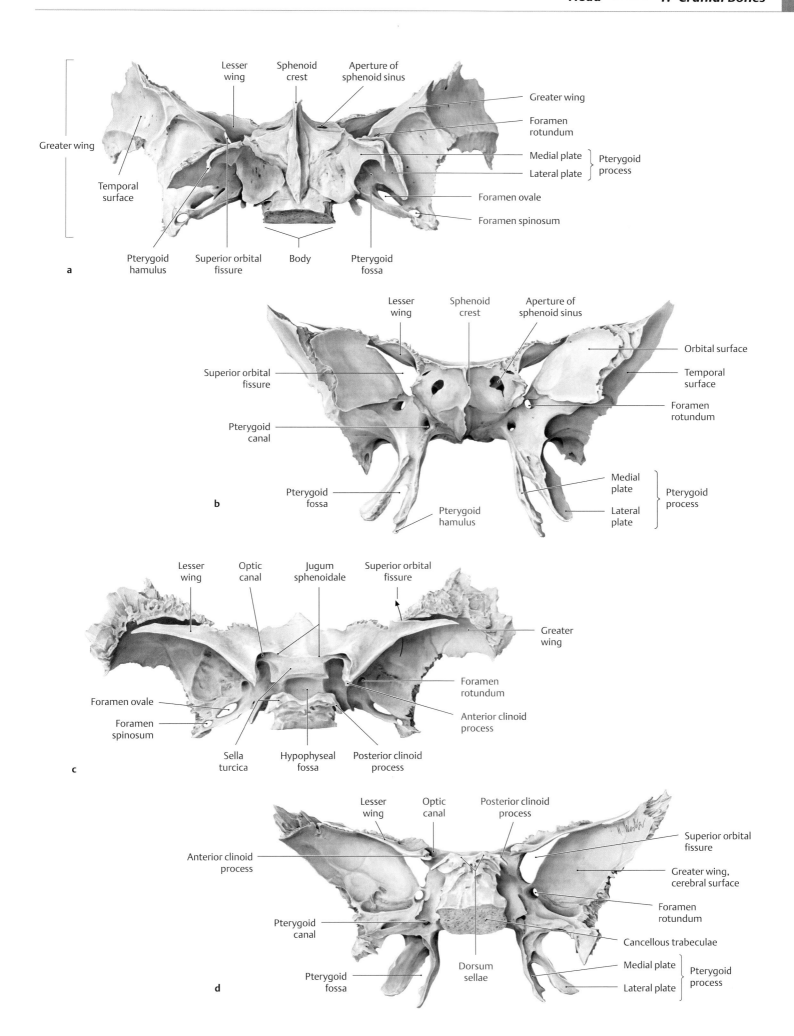

a

Greater wing

Lesser wing

Sphenoid crest

Aperture of sphenoid sinus

Greater wing

Foramen rotundum

Medial plate ⎫
Lateral plate ⎭ Pterygoid process

Foramen ovale

Foramen spinosum

Temporal surface

Pterygoid hamulus

Superior orbital fissure

Body

Pterygoid fossa

b

Lesser wing

Sphenoid crest

Aperture of sphenoid sinus

Orbital surface

Temporal surface

Foramen rotundum

Superior orbital fissure

Pterygoid canal

Pterygoid fossa

Pterygoid hamulus

Medial plate ⎫
Lateral plate ⎭ Pterygoid process

c

Lesser wing

Optic canal

Jugum sphenoidale

Superior orbital fissure

Greater wing

Foramen rotundum

Anterior clinoid process

Foramen ovale

Foramen spinosum

Sella turcica

Hypophyseal fossa

Posterior clinoid process

d

Lesser wing

Optic canal

Posterior clinoid process

Superior orbital fissure

Greater wing, cerebral surface

Foramen rotundum

Cancellous trabeculae

Anterior clinoid process

Pterygoid canal

Pterygoid fossa

Dorsum sellae

Medial plate ⎫
Lateral plate ⎭ Pterygoid process

1.13 Occipital Bone and Ethmoid Bones

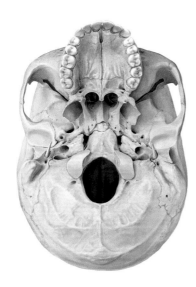

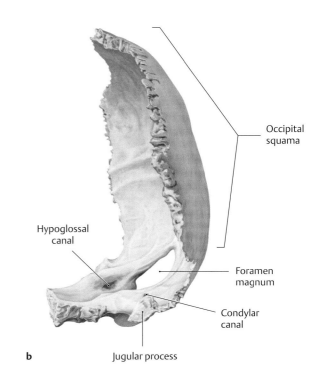

A Integration of the occipital bone into the external base of the skull
Inferior view. *Note* the relationship of the occipital bone to the adjacent bones.
The occipital bone fuses with the sphenoid bone during puberty to form the "tribasilar bone."

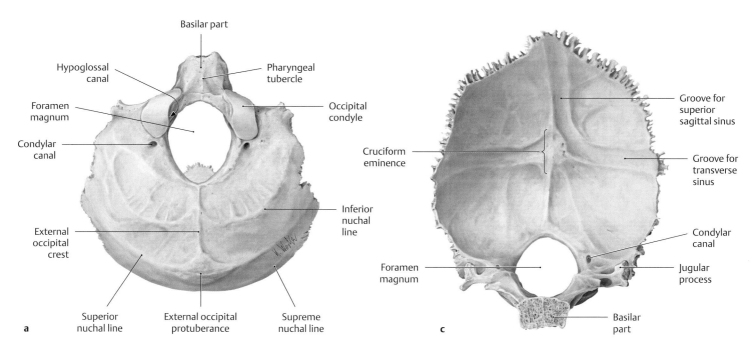

B Isolated occipital bone

a Inferior view. This view shows the basilar part of the occipital bone, whose anterior portion is fused to the sphenoid bone. The condylar canal terminates posterior to the occipital condyles, while the hypoglossal canal passes superior to the occipital condyles. The condylar canal is a venous channel that begins in the sigmoid sinus and ends in the occipital vein (emissary vein, see p. 9). The hypoglossal canal contains a venous plexus in addition to the hypoglossal nerve (CN XII). The pharyngeal tubercle gives attachment to the pharyngeal muscles, while the external occipital protuberance provides a palpable bony landmark on the occiput.

b Left lateral view. The extent of the occipital squama, which lies above the foramen magnum, is clearly appreciated in this view. The internal openings of the condylar canal and hypoglossal canal are visible along with the jugular process, which forms part of the wall of the jugular foramen (see p. 11). This process is analogous to the transverse process of a vertebra.

c Internal surface. The grooves for the dural venous sinuses of the brain can be identified in this view. The cruciform eminence overlies the confluence of the superior sagittal sinus and transverse sinuses. The configuration of the eminence shows that in some cases the sagittal sinus drains predominantly into the left transverse sinus.

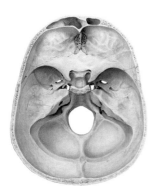

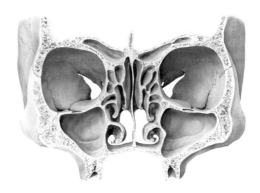

C Integration of the ethmoid bone into the internal base of the skull

Superior view. The upper portion of the ethmoid bone forms part of the anterior cranial fossa, while its lower portions contribute structurally to the nasal cavities. The ethmoid bone is bordered by the frontal and sphenoid bones.

D Integration of the ethmoid bone into the facial skeleton

Anterior view. The ethmoid bone is the central bone of the nose and paranasal sinuses.

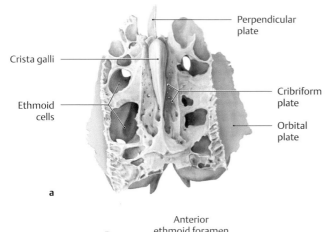

a

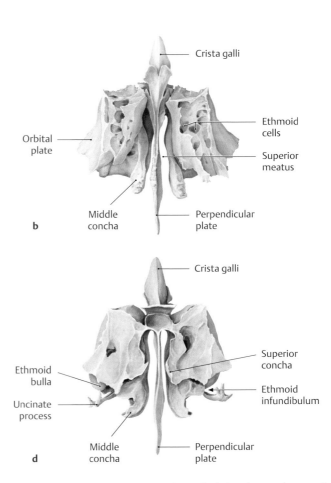

b

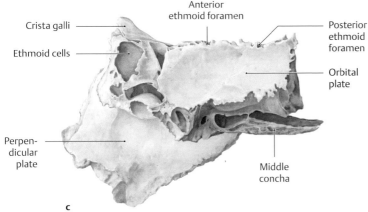

c

d

E Isolated ethmoid bone

a Superior view. This view demonstrates the crista galli, which gives attachment to the falx cerebri (see p. 188) and the horizontally directed cribriform plate. It is perforated by foramina through which the olfactory fibers pass from the nasal cavity into the anterior cranial fossa. With its numerous foramina, the cribriform plate is a mechanically weak structure that fractures easily in response to trauma. This type of fracture is manifested clinically by cerebrospinal fluid leakage from the nose ("runny nose" in a patient with head injury).

b Anterior view. The anterior view displays the midline structure that separates the two nasal cavities: the perpendicular plate (which resembles the pendulum of a grandfather clock). Note also the middle concha, which is part of the ethmoid bone (of the conchae, only the inferior concha is a separate bone), and the ethmoid cells, which are clustered on both sides of the middle conchae.

c Left lateral view. Viewing the bone from the left side, we observe the perpendicular plate and the opened anterior ethmoid cells. The orbit is separated from the ethmoid cells by a thin sheet of bone called the orbital plate.

d Posterior view. This is the only view that displays the uncinate process, which is almost completely covered by the middle concha when in situ. It partially occludes the entrance to the maxillary sinus, the semilunar hiatus, and it is an important landmark during endoscopic surgery of the maxillary sinus. The narrow depression between the middle concha and uncinate process is called the ethmoid infundibulum. The frontal sinus, maxillary sinus, and anterior ethmoid cells open into this "funnel." The superior concha is located at the posterior end of the ethmoid bone.

1.14 Hard Palate

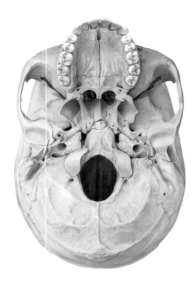

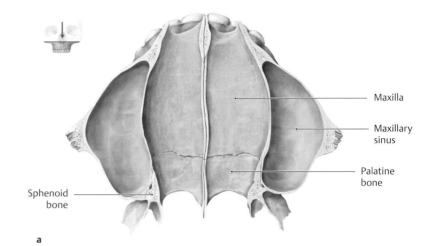

Maxilla

Maxillary sinus

Palatine bone

Sphenoid bone

a

A Integration of the hard palate into the base of the skull.
Inferior view.

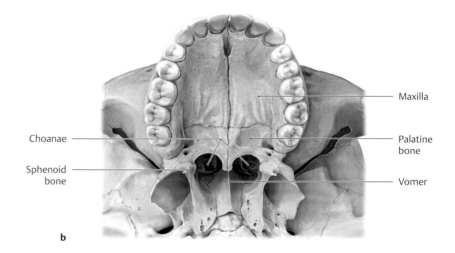

Maxilla

Choanae

Palatine bone

Sphenoid bone

Vomer

b

B Bones of the hard palate

a Superior view. The hard palate is a horizontal bony plate formed by parts of the maxilla and palatine bone. It serves as a partition between the oral and nasal cavities. In this view we are looking down at the floor of the nasal cavity, whose inferior surface forms the roof of the oral cavity. The upper portion of the maxilla has been removed. The palatine bone is bordered posteriorly by the sphenoid bone.

b Inferior view. The choanae, the posterior openings of the nasal cavity, begin at the posterior border of the hard palate.

c Oblique posterior view. This view demonstrates the close relationship between the oral and nasal cavities.
Note how the pyramidal process of the palatine bone is integrated into the lateral plate of the pterygoid process of the sphenoid bone.

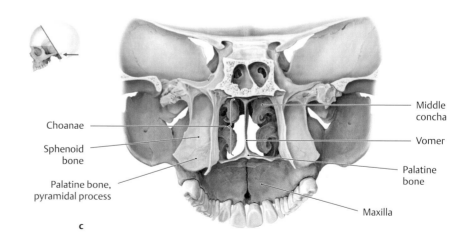

Middle concha

Choanae

Vomer

Sphenoid bone

Palatine bone

Palatine bone, pyramidal process

Maxilla

c

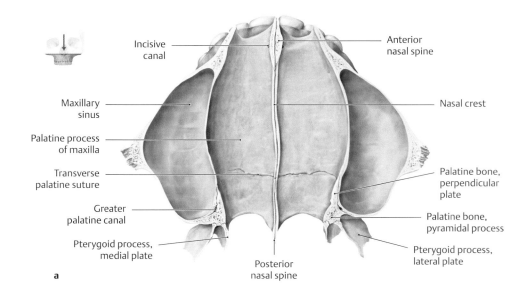

Incisive canal

Anterior nasal spine

Maxillary sinus

Palatine process of maxilla

Nasal crest

Transverse palatine suture

Palatine bone, perpendicular plate

Greater palatine canal

Palatine bone, pyramidal process

Pterygoid process, medial plate

Pterygoid process, lateral plate

Posterior nasal spine

a

C Hard palate

a **Superior view** of the floor of the nasal cavity (= upper portion of hard palate) with the upper part of the maxilla removed. The hard palate separates the oral cavity from the nasal cavities. The small canal that links the oral and nasal cavities, the incisive canal (present here on both sides), merges within the bone to form one canal, which opens on the inferior surface by a single orifice, the incisive foramen (see **b**).

b **Inferior view.** The two horizontal processes of the maxilla, the palatine processes, grow together during development and become fused at the median palatine suture. Failure of this fusion results in a *cleft palate*. The boundary line between anterior clefts (cleft lip, alone or combined with a cleft alveolus) and posterior clefts (cleft palate) is the incisive foramen. These anomalies may also take the form of cleft lip and palate (with a defect involving the lip, alveolus, and palate). *Note:* the nasal cavity (whose floor is formed by the hard palate) communicates with the nasopharynx by way of the choanae.

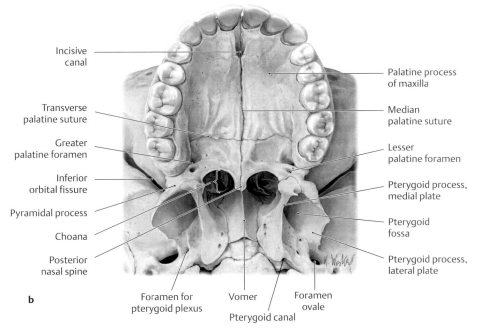

Incisive canal

Palatine process of maxilla

Transverse palatine suture

Median palatine suture

Greater palatine foramen

Lesser palatine foramen

Inferior orbital fissure

Pterygoid process, medial plate

Pyramidal process

Pterygoid fossa

Choana

Posterior nasal spine

Pterygoid process, lateral plate

Foramen for pterygoid plexus

Vomer

Foramen ovale

Pterygoid canal

b

c **Oblique posterior view** of the posterior part of the sphenoid bone at the level of the sphenoid body, displaying both sphenoid sinuses separated by a septum. The close topographical relationship between the nasal cavity and hard palate can be appreciated in this view. If the hard palate is unfused in a nursing infant due to a cleft anomaly (see **b**), some of the ingested milk will be diverted from the oral cavity and will enter the nose. This defect should be closed with a plate immediately after birth to permit satisfactory oral nutrition.

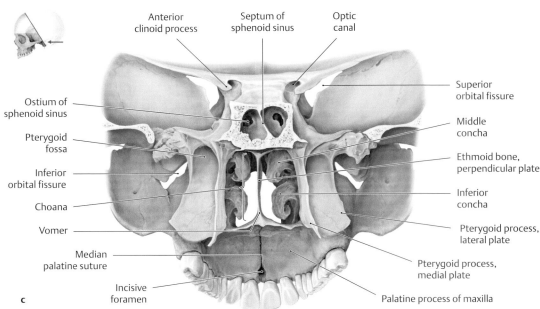

Anterior clinoid process

Septum of sphenoid sinus

Optic canal

Ostium of sphenoid sinus

Superior orbital fissure

Pterygoid fossa

Middle concha

Inferior orbital fissure

Ethmoid bone, perpendicular plate

Choana

Inferior concha

Vomer

Pterygoid process, lateral plate

Median palatine suture

Pterygoid process, medial plate

Incisive foramen

Palatine process of maxilla

c

1.15 Mandible and Hyoid Bone

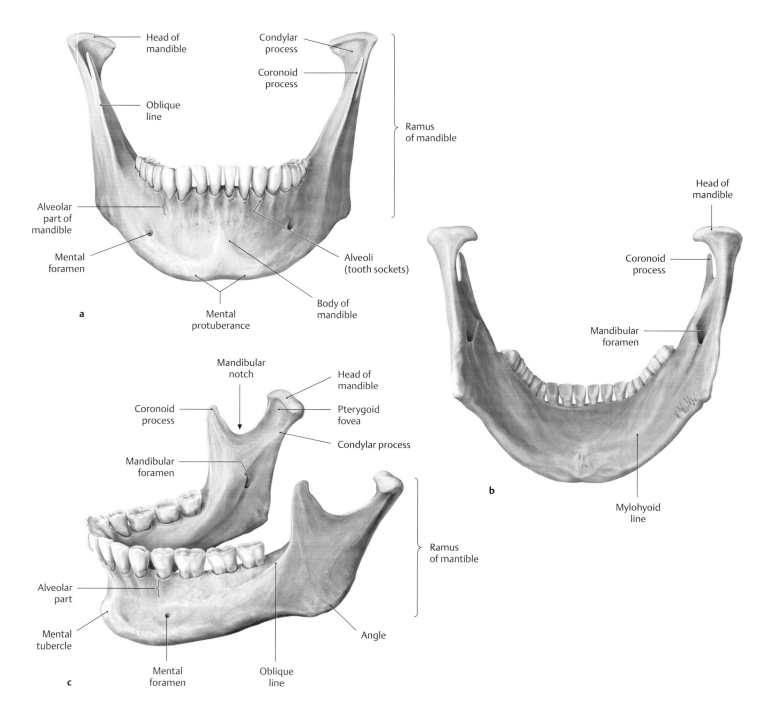

A Mandible

a Anterior view. The mandible is connected to the viscerocranium at the temporomandibular joint, whose convex surface is the head of the mandibular condyle. This "head of the mandible" is situated atop the vertical (ascending) ramus of the mandible, which joins with the body of the mandible at the mandibular angle. The teeth are set in the alveolar processes (alveolar part) along the upper border of the mandibular body. This part of the mandible is subject to typical age-related changes as a result of dental development (see **B**). The mental branch of the trigeminal nerve exits through the mental foramen to enter its bony canal. The location of this foramen is important in clinical examinations, as the tenderness of the nerve to pressure can be tested at that location (e.g., in trigeminal neuralgia, p. 77).

b Posterior view. The mandibular foramen is particularly well displayed in this view. It transmits the inferior alveolar nerve, which supplies sensory innervation to the mandibular teeth. Its terminal branch emerges from the mental foramen. The two mandibular foramina are interconnected by the mandibular canal.

c Oblique left lateral view. This view displays the coronoid process, the condylar process, and the mandibular notch between them. The coronoid process is a site for muscular attachments, while the condylar process bears the head of the mandible, which articulates with the mandibular fossa of the temporal bone. A depression on the medial side of the condylar process, the pterygoid fovea, gives attachment to portions of the lateral pterygoid muscle.

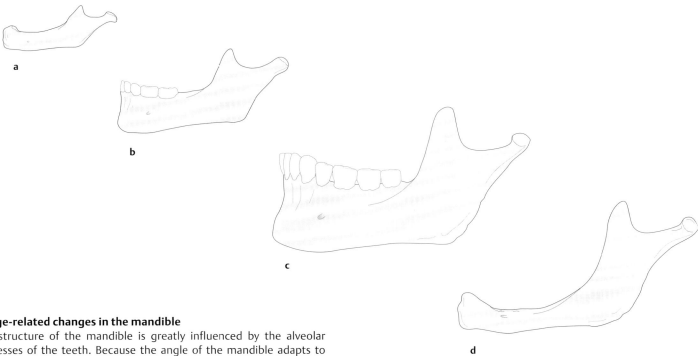

B Age-related changes in the mandible

The structure of the mandible is greatly influenced by the alveolar processes of the teeth. Because the angle of the mandible adapts to changes in the alveolar process, the angle between the body and ramus also varies with age-related changes in the dentition. The angle measures approximately 150° at birth, and approximately 120—130° in adults, decreasing to 140° in the edentulous mandible of old age.

a At birth the mandible is without teeth and the alveolar part has not yet formed.

b In children the mandible bears the deciduous teeth. The alveolar part is still relatively poorly developed because the deciduous teeth are considerably smaller than the permanent teeth.

c In adults the mandible bears the permanent teeth, and the alveolar part of the bone is fully developed.

d Old age is characterized by an edentulous mandible with resorption of the alveolar process.

Note: the resorption of the alveolar process with advanced age leads to a change in the position of the mental foramen (which is normally located below the second premolar tooth, as in **c**). This change must be taken into account in surgery or dissections involving the mental nerve.

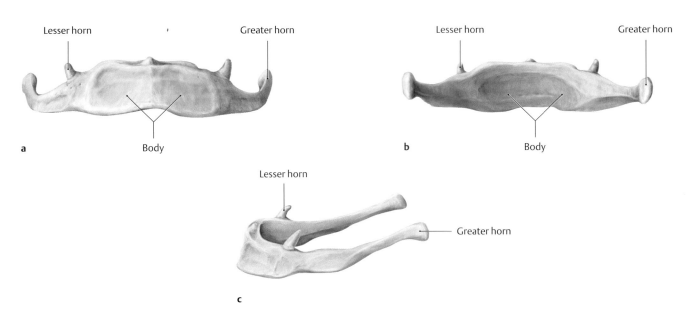

C Hyoid bone

a Anterior view, **b** posterior view, **c** oblique left lateral view. The hyoid bone is suspended by muscles between the oral floor and larynx in the neck, although it is listed among the cranial bones in the *Terminologia*

Anatomica. The greater horn and body of the hyoid bone are palpable in the neck. The physiological movement of the hyoid bone during swallowing is also palpable.

1.16 Temporomandibular Joint

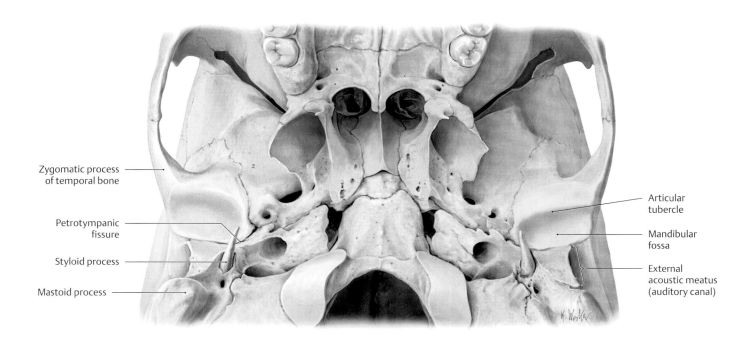

Zygomatic process
of temporal bone

Petrotympanic
fissure

Styloid process

Mastoid process

Articular
tubercle

Mandibular
fossa

External
acoustic meatus
(auditory canal)

A Mandibular fossa of the temporomandibular joint
Inferior view. The head of the mandible articulates with the mandibular fossa in the temporomandibular joint. The mandibular fossa is a depression in the squamous part of the temporal bone. The articular tubercle is located on the anterior side of the mandibular fossa. The head of the mandible (see **B**) is markedly smaller than the mandibular fossa, allow-

ing it to have an adequate range of movement (see p. 35). Unlike other articular surfaces, the mandibular fossa is covered by fibrocartilage rather than hyaline cartilage. As a result, it is not as clearly delineated on the skull as other articular surfaces. The external auditory canal lies just behind the mandibular fossa. This proximity explains why trauma to the mandible may damage the auditory canal.

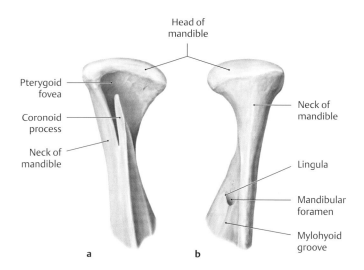

Head of
mandible

Pterygoid
fovea

Coronoid
process

Neck of
mandible

Neck of
mandible

Lingula

Mandibular
foramen

Mylohyoid
groove

a   b

B Head of the mandible in the right temporomandibular joint
a Anterior view, **b** posterior view. The head of the mandible is not only markedly smaller than the articular fossa but also has a cylindrical shape. This shape further increases the mobility of the mandibular head, as it allows rotational movements about a vertical axis.

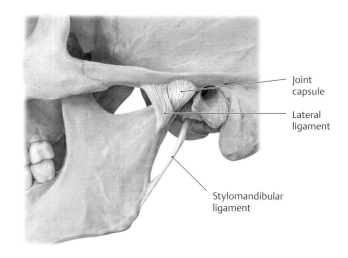

Joint
capsule

Lateral
ligament

Stylomandibular
ligament

C Ligaments of the left temporomandibular joint
Lateral view. The temporomandibular joint is surrounded by a relatively lax capsule, which permits physiological dislocation during jaw opening. The joint is stabilized by three ligaments (see **C** and **D**). This lateral view demonstrates the strongest of these ligaments, the lateral ligament, which stretches over the capsule and is blended with it. The weaker stylomandibular ligament is also shown.

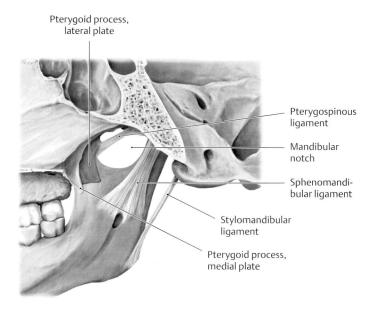

Pterygoid process, lateral plate

Pterygospinous ligament

Mandibular notch

Sphenomandibular ligament

Stylomandibular ligament

Pterygoid process, medial plate

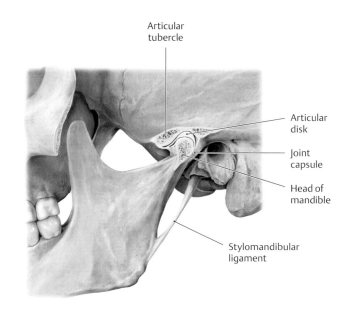

Articular tubercle

Articular disk

Joint capsule

Head of mandible

Stylomandibular ligament

D Right temporomandibular joint and ligaments
Medial view. The sphenomandibular ligament can also be identified in this view.

E Opened left temporomandibular joint
Lateral view. The capsule extends posteriorly to the petrotympanic fissure (not shown here). Interposed between the mandibular head and fossa is the articular disk, which is attached to the joint capsule on all sides.

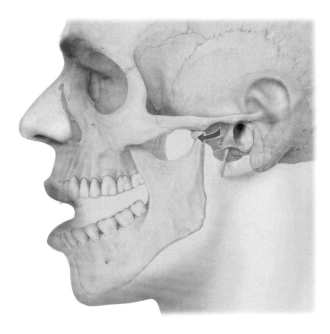

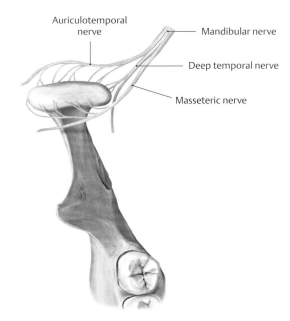

Auriculotemporal nerve

Mandibular nerve

Deep temporal nerve

Masseteric nerve

F Dislocation of the temporomandibular joint
The head of the mandible may slide past the articular tubercle when the mouth is opened, dislocating the temporomandibular joint. This may result from heavy yawning or a blow to the opened mandible. When the joint dislocates, the mandible becomes locked in a protruded position and can no longer be closed. This condition is easily diagnosed clinically and is reduced by pressing on the mandibular row of teeth.

G Sensory innervation of the temporomandibular joint capsule
 (after Schmidt)
Superior view. The temporomandibular joint capsule is supplied by articular branches arising from three branches of the mandibular division of the trigeminal nerve (CN V$_3$):

- Auriculotemporal nerve
- Deep temporal nerve
- Masseteric nerve

33

1.17 Tempororomandibular Joint, Biomechanics

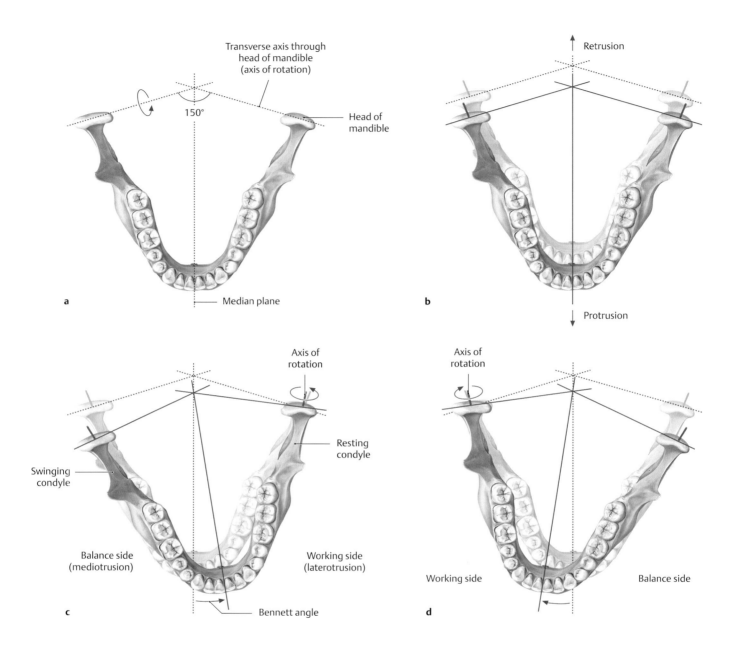

A Movements of the mandible in the temporomandibular joint
Superior view. Most of the movements in the temporomandibular joint are complex motions that have three main components:

- Rotation (opening and closing the mouth)
- Translation (protrusion and retrusion of the mandible)
- Grinding movements during mastication

a Rotation. The axis for joint rotation runs transversely through both heads of the mandible. The two axes intersect at an angle of approximately 150º (range of 110—180° between individuals). During this movement the temporomandibular joint acts as a hinge joint (abduction/depression and adduction/elevation of the mandible). In humans, pure rotation in the temporomandibular joint usually occurs only during sleep with the mouth slightly open (aperture angle up to approximately 15°, see **Bb**). When the mouth is opened past 15°, rotation is combined with translation (gliding) of the mandibular head.

b Translation. In this movement the mandible is advanced (protruded) and retracted (retruded). The axes for this movement are parallel to the median axes through the center of the mandibular heads.

c Grinding movements in the left temporomandibular joint. In describing these lateral movements, a distinction is made between the "resting condyle" and the "swinging condyle." The resting condyle on the left working side rotates about an almost vertical axis through the head of the mandible (also a rotational axis), while the swinging condyle on the right balance side swings forward and inward in a translational movement. The lateral excursion of the mandible is measured in degrees and is called the Bennett angle. During this movement the mandible moves in laterotrusion on the working side and in mediotrusion on the balance side.

d Grinding movements in the right temporomandibular joint. Here, the right temporomandibular joint is the working side. The right resting condyle rotates about an almost vertical axis, while the left condyle on the balance side swings forward and inward.

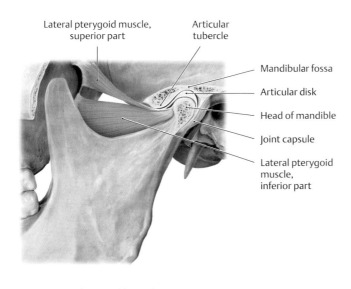

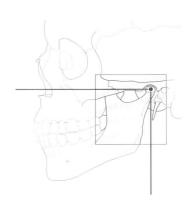

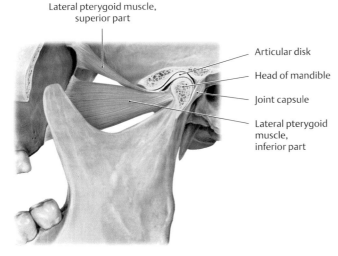

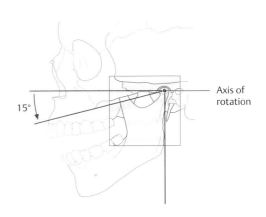

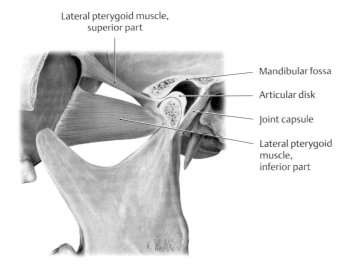

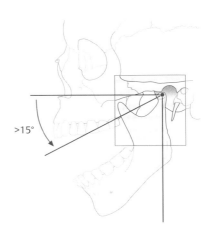

B Movements of the temporomandibular joint
Left lateral view. Each drawing shows the left temporomandibular joint including the articular disk and capsule and the lateral pterygoid muscle, and each schematic diagram at right shows the corresponding axis of joint movement. The muscle, capsule, and disk form a functionally coordinated musculo-disco-capsular system and work closely together when the mouth is opened and closed.

a Mouth closed. When the mouth is in a closed position, the head of the mandible rests against the mandibular fossa of the temporal bone.

b Mouth opened to 15°. Up to 15° of abduction, the head of the mandible remains in the mandibular fossa.

c Mouth opened past 15°. At this point the head of the mandible glides forward onto the articular tubercle. The joint axis that runs transversely through the mandibular head is shifted forward. The articular disk is pulled forward by the superior part of the lateral pterygoid muscle, and the head of the mandible is drawn forward by the inferior part of that muscle.

35

1.18 The Teeth in situ

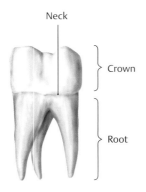

A Principal parts of the tooth

- Crown
- Neck
- Root

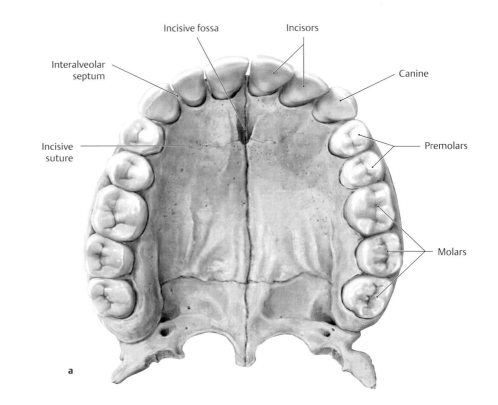

a

B Permanent teeth of an adult
a **Maxilla.** Inferior view displaying the occlusal surfaces of the teeth.
b **Mandible.** Superior view.

Each tooth is given an identification code (see p. 38) to describe the specific location of dental lesions such as caries.

Each half of the maxilla and mandible contains the following set of anterior and posterior (postcanine) teeth:

- Anterior teeth: two incisors and one canine tooth.
- Posterior teeth: two premolars and three molars.

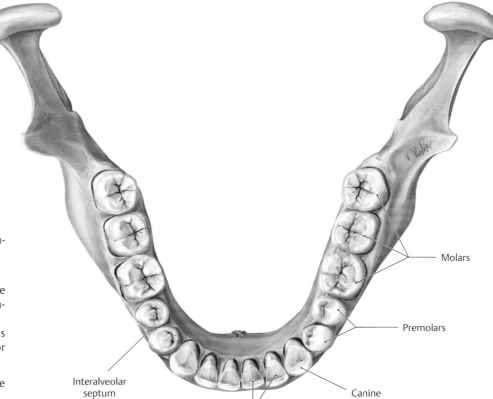

b

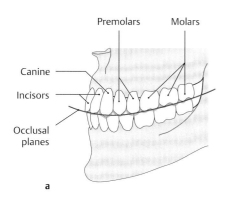

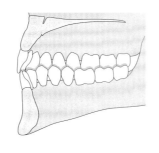

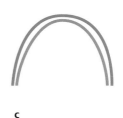

a

b

c

C Occlusal plane and dental arches

a, b Types of teeth and the occlusal plane. The maxilla and mandible present a symmetrical arrangement. With the mouth closed (occlusal position), the maxillary teeth are apposed to their mandibular counterparts. They are offset relative to one another so that the cusps of one tooth fit into the fissures of the two opposing teeth (cusp-and-fissure dentition). Because of this arrangement, every tooth comes into contact with two opposing teeth. This offset results from the slightly greater width of the maxillary incisors (see p. 39). The occlusal plane often forms a superiorly open arch (von Spee curve).

c Dental arches. The teeth of the maxilla (green) and mandible (blue) are arranged in superior and inferior arches. The superior dental arch forms a semi-ellipse while the inferior arch is shaped like a parabola.

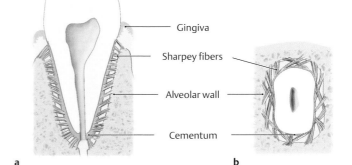

a

b

E Supporting structures of the tooth: the periodontium

The tooth is anchored in the alveolus by a special type of syndesmosis called a gomphosis. The tissues that invest and support the tooth, the periodontium, consist of:

- The periodontal ligament
- The cementum
- The alveolar wall
- The gingiva.

The Sharpey fibers are collagenous fibers that pass obliquely downward from the alveolar bone and insert into the cementum of the tooth. This downward obliquity of the fibers transforms masticatory pressures on the dental arch into tensile stresses acting on the fibers and anchored bone (pressure would lead to bony atrophy).

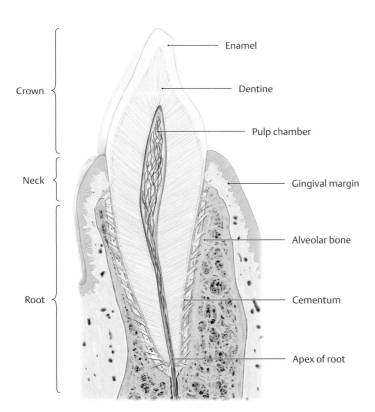

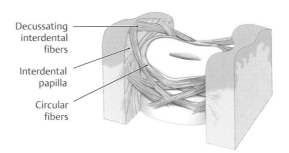

D Histology of a tooth

Illustrated here for a mandibular incisor. This diagram shows the hard tissues of the tooth (enamel, dentine, cementum) as well as the soft tissues (dental pulp).

F Connective tissue fibers in the gingiva

Many of the tough collagenous fiber bundles in the connective-tissue core of the gingiva above the alveolar bone are arranged in a screw-like pattern around the tooth, further strengthening its attachment.

1.19 Permanent Teeth and the Dental Panoramic Tomogram

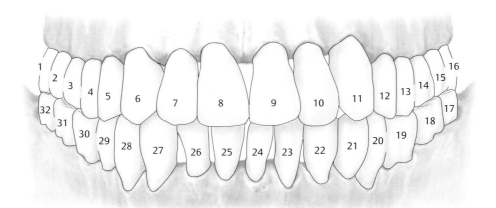

A Coding the permanent teeth

In the United States, the permanent teeth are numbered sequentially rather than being assigned to quadrants. Progressing in a clockwise fashion (from the perspecive of the viewer), the teeth of the upper arc are numbered 1 to 16, while those of the lower are considered 17 to 32. *Note:* The third upper molar (wisdom tooth) on the patient's right is considered 1.

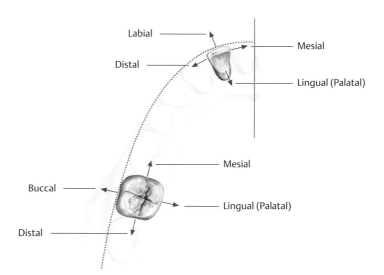

B Designation of tooth surfaces

Superior view of the mandibular dental arch. These designations are used in describing the precise location of small carious lesions. The term *labial* is used for incisors and canine teeth, and *buccal* is used for premolar and molar teeth. The term *lingual* is used for the mandibular teeth and *palatal* for the maxillary teeth.

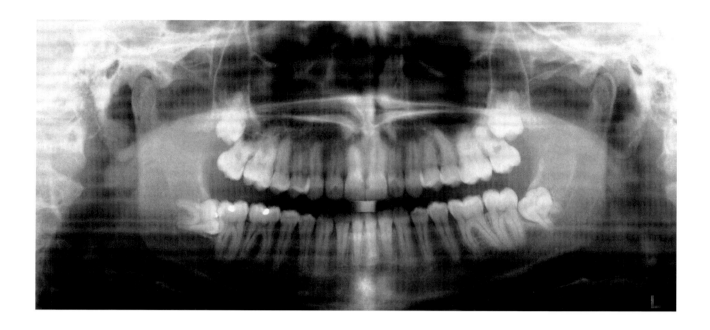

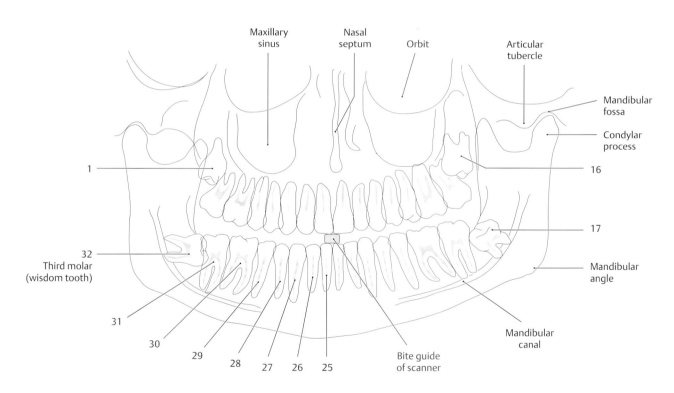

C Dental panoramic tomogram

The dental panoramic tomogram (DPT) is a survey radiograph that allows a preliminary assessment of the temporomandibular joints, maxillary sinuses, maxillomandibular bone, and dental status (carious lesions, location of the wisdom teeth). It is based on the principle of conventional tomography in which the X-ray tube and film are moved about the plane of interest to blur out the shadows of structures outside the sectional plane. The plane of interest in the DPT is shaped like a parabola, conforming to the shape of the jaws. In the case shown here, all four wisdom teeth (third molars) should be extracted: teeth 1, 16, and

17 are not fully erupted and tooth 32 is horizontally impacted (cannot erupt). If the DPT raises suspicion of caries or root disease, it should be followed with spot radiographs so that specific regions of interest can be evaluated at higher resolution.

(Tomogram courtesy of Prof. Dr. U. J. Rother, director of the Department of Diagnostic Radiology, Center for Dentistry and Oromaxillofacial Surgery, Eppendorf University Medical Center, Hamburg, Germany.)

Note: The upper incisors are broader than the lower incisors, leading to a "cusp-and-fissure" type of occlusion (see p. 37).

1.20 **Individual Teeth**

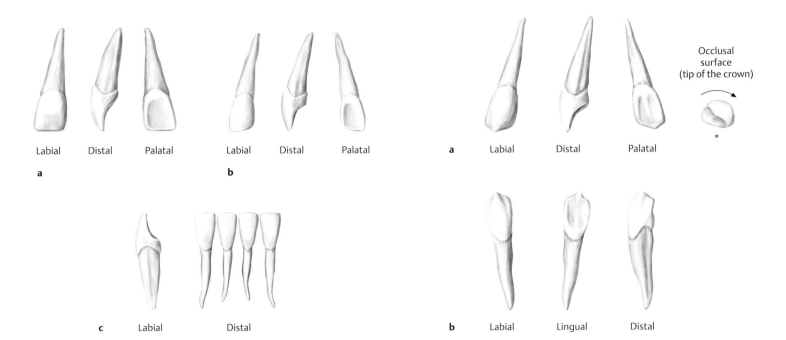

Labial   Distal   Palatal   Labial   Distal   Palatal

a   **b**

a   Labial   Distal   Palatal

Occlusal surface (tip of the crown)

*

c   Labial   Distal

b   Labial   Lingual   Distal

A Incisors
a Central incisor (9); **b** lateral incisor (10); **c** lower incisors (23–26; 24 and 25 central; see p. 38 for coding). The incisor teeth have a sharp-edged crown that is consistent with their function of biting off bits of food. The palatal surface often bears a blind pit, the foramen cecum (not shown here), which is a site of predilection for dental caries.

B Canines (Cuspids)
a Upper canine (11); **b** lower canine (22); * = the tip of the crown, which represents the occlusal surface. The crown is thicker mesially than distally, and has greater curvature (arrow). In dogs, these teeth (also known as cuspids or eye teeth) are developed into fangs for gripping the prey between the jaws—hence the term "canine."

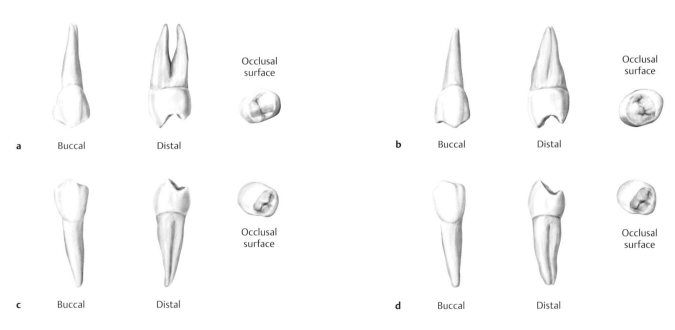

a   Buccal   Distal   Occlusal surface

b   Buccal   Distal   Occlusal surface

c   Buccal   Distal   Occlusal surface

d   Buccal   Distal   Occlusal surface

C Premolars (Bicuspids)
a First premolar (1st bicuspid, 12); **b** second premolar (2nd bicuspid, 13); **c** first premolar (21); **d** second premolar (20). The premolars represent a transitional form between the incisors and molars. Like the molars, they have cusps and fissures indicating that their primary function is the grinding of food, rather than biting and tearing. The upper left

first premolar (12, **a**) is the only premolar that has two roots. Its mesial surface which borders the neighboring proximal tooth often bears a small pit that is difficult to clean and vulnerable to caries. The other premolars have one root that is divided by a longitudinal groove and contains two root canals.

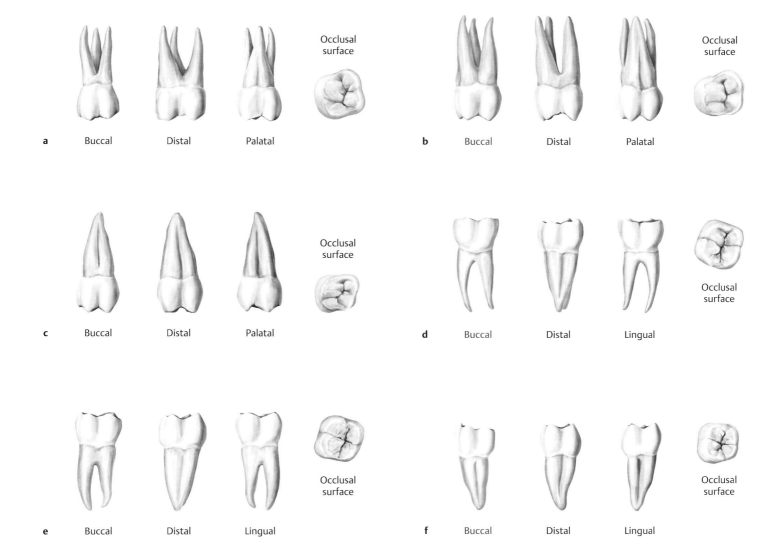

a | Buccal | Distal | Palatal | Occlusal surface
b | Buccal | Distal | Palatal | Occlusal surface
c | Buccal | Distal | Palatal | Occlusal surface
d | Buccal | Distal | Lingual | Occlusal surface
e | Buccal | Distal | Lingual | Occlusal surface
f | Buccal | Distal | Lingual | Occlusal surface

D Molars

a First molar (6-yr molar, 14); **b** second molar (12-yr molar, 15); **c** third molar (wisdom tooth, 16); **d** first molar (19); **e** second molar (18); **f** third molar (17). Most of the molars have three roots to withstand the greater masticatory pressures in the molar region. The roots of the third molars (the wisdom teeth, which erupt after 16 years of age,

if at all) are commonly fused together, particularly in the upper third molars. Because the molars crush and grind food, they have a crown with a plateau. The fissures between the cusps are a frequent site of caries formation in adolescents.

Note: The term *lingual* is used for the mandibular teeth, the term *palatal* for the maxillary teeth.

1.21 Deciduous Teeth

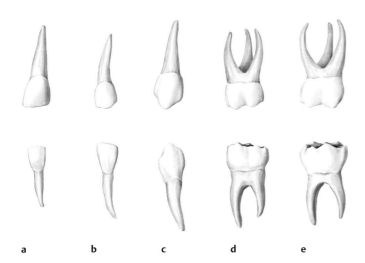

a   b   c   d   e

A Deciduous teeth of the left side
The deciduous dentition (baby teeth) consists of only 20 teeth. Each of the four quadrants contains the following teeth:

a   Central incisor (first incisor)
b   Lateral incisor (second incisor)
c   Canine (cuspid)
d   First molar (6-yr molar)
e   Second molar (12-yr molar)

To distinguish the deciduous teeth from the permanent teeth, they are coded with letters. The upper arch is labeled A to J, the lower is labeled K to T (see **D**).

B Eruption of the teeth
The eruptions of the deciduous and permanent teeth are called the first and second dentitions, respectively. The individual teeth are listed from left to right (viewer's perspective) and the types of teeth are ordered according to the time of eruption.

First dentition	Type of tooth	Individual tooth (see **D**)	Time of eruption
	Central incisor	E, F; P, O	6–8 months
	Lateral incisor	D, G; Q, N	8–12 months
	First molar	B, I; S, L	12–16 months
	Canines	C, H; R, M	15–20 months
	Second molar	A, J; T, K	20–40 months

Second dentition	Type of tooth	Individual tooth (see p. 38)	Time of eruption
	First molar	3, 14; 30, 19	6–8 years ("6-yr molar")
	Central incisor	8, 9; 25, 24	6–9 years
	Lateral incisor	7, 10; 26, 23	7–10 years
	First premolar	5, 12; 28, 21	9–13 years
	Canine	6, 11; 27, 22	9–14 years
	Second premolar	4, 13; 29, 20	11–14 years
	Second molar	2, 15; 31, 18	10–14 years ("12-yr molar")
	Third molar	1, 16; 32, 17	16–30 years ("wisdom tooth")

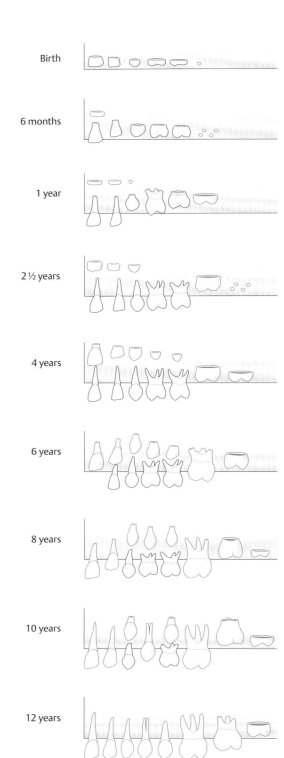

Birth

6 months

1 year

2 ½ years

4 years

6 years

8 years

10 years

12 years

C Eruption pattern of the deciduous and permanent teeth
   (after Meyer)
The eruption pattern is illustrated for the upper left teeth (deciduous teeth in black, permanent teeth in red). Knowing the times of eruption of the teeth is clinically important, as these data can provide a basis for diagnosing growth delays in children.

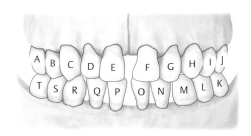

D Coding the deciduous teeth

The upper right molar is considered A. The lettering then proceeds clockwise along the upper arc and back across the lower.

E Dentition of a 6-year-old child

a, b Anterior view; **c, d** left lateral view. The anterior bony plate over the roots of the deciduous teeth has been removed to display the underlying permanent tooth buds (pale blue). This age was selected because all of the deciduous teeth have erupted by this time and are all still present. The first permanent tooth, the "6-year molar," also begins to erupt at this age (see **C**).

Anterior view of maxilla (**a**) and mandible (**b**); left lateral view of maxilla (**c**) and mandible (**d**).

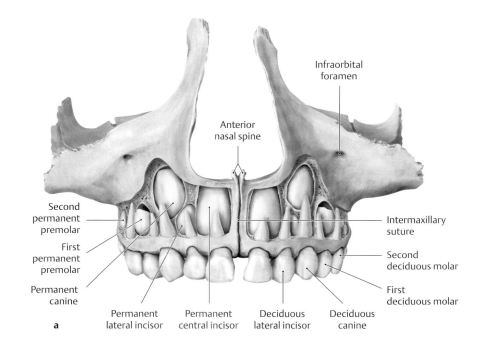

Infraorbital foramen
Anterior nasal spine
Second permanent premolar
First permanent premolar
Permanent canine
Intermaxillary suture
Second deciduous molar
First deciduous molar
Permanent lateral incisor
Permanent central incisor
Deciduous lateral incisor
Deciduous canine

a

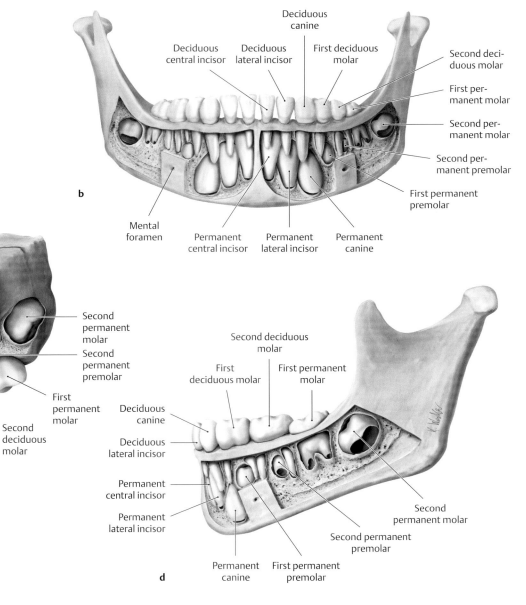

Deciduous canine
Deciduous central incisor
Deciduous lateral incisor
First deciduous molar
Second deciduous molar
First permanent molar
Second permanent molar
Second permanent premolar
First permanent premolar
Mental foramen
Permanent central incisor
Permanent lateral incisor
Permanent canine

b

Permanent canine
Permanent lateral incisor
First permanent premolar
Deciduous central incisor
Second permanent molar
Second permanent premolar
First permanent molar
Second deciduous molar
Deciduous lateral incisor
Deciduous canine
First deciduous molar

c

Second deciduous molar
First deciduous molar
First permanent molar
Deciduous canine
Deciduous lateral incisor
Permanent central incisor
Permanent lateral incisor
Second permanent molar
Second permanent premolar
Permanent canine
First permanent premolar

d

2.1 Muscles of Facial Expression, Overview

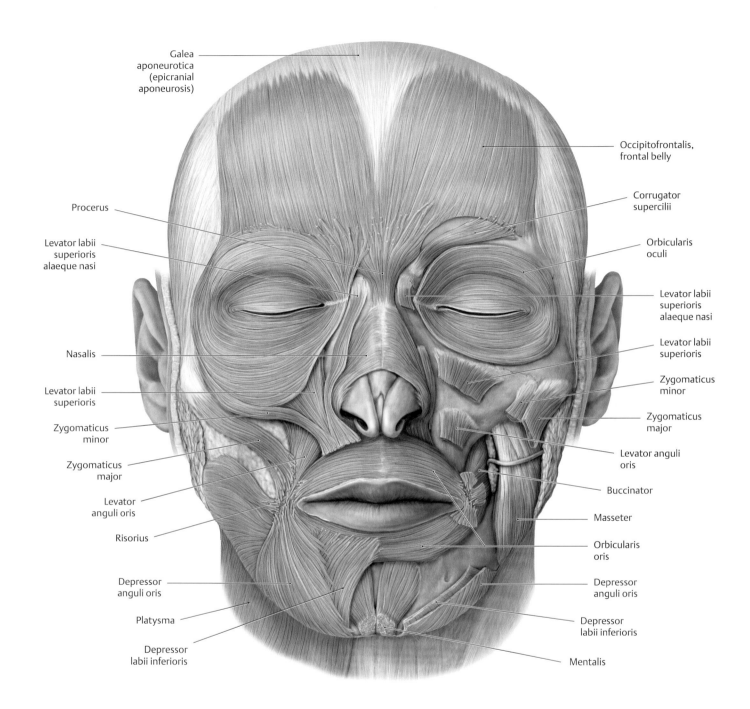

Galea aponeurotica (epicranial aponeurosis)

Procerus

Levator labii superioris alaeque nasi

Nasalis

Levator labii superioris

Zygomaticus minor

Zygomaticus major

Levator anguli oris

Risorius

Depressor anguli oris

Platysma

Depressor labii inferioris

Occipitofrontalis, frontal belly

Corrugator supercilii

Orbicularis oculi

Levator labii superioris alaeque nasi

Levator labii superioris

Zygomaticus minor

Zygomaticus major

Levator anguli oris

Buccinator

Masseter

Orbicularis oris

Depressor anguli oris

Depressor labii inferioris

Mentalis

A   Muscles of facial expression
Anterior view. The superficial layer of muscles is shown on the right half of the face, the deep layer on the left half. The muscles of facial expression represent the superficial muscle layer in the face and vary greatly in their development among different individuals. They arise either directly from the periosteum or from adjacent muscles to which they are connected, and they insert either onto other facial muscles or directly into the connective tissue of the skin. The classic scheme of classifying the other somatic muscles by their origins and insertions is not so easily adapted to the facial muscles. Because the muscles of facial expression terminate directly in the subcutaneous fat and because the superficial body fascia is absent in the face, the surgeon must be particularly careful when dissecting in this region. Because of their cutaneous attachments, the facial muscles are able to move the facial skin (e.g., they can wrinkle the skin, an action temporarily abolished by botulinum toxin injection) and produce a variety of facial expressions. They also serve a protective function (especially for the eyes) and are active during food ingestion (closing the mouth for swallowing). All of the facial muscles are innervated by branches of the facial nerve, while the muscles of mastication (see p. 48) are supplied by motor fibers from the trigeminal nerve (the masseter muscle has been left in place to represent these muscles). A thorough understanding of muscular anatomy in this region is facilitated by dividing the muscles into different groups (see p. 47).

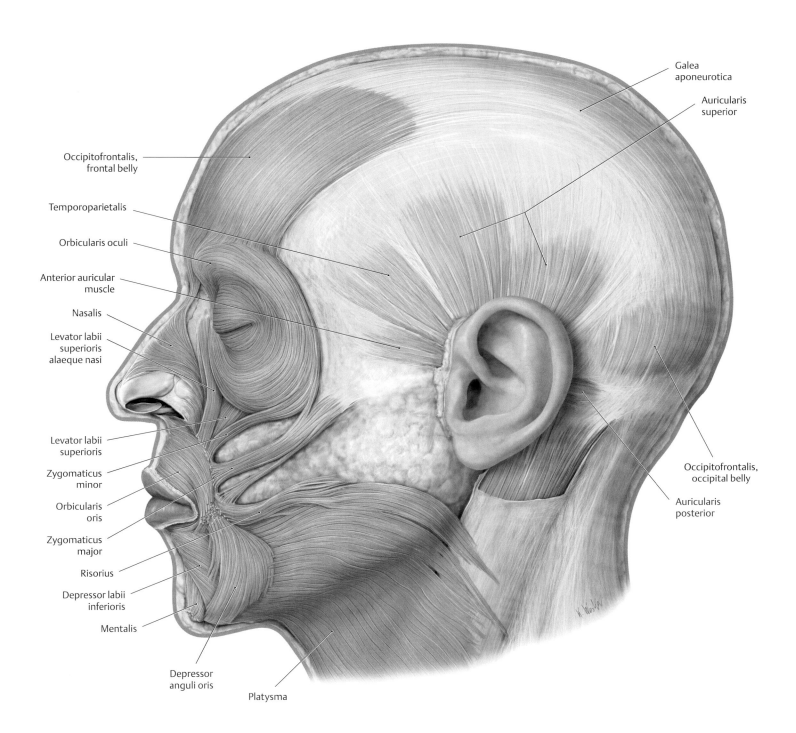

Galea
aponeurotica

Auricularis
superior

Occipitofrontalis,
frontal belly

Temporoparietalis

Orbicularis oculi

Anterior auricular
muscle

Nasalis

Levator labii
superioris
alaeque nasi

Levator labii
superioris

Zygomaticus
minor

Orbicularis
oris

Zygomaticus
major

Risorius

Depressor labii
inferioris

Mentalis

Depressor
anguli oris

Platysma

Occipitofrontalis,
occipital belly

Auricularis
posterior

B Muscles of facial expression
Left lateral view. The superficial muscles of the ear and neck are particularly well displayed from this perspective. A tough tendinous sheet, the galea aponeurotica, stretches over the calvaria and is loosely attached to the periosteum. The muscles of the calvaria that arise from the galea aponeurotica are known collectively as the "epicranial muscle." The two bellies of the occipitofrontalis (frontal and occipital) can be clearly identified. The temporoparietalis, whose posterior part is called the auricularis superior muscle, arises from the lateral part of the galea aponeurotica.

2.2 Muscles of Facial Expression, Actions

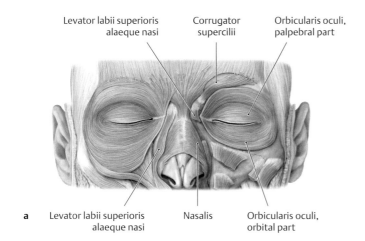

a | Levator labii superioris alaeque nasi | Nasalis | Orbicularis oculi, orbital part

Levator labii superioris alaeque nasi | Corrugator supercilii | Orbicularis oculi, palpebral part

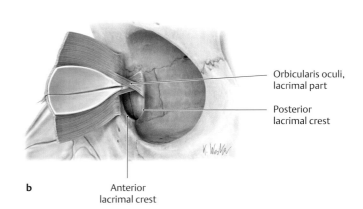

b | Anterior lacrimal crest

Orbicularis oculi, lacrimal part

Posterior lacrimal crest

A Muscles of facial expression: palpebral fissure and nose

a Anterior view. The most functionally important muscle is the *orbicularis oculi,* which closes the palpebral fissure (protective reflex against foreign matter). If the action of the orbicularis oculi is lost because of facial nerve paralysis (see also **D**), the loss of this protective reflex will be accompanied by drying of the eye from prolonged exposure to the air. The function of the orbicularis oculi is tested by asking the patient to squeeze the eyelids tightly shut.

b The orbicularis oculi has been dissected from the left orbit to the medial canthus of the eye and reflected anteriorly to demonstrate its lacrimal part (called the Horner muscle). This part of the orbicularis oculi arises mainly from the posterior lacrimal crest, and its action is a subject of debate (expand or empty the lacrimal sac).

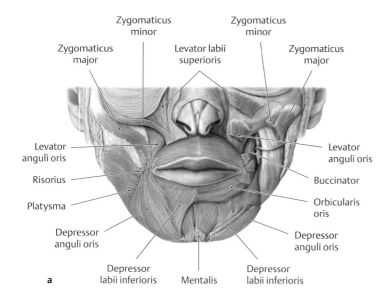

a | Depressor labii inferioris | Mentalis | Depressor labii inferioris

Zygomaticus major
Zygomaticus major | Zygomaticus minor | Levator labii superioris | Zygomaticus minor | Zygomaticus major
Levator anguli oris | Levator anguli oris
Risorius | Buccinator
Platysma | Orbicularis oris
Depressor anguli oris | Depressor anguli oris

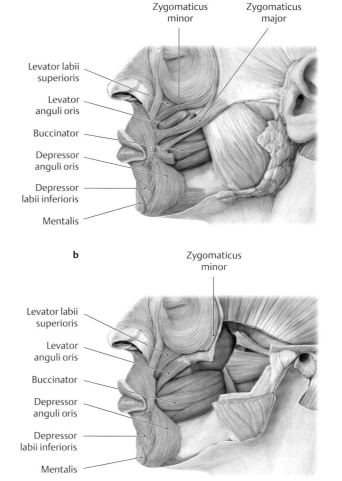

Zygomaticus minor | Zygomaticus major
Levator labii superioris
Levator anguli oris
Buccinator
Depressor anguli oris
Depressor labii inferioris
Mentalis
b

Zygomaticus minor
Levator labii superioris
Levator anguli oris
Buccinator
Depressor anguli oris
Depressor labii inferioris
Mentalis
c

B Muscles of facial expression: mouth

a Anterior view, **b** left lateral view, **c** left lateral view of the deeper lateral layer.

The *orbicularis oris* forms the muscular foundation of the lips, and its contraction closes the oral aperture. Its function can be tested by asking the patient to whistle. Facial nerve paralysis may lead to drinking difficulties because the liquid will trickle back out of the unclosed mouth during swallowing. The *buccinator* lies at a deeper level and forms the foundation of the cheek. During mastication, this muscle moves food in between the dental arches from the oral vestibule.

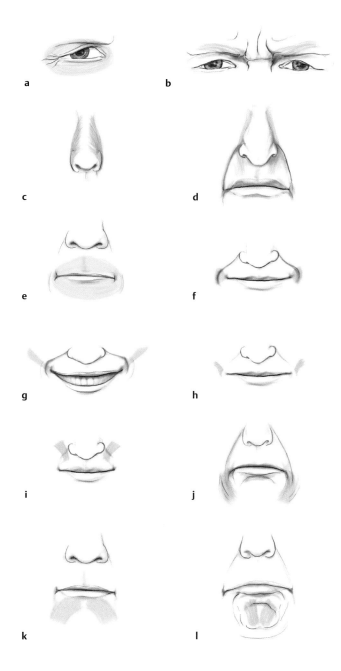

C Changes of facial expression

a Contraction of the orbicularis oculi at the lateral canthus of the eye expresses concern.

b Contraction of the corrugator supercilii occurs in response to bright sunlight: "thoughtful brow."

c Contraction of the nasalis constricts the naris and produces a cheery or lustful facial expression.

d Forceful contraction of the levator labii superioris alaeque nasi on both sides is a sign of disapproval.

e Contraction of the orbicularis oris expresses determination.

f Contraction of the buccinator signals satisfaction.

g The zygomaticus major contracts during smiling.

h Contraction of the risorius reflects purposeful action.

i Contraction of the levator anguli oris signals self-satisfaction.

j Contraction of the depressor anguli oris signals sadness.

k Contraction of the depressor labii inferioris depresses the lower lip and expresses perseverence.

l Contraction of the mentalis expresses indecision.

D Muscles of facial expression: functional groups

The various mimetic muscles are easier to learn when they are studied by regions. It is useful clinically to distinguish between the muscles of the forehead and palpebral fissure and the rest of the mimetic muscles. The muscles of the forehead and palpebral fissure are innervated by the superior branch of the facial nerve, while all the other mimetic muscles are supplied by other facial nerve branches. As a result, patients with central facial nerve paralysis can still close their eyes while patients with peripheral facial nerve paralysis cannot (see p. 79 for further details).

Region	Muscle	Remarks
Calvaria	Epicranial muscle, consisting of:	Muscle of the calvaria
	– Occipitofrontalis (frontal and occipital bellies)	Wrinkles the forehead
	– Temporoparietalis	Has no mimetic function
Palpebral fissure	Orbicularis oculi, consisting of:	Closes the eyelid (**a**)*
	– Orbital part	Tightly contracts the skin around the eye
	– Palpebral part	Palpebral reflex
	– Lacrimal part	Acts on the lacrimal sac
	Corrugator supercilii	Wrinkles the eyebrow (**b**)
	Depressor supercilii	Lowers the eyebrow
Nose	Procerus	Wrinkles the root of the nose
	Nasalis	Narrows the naris (**c**)
	Levator labii superioris alaeque nasi	Elevates the upper lip and nasal alae (**d**)
Mouth	Orbicularis oris	Closes the mouth (**e**)
	Buccinator	Muscle of the cheek (important during eating and drinking) (**f**)
	Zygomaticus major	Large muscle of the zygomatic arch (**g**)
	Zygomaticus minor	Small muscle of the zygomatic arch
	Risorius	Muscle of laughter (**h**)
	Levator labii superioris	Elevates the upper lip
	Levator anguli oris	Pulls the corner of the mouth upward (**i**)
	Depressor anguli oris	Pulls the corner of the mouth downward (**j**)
	Depressor labii inferioris	Pulls the lower lip downward (**k**)
	Mentalis	Pulls the skin of the chin upward (**l**)
Ear	Auricularis anterior	Anterior muscle of the auricle
	Auricularis superior	Superior muscle of the auricle
	Auricularis posterior	Posterior muscle of the auricle
Neck	Platysma	Cutaneous muscle of the neck

*Letters refer to sub-entries in **C**.

2.3 Muscles of Mastication, Overview and Superficial Muscles

Overview of the muscles of mastication

The muscles of mastication in the strict sense consist of four muscles: the masseter, temporalis, medial pterygoid, and lateral pterygoid.

The primary function of all these muscles is to close the mouth and move the upper teeth against the lower teeth in a grinding action during mastication. The lateral pterygoid muscle assists in opening the mouth. The two pterygoid muscles are also active during mastication (for the individual muscle actions, see **A–C**).

The mouth is opened primarily by the suprahyoid muscles and the force of gravity. The masseter and medial pterygoid form a muscular sling in which the mandible is suspended (see p. 50).

Note: all muscles of mastication are innervated by the mandibular nerve (third division of the trigeminal nerve), while the muscles of facial expression are innervated by the facial nerve.

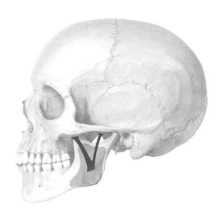

A Schematic of the masseter muscle

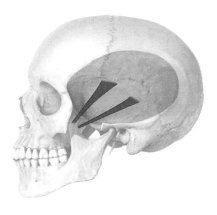

B Schematic of the temporalis muscle

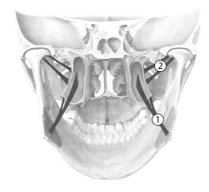

C Schematic of the medial and lateral pterygoid muscles

Masseter

Origin:	• Superficial part: zygomatic arch (anterior two-thirds)
	• Deep part: zygomatic arch (posterior third)
Insertion:	• Masseteric tuberosity on the mandibular angle
Actions:	• Elevates the mandible
	• Protrudes the mandible
Innervation:	Masseteric nerve, a branch of the mandibular division of the trigeminal nerve (CN V$_3$)

Temporalis

Origin:	Inferior temporal line of the temporal fossa
Insertion:	Apex and medial surface of the coronoid process of the mandible
Actions:	• Elevates the mandible, chiefly with its vertical fibers
	• Retracts the protruded mandible with its horizontal posterior fibers
	• Unilateral contraction: mastication (moves the mandibular head on the balance side forward)
Innervation:	Deep temporal nerves, branches of the mandibular division of the trigeminal nerve (CN V$_3$)

① Medial pterygoid

Origin:	Pterygoid fossa and lateral plate of the pterygoid process
Insertion:	Medial surface of the mandibular angle (pterygoid tuberosity)
Actions:	Elevates the mandible
Innervation:	Medial pterygoid nerve, a branch of the mandibular division of the trigeminal nerve (CN V$_3$)

② Lateral pterygoid

Origin:	• Superior part: infratemporal crest (greater wing of the sphenoid bone)
	• Inferior part: outer surface of the lateral plate of the pterygoid process
Insertion:	• Superior part: articular disk of the temporomandibular joint
	• Inferior part: condylar process of the mandible
Actions:	• Bilateral contraction: initiates mouth opening by protruding the mandible and moving the articular disk forward
	• Unilateral contraction: elevates the mandible to the opposite side during mastication
Innervation:	Lateral pterygoid nerve, a branch of the mandibular division of the trigeminal nerve (CN V$_3$)

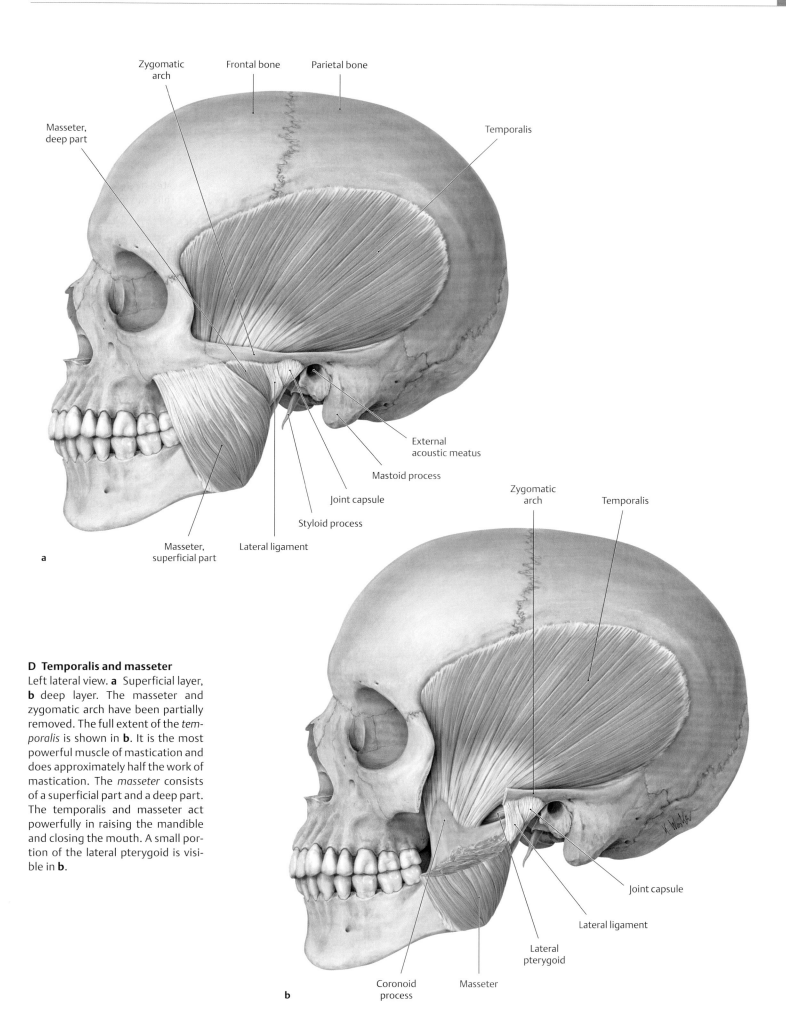

Zygomatic arch

Frontal bone

Parietal bone

Masseter, deep part

Temporalis

External acoustic meatus

Mastoid process

Joint capsule

Styloid process

Masseter, superficial part

Lateral ligament

a

Zygomatic arch

Temporalis

D Temporalis and masseter
Left lateral view. **a** Superficial layer, **b** deep layer. The masseter and zygomatic arch have been partially removed. The full extent of the *temporalis* is shown in **b**. It is the most powerful muscle of mastication and does approximately half the work of mastication. The *masseter* consists of a superficial part and a deep part. The temporalis and masseter act powerfully in raising the mandible and closing the mouth. A small portion of the lateral pterygoid is visible in **b**.

Joint capsule

Lateral ligament

Lateral pterygoid

Coronoid process

Masseter

b

49

2.4 Muscles of Mastication: Deep Muscles

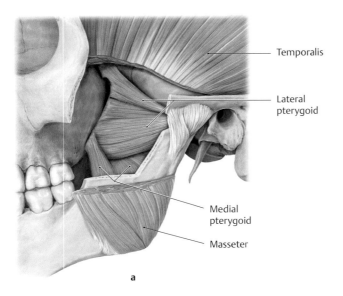

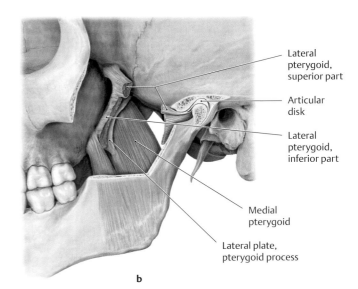

a

b

A Lateral and medial pterygoid muscles

Left lateral views.

a The coronoid process of the mandible has been removed here along with the lower part of the temporalis so that both pterygoid muscles can be seen (see p. 49 **Db**).

b Here the temporalis has been completely removed, and the inferior part of the lateral pterygoid has been windowed. The *lateral* pterygoid initiates mouth opening, which is then continued by the suprahyoid muscles. With the temporomandibular joint opened, we can

see that fibers from the lateral pterygoid blend with the articular disk. The lateral pterygoid functions as the guide muscle of the temporomandibular joint. Because its various parts (superior and inferior) are active during all movements, its actions are more complex than those of the other muscles of mastication. The *medial* pterygoid runs almost perpendicular to the lateral pterygoid and contributes to the formation of a muscular sling that partially encompasses the mandible (see **B**).

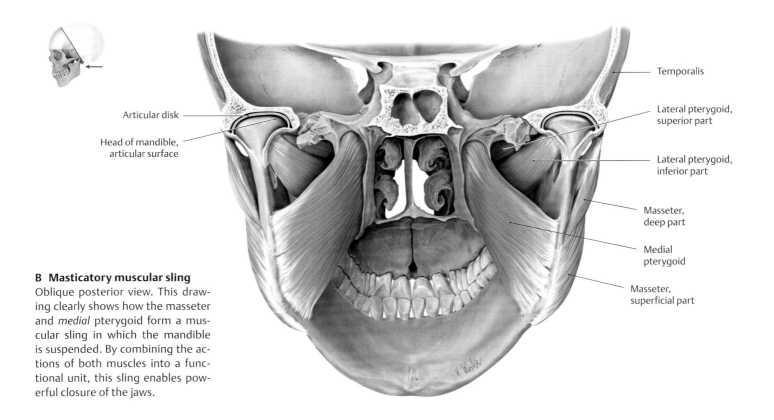

B Masticatory muscular sling

Oblique posterior view. This drawing clearly shows how the masseter and *medial* pterygoid form a muscular sling in which the mandible is suspended. By combining the actions of both muscles into a functional unit, this sling enables powerful closure of the jaws.

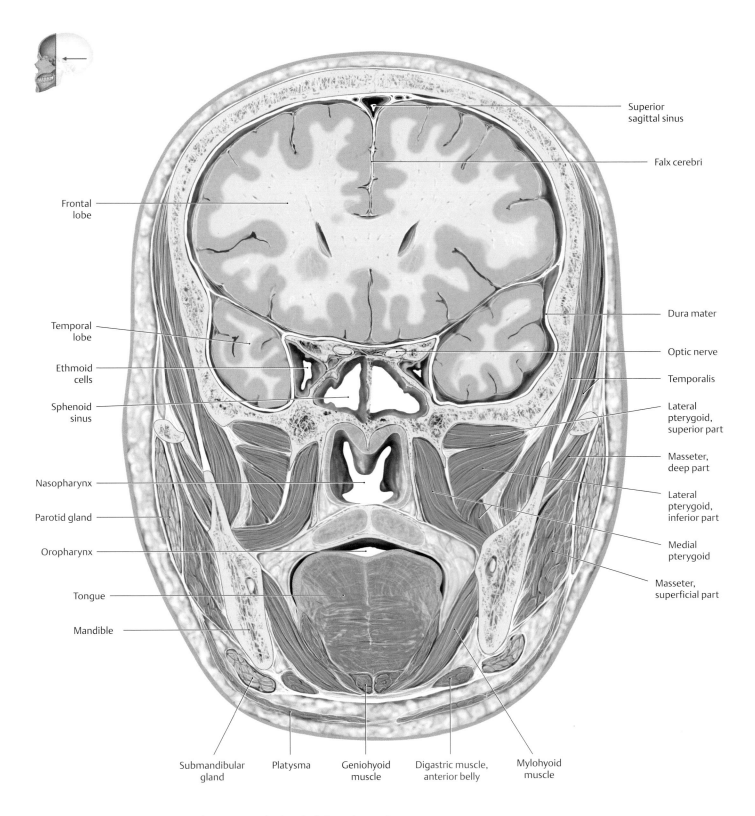

Superior
sagittal sinus

Falx cerebri

Frontal
lobe

Dura mater

Temporal
lobe

Optic nerve

Ethmoid
cells

Temporalis

Sphenoid
sinus

Lateral
pterygoid,
superior part

Masseter,
deep part

Nasopharynx

Lateral
pterygoid,
inferior part

Parotid gland

Oropharynx

Medial
pterygoid

Tongue

Masseter,
superficial part

Mandible

Submandibular
gland

Platysma

Geniohyoid
muscle

Digastric muscle,
anterior belly

Mylohyoid
muscle

C Muscles of mastication, coronal section at the level of the sphenoid sinus
Posterior view. The topography of the muscles of mastication and neighboring structures is particularly well displayed in this section.

2.5 Muscles of the Head, Origins and Insertions

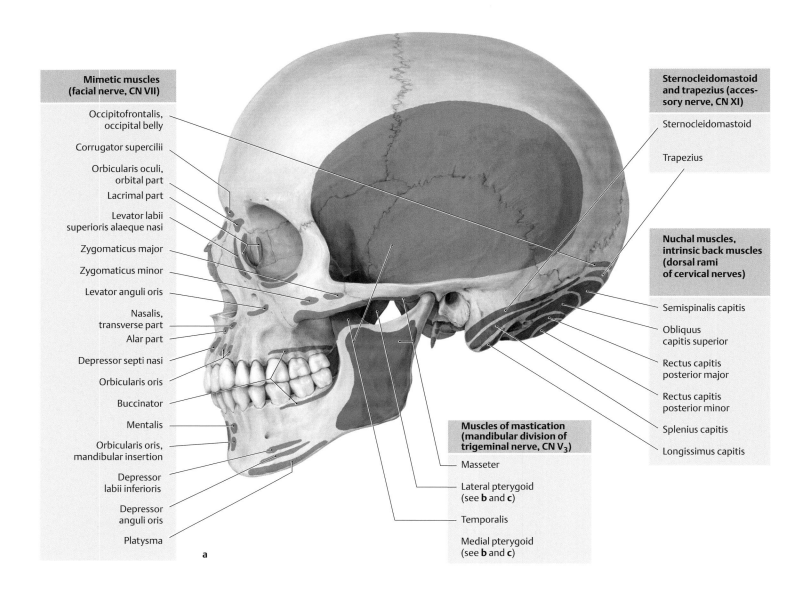

Mimetic muscles (facial nerve, CN VII)
- Occipitofrontalis, occipital belly
- Corrugator supercilii
- Orbicularis oculi, orbital part
- Lacrimal part
- Levator labii superioris alaeque nasi
- Zygomaticus major
- Zygomaticus minor
- Levator anguli oris
- Nasalis, transverse part
- Alar part
- Depressor septi nasi
- Orbicularis oris
- Buccinator
- Mentalis
- Orbicularis oris, mandibular insertion
- Depressor labii inferioris
- Depressor anguli oris
- Platysma

Sternocleidomastoid and trapezius (accessory nerve, CN XI)
- Sternocleidomastoid
- Trapezius

Nuchal muscles, intrinsic back muscles (dorsal rami of cervical nerves)
- Semispinalis capitis
- Obliquus capitis superior
- Rectus capitis posterior major
- Rectus capitis posterior minor
- Splenius capitis
- Longissimus capitis

Muscles of mastication (mandibular division of trigeminal nerve, CN V₃)
- Masseter
- Lateral pterygoid (see **b** and **c**)
- Temporalis
- Medial pterygoid (see **b** and **c**)

a

A Muscle origins and insertions on the skull

a Left lateral view, **b** view of the inner surface of the right hemimandible, **c** inferior view of the base of the skull.

The origins and insertions of the muscles are indicated by color shading (origin: red, insertion: blue).

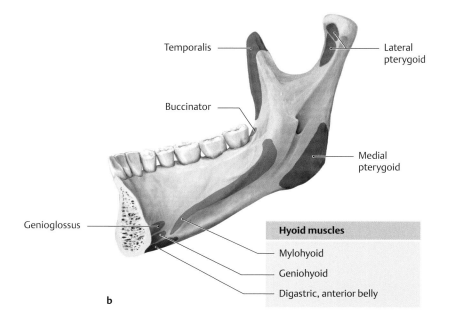

- Temporalis
- Lateral pterygoid
- Buccinator
- Medial pterygoid
- Genioglossus

Hyoid muscles
- Mylohyoid
- Geniohyoid
- Digastric, anterior belly

b

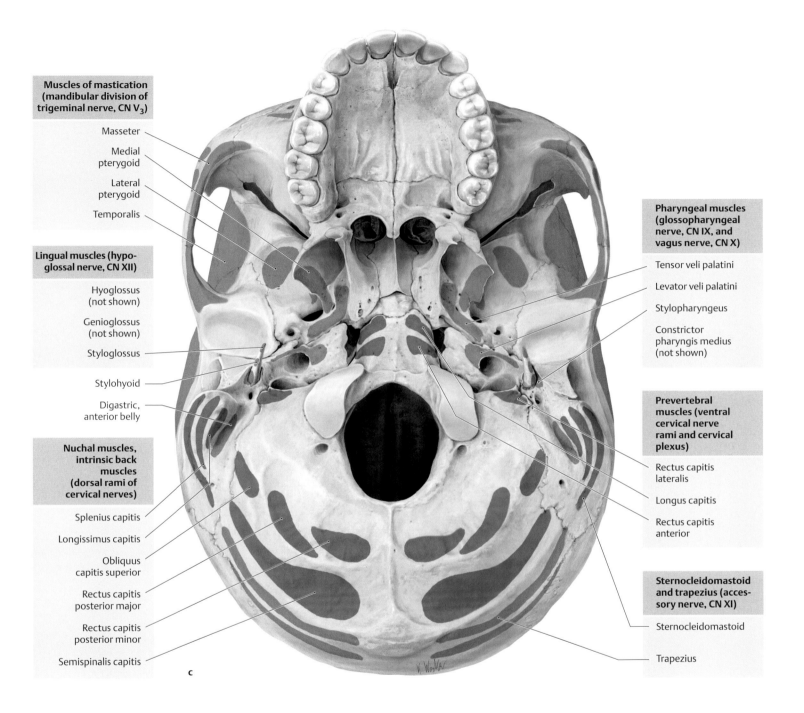

Muscles of mastication (mandibular division of trigeminal nerve, CN V₃)

Masseter

Medial pterygoid

Lateral pterygoid

Temporalis

Lingual muscles (hypoglossal nerve, CN XII)

Hyoglossus (not shown)

Genioglossus (not shown)

Styloglossus

Stylohyoid

Digastric, anterior belly

Nuchal muscles, intrinsic back muscles (dorsal rami of cervical nerves)

Splenius capitis

Longissimus capitis

Obliquus capitis superior

Rectus capitis posterior major

Rectus capitis posterior minor

Semispinalis capitis

Pharyngeal muscles (glossopharyngeal nerve, CN IX, and vagus nerve, CN X)

Tensor veli palatini

Levator veli palatini

Stylopharyngeus

Constrictor pharyngis medius (not shown)

Prevertebral muscles (ventral cervical nerve rami and cervical plexus)

Rectus capitis lateralis

Longus capitis

Rectus capitis anterior

Sternocleidomastoid and trapezius (accessory nerve, CN XI)

Sternocleidomastoid

Trapezius

c

3.1   Arteries of the Head, Overview and External Carotid Artery

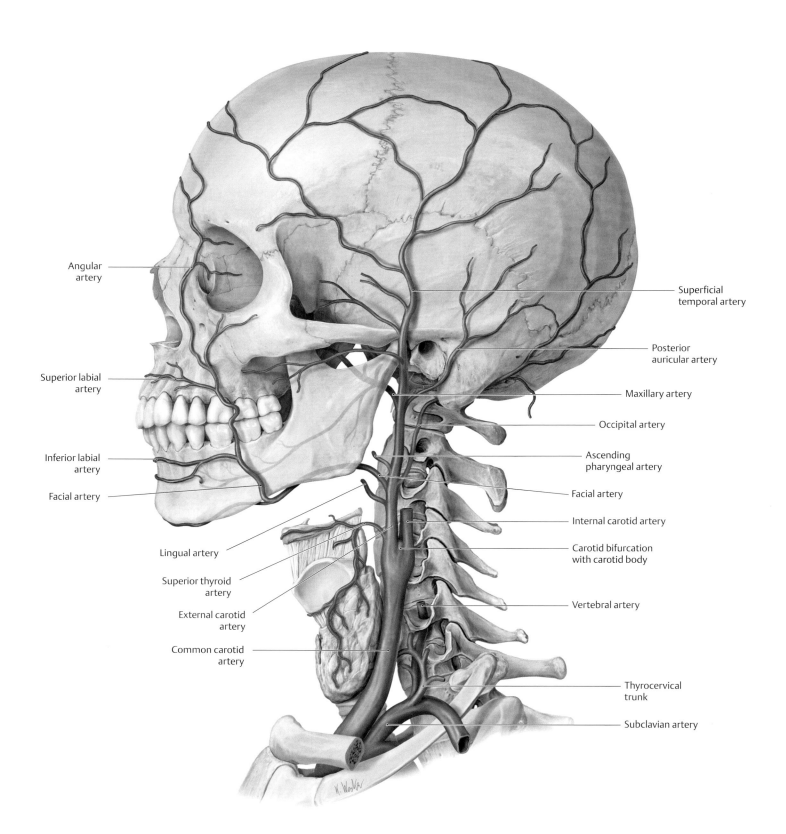

Angular artery

Superficial temporal artery

Superior labial artery

Posterior auricular artery

Maxillary artery

Occipital artery

Inferior labial artery

Ascending pharyngeal artery

Facial artery

Facial artery

Internal carotid artery

Lingual artery

Carotid bifurcation with carotid body

Superior thyroid artery

External carotid artery

Vertebral artery

Common carotid artery

Thyrocervical trunk

Subclavian artery

A Overview of the arteries of the head

Left lateral view. The common carotid artery divides into the internal carotid artery and external carotid artery at the carotid bifurcation, which is at the approximate level of the fourth cervical vertebra. The carotid body (not shown) is located at the carotid bifurcation. It contains chemoreceptors that respond to oxygen deficiency in the blood

(hypoxia) and to changes in pH (both are important in the regulation of breathing). While the external carotid artery divides into eight branches (see **D**), the internal carotid artery does not branch further before entering the skull (see p. 246, cerebral vessels), where it mainly supplies blood to the brain. It also gives off branches that supply areas of the facial skeleton (see p. 60).

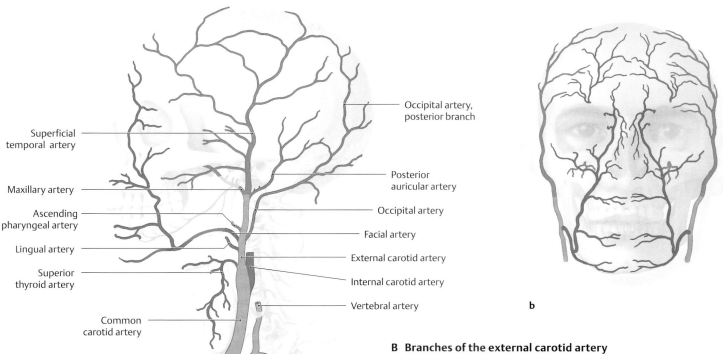

B Branches of the external carotid artery
a Left lateral view, **b** anterior view.
The four groups of branches of the external carotid artery are shown in different colors (anterior branches: red, medial branch: blue, posterior branches: green, terminal branches: brown).
Certain branches of the external carotid artery (facial artery, red) communicate with branches of the internal carotid artery (terminal branches of the ophthalmic artery, purple) through anastomoses in the facial region **b**. Extracerebral branches of the internal carotid artery are described on p. 60.

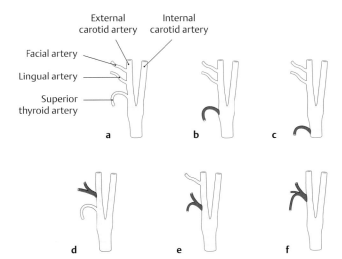

C Branches of the external carotid artery: typical anatomy and variants (after Lippert and Pabst)
a In **typical cases** (50 %) the facial artery, lingual artery, and superior thyroid artery arise from the external carotid artery above the carotid bifurcation.

b–f Variants:
b, c The superior thyroid artery arises at the level of the carotid bifurcation (20 %) or from the common carotid artery (10 %).
d–f Two or three branches combine to form a common trunk: linguofacial trunk (18 %), thyrolingual trunk (2 %), or thyrolinguofacial trunk (1 %).

D Overview of the branches of the external carotid artery
(more distal branches are described in the units below).
Subsequent units deal with the arteries of the head as they are grouped in the table below, followed by the branches of the internal carotid artery and the veins.

Name of the branches	Distribution
Anterior branches:	
• Superior thyroid artery	• Larynx, thyroid gland
• Lingual artery	• Oral floor, tongue
• Facial artery	• Superficial facial region
Medial branch:	
• Ascending pharyngeal artery	• Plexus to the skull base
Posterior branches:	
• Occipital artery	• Occiput
• Posterior auricular artery	• Ear
Terminal branches:	
• Maxillary artery	• Masticatory muscles, posteromedial part of the facial skeleton, meninges
• Superficial temporal artery	• Temporal region, part of the ear

3.2 External Carotid Artery: Anterior, Medial, and Posterior Branches

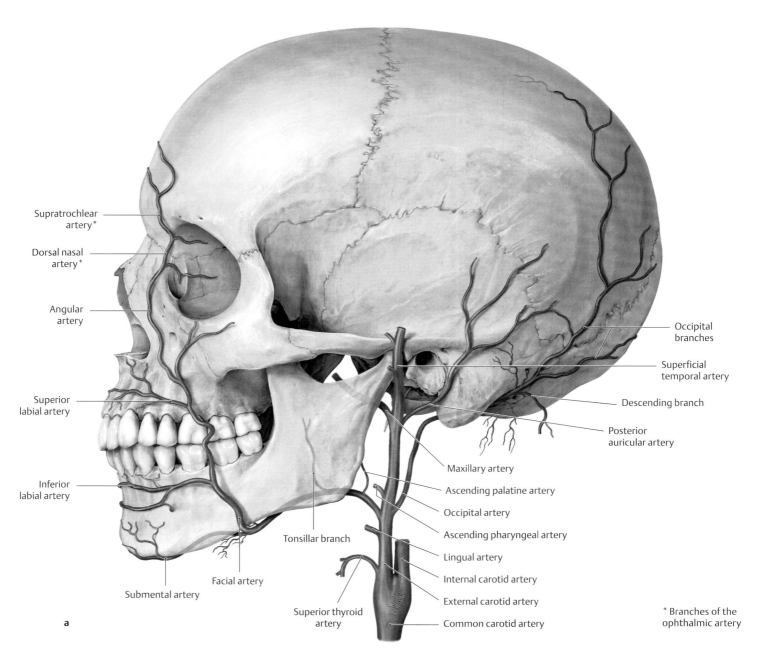

Supratrochlear artery*

Dorsal nasal artery*

Angular artery

Superior labial artery

Inferior labial artery

Occipital branches

Superficial temporal artery

Descending branch

Posterior auricular artery

Maxillary artery

Ascending palatine artery

Occipital artery

Ascending pharyngeal artery

Lingual artery

Internal carotid artery

External carotid artery

Common carotid artery

Tonsillar branch

Facial artery

Submental artery

Superior thyroid artery

a

* Branches of the ophthalmic artery

A Facial artery, occipital artery, and posterior auricular artery and their branches

Left lateral view. An important anterior branch of the external carotid artery is the **facial artery**, which gives off branches in the neck and face. The principal *cervical branch* is the ascending palatine artery; the *tonsillar branch* is ligated during tonsillectomy. Of the *facial branches*, the superior and inferior labial arteries combine to form an arterial circle around the mouth. The *terminal branch* of the facial artery, the angular artery, anastomoses with the dorsal nasal artery. The latter vessel is the terminal branch of the ophthalmic artery, which arises from the internal carotid artery. Because there are extensive arterial anastomoses, facial injuries have a tendency to bleed profusely but also tend to heal quickly and well owing to the copious blood supply. The pulse of the facial artery is palpable at the anterior border of the masseter muscle insertion on the mandibular ramus. The principal branches of the **posterior auricular artery** include the posterior tympanic artery and the parotid artery (**b**).

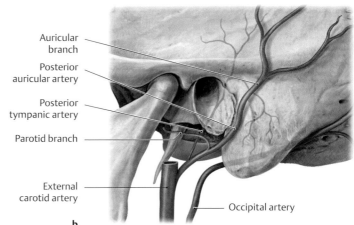

Auricular branch

Posterior auricular artery

Posterior tympanic artery

Parotid branch

External carotid artery

Occipital artery

b

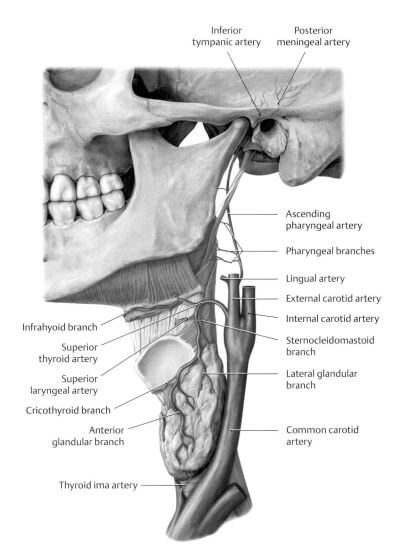

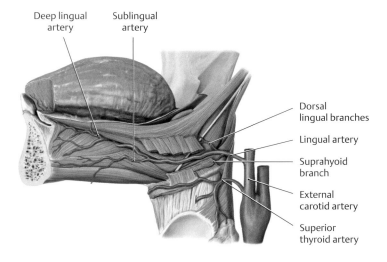

D Lingual artery and its branches

Left lateral view. The lingual artery is the second anterior branch of the external carotid artery. It has a relatively large caliber, providing the tongue with its rich blood supply. It also gives off branches to the plexus and tonsils.

B Superior thyroid artery, ascending pharyngeal artery and their branches

Left lateral view. The superior thyroid artery is typically the first branch to arise from the external carotid artery. One of the anterior branches, it supplies the larynx and thyroid gland. The ascending pharyngeal artery springs from the medial side of the external carotid artery, usually arising above the level of the superior thyroid artery. The level at which a vessel branches from the external carotid artery does not necessarily correlate with the course of the vessel.

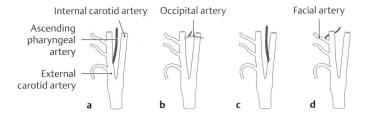

C Origin of the ascending pharyngeal artery: typical case and variants (after Lippert and Pabst)

a In **typical cases** (70%) the ascending pharyngeal artery arises from the external carotid artery.

b–d Variants:

The ascending pharyngeal artery arises from **b** the occipital artery (20%), **c** the internal carotid artery (8%), or **d** the facial artery (2%).

E Branches of the external carotid artery and their distribution: anterior, medial, and posterior branches with their principal distal branches

Branch	Distribution
Anterior branches:	
• Superior thyroid artery (see **B**)	
– Glandular branches	• Thyroid gland
– Superior laryngeal artery	• Larynx
– Sternocleidomastoid branch	• Sternocleidomastoid muscle
• Lingual artery (see **D**)	
– Dorsal lingual branches	• Base of tongue, epiglottis
– Sublingual artery	• Sublingual gland, tongue, oral floor, oral cavity
– Deep lingual artery	• Tongue
• Facial artery (see **A**)	
– Ascending palatine artery	• Pharyngeal wall, soft palate, pharyngotympanic tube
– Tonsillar branch	• Palatine tonsil (main branch)
– Submental artery	• Oral floor, submandibular gland
– Labial arteries	• Lips
– Angular artery	• Nasal root
Medial branch:	
• Ascending pharyngeal artery (see **B**)	
– Pharyngeal branches	• Pharyngeal wall
– Inferior tympanic artery	• Mucosa of middle ear
– Posterior meningeal artery	• Dura, posterior cranial fossa
Posterior branches:	
• Occipital artery (see **A**)	
– Occipital branches	• Scalp, occipital region
– Descending branch	• Posterior neck muscles
• Posterior auricular branch (see **A**)	
– Stylomastoid artery	• Facial nerve in the facial canal
– Posterior tympanic artery	• Tympanic cavity
– Auricular branch	• Posterior side of auricle
– Occipital branch	• Occiput
– Parotid branch	• Parotid gland

3.3 External Carotid Artery: Terminal Branches

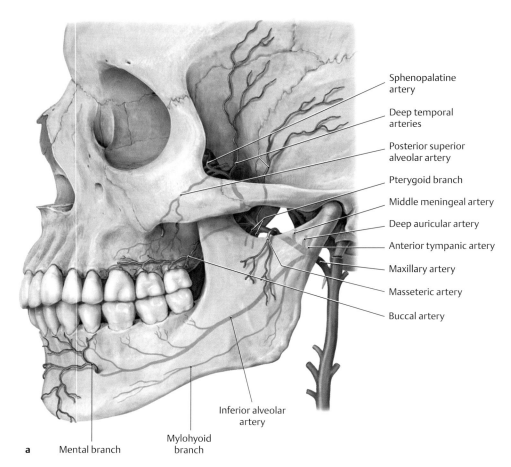

Sphenopalatine artery

Deep temporal arteries

Posterior superior alveolar artery

Pterygoid branch

Middle meningeal artery

Deep auricular artery

Anterior tympanic artery

Maxillary artery

Masseteric artery

Buccal artery

Inferior alveolar artery

Mylohyoid branch

Mental branch

a

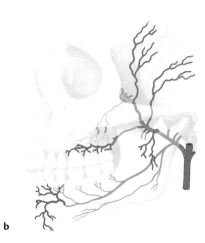

b

A Maxillary artery and its branches
Left lateral view. The maxillary artery is the larger of the two terminal branches of the external carotid artery. Its origin lies deep to the mandibular ramus (important landmark for locating the vessel). The maxillary artery consists of three parts:

- Mandibular part (blue)
- Pterygoid part (green)
- Pterygopalatine part (yellow)

B The two terminal branches of the external carotid artery with their principal branches

Branch		Distribution
Maxillary artery		
Mandibular part:	• Inferior alveolar artery	• Mandible, teeth, gingiva (the mental branch is its terminal branch)
	• Middle meningeal artery (see **C**)	• Calvaria, dura, anterior and middle cranial fossae
	• Deep auricular artery	• Temporomandibular joint, external auditory canal
	• Anterior tympanic artery	• Tympanic cavity
Pterygoid part:	• Masseteric artery	• Masseter muscle
	• Deep temporal branches	• Temporalis muscle
	• Pterygoid branches	• Pterygoid muscles
	• Buccal artery	• Buccal mucosa
Pterygopalatine part:	• Posterior superior alveolar artery	• Maxillary molars, maxillary sinus, gingiva
	• Infraorbital artery	• Maxillary alveoli
	• Descending palatine artery	
	– Greater palatine artery	• Hard palate
	– Lesser palatine artery	• Soft palate, palatine tonsil, pharyngeal wall
	• Sphenopalatine artery	
	– Lateral posterior nasal arteries	• Lateral wall of the nasal cavity, conchae
	– Posterior septal branches	• Nasal septum
Superficial temporal artery	• Transverse facial artery	• Soft tissues below the zygomatic arch
	• Frontal and parietal branches	• Scalp of the forehead and vertex
	• Zygomatico-orbital artery	• Lateral orbital wall

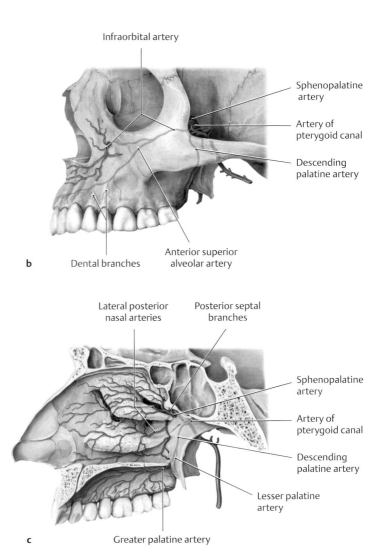

Anastomotic branch with lacrimal artery | Frontal branch | Parietal branch

Middle meningeal artery | Petrous branch

a

Infraorbital artery

Sphenopalatine artery

Artery of pterygoid canal

Descending palatine artery

Anterior superior alveolar artery

b | Dental branches

Lateral posterior nasal arteries | Posterior septal branches

Sphenopalatine artery

Artery of pterygoid canal

Descending palatine artery

Lesser palatine artery

c | Greater palatine artery

C Selected clinically important branches of the maxillary artery

a Right middle meningeal artery, **b** left infraorbital artery, **c** right sphenopalatine artery with its branches that supply the nasal cavity. The **middle meningeal artery** passes through the foramen spinosum into the middle cranial fossa. Despite its name, it supplies blood not just to the meninges but also to the overlying calvaria. Rupture of the middle meningeal artery by head trauma results in an epidural hematoma (see p. 262). The **infraorbital artery** is a branch of the maxillary artery and thus of the external carotid artery, while the supraorbital artery (a branch of the ophthalmic artery) is a terminal branch of the internal carotid artery. These vessels provide a path for a potential anastomosis between the external and internal carotid arteries. When severe naso-pharyngeal bleeding occurs from branches of the **sphenopalatine artery** (a branch of the maxillary artery), it may be necessary to ligate the maxillary artery in the pterygopalatine fossa (see pp. 100, 110; see also **C**, p. 61).

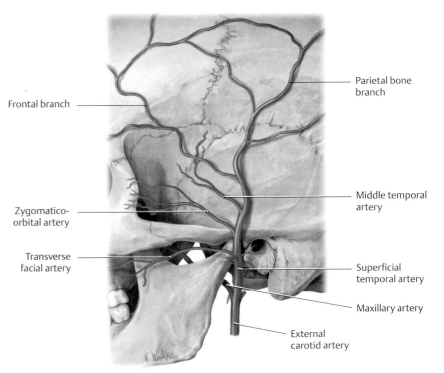

Parietal bone branch

Frontal branch

Middle temporal artery

Zygomatico-orbital artery

Transverse facial artery

Superficial temporal artery

Maxillary artery

External carotid artery

D Superficial temporal artery

Left lateral view. Particularly in elderly or ca-chectic patients, the often tortuous course of the frontal branch of this vessel can easily be traced across the temple. The superficial temporal artery may be involved in an in-flammatory autoimmune disease (temporal arteritis), which can be confirmed by biopsy of the vessel. The patients, usually elderly males, complain of severe headaches.

3.4 Internal Carotid Artery: Branches to Extracerebral Structures

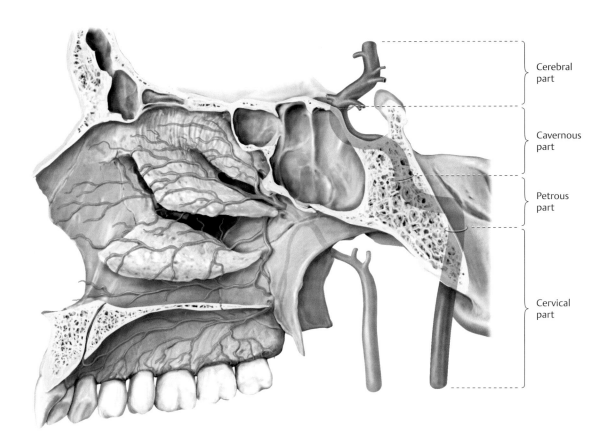

Cerebral part

Cavernous part

Petrous part

Cervical part

a

A Subdivisions of the internal carotid artery and branches that supply extracerebral structures of the head

a Medial view of the right internal carotid artery in its passage through the bones of the skull. **b** Anatomical segments of the internal carotid artery and their branches. The internal carotid artery is distributed chiefly to the brain but also supplies extracerebral regions of the head. It consists of four parts (listed from bottom to top):

- Cervical part
- Petrous part
- Cavernous part
- Cerebral part

The petrous part of the internal carotid artery (traversing the carotid canal) and the cavernous part (traversing the cavernous sinus) have a role in supplying extracerebral structures of the head. They give off additional small branches that supply local structures and are usually named for the areas they supply. Only specialists may be expected to have a detailed knowledge of these branches. Of special importance is the ophthalmic artery, which arises from the cerebral part of the internal carotid artery (see **B**).

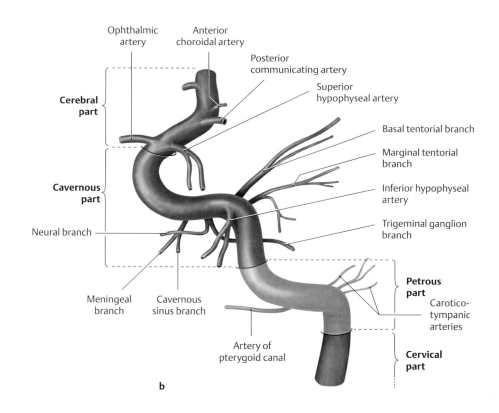

Ophthalmic artery

Anterior choroidal artery

Posterior communicating artery

Superior hypophyseal artery

Cerebral part

Basal tentorial branch

Marginal tentorial branch

Inferior hypophyseal artery

Cavernous part

Trigeminal ganglion branch

Neural branch

Meningeal branch

Cavernous sinus branch

Petrous part

Caroticotympanic arteries

Artery of pterygoid canal

Cervical part

b

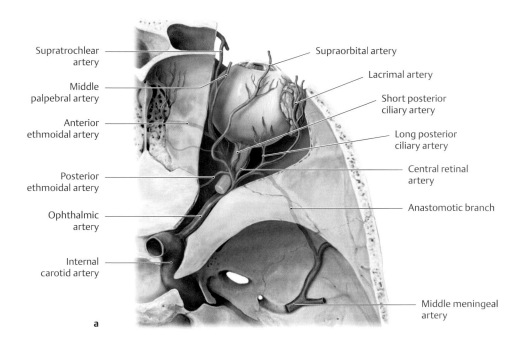

Supratrochlear artery
Middle palpebral artery
Anterior ethmoidal artery
Posterior ethmoidal artery
Ophthalmic artery
Internal carotid artery

Supraorbital artery
Lacrimal artery
Short posterior ciliary artery
Long posterior ciliary artery
Central retinal artery
Anastomotic branch
Middle meningeal artery

a

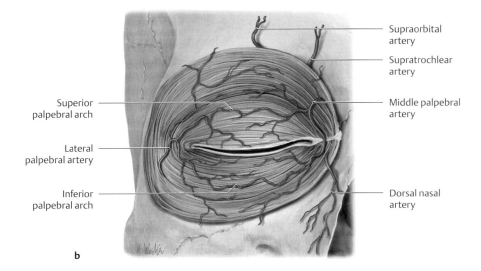

Superior palpebral arch
Lateral palpebral artery
Inferior palpebral arch

Supraorbital artery
Supratrochlear artery
Middle palpebral artery
Dorsal nasal artery

b

B Ophthalmic artery

a Superior view of the right orbit. **b** Anterior view of the facial branches of the right ophthalmic artery.

Panel **a** shows the origin of the ophthalmic artery at the internal carotid artery. The ophthalmic artery supplies blood to the eyeball itself and to the orbital structures. Some of its terminal branches are distributed to the eyelid and portions of the forehead (**b**). Other terminal branches (anterior and posterior ethmoidal arteries) contribute to the supply of the nasal septum (see **C**).

Note: Branches of the lateral palpebral artery and supraorbital artery (**b**) may form an anastomosis with the frontal branch of the superficial temporal artery (territory of the external carotid artery) (see p. 55). With atherosclerosis of the internal carotid artery, this anastomosis may become an important alternative route for blood to the brain.

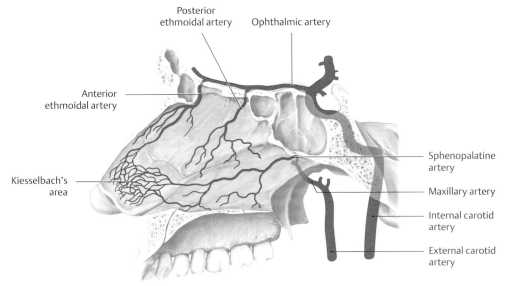

Posterior ethmoidal artery
Ophthalmic artery
Anterior ethmoidal artery
Kiesselbach's area

Sphenopalatine artery
Maxillary artery
Internal carotid artery
External carotid artery

C Vascular supply of the nasal septum

Left lateral view. The nasal septum is another region in which the internal carotid artery (anterior and posterior ethmoidal arteries, green) meets the external carotid artery (sphenopalatine artery, yellow). A richly vascularized area on the anterior part of the nasal septum, called Kiesselbach's area (blue), is the most common site of nosebleed. Since Kiesselbach's area is an area of anastamosis, it may be necessary to ligate the sphenopalatine/maxillary artery and/or the ethmoidal arteries through an orbital approach, depending on the source of the bleeding.

61

3.5 Veins of the Head and Neck: Superficial Veins

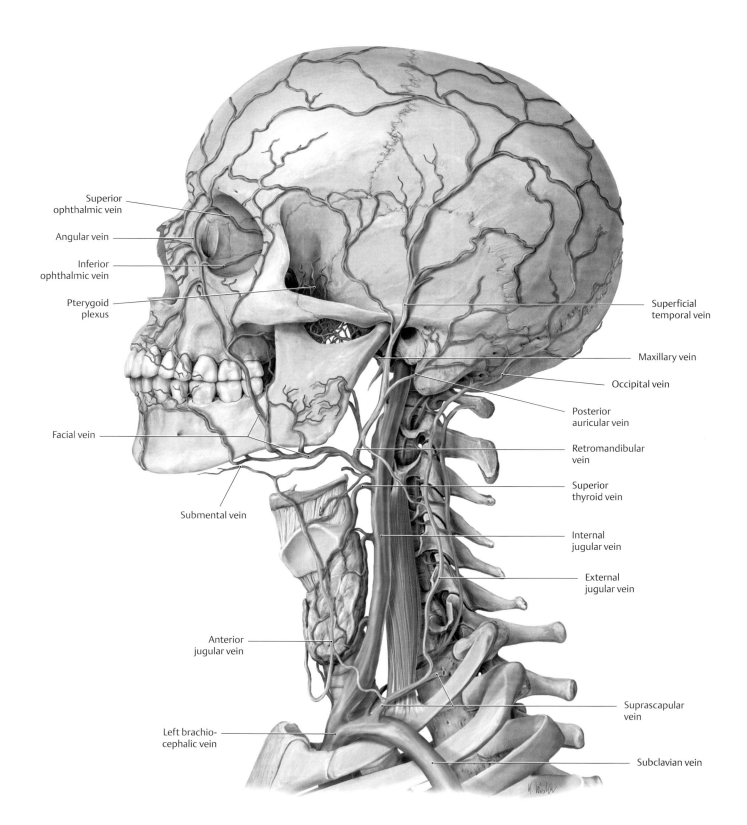

Superior ophthalmic vein

Angular vein

Inferior ophthalmic vein

Pterygoid plexus

Facial vein

Submental vein

Anterior jugular vein

Left brachio-cephalic vein

Superficial temporal vein

Maxillary vein

Occipital vein

Posterior auricular vein

Retromandibular vein

Superior thyroid vein

Internal jugular vein

External jugular vein

Suprascapular vein

Subclavian vein

A Superficial head and neck veins and their drainage to the brachiocephalic vein

Left lateral view. The principal vein of the neck is the *internal jugular vein,* which drains blood from the interior of the skull (including the brain). Enclosed in the carotid sheath, the left internal jugular vein descends from the jugular foramen to its union with the subclavian vein to form the brachiocephalic vein. The main tributaries of the internal jugular vein in the head region are the facial and thyroid veins. The *external jug-*

ular vein drains blood from the occiput (occipital vein) and nuchal region to the subclavian vein, while the *anterior jugular vein* drains the superficial anterior neck region. Besides these superficial veins, there are more deeply situated venous plexuses (orbit, pterygoid plexus, middle cranial fossa) that are described in the next unit. *Note:* The superficial veins are most closely related to the deep veins in the area of the angular vein, with an associated risk of spreading infectious organisms intracranially (see p. 65).

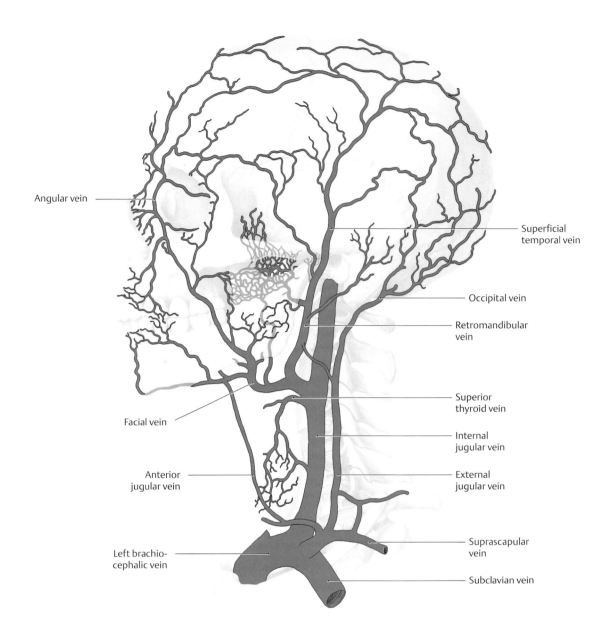

Angular vein

Superficial temporal vein

Occipital vein

Retromandibular vein

Facial vein

Superior thyroid vein

Internal jugular vein

Anterior jugular vein

External jugular vein

Suprascapular vein

Left brachio-cephalic vein

Subclavian vein

B Overview of the principal veins in the head and neck
Left lateral view. Only the more important veins are labeled in the diagram. As at many other sites in the body, the course and caliber of the veins in the head and neck are variable to a certain degree, except for the largest venous trunk. The veins interconnect to form extensive anastomoses, some of which extend to the deep veins (see **A**, pterygoid plexus).

C Drainage of blood from the head and neck
Blood from the head and neck is drained chiefly by three jugular veins: the internal, external and anterior jugular veins. These veins have a variable size and course, but the anterior jugular vein is usually the smallest and most variable of the three. The external and internal jugular veins communicate by valveless anastomoses that allow blood to drain from the external jugular vein back into the internal jugular vein. This reflux is clinically significant, as it provides a route by which bacteria from the skin of the head may gain access to the meninges (see p. 65 for details). The neck is subdivided into spaces by multiple layers of cervical fascia. One fascia-enclosed space is the carotid sheath, whose contents include the internal jugular vein. The other two jugular veins lie within the superficial cervical fascia.

Vein	Region drained	Relationship to deep cervical fasciae
• Internal jugular vein	• Interior of the skull (including the brain)	• Within the carotid sheath
• External jugular vein	• Head (superficial)	• Within the superficial cervical fascia
• Anterior jugular vein	• Neck, portions of the head	• Within the superficial cervical fascia

3.6 Veins of the Head and Neck: Deep Veins

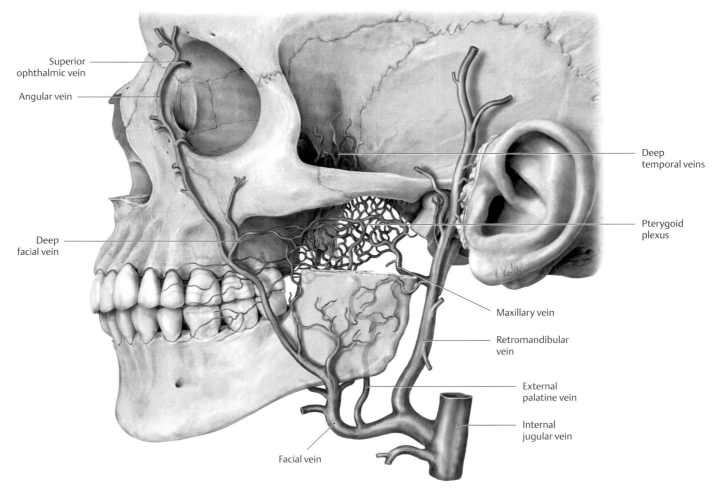

A Deep veins of the head: pterygoid plexus
Left lateral view. The pterygoid plexus is a venous network situated behind the mandibular ramus between the muscles of mastication. It has extensive connections with the adjacent veins.

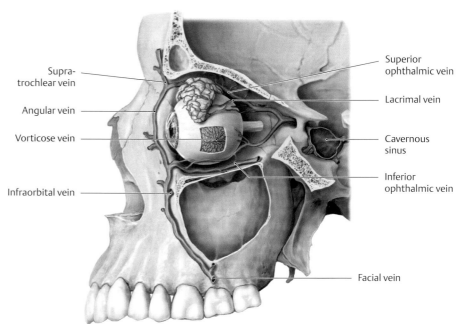

B Deep veins of the head: orbit and middle cranial fossa
Left lateral view. There are two relatively large venous trunks in the orbit, the superior and inferior ophthalmic vein. They do not run parallel to the arteries. The veins of the orbit drain predominantly into the cavernous sinus. Orbital blood can also drain externally via the angular vein and facial vein. Because the veins are valveless, extracranial bacteria may migrate to the cavernous sinus and cause thrombosis in that venous channel (see **E** and p. 93).

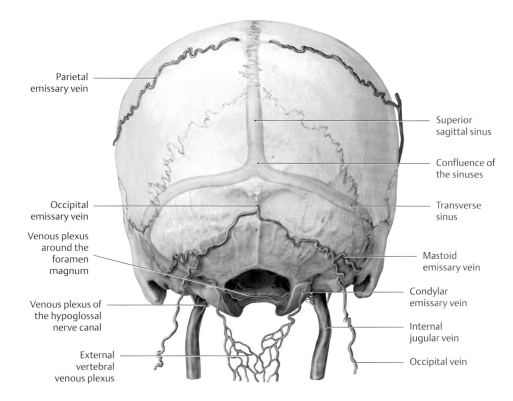

C Veins of the occiput
Posterior view. The superficial veins of the occiput communicate with the dural sinuses by way of the diploic veins. These vessels, called emissary veins, provide a potential route for the spread of infectious organisms into the dural sinuses.

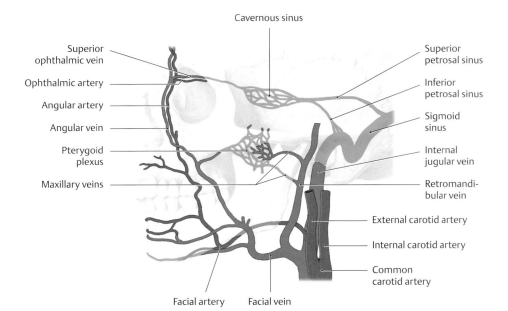

D Clinically important vascular relationships in the facial region
The facial artery and its branches and the terminal branch of the ophthalmic artery, the dorsal nasal artery, are clinically important vessels in the facial region because they may bleed profusely in patients who sustain midfacial fractures. The veins in this region are clinically important because they may allow infectious organisms to enter the cranial cavity. Bacteria from furuncles (boils) on the upper lip or nose may gain access to the cavernous sinus by way of the angular vein (see **E**).

E Venous anastomoses as portals of infection

* Very important clinically because the deep spread of bacterial infection from the facial region may result in cavernous sinus thrombosis (infection leading to clot formation that may occlude the sinus). Bacterial thrombosis is less common at other sites.

Extracranial vein	Connecting vein	Venous sinus
• Angular vein	• Superior ophthalmic vein	• Cavernous sinus *
• Veins of palatine tonsil	• Pterygoid plexus, inferior ophthalmic vein	• Cavernous sinus *
• Superficial temporal vein	• Parietal emissary vein	• Superior sagittal sinus
• Occipital vein	• Occipital emissary vein	• Transverse sinus, confluence of the sinuses
• Occipital vein, posterior auricular vein	• Mastoid emissary vein	• Sigmoid sinus
• External vertebral venous plexus	• Condylar emissary vein	• Sigmoid sinus

4.1 Overview of the Cranial Nerves

A Functional components of the cranial nerves

The twelve pairs of cranial nerves are designated by Roman numerals according to the order of their emergence from the brainstem (see topographical organization in **C**).

Note: The first two cranial nerves, the olfactory nerve (CN I) and optic nerve (CN II), are not peripheral nerves in the true sense but rather extensions of the brain, i.e., they are CNS pathways that are covered by meninges and contain cell types occurring exclusively in the CNS (oligodendrocytes and microglial cells).

Like the spinal nerves, the cranial nerves may contain both *afferent* and *efferent* axons. These axons belong either to the somatic nervous system, which enables the organism to interact with its environment *(somatic fibers)*, or to the autonomic nervous system, which regulates the activity of the internal organs *(visceral fibers)*. The combinations of these different *general* fiber types in spinal nerves result in four possible compositions that are found chiefly in spinal nerves but also occur in cranial nerves (see functional organization in **C**):

General somatic afferents (somatic sensation):
→ E.g., fibers convey impulses from the skin and striated muscle spindles

General visceral afferents (visceral sensation):
→ E.g., fibers convey impulses from the viscera and blood vessels

General visceral efferents (visceromotor function):
→ Fibers innervate the smooth muscle of the viscera, intraocular muscles, heart, salivary glands, etc.

General somatic efferents (somatomotor function):
→ Fibers innervate striated muscles

Additionally, cranial nerves may contain special fiber types that are associated with particular structures in the head:

Special somatic afferents:
→ E.g., fibers conduct impulses from the retina and from the auditory and vestibular apparatus

Special visceral afferents:
→ E.g., fibers conduct impulses from the taste buds of the tongue and from the olfactory mucosa

Special visceral efferents:
→ E.g., fibers innervate striated muscles derived from the branchial arches *(branchiogenic efferents and branchiogenic muscles)*

B Color coding used in subsequent units to indicate different fiber types

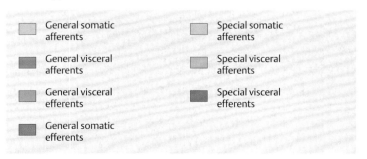

General somatic afferents	Special somatic afferents
General visceral afferents	Special visceral afferents
General visceral efferents	Special visceral efferents
General somatic efferents	

C Topographical and functional organization of the cranial nerves

Topographical origin	Name	Functional fiber type
Telencephalon	• Olfactory nerve (CN I)	• Special visceral afferent
Diencephalon	• Optic nerve (CN II)	• Special somatic afferent
Mesencephalon	• Oculomotor nerve (CN III)*	• Somatic efferent • Visceral efferent (parasympathetic)
	• Trochlear nerve (CN IV)*	• Somatic efferent
Pons	• Trigeminal nerve (CN V)	• Special visceral efferent *(first branchial arch)* • Somatic efferent
	• Abducent nerve (CN VI)*	• Somatic efferent
	• Facial nerve (CN VII)	• Special visceral efferent *(second branchial arch)* • Special visceral afferent • Visceral efferent (parasympathetic) • Somatic afferent
Medulla oblongata	• Vestibulocochlear nerve (CN VIII)	• Special somatic afferent
	• Glossopharyngeal nerve (CN IX)	• Special visceral efferent *(third branchial arch)* • Special visceral afferent • Visceral afferent (parasympathetic) • Somatic afferent
	• Vagus nerve (CN X)	• Special visceral efferent *(fourth branchial arch)* • Special visceral afferent • Visceral efferent (parasympathetic) • Visceral afferent • Somatic afferent
	• Accessory nerve (CN XI)*	• Special visceral efferent *(fifth branchial arch)* • Somatic efferent
	• Hypoglossal nerve (CN XII)*	• Somatic efferent

* Note: Cranial nerves with somatic efferent fibers innervating the striated muscles also have somatic afferent fibers that conduct proprioceptive impulses from the muscle spindles and other structures (for clarity, not listed above).

A characteristic feature of the cranial nerves is that their sensory and motor fibers enter and exit the brainstem at the same sites. This differs from the spinal nerves, in which the sensory fibers enter the spinal cord through the dorsal roots while the motor fibers leave the spinal cord through the ventral roots.

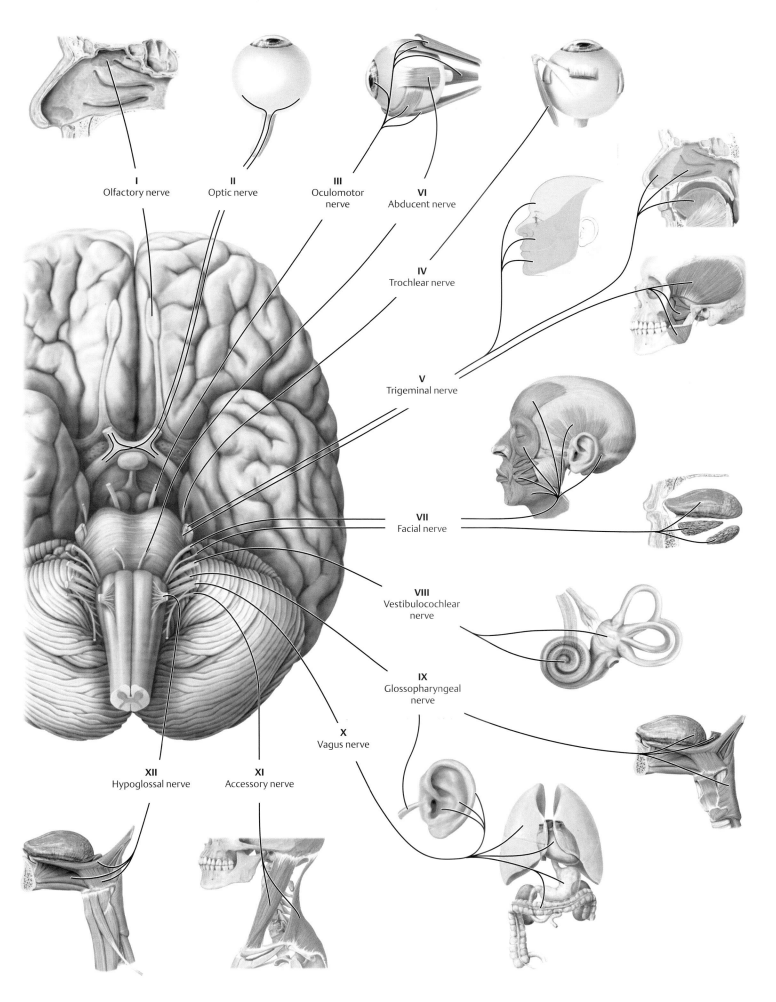

I
Olfactory nerve

II
Optic nerve

III
Oculomotor nerve

VI
Abducent nerve

IV
Trochlear nerve

V
Trigeminal nerve

VII
Facial nerve

VIII
Vestibulocochlear nerve

IX
Glossopharyngeal nerve

X
Vagus nerve

XII
Hypoglossal nerve

XI
Accessory nerve

4.2 Cranial Nerves: Brainstem Nuclei and Peripheral Ganglia

A Overview of the nuclei of cranial nerves III – XII

Just as different fiber types can be distinguished in the cranial nerves (**C**, p. 66), the nuclei of origin and nuclei of termination of the cranial nerves can also be classified according to different sensory and motor types and modalities. According to this scheme, the nuclei that belong to the parasympathetic nervous system are classified as *general* visceral efferent nuclei, while the nuclei of the branchial arch nerves are classified as *special* visceral efferent nuclei. The visceral afferent nuclei are considered either *general* (lower part of the solitary nuclei) or *special* (upper part, gustatory fibers). The somatic afferent nuclei can be differentiated in a similar way: the principal sensory nucleus of the trigeminal nerve is classified as *general* somatic afferent, while the nucleus of the vestibulocochlear nerve is *special* somatic afferent.

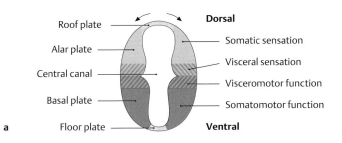

Motor nuclei: (give rise to efferent [motor] fibers, left in **C**)

Somatic efferent (somatic motor) nuclei (red):
- Nucleus of oculomotor nerve (CN III: eye muscles)
- Nucleus of trochlear nerve (CN IV: eye muscles)
- Nucleus of abducent nerve (CN VI: eye muscles)
- Nucleus of accessory nerve (CN XI, spinal root: shoulder muscles)
- Nucleus of hypoglossal nerve (CN XII: lingual muscles)

Visceral efferent (visceral motor) nuclei (blue):
Nuclei associated with the parasympathetic nervous system (light blue):
- Visceral oculomotor (Edinger-Westphal) nucleus (CN III: papillary sphincter and ciliary muscle)
- Superior salivatory nucleus (CN VII, facial nerve: submandibular and sublingual glands)
- Inferior salivatory nucleus (CN IX, glossopharyngeal nerve: parotid gland)
- Dorsal vagal nucleus (CN X: viscera)

Nuclei of the branchial arch nerves (dark blue):
- Trigeminal motor nucleus (CN V: muscles of mastication)
- Facial nucleus (CN VII: facial muscles)
- Nucleus ambiguus (CN IX, glossopharyngeal nerve; CN X, vagus nerve; CN XI, accessory nerve [cranial root]: pharyngeal and laryngeal muscles)

Sensory nuclei: (where afferent [sensory] fibers terminate, right in **C**)

Somatic afferent (somatic sensory) and vestibulocochlear nuclei (yellow):
Sensory nuclei associated with the trigeminal nerve (CN V):
- Mesencephalic nucleus (proprioceptive afferents from muscles of mastication)
- Principal (pontine) sensory nucleus (touch, vibration, joint position)
- Spinal nucleus (pain and temperature sensation in the head)

Nuclei of the vestibulocochlear nerve (CN VIII):
- Vestibular part (sense of balance):
  — Medial vestibular nucleus
  — Lateral vestibular nucleus
  — Superior vestibular nucleus
  — Inferior vestibular nucleus
- Cochlear part (hearing):
  — Anterior cochlear nucleus
  — Posterior cochlear nucleus

Visceral afferent (visceral sensory) nuclei (green):
- Nucleus of the solitary tract (nuclear complex):
  — Superior part (special visceral afferents [taste] from CN VII [facial], CN IX [glossopharyngeal], and CN X [vagus] nerves)
  — Inferior part (general visceral afferents from CN IX [glossopharyngeal] and CN X [vagus] nerves)

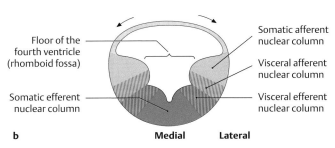

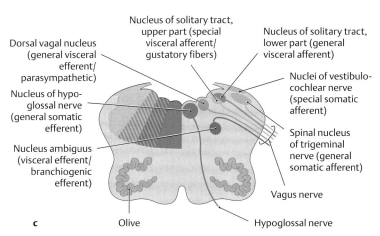

B Arrangement of brainstem nuclear columns during embryonic development (after Herrick)

Cross-sections through the spinal cord and brainstem, superior view. The functional organization of the brainstem is determined by the location of the cranial nerve nuclei, which can be explained in terms of the embryonic migration of neuron populations.

a Initial form as seen in the spinal cord: The motor (efferent) neurons are ventral, and the sensory (afferent) neurons are dorsal (= dorsoventral arrangement).

b early embryonic stage of brainstem development: the neurons of the alar plate (sensory nuclei) migrate laterally while the neurons of the basal plate (motor nuclei) migrate medially. This gives rise to a general mediolateral arrangement of the nuclear columns. The arrows indicate the directions of cell migration.

c adult brainstem: features a medial-to-lateral arrangement of four longitudinal nuclear columns (one *somatic efferent,* one *visceral efferent,* one *visceral afferent,* and one *somatic afferent*). In each of these columns, nuclei that have the same function are arranged one above the other in a craniocaudal direction (see **C**). The nuclei in the *somatic afferent* and *visceral afferent* columns are differentiated into general and special afferent nuclei. Similarly, the *visceral efferent nuclear column* is differentiated into general (parasympathetic) and special (branchiogenic) efferent nuclei. This general/special subdivision is not present in the *somatic efferent nuclear column.*

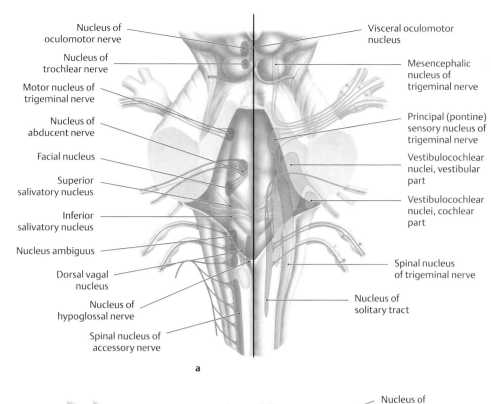

Nucleus of oculomotor nerve

Nucleus of trochlear nerve

Motor nucleus of trigeminal nerve

Nucleus of abducent nerve

Facial nucleus

Superior salivatory nucleus

Inferior salivatory nucleus

Nucleus ambiguus

Dorsal vagal nucleus

Nucleus of hypoglossal nerve

Spinal nucleus of accessory nerve

Visceral oculomotor nucleus

Mesencephalic nucleus of trigeminal nerve

Principal (pontine) sensory nucleus of trigeminal nerve

Vestibulocochlear nuclei, vestibular part

Vestibulocochlear nuclei, cochlear part

Spinal nucleus of trigeminal nerve

Nucleus of solitary tract

a

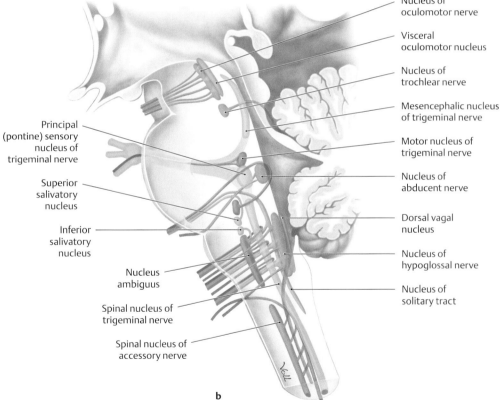

Nucleus of oculomotor nerve

Visceral oculomotor nucleus

Nucleus of trochlear nerve

Mesencephalic nucleus of trigeminal nerve

Motor nucleus of trigeminal nerve

Nucleus of abducent nerve

Dorsal vagal nucleus

Nucleus of hypoglossal nerve

Nucleus of solitary tract

Principal (pontine) sensory nucleus of trigeminal nerve

Superior salivatory nucleus

Inferior salivatory nucleus

Nucleus ambiguus

Spinal nucleus of trigeminal nerve

Spinal nucleus of accessory nerve

b

C Location of cranial nerves III – XII in the brainstem

a Posterior view (with cerebellum removed).
b Midsagittal section, left lateral view.

Except for cranial nerves I and II, which are extensions of the brain rather than true nerves, all pairs of cranial nerves are associated with corresponding nuclei in the brainstem. The diagrams show the nerve pathways leading *to* and *from* these nuclei. The arrangement of the cranial nerve nuclei is easier to understand when we classify them into functional nuclear columns (see **B**). The *efferent (motor) nuclei* where the *efferent* fibers arise are shown on the left side in **a**. The *afferent (sensory) nuclei* where the *afferent* fibers end are shown on the right side.

■	Somatic efferent nuclei
■	General visceral efferent nuclei
■	Special visceral efferent nuclei
☐	Somatic afferent nuclei
■	General visceral afferent nuclei
■	Special visceral afferent nuclei

D Ganglia associated with cranial nerves

Ganglia fall into two main categories: sensory and autonomic (parasympathetic). The **sensory ganglia** are analogous to the spinal ganglia in the dorsal roots of the spinal cord. They contain the perikarya of the *pseudounipolar* nerve cells (= primary afferent neuron). Their peripheral process comes from a receptor, and their central process terminates in the CNS. Synaptic relays do not occur in the sensory ganglia. The **autonomic ganglia** in the head are entirely parasympathetic. They contain the perikarya of the *multipolar* nerve cells (= second efferent, or postsynaptic, neuron). Unlike the sensory ganglia, these ganglia synapse with parasympathetic fibers from the brainstem (= first efferent, or *preganglionic,* neuron). Specifically they synapse with the perikarya of the second efferent (or *postsynaptic*) neuron, whose fibers are distributed to the target organ.

Cranial nerves	Sensory ganglia	Autonomic ganglia
Oculomotor nerve (CN III)		• Ciliary ganglion
Trigeminal nerve (CN V)	• Trigeminal ganglion	
Facial nerve (CN VII)	• Geniculate ganglion	• Pterygo-palatine ganglion • Subman-dibular ganglion
Vestibuloco-chlear nerve (CN VIII)	• Spiral ganglion • Vestibular ganglion	
Glosso-pharyngeal nerve (CN IX)	• Superior ganglion • Inferior (petrosal) ganglion	• Otic ganglion
Vagus nerve (CN X)	• Superior (jugular) ganglion • Inferior (nodose) ganglion	• Prevertebral and intramural ganglia

4.3 Cranial Nerves: Olfactory (CN I) and Optic (CN II)

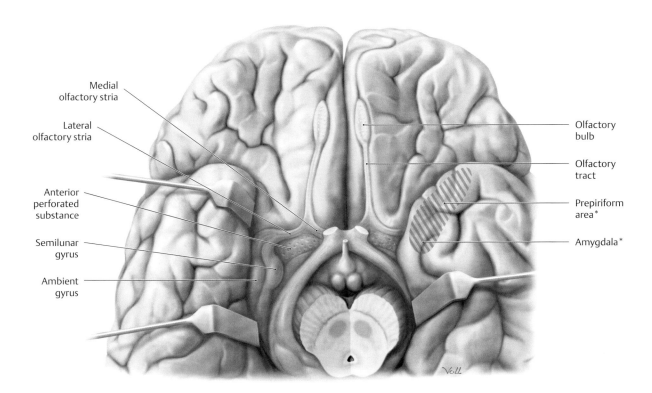

A Olfactory bulb and olfactory tract on the basal surface of the frontal lobes of the brain

The unmyelinated axons of the primary bipolar sensory neurons in the olfactory mucosa are collected into approximately 20 fiber bundles (see **B**), which are referred to collectively as the *olfactory nerve*. These axon bundles pass from the nasal cavity through the cribriform plate of the ethmoid bone into the anterior cranial fossa (see **B**), and synapse in the *olfactory bulb*. The *olfactory bulb* and associated *olfactory tract* are not parts of a peripheral nerve but instead constitute an extension of the telencephalon that contains CNS-specific cell types (oligodendrocytes and microglia). The olfactory bulb and tract share with the telencephalon a meningeal covering that is removed here. Axons from second-order afferent neurons in the olfactory bulb pass through the olfactory tract and medial or lateral olfactory stria, ending in the cerebral cortex of the prepiriform area, in the amygdala, or in neighboring areas. By this short route, olfactory information is thus transmitted into the CNS and can be relayed directly to the cerebral cortex.

The primary sensory neurons of the olfactory mucosa have several unusual properties that should be noted. These neurons have a limited lifespan of up to several months, but are continuously replenished from a pool of precursor cells in the olfactory mucosa that undergo periodic mitosis. New olfactory receptors are thus generated throughout adult life, and their axons enter the olfactory bulb to form new synapses with existing CNS neurons. The regenerative capacity of the olfactory mucosa gradually diminishes with advancing age, however, resulting in a net loss of receptors and a slow decline in overall sensory function.

Note: Injuries to the cribriform plate may damage the meningeal covering of the olfactory fibers, resulting in olfactory disturbances and cerebrospinal fluid leakage from the nose ("runny nose" after head trauma). There is an associated risk of ascending bacterial infection causing meningitis.

* The shaded structures are deep to the basal surface of the brain.

B Extent of the olfactory mucosa (olfactory region)

Portion of the left nasal septum and lateral wall of the right nasal cavity, viewed from the left side. The olfactory fibers on the septum and superior concha define the extent of the olfactory region (2–4 cm²). The thin, unmyelinated olfactory fibers enter the skull through the cribriform plate of the ethmoid bone (see p. 27) and pass to the olfactory bulb (see also pp. 116, 204, and 372).

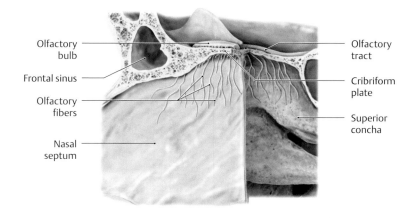

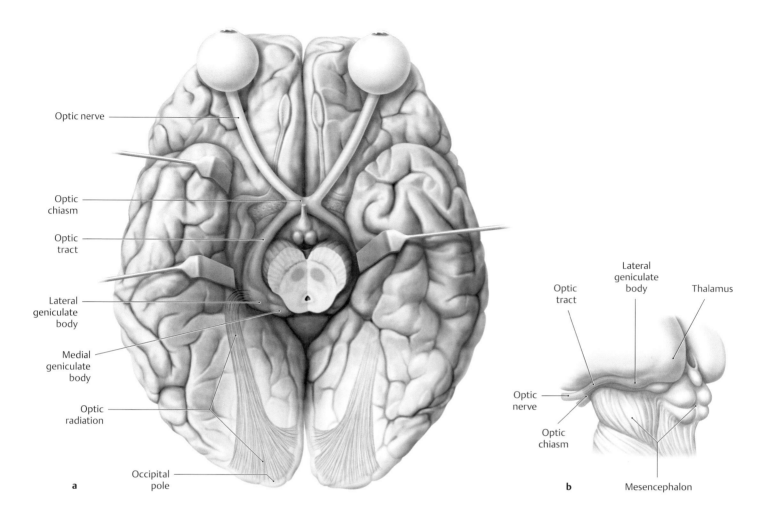

Optic nerve

Optic chiasm

Optic tract

Lateral geniculate body

Medial geniculate body

Optic radiation

Occipital pole

a

Optic tract

Optic nerve

Lateral geniculate body

Thalamus

Optic chiasm

b

Mesencephalon

C Eye, optic nerve, optic chiasm, and optic tract

a View of the base of the brain, **b** posterolateral view of the left side of the brainstem. The termination of the optic tract in the lateral geniculate body is shown.

The optic nerve is not a true nerve but an extension of the brain, in this case of the diencephalon. Analogously to the olfactory bulb and tract (see **A**), the optic nerve is sheathed by meninges (removed here) and contains CNS-specific cells (see **A**). The optic nerve contains the axons of retinal ganglion cells. These axons terminate mainly in the lateral geniculate body of the diencephalon and in the mesencephalon (superior colliculus, pp. 234–235).

Note: Because the optic nerve is an extension of the brain, the clinician can directly inspect a portion of the brain with an ophthalmoscope. This examination is important in the diagnosis of many neurological diseases (ophthalmoscopy is described on p. 133).

The optic nerve passes from the eyeball through the optic canal into the middle cranial fossa (see **D**). Many, but not all, retinal cell ganglion axons cross the midline to the contralateral side of the brain in the optic chiasm (**a**). The optic tract extends from the optic chiasm to the lateral geniculate body (see also **b**).

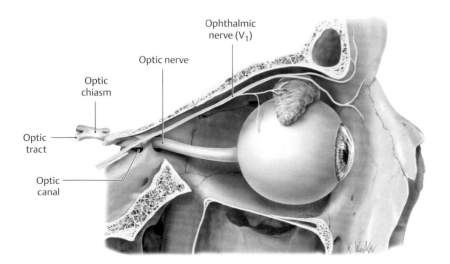

Ophthalmic nerve (V₁)

Optic nerve

Optic chiasm

Optic tract

Optic canal

D Course of the optic nerve in the right orbit

Lateral view. The optic nerve extends through the optic canal from the orbit into the middle cranial fossa. It exits the posterior side of the eyeball within the retro-orbital fat (removed here). The other cranial nerves enter the orbit through the superior orbital fissure (only CN V₁ is shown here).

4.4 Cranial Nerves of the Extraocular Muscles: Oculomotor (CN III), Trochlear (CN IV), and Abducent (CN VI)

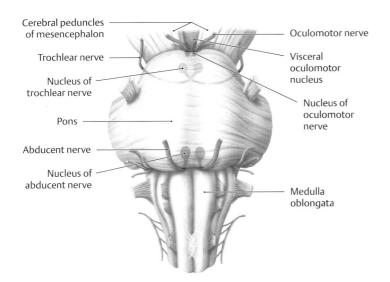

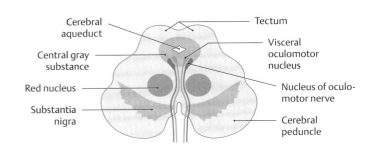

C Topography of the oculomotor nucleus

Cross-section through the brainstem at the level of the oculomotor nucleus, superior view.

Note: the visceral efferent, parasympathetic nuclear complex (visceral oculomotor [Edinger-Westphal] nucleus) can be distinguished from the somatic efferent nuclear complex (nucleus of the oculomotor nerve).

D Overview of the trochlear nerve (CN IV)

The trochlear nerve contains only *somatic efferent* fibers.

Course: The trochlear nerve emerges from the posterior surface of the brainstem near the midline, courses anteriorly around the cerebral peduncle, and enters the orbit through the superior orbital fissure.

Special features:
- The trochlear nerve is the only cranial nerve in which all the fibers cross to the opposite side (see **A**). Consequently, lesions of the nucleus or of nerve fibers very close to the nucleus, before they cross the midline, result in tochlear nerve palsy on the side opposite to the lesion (contralateral palsy). A lesion past the site where the nerve crosses the midline leads to tochlear nerve palsy on the same side as the lesion (ipsilateral palsy).
- The trochlear nerve is the only cranial nerve that emerges from the *dorsal* side of the brainstem.
- It has the longest intradural course of the three extraocular motor nerves.

Nucleus and distribution: The nucleus of the trochlear nerve is located in the midbrain (mesencephalon). Its efferents supply motor innervation to one muscle, the superior oblique.

Effects of trochlear nerve injury:
- The affected eye is higher and is also deviated medially because the inferior oblique (responsible for elevation and abduction) becomes dominant due to loss of the superior oblique.
- Diplopia.

E Overview of the abducent nerve (CN VI)

The abducent nerve contains only *somatic efferent* fibers.

Course: The nerve follows a long *extradural* path before entering the orbit through the superior orbital fissure.

Nucleus and distribution:
- The nucleus of the abducent nerve is located in the pons (= midlevel brainstem), its fibers emerging at the inferior border of the pons.
- Its efferent fibers supply somatomotor innervation to a single muscle, the lateral rectus.

Effects of abducent nerve injury:
- The affected eye is deviated medially.
- Diplopia.

A Emergence of the nerves from the brainstem

Anterior view. All three nerves that supply the extraocular muscles emerge from the brainstem. The nuclei of the oculomotor nerve and trochlear nerve are located in the midbrain (mesencephalon), while the nucleus of the abducent nerve is located in the pons.

Note: Of these three nerves, the oculomotor (CN III) is the only one that contains somatic efferent and visceral efferent fibers and supplies several extraocular muscles (see **C**).

B Overview of the oculomotor nerve (CN III)

The oculomotor nerve contains *somatic efferent* and *visceral efferent* fibers.

Course: The nerve runs anteriorly from the mesencephalon (midbrain = highest level of the brainstem; see pp. 226, 228) and enters the orbit through the superior orbital fissure

Nuclei and distribution, *ganglia:*
- *Somatic efferents:* Efferents from a nuclear complex (oculomotor nucleus) in the midbrain (see **C**) supply the following muscles:
  - Levator palpebrae superioris (acts on the upper eyelid)
  - Superior, medial, and inferior rectus and inferior oblique (= extraocular muscles, all act on the eyeball).
- *Visceral efferents:* Parasympathetic preganglionic efferents from the visceral oculomotor (Edinger-Westphal) nucleus synapse with neurons in the ciliary ganglion that innervate the following intraocular muscles:
  - Pupillary sphincter
  - Ciliary muscle

Effects of oculomotor nerve injury:
Oculomotor palsy, severity depending on the extent of the injury.
- Effects of complete oculomotor palsy (paralysis of the extraocular *and* intraocular muscles and levator palpebrae):
  - Ptosis (drooping of the lid)
  - Downward and lateral gaze deviation in the affected eye
  - Diplopia (in the absence of complete ptosis)
  - Mydriasis (pupil dilated due to sphincter pupillae paralysis)
  - Accommodation difficulties (ciliary paralysis – lens cannot focus).

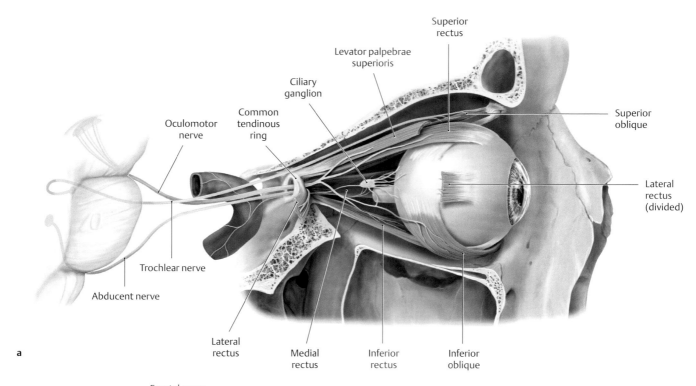

a Lateral view. Right orbit.

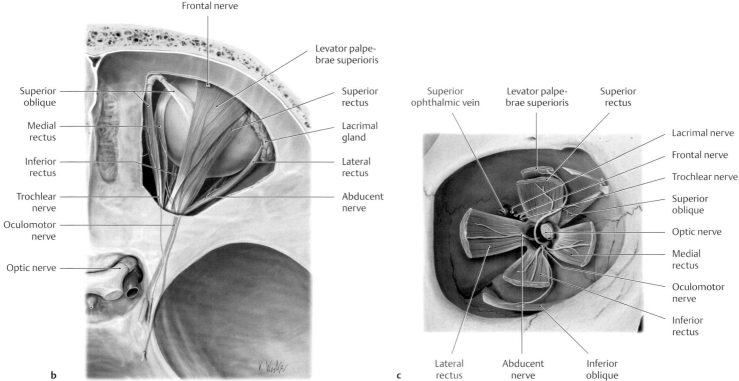

F Course of the nerves supplying the ocular muscles

a Lateral view. Right orbit. **a** Lateral view, **b** superior view (opened), **c** anterior view. All three cranial nerves leave the brainstem and enter the orbit through the superior orbital fissure, passing through the common tendinous ring of the extraocular muscles. The *abducent nerve* has the longest *extradural* course. Because of this, abducent nerve palsy may develop in association with meningitis and subarachnoid hemorrhage. Transient palsy may even occur in cases where lumbar puncture has caused an excessive fall of CSF pressure, with descent of the brainstem exerting traction on the nerve. The *oculomotor nerve* supplies para-

sympathetic innervation to intraocular muscles (its parasympathetic fibers synapse in the ciliary ganglion) as well as somatic motor innervation to most of the extraocular muscles and the levator palpebrae superioris. Oculomotor nerve palsy may affect the parasympathetic fibers exclusively, the somatic motor fibers exclusively, or both at the same time (see **B**). Because the preganglionic parasympathetic fibers for the pupil lie directly beneath the epineurium after emerging from the brainstem, they are often the first structures to be affected by pressure due to trauma, tumors, or aneurysms.

4.5 Cranial Nerves: Trigeminal (CN V), Nuclei and Distribution

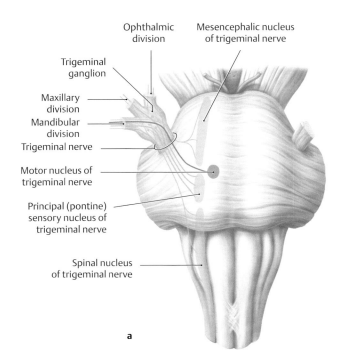

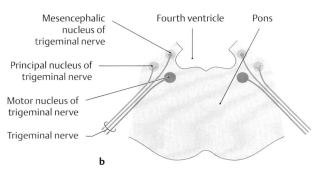

A Nuclei and emergence from the pons.

a Anterior view. The larger sensory nuclei of the trigeminal nerve are distributed along the brainstem and extend downward into the spinal cord. The *sensory root (portio major)* of the trigeminal nerve thus forms the bulk of the fibers, while the *motor root (portio minor)* is formed by fibers arising from the small motor nucleus in the pons. They supply motor innervation to the muscles of mastication (see **B**). The following *somatic afferent* nuclei are distinguished:

- *Mesencephalic nucleus of the trigeminal nerve:* proprioceptive fibers from the muscles of mastication. Special feature: the neurons of this nucleus are pseudounipolar ganglion cells that have migrated into the brain.
- *Principal (pontine) sensory nucleus of the trigeminal nerve:* chiefly mediates touch.
- *Spinal nucleus of the trigeminal nerve:* pain and temperature sensation, also touch. A small, circumscribed lesion of the trigeminal spinal sensory nucleus leads to characteristic sensory disturbances in the face (see **D**).

b Cross-section through the pons at the level of emergence of the trigeminal nerve, superior view.

B Overview of the trigeminal nerve (CN V)

The trigeminal nerve, the sensory nerve of the head, contains mostly *somatic afferent* fibers with a smaller proportion of special *visceral efferent* fibers. Its three major somatic **divisions** have the following **sites of emergence** from the middle cranial fossa:
- *Ophthalmic division (CN V₁):* enters the orbit through the superior orbital fissure.
- *Maxillary division (CN V₂):* enters the pterygopalatine fossa through the foramen rotundum.
- *Mandibular division (CN V₃):* passes through the foramen ovale to the inferior surface of the base of the skull; only division containing motor fibers.

Nuclei and distribution:
- *Special visceral efferent:* Efferent fibers from the motor nucleus of the trigeminal nerve pass in the mandibular division (CN V₃) to:
  - Muscles of mastication (temporalis, masseter, medial and lateral pterygoid)
  - Oral floor muscles: mylohyoid and anterior belly of the digastric
  - Middle ear muscle: tensor tympani
  - Pharyngeal muscle: tensor veli palatini
- *Somatic afferent:* The trigeminal ganglion contains pseudounipolar ganglion cells whose central fibers pass to the sensory nuclei of the trigeminal nerve (see **A a**). Their peripheral fibers innervate the facial skin, large portions of the nasopharyngeal mucosa, and the anterior two-thirds of the tongue (somatic sensation, see **C**).
- *"Visceral efferent pathway":* The visceral efferent fibers of some cranial nerves adhere to branches or sub-branches of the trigeminal nerve, by which they travel to their destination:
  - The lacrimal nerve (branch of CN V₁) conveys parasympathetic fibers from the facial nerve along the zygomatic nerve (branch of CN V₂) to the lacrimal gland.
  - The auriculotemporal nerve (branch of CN V₃) conveys parasympathetic fibers from the glossopharyngeal nerve to the parotid gland.
  - The lingual nerve (branch of CN V₃) conveys parasympathetic fibers from the facial nerve along the chorda tympani to the submandibular and sublingual glands.
- *"Visceral afferent pathway":* Gustatory fibers from the facial nerve (chorda tympani) travel by the lingual nerve (branch of CN V₃) to supply the anterior two-thirds of the tongue.

Developmentally, the trigeminal nerve is the nerve of the first branchial arch.

Clinical disorders of the trigeminal nerve:
Sensory disturbances and deficits may arise in various conditions:
- Sensory loss due to traumatic nerve lesions.
- Herpes zoster ophthalmicus (involvement of the territory of the first division of the trigeminal nerve, including the skin and/or the eye, by the varicella-zoster virus); herpes zoster of the face.

The afferent fibers of the trigeminal nerve (like the facial nerve, see p. 78) are involved in the *corneal reflex* (reflex closure of the eyelid; see **C**, p. 361).

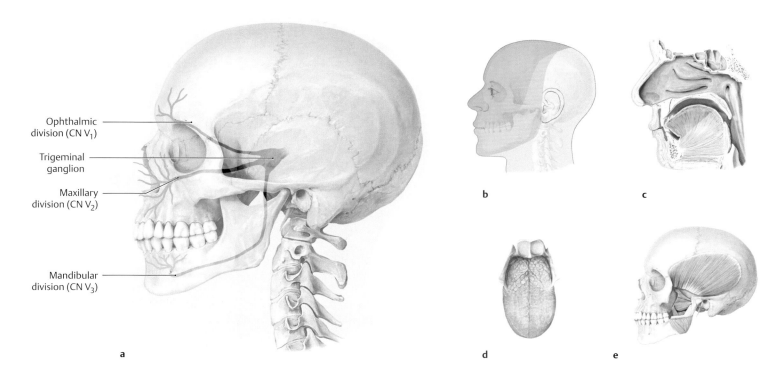

b

c

d

e

a

C Course and distribution of the trigeminal nerve

a Left lateral view. The three divisions of the trigeminal nerve and clinically important terminal branches are shown.

All three divisions of the trigeminal nerve supply the skin of the face (**b**) and the mucosa of the nasopharynx (**c**). The anterior two-thirds of the tongue (**d**) receives sensory innervation (touch, pain and thermal sensation, but not taste) via the lingual nerve, which is a branch of the mandibular division (CN V$_3$). The muscles of mastication are supplied by the motor root of the trigeminal nerve, whose axons enter the mandibular division (**e**).

Note: The efferent fibers course exclusively in the mandibular division. A *peripheral trigeminal nerve lesion* involving one of its divisions—ophthalmic (CN V$_1$), maxillary (CN V$_2$), or mandibular (CN V$_3$)—may cause loss of somatic sensation (touch, pain, and temperature) in the area innervated by the afferent nerve (see **b**). This contrasts with the more concentric pattern, and more restricted modality, of sensory deficit produced by a central (CNS) lesion involving trigeminal nuclei and pathways (see **D**).

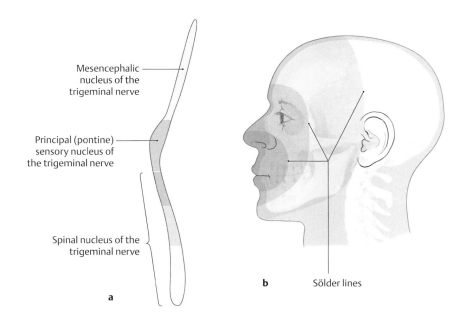

a

b Sölder lines

D Central trigeminal lesion

a Somatotopic organization of the spinal nucleus of the trigeminal nerve. **b** Facial zones in which sensory deficits (pain and temperature) arise when certain regions of the trigeminal spinal nucleus are destroyed. These zones follow the concentric Sölder lines in the face. Their pattern indicates the corresponding portion of the trigeminal nucleus in which the lesion is located (matching color shades).

4.6 Cranial Nerves: Trigeminal (CN V), Divisions

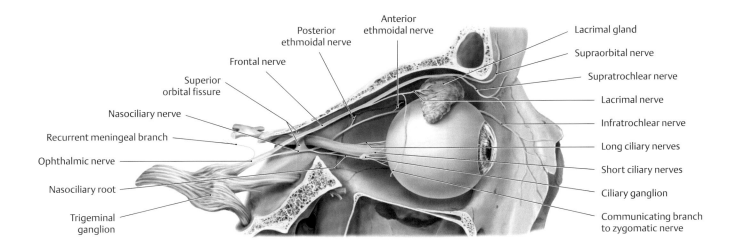

A Branches of the ophthalmic division (= first division of the trigeminal nerve, CN V₁) in the orbital region

Lateral view of the partially-opened right orbit. The first small branch arising from the ophthalmic division is the recurrent meningeal branch, which supplies sensory innervation to the dura mater. The bulk of the ophthalmic division fibers enter the orbit from the middle cranial fossa by passing through the *superior orbital fissure*. The ophthalmic division divides into three branches whose names indicate their distribution: the **lacrimal nerve**, **frontal nerve**, and **nasociliary nerve**.

Note: The lacrimal nerve receives postganglionic, parasympathetic secretomotor fibers from the zygomatic nerve (maxillary division) via a *communicating branch*. These fibers travel to the lacrimal gland by the lacrimal nerve. Sympathetic fibers cleave to the long ciliary nerves that arise from the nasociliary nerve, traveling in these nerves to the pupil. The ciliary nerves also contain afferent fibers that mediate the corneal reflex. Sensory fibers from the eyeball course in the nasociliary root, passing through the ciliary ganglion to the nasociliary nerve.

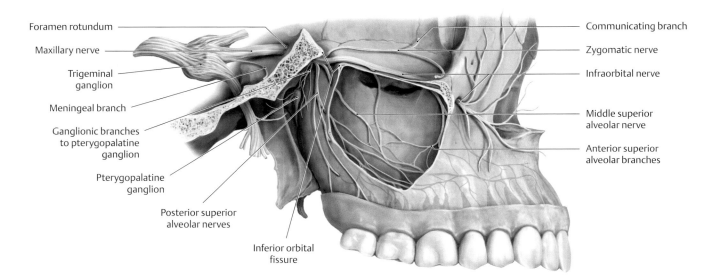

B Branches of the maxillary division (= second division of the trigeminal nerve, CN V₂) in the maxillary region

Lateral view of the partially opened right maxillary sinus with the zygomatic arch removed. After giving off a meningeal branch, the maxillary division leaves the middle cranial fossa through the foramen rotundum and enters the pterygopalatine fossa, where it divides into the following branches:

- Zygomatic nerve
- Ganglionic branches to the pterygopalatine ganglion (sensory root of the pterygopalatine ganglion)
- Infraorbital nerve

The **zygomatic nerve** enters the orbit through the *inferior orbital fissure*. Its two terminal branches, the zygomaticofacial branch and zygomati-

cotemporal branch (not shown here), supply sensory innervation to the skin over the zygomatic arch and temple. Parasympathetic, postsynaptic fibers from the pterygopalatine ganglion are carried to the lacrimal nerve by the communicating branch (see p. 81). The preganglionic fibers originally arise from the facial nerve. The **infraorbital nerve** also passes through the inferior orbital fissure into the orbit, from which it enters the infraorbital canal. Its fine terminal branches supply the skin between the lower eyelid and upper lip. Its other terminal branches form the *superior dental plexus*, which supplies sensory innervation to the maxillary teeth:

- Anterior superior alveolar branches to the incisors
- Middle superior alveolar branch to the premolars
- Posterior superior alveolar branches to the molars

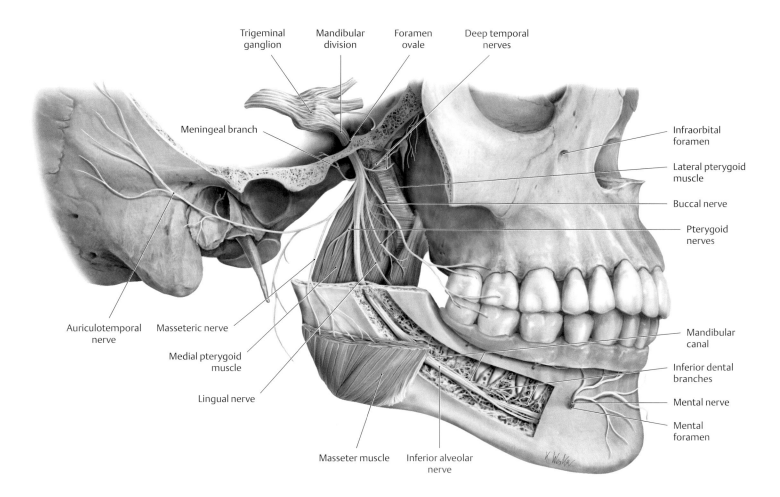

Trigeminal ganglion · **Mandibular division** · **Foramen ovale** · **Deep temporal nerves** · Meningeal branch · Infraorbital foramen · Lateral pterygoid muscle · Buccal nerve · Pterygoid nerves · Auriculotemporal nerve · Masseteric nerve · Medial pterygoid muscle · Lingual nerve · Masseter muscle · Inferior alveolar nerve · Mandibular canal · Inferior dental branches · Mental nerve · Mental foramen

C Branches of the mandibular division (= third division of the trigeminal nerve, CN V₃) in the mandibular region

Right lateral view of the partially opened mandible with the zygomatic arch removed. The mixed afferent-efferent mandibular division leaves the middle cranial fossa through the foramen ovale and enters the infra-temporal fossa on the external aspect of the base of the skull. Its menin-geal branch reenters the middle cranial fossa to supply sensory innerva-tion to the dura. Its **sensory branches** are as follows:

- Auriculotemporal nerve
- Lingual nerve
- Inferior alveolar nerve (also carries motor fibers, see below)
- Buccal nerve

The branches of the *auriculotemporal nerve* supply the temporal skin, the external auditory canal, and the tympanic membrane. The *lingual nerve* supplies sensory fibers to the anterior two-thirds of the tongue, and gustatory fibers from the chorda tympani (facial nerve branch) travel with it. The *afferent* fibers of the *inferior alveolar nerve* pass through the mandibular foramen into the mandibular canal, where they give off inferior dental branches to the mandibular teeth. The mental nerve is a terminal branch that supplies the skin of the chin, lower lip, and the body of the mandible. The *efferent* fibers that branch from the inferior alveolar nerve supply the mylohyoid muscle and the anterior belly of the digastric (not shown). The *buccal nerve* pierces the buccinator mus-cle and supplies sensory innervation to the mucous membrane of the cheek. The pure **motor branches** leave the main nerve trunk just distal to the origin of the meningeal branch. They are:

- Masseteric nerve (masseter muscle)
- Deep temporal nerves (temporalis muscle)
- Pterygoid nerves (pterygoid muscles)
- Nerve of the tensor tympani muscle
- Nerve of the tensor veli palatini muscle (not shown)

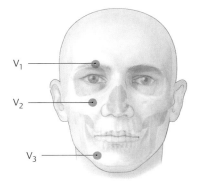

V₁ · V₂ · V₃

D Clinical assessment of trigeminal nerve function

Each of the three main divisions of the trigeminal nerve is tested sepa-rately during the physical examination. This is done by pressing on the *nerve exit points* with one finger to test the sensation there (local tender-ness to pressure). The characteristic nerve exit points are as follows:

- For CN V₁: the supraorbital foramen or supraorbital notch
- For CN V₂: the infraorbital foramen
- For CN V₃: the mental foramen

4.7 Cranial Nerves: Facial (CN VII), Nuclei and Distribution

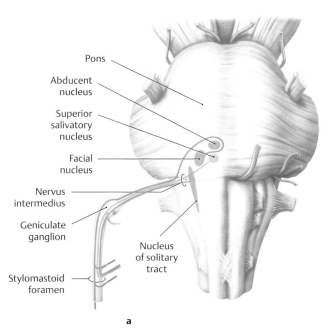

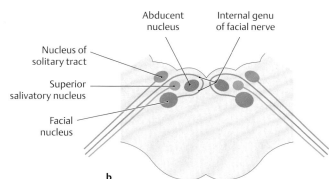

a

b

A Nuclei and principal branches of the facial nerve

a Anterior view of the brainstem, showing the site of emergence of the facial nerve from the lower pons. **b** Cross-section through the pons at the level of the internal genu of the facial nerve.

Note: each of the different fiber types (different sensory modalities) is associated with a particular nucleus.

From the **facial nucleus**, the *special visceral efferent* axons that innervate the muscles of facial expression first loop backward around the abducent nucleus, where they form the internal genu of the facial nerve. Then they run forward and emerge at the lower border of the pons. The **superior salivatory nucleus** contains *visceromotor*, presynaptic *parasympathetic* neurons. Together with *viscerosensory* (= gustatory) fibers from the nucleus of the solitary tract (superior part), they emerge from the pons as the nervus intermedius and then are bundled with the *visceromotor* axons from the facial motor nucleus to together form the facial nerve.

B Overview of the facial nerve (CN VII)

The facial nerve mainly conveys *special visceral efferent* (branchiogenic) fibers from the facial nerve nucleus which innervate the striated muscles of facial expression. The other visceral efferent (parasympathetic) fibers from the superior salivatory nucleus are grouped with the *visceral afferent* (gustatory) fibers from the nucleus of the solitary tract to form the *nervus intermedius* and aggregate with the visceral efferent fibers from the facial nerve nucleus.

Sites of emergence: The facial nerve emerges in the cerebellopontine angle between the pons and olive. It passes through the internal acoustic meatus into the petrous part of the temporal bone, where it divides into its branches:

- The visceral efferent fibers pass through the *stylomastoid foramen* to the base of the skull to form the intraparotid plexus (see **C**).
- The parasympathetic, visceral efferent, and visceral afferent fibers pass through the *petrotympanic fissure* to the base of the skull (see **A**, p. 80). While still in the petrous bone, the facial nerve gives off the greater petrosal nerve, stapedial nerve, and chorda tympani.

Nuclei and distribution, *ganglia:*

- *Special visceral efferent:* Efferents from the facial nucleus supply the following muscles:
  - Muscles of facial expression
  - Stylohyoid
  - Posterior belly of the digastric
  - Stapedius (stapedial nerve)
- *Visceral efferent (parasympathetic):* Parasympathetic presynaptic fibers arising from the superior salivatory nucleus synapse with neurons in the *pterygopalatine ganglion* or *submandibular ganglion.* They innervate the following structures:
  - Lacrimal gland
  - Small glands of the nasal mucosa and of the hard and soft palate
  - Submandibular gland
  - Sublingual gland
  - Small salivary glands on the dorsum of the tongue
- *Special visceral efferent:* Central fibers of pseudounipolar ganglion cells from the geniculate ganglion (corresponds to a spinal ganglion) synapse in the nucleus of the solitary tract. The peripheral processes of these neurons form the *chorda tympani* (gustatory fibers from the anterior two-thirds of the tongue).
- *Somatic afferent neurons:* Some sensory fibers that supply the auricle, the skin of the auditory canal, and the outer surface of the tympanic membrane travel by the facial nerve and *geniculate ganglion* to the trigeminal sensory nuclei. Their precise course is unknown.

Developmentally, the facial nerve is the nerve of the second branchial arch.

Effects of facial nerve injury: A peripheral facial nerve injury is characterized by paralysis of the muscles of expression on the affected side of the face (see **D**). Because the facial nerve conveys various fiber components that leave the main trunk of the nerve at different sites, the clinical presentation of facial paralysis is subject to subtle variations marked by associated disturbances of taste, lacrimation, salivation, etc. (see **B**, p. 80).

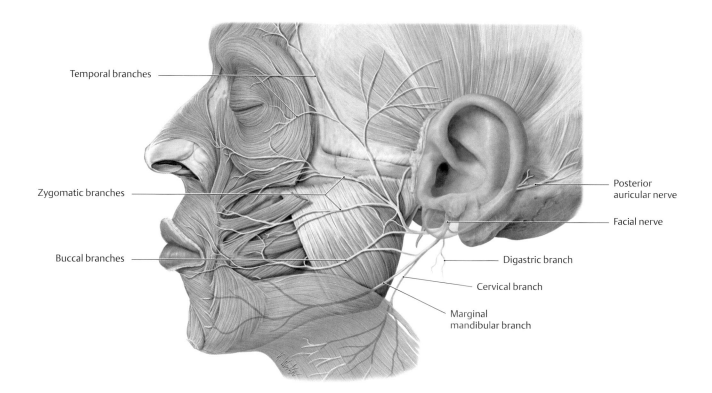

Temporal branches

Zygomatic branches

Buccal branches

Posterior auricular nerve

Facial nerve

Digastric branch

Cervical branch

Marginal mandibular branch

C Facial nerve branches for the muscles of expression

Note the different fiber types. This unit focuses almost exclusively on the *visceral efferent* (branchiogenic) fibers for the muscles of facial expression. (The other fiber types are described on p. 80.)

The stapedial nerve (to the stapedius muscle) branches from the facial nerve while still in the petrous part of the temporal bone and is mentioned here only because it also contains visceral efferent fibers (its course is shown on p. 80). The first branch that arises from the facial nerve after its emergence from the stylomastoid foramen is the **posterior auricular nerve**; it supplies *visceral efferent* fibers to the posterior auricular muscles and the posterior belly of the occipitofrontalis. It also conveys *somatosensory* fibers from the external ear, whose pseudounipolar nerve cells are located in the geniculate ganglion (see p. 80). After

leaving the petrous bone, the bulk of the remaining visceral efferent fibers of the facial nerve form the **intraparotid plexus** in the parotid gland, from which successive branches *(temporal, zygomatic, buccal,* and *marginal mandibular)* are distributed to the muscles of facial expression. These facial nerve branches must be protected during the removal of a benign parotid tumor in order to preserve muscle function. Additionally, there are even smaller branches such as the digastric branch to the posterior belly of the digastric muscle and the stylohyoid branch to the stylohyoid muscle (not shown). The lowest branch arising from the intraparotid plexus is the *cervical branch*. It joins with the transverse cervical nerve, an anterior branch of the C3 spinal nerve.

Precentral gyrus

Cortico-nuclear fibers

Facial nerve

Facial nucleus

a

b

c

D Central and peripheral facial paralysis

a The facial motor nucleus contains the cell bodies of lower motor neurons which innervate ipsilateral muscles of facial expression. The axons (special visceral efferent) of these neurons reach their muscle

targets through the facial nerve. These motor neurons are innervated in turn by upper motor neurons in the primary somatomotor cortex (precentral gyrus), whose axons enter corticonuclear fiber bundles to reach the facial motor nucleus in the brainstem.

Note: the facial nucleus has a "bipartite" structure, its upper part supplying the muscles of the forehead and eyes (temporal branches) while its lower part supplies the muscles in the lower half of the face. The upper part of the facial nerve nucleus receives bilateral innervation, the lower part contralateral innervation from cortical (upper) motor neurons.

b Central (supranuclear) paralysis (loss of the upper motor neurons, in this case on the left side) presents clinically with paralysis of the contralateral muscles of facial expression in the lower half of the face, while the contralateral forehead and extra-ocular muscles remain functional. Thus, the corner of the mouth sags on the right (contralateral) side, but the patient can still wrinkle the forehead and close the eyes on both sides. Speech articulation is impaired.

c Peripheral (infranuclear) paralysis (loss of lower motor neurons, in this case on the right side) is characterized by complete paralysis of the ipsilateral muscles. The patient cannot wrinkle the forehead, the corner of the mouth sags, articulation is impaired, and the eyelid cannot be fully closed. A Bell phenomenon is present (the eyeball turns upward and outward, exposing the sclera, when the patient attempts to close the eyelid), and the eyelid closure reflex is abolished. Depending on the site of the lesion, additional deficits may be present such as decreased lacrimation and salivation or loss of taste sensation in the anterior two-thirds of the tongue.

4.8 Cranial Nerves: Facial (CN VII), Branches

A Facial nerve branches in the temporal bone

Lateral view of the right temporal bone, petrous portion (petrous bone). The facial nerve, accompanied by the vestibulocochlear nerve (CN VIII, not shown), passes through the internal acoustic meatus (not shown) to enter the petrous bone. Shortly thereafter it forms the *external genu* of the facial nerve, which marks the location of the geniculate ganglion. The bulk of the visceral efferent fibers for the muscles of expression pass through the petrous bone and leave it at the stylomastoid foramen (see p. 79). The facial nerve gives off three branches between the geniculate ganglion and stylomastoid foramen:

- The parasympathetic **greater petrosal nerve** arises directly at the geniculate ganglion. This nerve leaves the anterior surface of the petrous pyramid at the hiatus of the canal for the greater petrosal nerve. It continues through the foramen lacerum (not shown), enters the pterygoid canal (see **C**), and passes to the pterygopalatine ganglion.
- The **stapedial nerve** passes to the muscle of the same name.
- The **chorda tympani** branches from the facial nerve above the stylomastoid foramen. It contains gustatory fibers as well as presynaptic parasympathetic fibers. It runs through the tympanic cavity and petrotympanic fissure and unites with the lingual nerve.

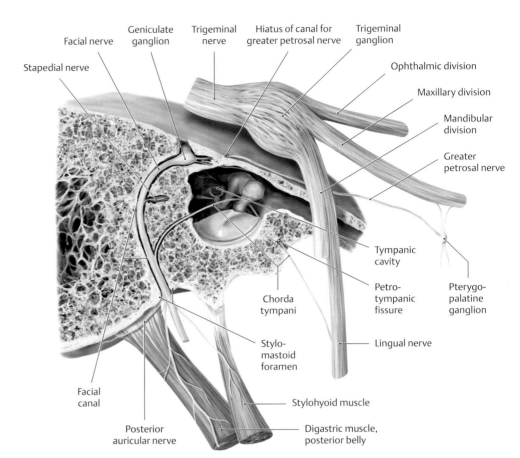

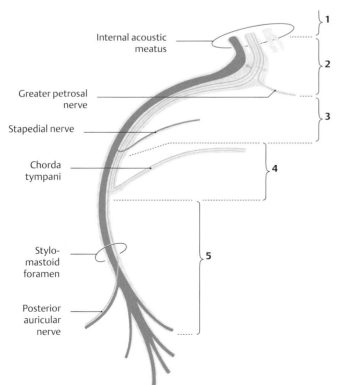

B Branching pattern of the facial nerve: diagnostic significance in temporal bone fractures

The principal signs and symptoms are different depending upon the exact site of the lesion in the course of the facial nerve through the bone. *Note:* only the *principal* signs and symptoms associated with a particular lesion site are described. The more peripheral the site of the nerve injury, the less diverse the signs and symptoms become.

1 A lesion at this level affects the facial nerve in addition to the vestibulochochlear nerve. As a result, peripheral motor facial paralysis is accompanied by hearing loss (deafness) and vestibular dysfunction (dizziness).
2 Peripheral motor facial paralysis is accompanied by disturbances of taste sensation (chorda tympani), lacrimation, and salivation.
3 Motor paralysis is accompanied by disturbances of salivation and taste. Hyperacusis due to paralysis of the stapedius muscle has little clinical importance.
4 Peripheral motor paralysis is accompanied by disturbances of taste and salivation.
5 Peripheral motor (facial) paralysis is the only manifestation of a lesion at this level.

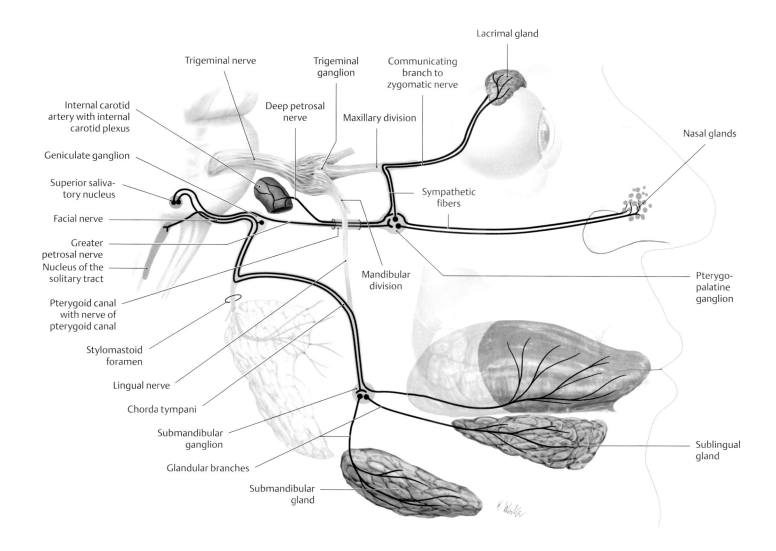

Lacrimal gland

Trigeminal nerve

Trigeminal ganglion

Communicating branch to zygomatic nerve

Deep petrosal nerve

Maxillary division

Internal carotid artery with internal carotid plexus

Nasal glands

Geniculate ganglion

Superior salivatory nucleus

Sympathetic fibers

Facial nerve

Greater petrosal nerve

Nucleus of the solitary tract

Mandibular division

Pterygoid canal with nerve of pterygoid canal

Pterygo-palatine ganglion

Stylomastoid foramen

Lingual nerve

Chorda tympani

Submandibular ganglion

Glandular branches

Sublingual gland

Submandibular gland

C Parasympathetic visceral efferents and visceral afferents (gustatory fibers) of the facial nerve

The presynaptic, parasympathetic, visceral efferent neurons are located in the superior salivatory nucleus. Their axons enter and leave the pons with the visceral efferent axons as the nervus intermedius, then travel with the visceral efferent fibers arising from the facial motor nucleus. These preganglionic parasympathetic axons exit the brainstem in the facial nerve and branch from it in the greater petrosal nerve, then mingle with *postganglionic sympathetic axons* (from the superior cervical ganglion, via the deep petrosal nerve) in the nerve of the pterygoid canal. This nerve enters the **pterygopalatine ganglion**, where the preganglionic parasympathetic motor axons synapse; the sympathetic axons pass through uninterrupted to innervate local blood vessels. The pterygopalatine ganglion supplies the lacrimal gland, nasal glands, and nasal,

palatine, and pharyngeal mucosa. Fibers from this ganglion enter the maxillary division and travel with it to innervate the lacrimal gland. *Visceral afferent* axons (gustatory fibers) for the anterior two-thirds of the tongue run in the chorda tympani. The gustatory fibers originate from pseudounipolar sensory neurons in the **geniculate ganglion**, which corresponds to a spinal sensory (dorsal root) ganglion. The chorda tympani also conveys the presynaptic *parasympathetic visceral efferent fibers* for the submandibular gland, sublingual gland, and small salivary glands in the anterior two-thirds of the tongue. These fibers travel with the lingual nerve (CN V$_3$) and are relayed in the submandibular ganglion. Glandular branches are then distributed to the respective glands.

D Nerves of the petrous bone

Greater petrosal nerve	Presynaptic parasympathetic branch from CN VII to the pterygopalatine ganglion (lacrimal gland, nasal glands)	Deep petrosal nerve	Postsynaptic sympathetic branch from the internal carotid plexus; unites with the greater petrosal nerve to form the nerve of the pterygoid canal, then continues to the pterygopalatine ganglion and supplies the same territory as the greater petrosal nerve (see **C**).
Lesser petrosal nerve	Presynaptic parasympathetic branch from CN IX to the otic ganglion (parotid gland, buccal and labial glands, see p. 85)		

4.9 Cranial Nerves: Vestibulocochlear (CN VIII)

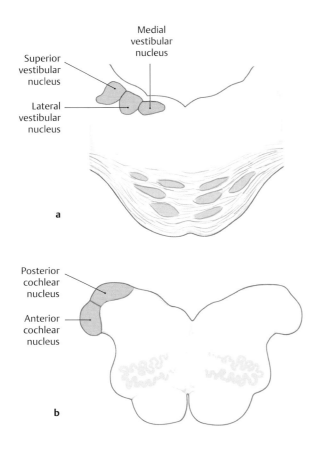

A Nuclei of the vestibulocochlear nerve (CN VIII)
Cross-sections through the upper medulla oblongata.

a Vestibular nuclei. Four nuclear complexes are distinguished:

- Superior vestibular nucleus (of Bechterew)
- Lateral vestibular nucleus (of Deiters)
- Medial vestibular nucleus (of Schwalbe)
- Inferior vestibular nucleus (of Roller)

Note: The inferior vestibular nucleus does not appear in a cross-section at this level (see the location of the cranial nerve nuclei in the brainstem, p. 228).
Most of the axons from the vestibular ganglion terminate in these four nuclei, but a smaller number pass directly through the inferior cerebellar peduncle into the cerebellum (see **Ea**). The vestibular nuclei appear as eminences on the floor of the rhomboid fossa (see **Eb**, p. 227). Their central connections are shown in **Ea**.

b Cochlear nuclei. Two nuclear complexes are distinguished:

- Anterior cochlear nucleus
- Posterior cochlear nucleus

Both nuclei are located lateral to the vestibular nuclei (see **Aa**, p. 228). Their central connections are shown in **Eb**.

B Overview of the vestibulocochlear nerve (CN VIII)

The vestibulocochlear nerve is a *special somatic afferent* (sensory) nerve that consists anatomically and functionally of two components:
- The *vestibular root* transmits impulses from the vestibular apparatus.
- The *cochlear root* transmits impulses from the auditory apparatus.

These roots are surrounded by a common connective-tissue sheath. They pass from the inner ear through the internal acoustic meatus to the cerebellopontine angle, where they enter the brain.

Nuclei and distribution, *ganglia:*
- *Vestibular root:* The *vestibular ganglion* contains bipolar ganglion cells whose central processes pass to the four vestibular nuclei on the floor of the rhomboid fossa of the medulla oblongata. Their peripheral processes begin at the sensory cells of the semicircular canals, saccule, and utricle.
- *Cochlear root:* The *spiral ganglion* contains bipolar ganglion cells whose central processes pass to the two cochlear nuclei, which are lateral to the vestibular nuclei in the rhomboid fossa. Their peripheral processes begin at the hair cells of the organ of Corti.

Every thorough physical examination should include a rapid assessment of both nerve components (hearing and balance tests). A lesion of the vestibular root leads to dizziness, while a lesion of the cochlear root leads to hearing loss (ranging to deafness).

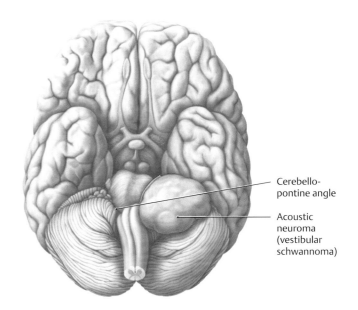

C Acoustic neuroma in the cerebellopontine angle
Acoustic neuromas (more accurately, vestibular schwannomas) are benign tumors of the cerebellopontine angle arising from the Schwann cells of the vestibular root of CN VIII. As they grow, they compress and displace the adjacent structures and cause slowly progressive hearing loss and gait ataxia. Large tumors can impair the egress of CSF from the fourth ventricle, causing hydrocephalus and symptomatic intracranial hypertension (vomiting, impairment of consciousness).

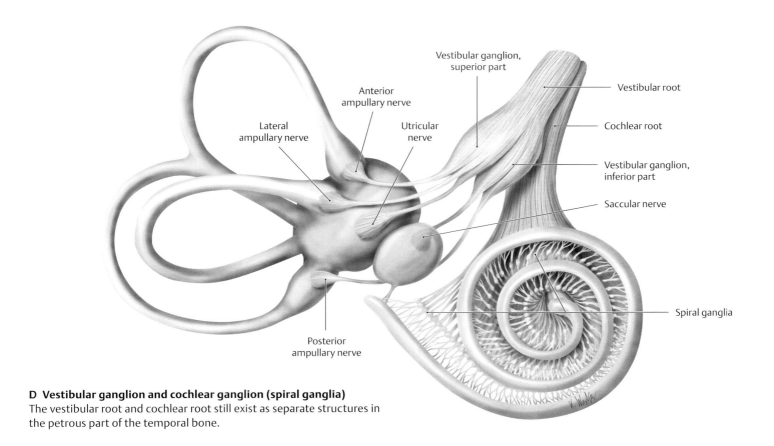

D Vestibular ganglion and cochlear ganglion (spiral ganglia)
The vestibular root and cochlear root still exist as separate structures in the petrous part of the temporal bone.

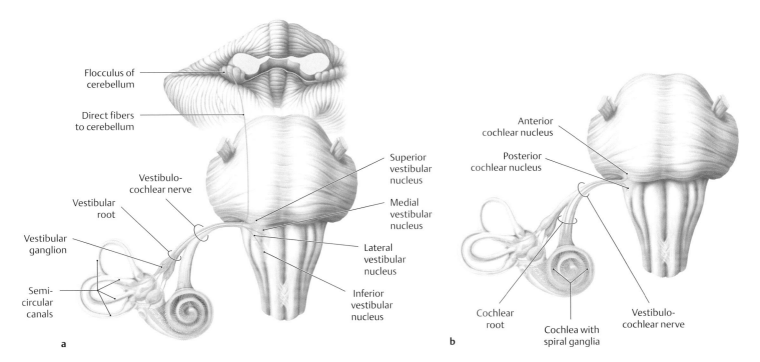

E Nuclei of the vestibulocochlear nerve in the brainstem
Anterior view of the medulla oblongata and pons. The inner ear and its connections with the nuclei are shown schematically.

a Vestibular part: The vestibular ganglion contains bipolar sensory cells whose peripheral processes pass to the semicircular canals, saccule, and utricle. Their axons travel as the vestibular root to the four vestibular nuclei on the floor of the rhomboid fossa (further connections are shown on p. 368). The vestibular organ processes information concerning orientation in space. An acute lesion of the vestibular organ is manifested clinically by dizziness (vertigo).

b Cochlear part: The spiral ganglia form a band of nerve cells that follows the course of the bony core of the cochlea. It contains bipolar sensory cells whose peripheral processes pass to the hair cells of the organ of Corti. Their central processes unite on the floor of the internal auditory canal to form the cochlear root and are distributed to the two nuclei that are posterior to the vestibular nuclei. Other connections of the nuclei are shown on p. 366.

83

4.10 Cranial Nerves: Glossopharyngeal (CN IX)

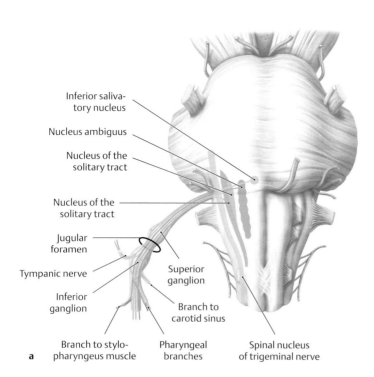

Inferior saliva-tory nucleus

Nucleus ambiguus

Nucleus of the solitary tract

Nucleus of the solitary tract

Jugular foramen

Tympanic nerve

Inferior ganglion

Branch to stylo-pharyngeus muscle

Superior ganglion

Branch to carotid sinus

Pharyngeal branches

Spinal nucleus of trigeminal nerve

a

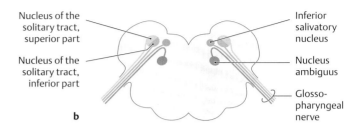

Nucleus of the solitary tract, superior part

Nucleus of the solitary tract, inferior part

Inferior salivatory nucleus

Nucleus ambiguus

Glosso-pharyngeal nerve

b

A Nuclei of the glossopharyngeal nerve

a Medulla oblongata, anterior view. **b** Cross-section through the medulla oblongata at the level of emergence of the glossopharyngeal nerve. For clarity, the nuclei of the trigeminal nerve are not shown (see **B** for further details on the nuclei).

B Overview of the glossopharyngeal nerve (CN IX)

The glossopharyngeal nerve contains *general* and *special visceral efferent fibers* in addition to *visceral afferent* and *somatic afferent fibers*.

Sites of emergence: The glossopharyngeal nerve emerges from the medulla oblongata and leaves the cranial cavity through the jugular foramen.

Nuclei and distribution, *ganglia:*
* *Special visceral efferent (branchiogenic):* The nucleus ambiguus sends its axons to the constrictor muscles of the pharynx (= pharyngeal branches, join with the vagus nerve to form the pharyngeal plexus) and to the stylopharyngeus (see **C**).
* *General visceral efferent (parasympathetic):* The inferior salivatory nucleus sends parasympathetic presynaptic fibers to the otic ganglion. Postsynaptic axons from the otic ganglion are distributed to the parotid gland and to the buccal and labial glands (see **a** and **E**).
* *Somatic afferent:* Central processes of pseudounipolar sensory ganglion cells located in the *intracranial superior ganglion* or *extracranial inferior ganglion* of the glossopharyngeal nerve terminate in the spinal nucleus of the trigeminal nerve. The peripheral processes of these cells arise from:
  – the posterior third of the tongue, soft palate, pharyngeal mucosa, and tonsils (afferent fibers for the gag reflex), see **b** and **c**
  – the mucosa of the tympanic cavity and eustachian tube (tympanic plexus), see **d**
  – the skin of the external ear and auditory canal (blends with the territory supplied by the vagus nerve) and the internal surface of the tympanic membrane (part of the tympanic plexus).
* *Special visceral afferent:* Central processes of pseudounipolar ganglion cells from the inferior ganglion terminate in the superior part of the nucleus of the solitary tract. Their peripheral processes originate in the posterior third of the tongue (gustatory fibers, see **e**).
* *Visceral efferent:* Sensory fibers from the following receptors terminate in the inferior part of the nucleus of the solitary tract:
  – Chemoreceptors in the carotid body
  – Pressure receptors in the carotid sinus (see **f**)

Developmentally, the glossopharyngeal nerve is the nerve of the third branchial arch.

Isolated **lesions** of the glossopharyngeal nerve are rare. Lesions of this nerve are usually accompanied by lesions of CN X and XI (vagus nerve and accessory nerve, cranial part) because all three nerves emerge jointly from the jugular foramen and are all susceptible to injury in basal skull fractures.

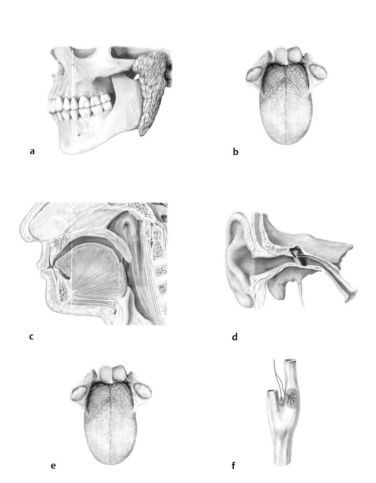

a

b

c

d

e

f

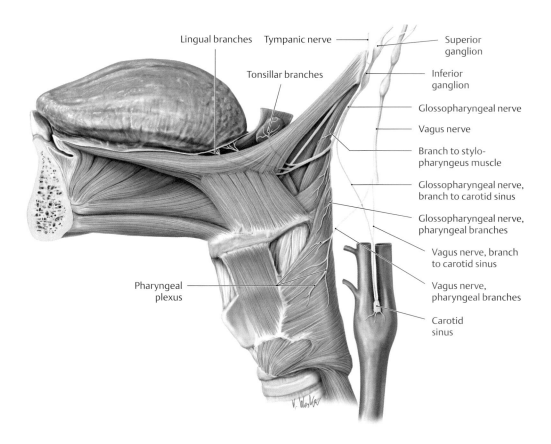

Lingual branches Tympanic nerve Superior ganglion

Tonsillar branches Inferior ganglion

Glossopharyngeal nerve

Vagus nerve

Branch to stylopharyngeus muscle

Glossopharyngeal nerve, branch to carotid sinus

Glossopharyngeal nerve, pharyngeal branches

Vagus nerve, branch to carotid sinus

Vagus nerve, pharyngeal branches

Pharyngeal plexus

Carotid sinus

C Branches of the glossopharyngeal nerve beyond the skull base

Left lateral view.

Note the close relationship of the glossopharyngeal nerve to the vagus nerve (CN X). The carotid sinus is supplied by both nerves.

The most important branches of CN IX seen in the diagram are as follows:

- Pharyngeal branches: three or four branches for the pharyngeal plexus.
- Branch to the stylopharyngeus muscle.
- Branch to the carotid sinus: supplies the carotid sinus and carotid body.
- Tonsillar branches: for the mucosa of the pharyngeal tonsil and its surroundings.
- Lingual branches: somatosensory fibers and gustatory fibers for the posterior third of the tongue.

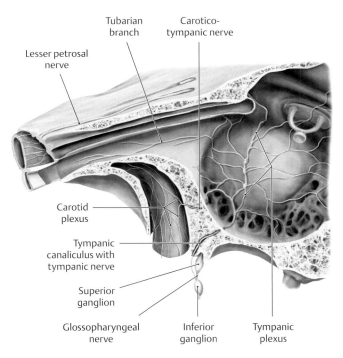

Tubarian branch Caroticotympanic nerve

Lesser petrosal nerve

Carotid plexus

Tympanic canaliculus with tympanic nerve

Superior ganglion

Glossopharyngeal nerve Inferior ganglion Tympanic plexus

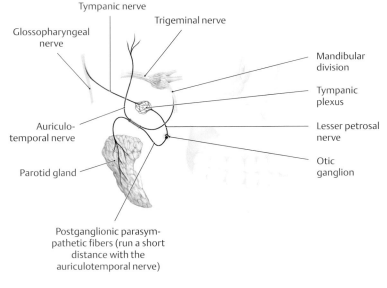

Tympanic nerve Trigeminal nerve

Glossopharyngeal nerve

Mandibular division

Tympanic plexus

Auriculotemporal nerve

Lesser petrosal nerve

Otic ganglion

Parotid gland

Postganglionic parasympathetic fibers (run a short distance with the auriculotemporal nerve)

E Visceral efferent (parasympathetic) fibers of the glossopharyngeal nerve

The presynaptic parasympathetic fibers from the inferior salivatory nucleus leave the medulla oblongata with the glossopharyngeal nerve and branch off as the tympanic nerve immediately after emerging from the base of the skull. The tympanic nerve divides within the tympanic cavity to form the tympanic plexus (see A, p. 144), which is joined by postsynaptic sympathetic fibers from the plexus on the middle meningeal artery (not shown). The tympanic plexus gives rise to the lesser petrosal nerve, which leaves the petrous bone through the hiatus of the canal for the lesser petrosal nerve and enters the middle cranial fossa. Coursing beneath the dura, it passes through the foramen lacerum to the otic ganglion. Its fibers enter the auriculotemporal nerve, pass to the facial nerve, and its autonomic fibers are distributed to the parotid gland via facial nerve branches.

D Branches of the glossopharyngeal nerve in the tympanic cavity

Left anterolateral view. The tympanic nerve, which passes through the tympanic canaliculus into the tympanic cavity, is the first branch of the glossopharyngeal nerve. It contains visceral efferent (presynaptic parasympathetic) fibers for the otic ganglion and somatic afferent fibers for the tympanic cavity and pharyngotympanic (Eustachian) tube. It joins with sympathetic fibers from the carotid plexus (via the caroticotympanic nerve) to form the tympanic plexus. The parasympathetic fibers travel as the lesser petrosal nerve to the otic ganglion (see p. 99), which provides parasympathetic innervation to the parotid gland.

4.11 Cranial Nerves: Vagus (CN X)

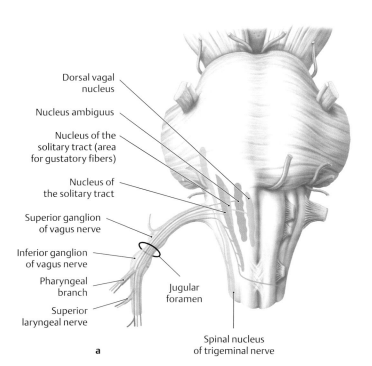

Dorsal vagal nucleus

Nucleus ambiguus

Nucleus of the solitary tract (area for gustatory fibers)

Nucleus of the solitary tract

Superior ganglion of vagus nerve

Inferior ganglion of vagus nerve

Pharyngeal branch

Jugular foramen

Superior laryngeal nerve

Spinal nucleus of trigeminal nerve

a

Dorsal vagal nucleus

Nucleus of the solitary tract, superior part

Nucleus of the solitary tract, inferior part

Spinal nucleus of trigeminal nerve

Nucleus ambiguus

b   Olive

A Nuclei of the vagus nerve.

a Medulla oblongata, anterior view showing the site of emergence of the vagus nerve.

b Cross-section through the medulla oblongata at the level of the superior olive. *Note* the various nuclei of the vagus nerve and their functions.

The *nucleus ambiguus* contains the *somatic efferent* (branchiogenic) fibers for the superior and inferior laryngeal nerves. It has a somatotopic organization, i.e., the neurons for the *superior* laryngeal nerve are above, and those for the *inferior* laryngeal nerve are below. The *dorsal nucleus of the vagus nerve* is located on the floor of the rhomboid fossa and contains presynaptic, parasympathetic visceral efferent neurons. The somatic afferent fibers whose pseudounipolar ganglion cells are located in the superior (jugular) ganglion of the vagus nerve terminate in the *spinal nucleus of the trigeminal nerve.* They use the vagus nerve only as a means of conveyance. The central processes of the pseudounipolar ganglion cells from the inferior (nodose) ganglion are gustatory fibers and visceral afferent fibers. They terminate in the *nucleus of the solitary tract .*

B Overview of the vagus nerve (CN X)

The vagus nerve contains general and special visceral efferent fibers as well as visceral afferent and somatic afferent fibers. It has the most extensive distribution of all the cranial nerves (vagus = "vagabond") and consists of cranial, cervical, thoracic, and abdominal parts. This unit deals mainly with the vagus nerve in the head and neck (its thoracic and abdominal parts are described in the volume on the Neck and Internal Organs).

Site of emergence: The vagus nerve emerges from the medulla oblongata and leaves the cranial cavity through the jugular foramen.

Nuclei and distribution, *ganglia:*
- *Special visceral efferent (branchiogenic):* Efferent fibers from the nucleus ambiguus supply the following muscles:
  - Pharyngeal muscles (pharyngeal branch, joins with glosso-pharyngeal nerve to form the pharyngeal plexus) and muscles of the soft palate (levator veli palatini, muscle of uvula).
  - All laryngeal muscles: The superior laryngeal nerve supplies the cricothyroid, while the inferior laryngeal nerve supplies the other laryngeal muscles (the origin of the fibers is described on p. 88).
- *General visceral efferent (parasympathetic, see* **Dg**): Parasympathetic presynaptic efferents from the dorsal vagal nucleus nerve synapse in prevertebral or intramural ganglia with postsynaptic fibers to supply smooth muscles and glands of:
  - thoracic viscera and
  - abdominal viscera as far as the left colic flexure (Cannon-Böhm point).
- *Somatic afferent:* Central processes of pseudounipolar ganglion cells located in the *superior (jugular) ganglion* of the vagus nerve terminate in the spinal nucleus of the trigeminal nerve. The peripheral fibers originate from:
  - the dura in the posterior cranial fossa (meningeal branch, see **Df**),
  - a small area of skin behind the ear (see **Db**) and external auditory canal (auricular branch, see **Dc**). The auricular branch is the only cutaneous branch of the vagus nerve.
- *Special visceral afferent:* Central processes of pseudounipolar ganglion cells from the inferior nodose ganglion terminate in the superior part of the nucleus of the solitary tract. Their peripheral processes supply the taste buds on the epiglottis (see **Dd**).
- *General visceral afferent:* The perikarya of these afferents are also located in the inferior ganglion. Their central processes terminate in the inferior part of the nucleus of the solitary tract. Their peripheral processes supply the following areas:
  - Mucosa of the lower pharynx at its junction with the esophagus (see **Da**)
  - Laryngeal mucosa above (superior laryngeal nerve) and below (inferior laryngeal nerve) the glottic aperture (see **Da**)
  - Pressure receptors in the aortic arch (see **De**)
  - Chemoreceptors in the para-aortic body (see **De**)
  - Thoracic and abdominal viscera (see **Dg**)

Developmentally, the vagus nerve is the nerve of the fourth and sixth branchial arch.

A structure of major **clinical** importance is the *recurrent laryngeal nerve,* which supplies visceromotor innervation to the only muscle that abducts the vocal cords, the posterior cricoarytenoid. Unilateral destruction of this nerve leads to hoarseness, and bilateral destruction leads to respiratory distress (dyspnea).

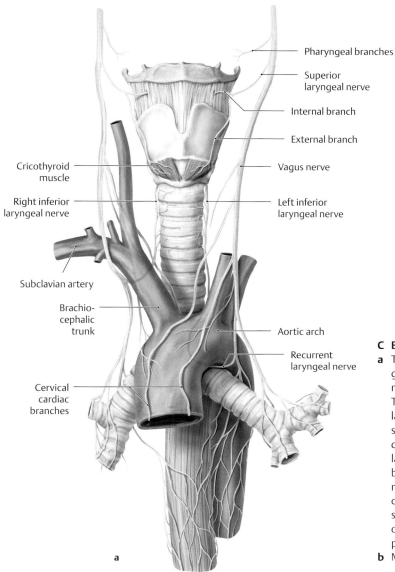

Pharyngeal branches
Superior laryngeal nerve
Internal branch
External branch
Vagus nerve
Left inferior laryngeal nerve
Cricothyroid muscle
Right inferior laryngeal nerve
Subclavian artery
Brachio-cephalic trunk
Aortic arch
Recurrent laryngeal nerve
Cervical cardiac branches

a

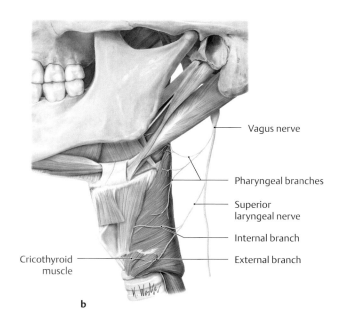

Vagus nerve
Pharyngeal branches
Superior laryngeal nerve
Internal branch
External branch
Cricothyroid muscle

b

C Branches of the vagus nerve (CN X) in the neck

a The vagus nerve gives off four sets of branches in the neck: pharyngeal branches, the superior laryngeal nerve, the recurrent laryngeal nerve, and the cervical cardiac branches.

The inferior laryngeal nerve is the terminal branch of the recurrent laryngeal nerve. It winds around the subclavian artery on the right side and around the aortic arch on the left side. On that side it is in close relationship to the left main bronchus. A lesion of the inferior laryngeal nerve (e.g., due to pressure from a nodal metastasis of bronchial carcinoma or from an aortic aneurysm) may lead to hoarseness (intrinsic laryngeal muscles). The inferior laryngeal nerve passes close to the posterolateral aspect of the thyroid gland, making it susceptible to injury during thyroid operations. For this reason, an otolaryngologist should assess the function of the laryngeal muscles prior to thyroid surgery.

b Muscles supplied by the superior laryngeal nerve.

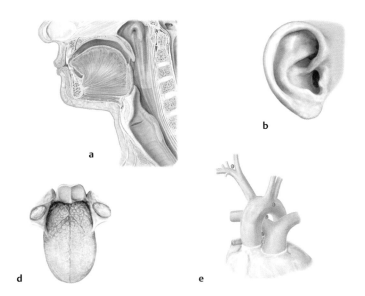

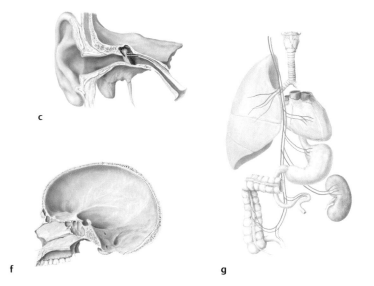

a

b

c

d

e

f

g

D Visceral and sensory distribution of the vagus nerve (CN X)

4.12 Cranial Nerves: Accessory (CN XI) and Hypoglossal (CN XII)

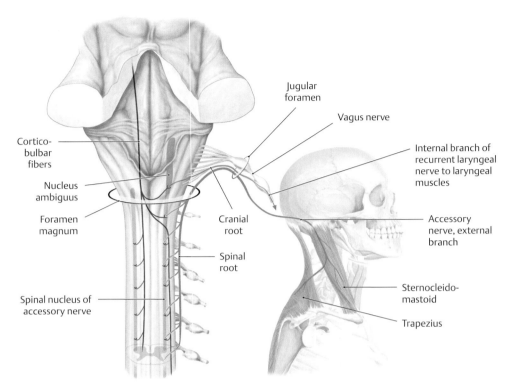

A Nucleus and course of the accessory nerve
Posterior view of the brainstem (with the cerebellum removed). For didactic reasons, the muscles are displayed from the right side (see **C** for further details).

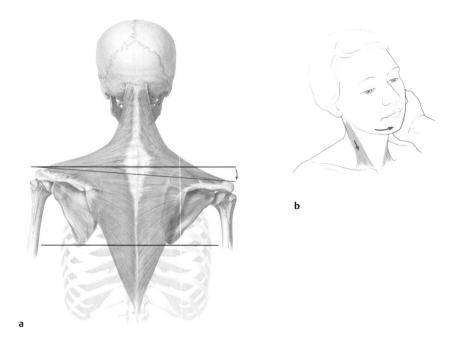

B Lesion of the accessory nerve (on the right side)

a Posterior view. Paralysis of the trapezius muscle causes drooping of the shoulder on the affected side.

b Right anterolateral view. With paralysis of the sternocleidomastoid muscle, it is difficult for the patient to turn the head to the opposite side against a resistance.

C Overview of the accessory nerve (CN XI)

The accessory nerve is considered by some authors to be an *independent* part of the vagus nerve (CN X). It contains both visceral and somatic efferent fibers, and has one cranial and one spinal root.

Sites of emergence: The spinal root emerges from the spinal cord, passes superiorly, and enters the skull through the *foramen magnum,* where it joins with the cranial root from the medulla oblongata. Both roots then leave the skull together through the *jugular foramen.* While still within the jugular foramen, fibers from the cranial root pass to the vagus nerve (internal branch). The spinal portion descends to the nuchal region as the external branch of the accessory nerve.

Nuclei and distribution:
- *Cranial root:* The special visceral efferent fibers of the accessory nerve that arise from the caudal part of the nucleus ambiguus join the vagus nerve and are distributed with the recurrent laryngeal nerve. They innervate all of the laryngeal muscles except the cricothyroid.
- *Spinal root:* The spinal nucleus of the accessory nerve forms a narrow column of cells in the anterior horn of the spinal cord at the level of C2—C5/6. After emerging from the spinal cord, its somatic efferent fibers form the external branch of the accessory nerve, which supplies the trapezius and sternocleidomastoid muscles.

Effects of accessory nerve injury
A unilateral lesion results in the following deficits:
- *Trapezius paralysis,* characterized by drooping of the shoulder and difficulty raising the arm above the horizontal (the trapezius supports the serratus anterior in elevating the arm past 90°). The part of the accessory nerve that supplies the trapezius is vulnerable during operations in the neck (e.g., lymph node biopsies). Because the lower portions of the muscle are also innervated by segments C3 and C4/5, an injury of the accessory nerve will not result in complete trapezius paralysis.
- *Sternocleidomastoid paralysis,* characterized by torticollis (wry neck, i.e., difficulty turning the head to the opposite side). Because this muscle is supplied exclusively by the accessory nerve, an injury to that nerve causes flaccid paralysis. With bilateral lesions, it is difficult for the patient to hold the head in an upright position.

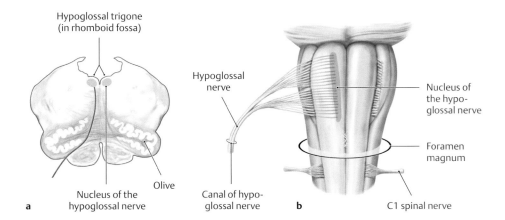

a

Hypoglossal trigone
(in rhomboid fossa)

Hypoglossal
nerve

Nucleus of
the hypo-
glossal nerve

Foramen
magnum

Olive

Nucleus of the
hypoglossal nerve

Canal of hypo-
glossal nerve

b

C1 spinal nerve

D Nuclei of the hypoglossal nerve

a Cross-section through the medulla oblongata at the level of the olive. This section passes through the nucleus of the hypoglossal nerve. It can be seen that the nucleus lies just beneath the rhomboid fossa and raises the floor of the fossa to form the hypoglossal trigone. Because each nucleus

is close to the midline, it is common for more extensive lesions to involve the nuclei on both sides, producing the clinical manifestations of a bilateral nuclear lesion.

b Anterior view. The neurons contained in this nuclear column correspond to the alpha motor neurons of the spinal cord.

E Overview of the hypoglossal nerve (CN XII)

The hypoglossal nerve is a purely somatic efferent nerve that supplies the musculature of the tongue.

Nucleus and site of emergence: The nucleus of the hypoglossal nerve is located in the floor of the rhomboid fossa. Its somatic efferent fibers emerge from the medulla oblongata, leaving the cranial cavity through the hypoglossal canal and descending lateral to the vagus nerve. The hypoglossal nerve enters the root of the tongue above the hyoid bone and distributes its fibers there.

Distribution: The hypoglossal nerve supplies all intrinsic and extrinsic muscles of the tongue (except for the palatoglossus, CN X). It can be considered a "zeroth" ventral root rather than a true cranial nerve. The ventral fibers of C1 and C2 travel with the hypoglossal nerve but leave it again after a short distance to form the superior root of the (deep) ansa cervicalis.

Effects of hypoglossal nerve injury:

- Central hypoglossal paralysis (supranuclear): The tongue deviates away from the side of the lesion.
- Nuclear or peripheral paralysis: The tongue deviates toward the affected side due to a preponderance of muscular action on the healthy side.

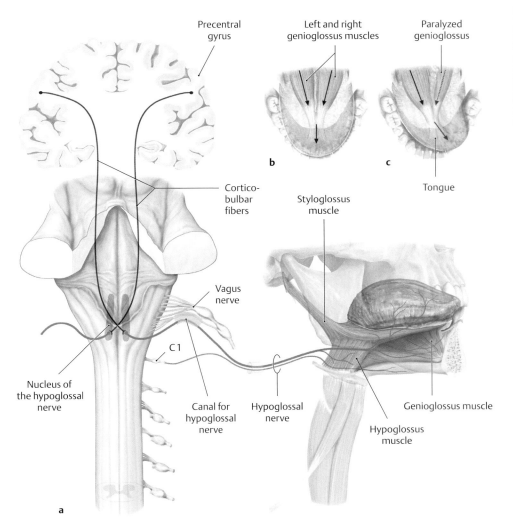

Precentral
gyrus

Left and right
genioglossus muscles

Paralyzed
genioglossus

b

c

Tongue

Cortico-
bulbar
fibers

Styloglossus
muscle

Vagus
nerve

C1

Nucleus of
the hypoglossal
nerve

Canal for
hypoglossal
nerve

Hypoglossal
nerve

Hypoglossus
muscle

Genioglossus muscle

a

F Distribution of the hypoglossal nerve

a Central and peripheral course.

b Function of the genioglossus muscle.

c Deviation of the tongue toward the paralyzed side.

The nucleus of the hypoglossal nerve is innervated (upper motor neurons) by cortical neurons from the contralateral side. With a unilateral *nuclear or peripheral* lesion of the hypoglossal nerve, the tongue deviates toward the side of the lesion when protruded because of the relative dominance of the healthy genioglossus muscle (**c**). When both nuclei are injured, the tongue cannot be protruded (flaccid paralysis).

89

4.13 Neurovascular Pathways through the Base of the Skull, Synopsis

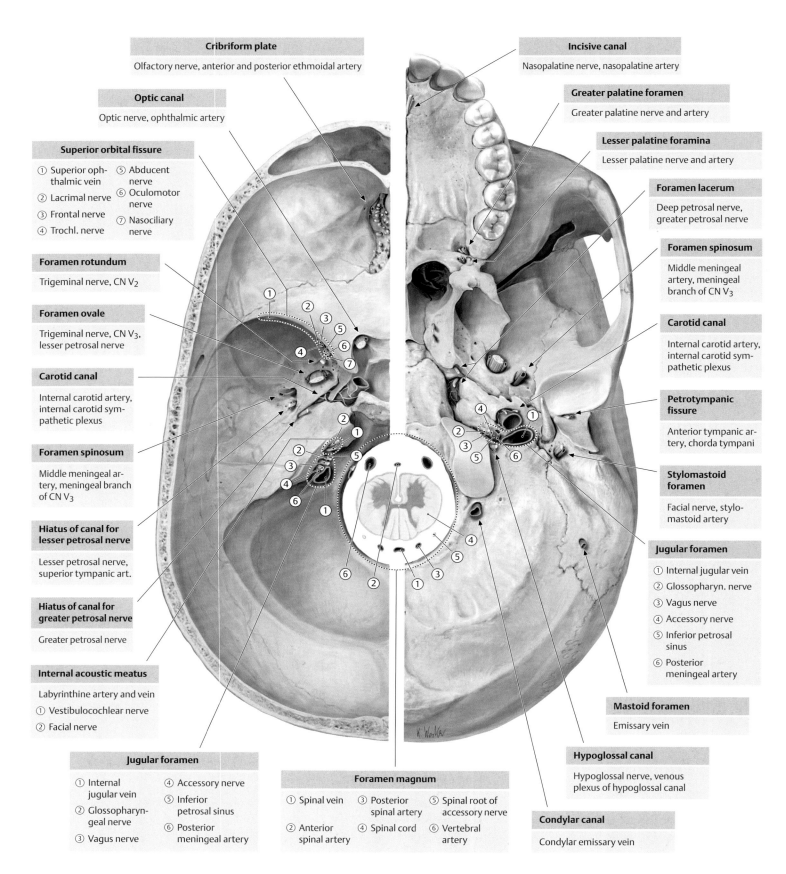

Cribriform plate
Olfactory nerve, anterior and posterior ethmoidal artery

Optic canal
Optic nerve, ophthalmic artery

Superior orbital fissure
① Superior oph-　⑤ Abducent
　thalmic vein　　　nerve
② Lacrimal nerve　⑥ Oculomotor
③ Frontal nerve　　nerve
④ Trochl. nerve　　⑦ Nasociliary
　　　　　　　　　　nerve

Foramen rotundum
Trigeminal nerve, CN V₂

Foramen ovale
Trigeminal nerve, CN V₃,
lesser petrosal nerve

Carotid canal
Internal carotid artery,
internal carotid sym-
pathetic plexus

Foramen spinosum
Middle meningeal ar-
tery, meningeal branch
of CN V₃

**Hiatus of canal for
lesser petrosal nerve**
Lesser petrosal nerve,
superior tympanic art.

**Hiatus of canal for
greater petrosal nerve**
Greater petrosal nerve

Internal acoustic meatus
Labyrinthine artery and vein
① Vestibulocochlear nerve
② Facial nerve

Jugular foramen
① Internal　　④ Accessory nerve
　jugular vein　⑤ Inferior
② Glossopharyn-　petrosal sinus
　geal nerve　　⑥ Posterior
③ Vagus nerve　　meningeal artery

Foramen magnum
① Spinal vein　③ Posterior　⑤ Spinal root of
　　　　　　　　spinal artery　accessory nerve
② Anterior　　④ Spinal cord　⑥ Vertebral
　spinal artery　　　　　　　　artery

Incisive canal
Nasopalatine nerve, nasopalatine artery

Greater palatine foramen
Greater palatine nerve and artery

Lesser palatine foramina
Lesser palatine nerve and artery

Foramen lacerum
Deep petrosal nerve,
greater petrosal nerve

Foramen spinosum
Middle meningeal
artery, meningeal
branch of CN V₃

Carotid canal
Internal carotid artery,
internal carotid sym-
pathetic plexus

**Petrotympanic
fissure**
Anterior tympanic ar-
tery, chorda tympani

**Stylomastoid
foramen**
Facial nerve, stylo-
mastoid artery

Jugular foramen
① Internal jugular vein
② Glossopharyn. nerve
③ Vagus nerve
④ Accessory nerve
⑤ Inferior petrosal
　sinus
⑥ Posterior
　meningeal artery

Mastoid foramen
Emissary vein

Hypoglossal canal
Hypoglossal nerve, venous
plexus of hypoglossal canal

Condylar canal
Condylar emissary vein

A Sites where nerves and vessels pass through the skull base
Left half of drawing: internal view of the base of the skull. Right half of drawing: external view of the base of the skull. Because the opening into the cranium is not identical to the site of emergence on the external aspect of the base of the skull for some neurovascular structures, the site of entry into the cranuim is shown on the left side and the site of emergence is shown on the right side.

	Opening	Transmitted structures
Internal view, base of the skull		
Anterior cranial fossa	• Cribriform plate	• Olfactory fibers (collected to form CN I) • Anterior and posterior ethmoidal artery
Middle cranial fossa	• Optic canal	• Optic nerve (CN II) • Ophthalmic artery
	• Superior orbital fissure	• Oculomotor nerve (CN III) • Trochlear nerve (CN IV) • Ophthalmic nerve (CN V$_1$) • Abducent nerve (CN VI) • Superior ophthalmic vein
	• Foramen rotundum	• Maxillary nerve (CN V$_2$)
	• Foramen ovale*	• Mandibular nerve (CN V$_3$)
	• Foramen spinosum	• Middle meningeal artery • Meningeal branch of CN V$_3$
	• Carotid canal	• Internal carotid artery • Carotid sympathetic plexus
	• Hiatus of canal for greater petrosal nerve	• Greater petrosal nerve
	• Hiatus of canal for lesser petrosal nerve	• Lesser petrosal nerve • Superior tympanic artery
Posterior cranial fossa	• Internal acoustic meatus	• Facial nerve (CN VII) • Vestibulocochlear nerve (CN VIII) • Labyrinthine artery • Labyrinthine veins
	• Jugular foramen	• Superior bulb of internal jugular vein • Glossopharyngeal nerve (CN IX) • Vagus nerve (CN X) • Accessory nerve (CN XI) • Posterior meningeal artery
	• Hypoglossal canal	• Hypoglossal nerve (CN XII)
	• Foramen magnum	• Meninges • Medulla oblongata, spinal cord • Vertebral arteries • Anterior spinal artery • Posterior spinal arteries • Accessory nerve (CN XI): entering spinal roots • Spinal vein
External aspect, base of the skull (where different from internal aspect)	• Incisive canal	• Nasopalatine nerve
	• Greater palatine foramen	• Greater palatine nerve • Greater palatine artery
	• Lesser palatine foramen	• Lesser palatine nerves • Lesser palatine arteries
	• Foramen lacerum	• Deep petrosal nerve • Greater petrosal nerve
	• Petrotympanic fissure	• Chorda tympani • Anterior tympanic artery
	• Stylomastoid foramen	• Facial nerve • Stylomastoid artery
	• Condylar canal	• Condylar emissary vein
	• Mastoid foramen	• Emissary vein

B Principal sites where neurovascular structures pass through the skull base

Note: The external opening of the foramen rotundum is located in the pterygopalatine fossa, which is located deep on the lateral surface of the base of the skull and is not visible here.

* This foramen has an oval shape because it transmits the motor roots of the trigeminal nerve (CN V) for the muscles of mastication.

5.1 Face: Nerves and Vessels

This chapter describes the topographical anatomy of the anterior and lateral aspects of the head. It is assumed that the reader is already familiar with the skeletal, muscular, and neurovascular anatomy illustrated in previous chapters. The most clinically important regions around the eyes, nose, and ears are described in separate chapters. In this chapter the various regions of the face, head, and neck are displayed on the even-numbered pages (left-hand side), while the odd-numbered pages (right-hand side) provide information on functional groups of specific anatomical structures and their clinical importance.

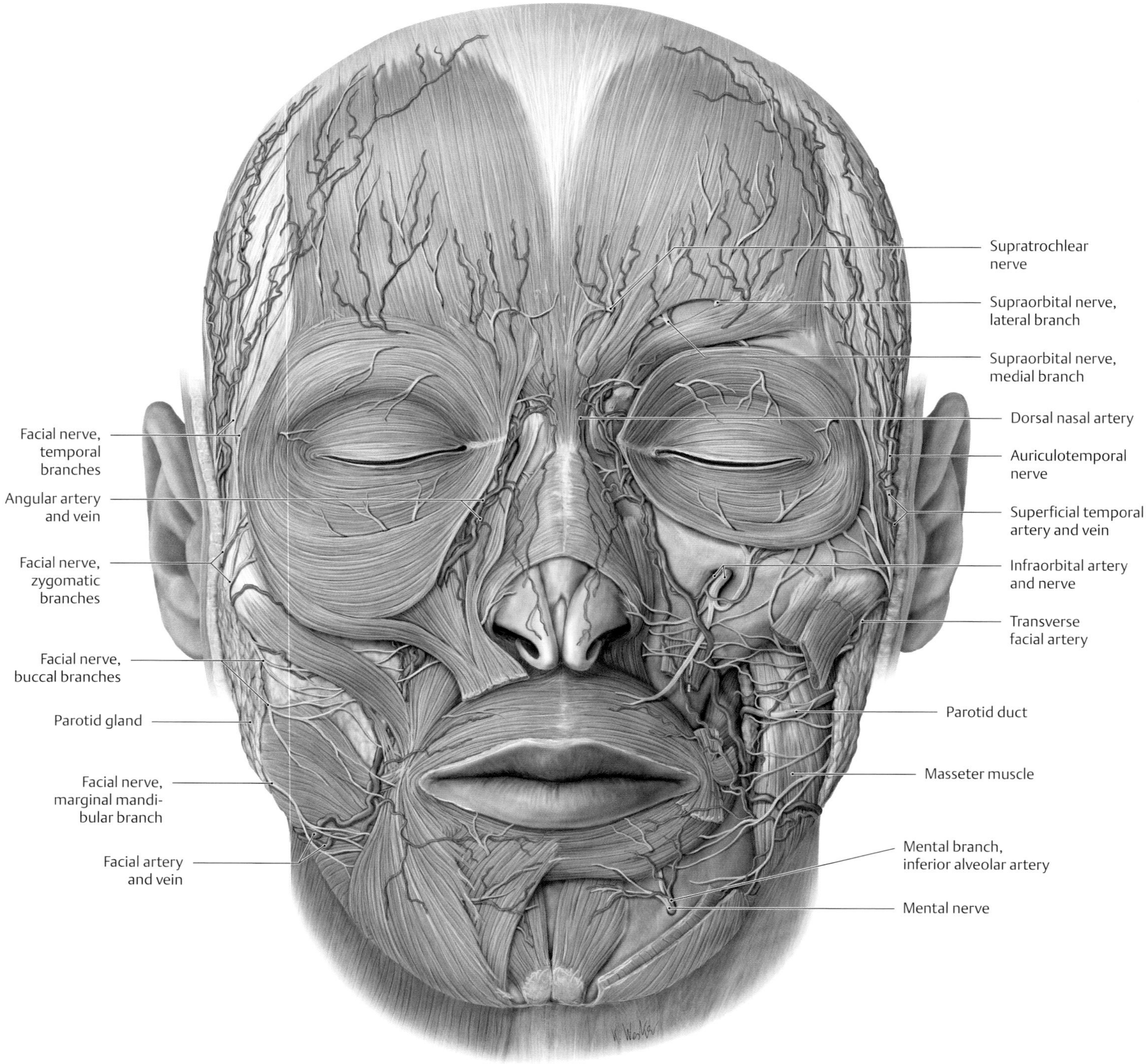
Supratrochlear nerve
Supraorbital nerve, lateral branch
Supraorbital nerve, medial branch
Dorsal nasal artery
Auriculotemporal nerve
Superficial temporal artery and vein
Infraorbital artery and nerve
Transverse facial artery
Parotid duct
Masseter muscle
Mental branch, inferior alveolar artery
Mental nerve
Facial nerve, temporal branches
Angular artery and vein
Facial nerve, zygomatic branches
Facial nerve, buccal branches
Parotid gland
Facial nerve, marginal mandibular branch
Facial artery and vein

A Superficial nerves and vessels of the anterior facial region
The skin and fatty tissue have been removed to demonstrate the superficial muscular layer, the muscles of facial expression. This layer has been partially removed on the left side of the face to display underlying portions of the muscles of mastication. The muscles of expression receive their motor innervation from the *facial nerve,* which emerges laterally from the parotid gland. The face receives its sensory innervation from the *trigeminal nerve,* whose three terminal branches are shown here (see **E**). Branches from the third division of the trigeminal nerve additionally supply motor innervation to the muscles of mastication. The face receives most of its blood supply from the *external carotid artery.* Only small areas around the medial and lateral canthi of the eyes and in the forehead are supplied by the *internal carotid artery* (see **B**).

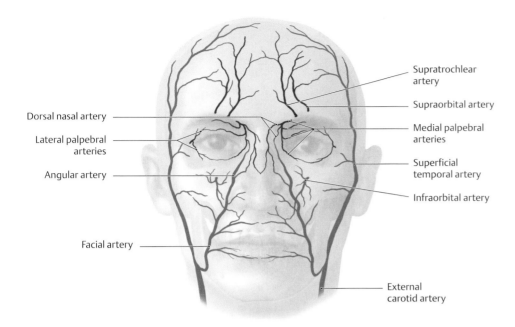

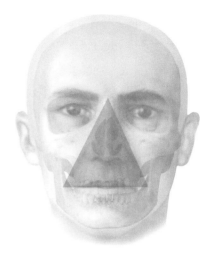

B Distribution of the external carotid artery (red) and internal carotid artery (brown) in the face

Hemodynamically significant anastomoses may develop between these two arterial territories. Even a marked reduction of flow in the internal carotid artery by atherosclerosis may not lead to cerebral ischemia, as long as there is adequate compensatory flow through the superficial temporal artery. If this is the case, then ligation of the superficial temporal artery is contraindicated (the artery might otherwise be ligated, for example, in a biopsy to confirm the diagnosis of temporal arteritis; see p. 59).

C Triangular danger zone in the face

This zone is marked by the presence of venous connections from the face to the dural venous sinuses. Because the veins in this region are valveless, there is a particularly high risk of bacterial dissemination into the cranial cavity (a boil may lead to meningitis—see p. 65).

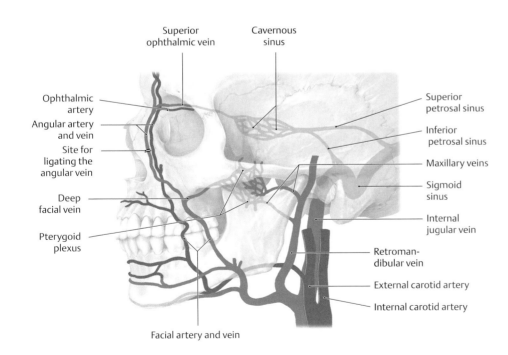

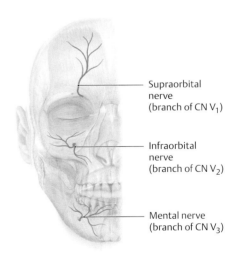

D Clinically important vascular relationships in the face

Note the connections between the exterior of the face and the dural sinuses.

If a purulent inflammation develops in the "danger zone" (see **C**), the angular vein can be ligated at a standard site to prevent the transmission of infectious organisms to the cavernous sinus.

E Clinically important sites of emergence of the three trigeminal nerve branches

The trigeminal nerve (CN V) is the major somatic sensory nerve of the head. The diagram shows the sites of emergence of its three large sensory branches:

- branch of CN V_1: supraorbital nerve (supraorbital foramen)
- branch of CN V_2: infraorbital nerve (infraorbital foramen)
- branch of CN V_3: mental nerve (mental foramen); see also p. 77.

5.2 Head, Lateral View: Superficial Layer

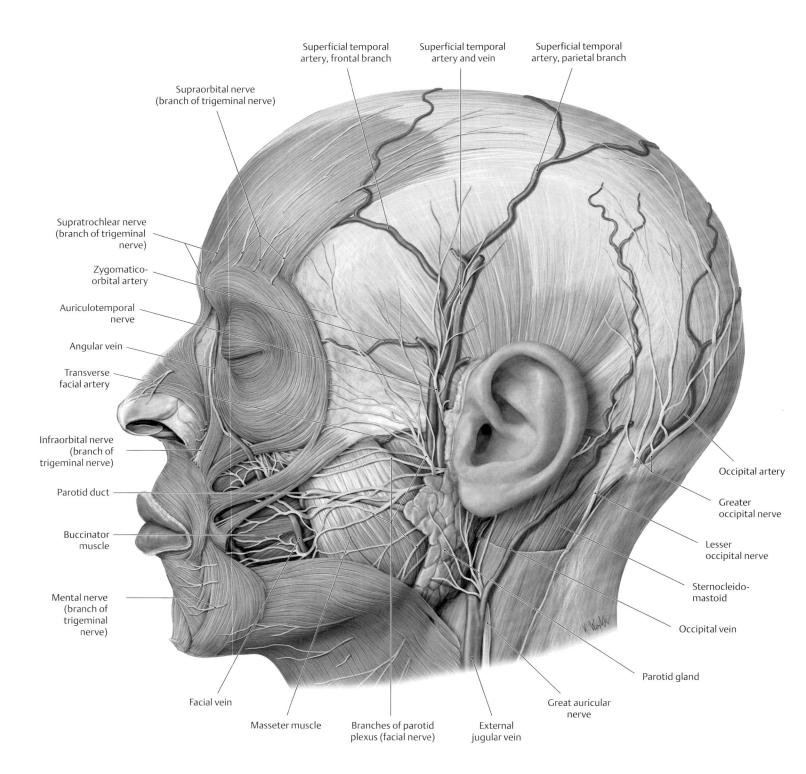

Superficial temporal artery, frontal branch

Superficial temporal artery and vein

Superficial temporal artery, parietal branch

Supraorbital nerve (branch of trigeminal nerve)

Supratrochlear nerve (branch of trigeminal nerve)

Zygomatico-orbital artery

Auriculotemporal nerve

Angular vein

Transverse facial artery

Infraorbital nerve (branch of trigeminal nerve)

Parotid duct

Buccinator muscle

Mental nerve (branch of trigeminal nerve)

Occipital artery

Greater occipital nerve

Lesser occipital nerve

Sternocleido-mastoid

Occipital vein

Parotid gland

Facial vein

Masseter muscle

Branches of parotid plexus (facial nerve)

External jugular vein

Great auricular nerve

A Superficial vessels and nerves of the head

Left lateral view. All the arteries visible in this diagram arise from the *external carotid artery,* which is too deep to be visible in this superficial dissection. The lateral head region is drained by the *external jugular vein.* The facial vein, however, drains into the deeper internal jugular vein (not shown here). The *facial nerve* has divided in the parotid gland to form the parotid plexus, whose branches leave the parotid gland at its anterior border and are distributed to the facial muscles (see **C**). This lateral head region also receives sensory innervation from branches of the *trigeminal nerve* (see **D**), while the portion of the occiput visible in the drawing is supplied by the *greater* and *lesser occipital nerves.* Unlike the trigeminal nerve, the occipital nerves originate from the spinal nerves of the cervical plexus (see **E**). The secretory duct of the parotid gland (the parotid duct) is easy to identify at dissection. It passes forward on the masseter muscle, pierces the buccinator, and terminates in the oral vestibule opposite the second upper molar (not shown).

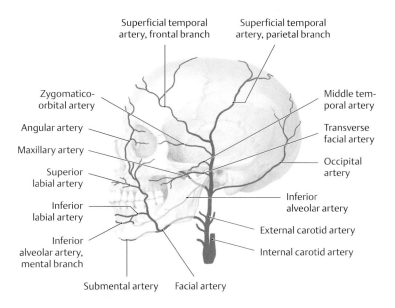

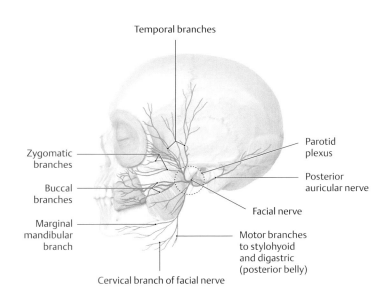

B Superficial branches of the external carotid artery
Left lateral view. This diagram shows the arteries in isolation to demonstrate their branches and their relationships to one another (compare with **A**; see p. 54 for details).

C Facial nerve (CN VII)
Left lateral view. The muscles of facial expression receive all of their motor innervation from the seventh cranial nerve (see p. 79).

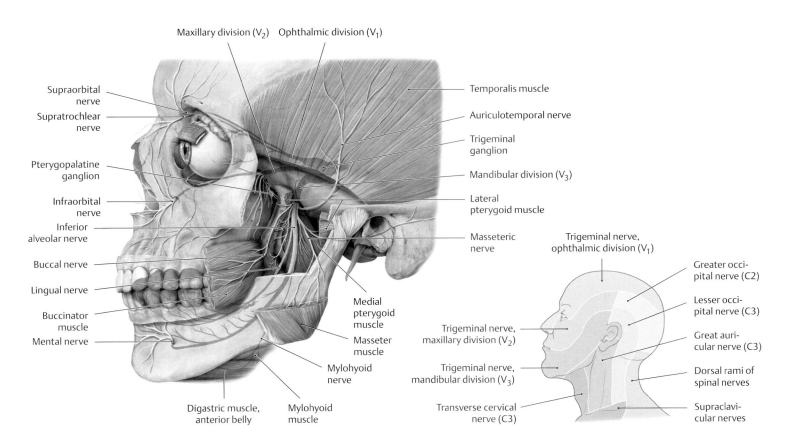

D Trigeminal nerve (CN V)
Left lateral view. In the region shown here, the head derives its somatic sensory supply from three large branches of the trigeminal nerve (supraorbital nerve, infraorbital nerve, and mental nerve). The diagram illustrates their course in the skull and their sites of emergence in the anterior facial region (see the anterior view on p. 92). The trigeminal nerve is partly a mixed nerve because motor fibers travel with the mandibular nerve (= third division of the trigeminal nerve) to supply the muscles of mastication.

E Nerve territories of the lateral head and neck
Left lateral view.
Note: The lateral head and neck region receives its sensory supply from one cranial nerve (trigeminal nerve and its branches), and from the dorsal rami (greater occipital nerve) and ventral rami (lesser occipital nerve, great auricular nerve, transverse cervical nerve) of spinal nerves. The C1 spinal nerve has a ventral root, containing motor fibers, but no dorsal root; it therefore provides no sensory innervation to the skin (i.e., it has no dermatome).

5.3   Head, Lateral View: Middle and Deep Layers

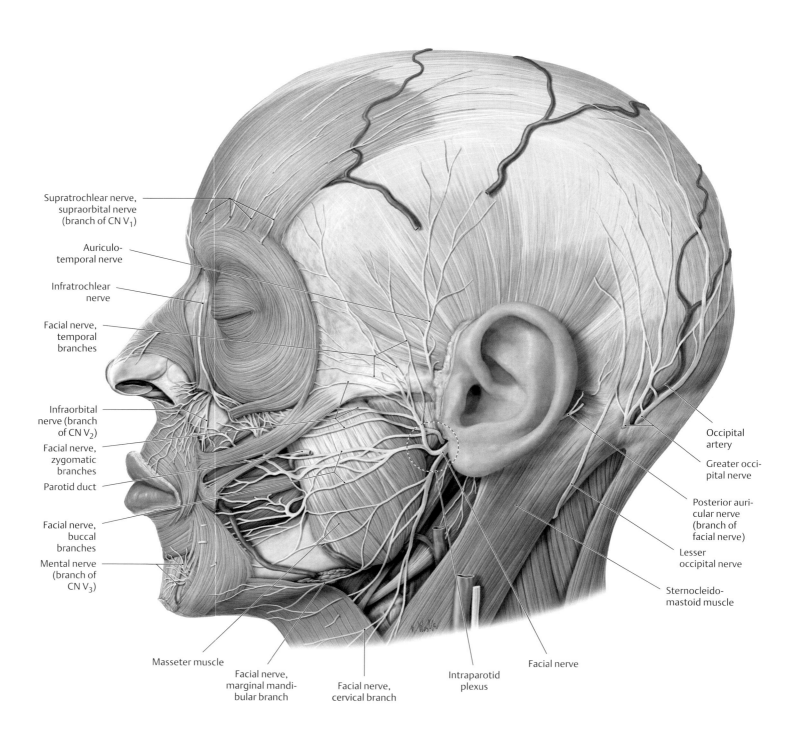

Supratrochlear nerve, supraorbital nerve (branch of CN V₁)

Auriculo-temporal nerve

Infratrochlear nerve

Facial nerve, temporal branches

Infraorbital nerve (branch of CN V₂)

Facial nerve, zygomatic branches

Parotid duct

Facial nerve, buccal branches

Mental nerve (branch of CN V₃)

Occipital artery

Greater occipital nerve

Posterior auricular nerve (branch of facial nerve)

Lesser occipital nerve

Sternocleido-mastoid muscle

Masseter muscle

Facial nerve, marginal mandibular branch

Facial nerve, cervical branch

Intraparotid plexus

Facial nerve

A Vessels and nerves of the intermediale layer
Left lateral view. The parotid gland has been removed to demonstrate the structure of the intraparotid plexus of the facial nerve.
Note: certain nerves have been described in previous units.
The veins have been removed for clarity.

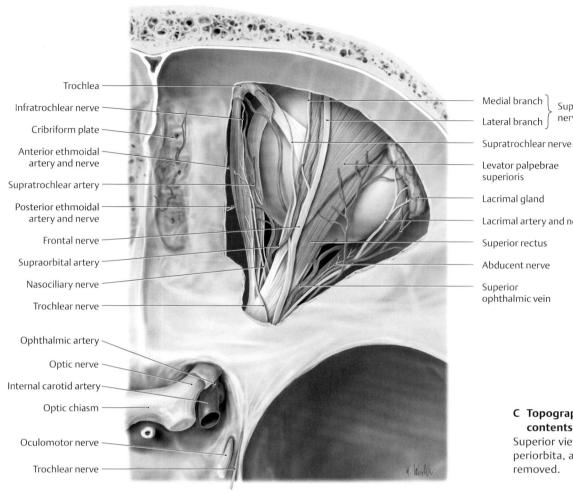

Trochlea
Infratrochlear nerve
Cribriform plate
Anterior ethmoidal artery and nerve
Supratrochlear artery
Posterior ethmoidal artery and nerve
Frontal nerve
Supraorbital artery
Nasociliary nerve
Trochlear nerve

Ophthalmic artery
Optic nerve
Internal carotid artery
Optic chiasm
Oculomotor nerve
Trochlear nerve

Medial branch ⎱ Supraorbital
Lateral branch ⎰ nerve
Supratrochlear nerve
Levator palpebrae superioris
Lacrimal gland
Lacrimal artery and nerve
Superior rectus
Abducent nerve
Superior ophthalmic vein

C Topography of the right orbit: contents of the upper level
Superior view. The bony roof of the orbit, the periorbita, and the retro-orbital fat have been removed.

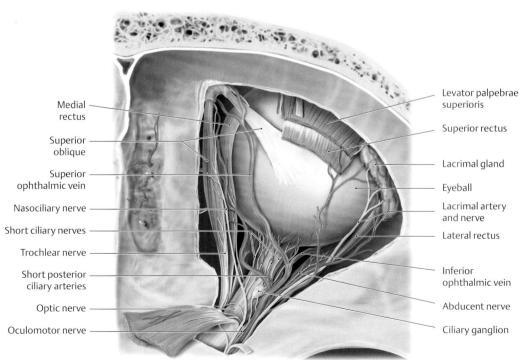

Medial rectus
Superior oblique
Superior ophthalmic vein
Nasociliary nerve
Short ciliary nerves
Trochlear nerve
Short posterior ciliary arteries
Optic nerve
Oculomotor nerve

Levator palpebrae superioris
Superior rectus
Lacrimal gland
Eyeball
Lacrimal artery and nerve
Lateral rectus
Inferior ophthalmic vein
Abducent nerve
Ciliary ganglion

D Topography of the right orbit: contents of the middle level
Superior view. The levator palpebrae superioris and the superior rectus have been divided and reflected backward, and all fatty tissue has been removed to better expose the optic nerve.
Note: The ciliary ganglion is approximately 2 mm in diameter and lies lateral to the optic nerve approximately 2 cm behind the eyeball. The parasympathetic innervation for the intraocular muscles (ciliary muscle and pupillary sphincter) is relayed in the ciliary ganglion. The postsynaptic sympathetic fibers for the pupillary dilator, from the superior cervical ganglion, also pass through this ganglion.

9.1 Ear, Overview

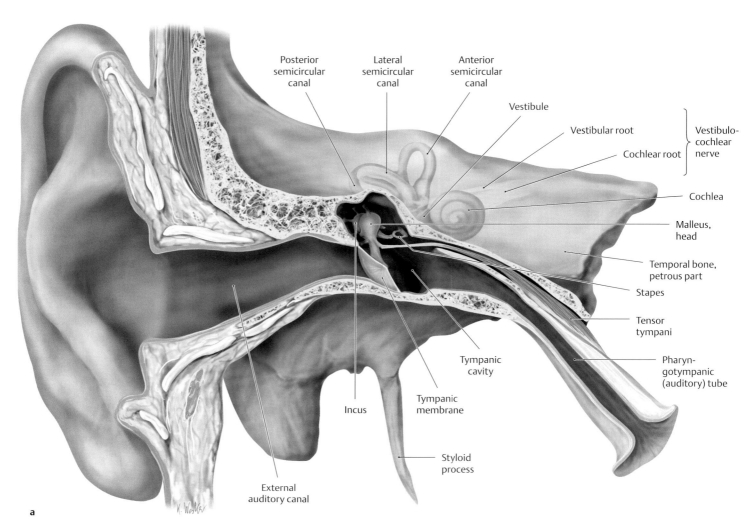

Posterior semicircular canal

Lateral semicircular canal

Anterior semicircular canal

Vestibule

Vestibular root

Cochlear root

Vestibulo-cochlear nerve

Cochlea

Malleus, head

Temporal bone, petrous part

Stapes

Tensor tympani

Pharyn-gotympanic (auditory) tube

Tympanic cavity

Tympanic membrane

Incus

Styloid process

External auditory canal

a

A Auditory and vestibular apparatus in situ

a Coronal section through the right ear, anterior view. **b** Main parts of the auditory apparatus: external ear (yellow), middle ear (blue), and inner ear (green).

The auditory and vestibular apparatus are located deep in the petrous part of the temporal bone (petrous bone). The **auditory apparatus** consists of the external ear, middle ear, and inner ear (see **b**). Sound waves are captured by the *external* ear (auricle, see **B**) and travel through the external auditory canal to the tympanic membrane, which marks the lateral boundary of the *middle ear*. The sound waves set the tympanic membrane into motion, and these mechanical vibrations are transmitted by the chain of auditory ossicles in the middle ear to the oval window, which leads into the *inner* ear (see p. 144). The ossicular chain induces vibrations in the membrane covering the oval window, and these in turn cause a fluid column in the inner ear to vibrate, setting receptor cells in motion (see p. 150). The transformation of sound waves into electrical impulses takes place in the inner ear, which is the actual organ of hearing. The external ear and middle ear, on the other hand, constitute the *sound conduction apparatus*. The organ of balance is the **vestibular apparatus**, which is also located in the auditory apparatus and will be described after the units that deal with the auditory apparatus. It contains

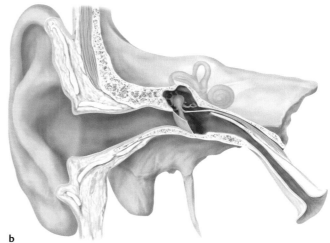

b

the *semicircular canals* for the perception of angular acceleration (rotational head movements) and the *saccule* and *utricle* for the perception of linear acceleration. Diseases of the vestibular apparatus produce dizziness (vertigo).

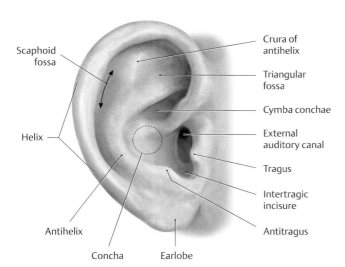

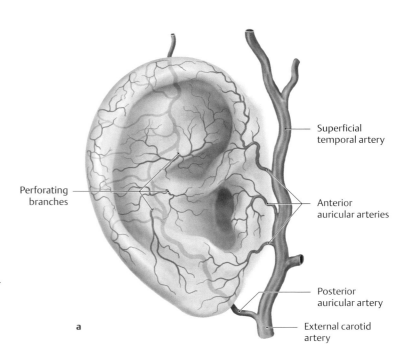

B Right auricle

The auricle of the ear encloses a cartilaginous framework (auricular cartilage) that forms a funnel-shaped receptor for acoustic vibrations.

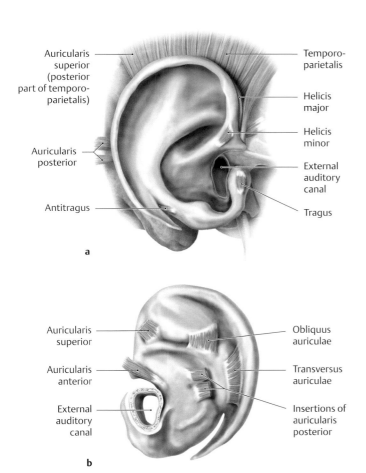

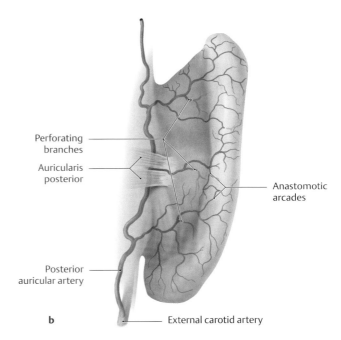

C Cartilage and muscles of the auricle

a Lateral view of the external surface. **b** Medial view of the posterior surface of the right ear.

The skin (removed here) is closely applied to the elastic cartilage of the auricle (shown in light blue). The muscles of the ear are classified as muscles of facial expression and, like the other members of this group, are supplied by the facial nerve. Prominent in other mammals, the auricular muscles are vestigial in humans, with no significant function.

D Arterial supply of the right auricle

Lateral view (**a**) and posterior view (**b**).

The proximal and medial portions of the laterally directed anterior surface of the ear are supplied by the anterior auricular arteries, which arise from the superficial temporal artery (see p. 59). The other parts of the ear are supplied by branches of the posterior auricular artery, which arises from the external carotid artery. These vessels are linked by extensive anastomoses, so operations on the external ear are unlikely to compromise the auricular blood supply. The copious blood flow through the auricle contributes to temperature regulation: dilation of the vessels helps dissipate heat through the skin. The lack of insulating fat predisposes the ear to frostbite, which is particularly common in the upper third of the auricle. The lymphatic drainage and innervation of the auricle are covered in the next unit.

9.2 External Ear: Auricle, Auditory Canal, and Tympanic Membrane

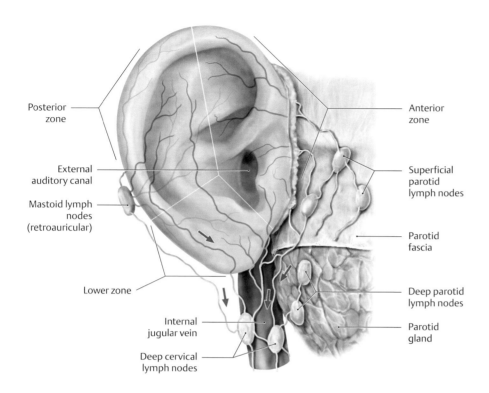

A Auricle and external auditory canal: lymphatic drainage and regional groups of lymph nodes

Right ear, oblique lateral view. The cartilaginous framework and blood supply of the ear were described in the previous unit. The lymphatic drainage of the ear is divided into three zones, all of which drain directly or indirectly into the deep cervical lymph nodes along the internal jugular vein. The lower zone drains directly into the deep cervical lymph nodes. The anterior zone first drains into the parotid lymph nodes, the posterior zone into the mastoid lymph nodes.

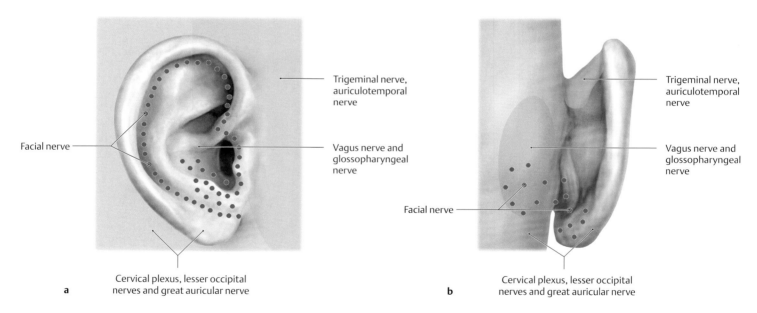

B Sensory innervation of the auricle

Right ear, lateral view (**a**) and posterior view (**b**). The auricular region has a complex nerve supply because, developmentally, it is located at the boundary between the cranial nerves (pharyngeal arch nerves) and branches of the cervical plexus. Four cranial nerves contribute to the innervation of the auricle:

- Trigeminal nerve (CN V)
- Facial nerve (CN VII; the skin area that receives sensory innervation from the facial nerve is not precisely known)
- Glossopharyngeal nerve (CN IX) and vagus nerve (CN X)

Two branches of the **cervical plexus** are involved:

- Lesser occipital nerve (C 2)
- Great auricular nerve (C 2, C 3)

Note: Because the vagus nerve contributes to the innervation of the external auditory canal (auricular branch, see below), mechanical cleaning of the ear canal (by inserting an aural speculum or by irrigating the ear) may evoke coughing and nausea. The auricular branch of the vagus nerve passes through the mastoid canaliculus and through a space between the mastoid process and the tympanic part of the temporal bone (tympanomastoid fissure, see p. 23) to the external ear and external auditory canal. The ear canal receives sensory fibers from the glossopharyngeal nerve through its communicating branch with the vagus nerve.

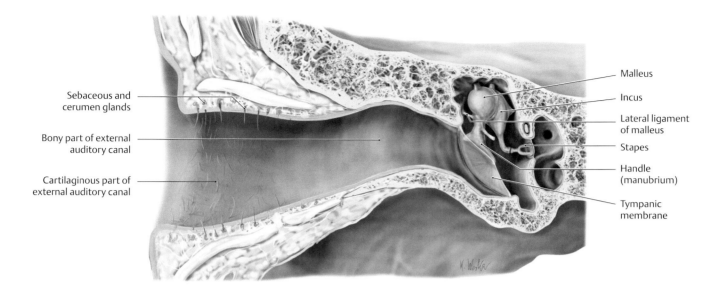

Sebaceous and cerumen glands
Bony part of external auditory canal
Cartilaginous part of external auditory canal

Malleus
Incus
Lateral ligament of malleus
Stapes
Handle (manubrium)
Tympanic membrane

C External auditory canal, tympanic membrane, and tympanic cavity

Right ear, coronal section, anterior view. The tympanic membrane (eardrum, see **E**) separates the external auditory canal from the tympanic cavity, which is part of the middle ear (see p. 144). The external auditory canal is an S-shaped tunnel (see **D**) that is approximately 3 cm long with an average diameter of 0.6 cm. The outer third of the ear canal is cartilaginous. The inner two-thirds of the canal are osseous, the wall being formed by the tympanic part of the temporal bone. The cartilaginous part in particular bears numerous sebaceous and cerumen glands beneath the keratinized stratified squamous epithelium. The cerumen glands produce a watery secretion that combines with the sebum and sloughed epithelial cells to form a protective barrier (cerumen, "earwax") that screens out foreign bodies and keeps the epithelium from drying out. If the cerumen absorbs water (e.g., water in the ear canal after swimming), it may obstruct the ear canal (cerumen impaction), temporarily causing a partial loss of hearing.

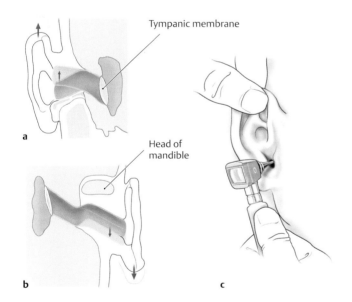

Tympanic membrane

Head of mandible

a

b

c

D Curvature of the external auditory canal

Right ear, anterior view (**a**) and transverse section (**b**).
The external auditory canal is most curved in its cartilaginous portion. It is important for the clinician to know how the ear canal is curved. When the tympanic membrane is inspected with an otoscope, the auricle should be pulled backward and upward in order to straighten the cartilaginous part of the ear canal so that the speculum of the otoscope can be introduced (**c**).

Note the proximity of the cartilaginous anterior wall of the external auditory canal to the temporomandibular joint. This allows the examiner to palpate movements of the mandibular head by inserting the small finger into the outer part of the ear canal.

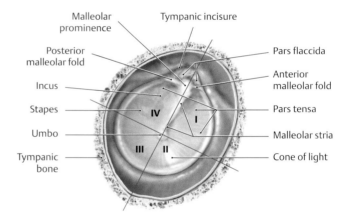

Malleolar prominence
Posterior malleolar fold
Incus
Stapes
Umbo
Tympanic bone

Tympanic incisure
Pars flaccida
Anterior malleolar fold
Pars tensa
Malleolar stria
Cone of light

IV I III II

E Tympanic membrane

Right tympanic membrane, lateral view. The healthy tympanic membrane has a pearly gray color and an oval shape with an average surface area of approximately 75 mm². It consists of a lax portion, the *pars flaccida* (Shrapnell membrane), and a larger taut portion, the *pars tensa*, which is drawn inward at its center to form the umbo ("navel"). The umbo marks the lower tip of the handle (manubrium) of the malleus, which is attached to the tympanic membrane all along its length. It is visible through the pars tensa as a light-colored streak (malleolar stria). The tympanic membrane is divided into four quadrants in a clockwise direction: anterosuperior (I), anteroinferior (II), posteroinferior (III), posterosuperior (IV). The boundary lines of the quadrants are the malleolar stria and a line intersecting it perpendicularly at the umbo. The quadrants of the tympanic membrane are clinically important because they are used in describing the location of lesions. The function of the tympanic membrane is reviewed on pp. 140 and 146. A triangular area of reflected light can be seen in the anteroinferior quadrant of a normal tympanic membrane. The location of this "cone of light" is helpful in evaluating the tension of the tympanic membrane.

9.3　Middle Ear: Tympanic Cavity and Pharyngotympanic Tube

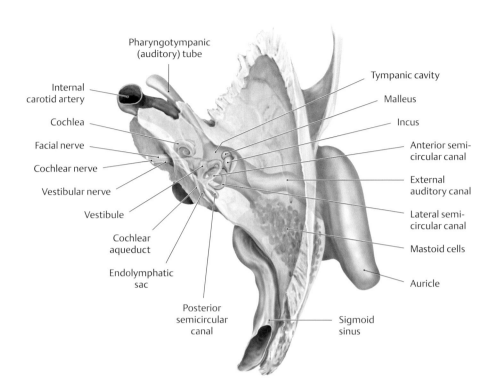

Pharyngotympanic (auditory) tube
Internal carotid artery
Cochlea
Facial nerve
Cochlear nerve
Vestibular nerve
Vestibule
Cochlear aqueduct
Endolymphatic sac
Posterior semicircular canal

Tympanic cavity
Malleus
Incus
Anterior semicircular canal
External auditory canal
Lateral semicircular canal
Mastoid cells
Auricle
Sigmoid sinus

A　The middle ear and associated structures

Right petrous bone, superior view. The middle ear (light blue) is located within the petrous part of the temporal bone between the external ear (yellow) and inner ear (green). The tympanic cavity of the middle ear contains the chain of auditory ossicles, of which the malleus (hammer) and incus (anvil) are visible here. The tympanic cavity communicates anteriorly with the pharynx via the pharyngotympanic (auditory) tube, and it communicates posteriorly with the mastoid air cells. Infections can spread from the phyynx to the mastoid cells by this route (see **C**).

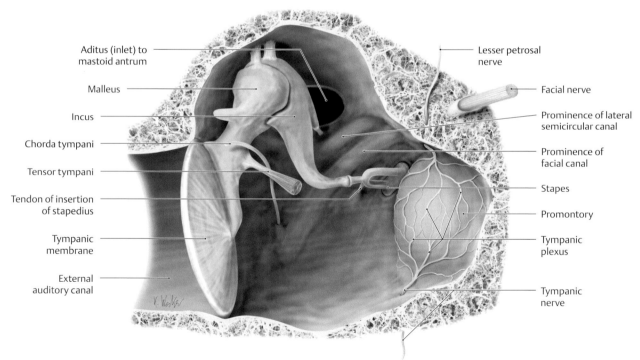

Aditus (inlet) to mastoid antrum
Malleus
Incus
Chorda tympani
Tensor tympani
Tendon of insertion of stapedius
Tympanic membrane
External auditory canal

Lesser petrosal nerve
Facial nerve
Prominence of lateral semicircular canal
Prominence of facial canal
Stapes
Promontory
Tympanic plexus
Tympanic nerve

B　Walls of the tympanic cavity

Anterior view with the anterior wall removed. The tympanic cavity is a slightly oblique space that is bounded by six walls:

- Lateral (membranous) wall: boundary with the external ear; formed largely by the tympanic membrane.
- Medial (labyrinthine) wall: boundary with the inner ear; formed largely by the promontory, or the bony eminence, overlying the basal turn of the cochlea.
- Inferior (jugular) wall: forms the floor of the tympanic cavity and borders on the bulb of the jugular vein.
- Posterior (mastoid) wall: borders on the air cells of the mastoid process, communicating with the cells through the aditus (inlet) of the mastoid antrum.
- Superior (tegmental) wall: forms the roof of the tympanic cavity.
- Anterior (carotid) wall (removed here): includes the opening to the pharyngotympanic (auditory) tube and borders on the carotid canal.

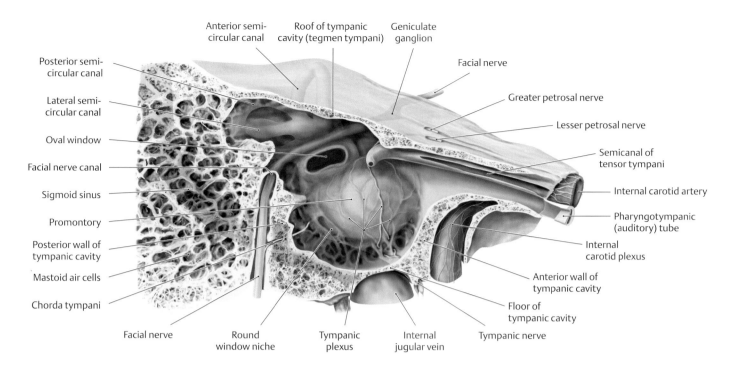

Posterior semi-circular canal

Lateral semi-circular canal

Oval window

Facial nerve canal

Sigmoid sinus

Promontory

Posterior wall of tympanic cavity

Mastoid air cells

Chorda tympani

Anterior semi-circular canal

Roof of tympanic cavity (tegmen tympani)

Geniculate ganglion

Facial nerve

Greater petrosal nerve

Lesser petrosal nerve

Semicanal of tensor tympani

Internal carotid artery

Pharyngotympanic (auditory) tube

Internal carotid plexus

Anterior wall of tympanic cavity

Floor of tympanic cavity

Facial nerve

Round window niche

Tympanic plexus

Internal jugular vein

Tympanic nerve

C Tympanic cavity: clinically important anatomical relationships
Oblique sagittal section showing the medial wall of the tympanic cavity (see **B**). The anatomical relationships of the tympanic cavity are particularly important in treating chronic suppurative otitis media. During this inflammation of the middle ear, pathogenic bacteria may spread upward to adjacent regions. For example, bacteria may spread upward through the roof of the tympanic cavity into the middle cranial fossa (inciting meningitis or a cerebral abscess, especially of the temporal lobe); they may invade the mastoid air cells (mastoiditis) or sigmoid sinus (sinus thrombosis); they may pass through the air cells of the petrous apex and enter the CSF space, causing abducent paralysis, trigeminal nerve irritation, or visual disturbances (Gradenigo syndrome); or they may invade the facial nerve canal, resulting in facial paralysis.

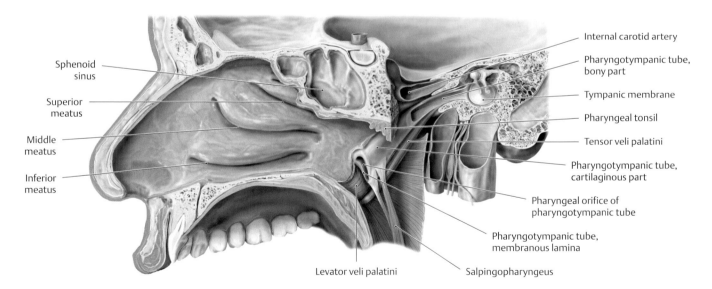

Sphenoid sinus

Superior meatus

Middle meatus

Inferior meatus

Internal carotid artery

Pharyngotympanic tube, bony part

Tympanic membrane

Pharyngeal tonsil

Tensor veli palatini

Pharyngotympanic tube, cartilaginous part

Pharyngeal orifice of pharyngotympanic tube

Pharyngotympanic tube, membranous lamina

Levator veli palatini

Salpingopharyngeus

D Pharyngotympanic (auditory) tube
Medial view of the right half of the head. The pharyngotympanic tube (auditory tube) creates an open channel between the middle ear and pharynx. One-third of the tube is bony and two-thirds are cartilaginous. The bony part of the tube is located in the petrous bone, and the cartilaginous part continues onward to the pharynx, where it expands into a funnel-shaped orifice. As it expands, it forms a kind of hook (hamulus) which is attached to a membranous part (membranous lamina) that enlarges toward the pharynx. The pharyngotympanic tube also opens during swallowing. Air passing through the tube serves to equalize the air pressure on the two sides of the tympanic membrane. This equalization is essential for maintaining normal tympanic membrane mobility, which, in turn, is necessary for normal hearing. The pharyngotympanic tube is opened by the muscles of the soft palate (tensor veli palatini and levator veli palatini) and by the salpingopharyngeus, which is part of the superior pharyngeal muscle. The fibers of the tensor veli palatini arising from the membranous lamina of the pharyngotympanic tube are of special significance: When the tensor veli palatini tenses the soft palate during swallowing, its fibers attached to the membranous lamina simultaneously open the pharyngotympanic tube. The tube is lined with ciliated respiratory epithelium whose cilia beat toward the pharynx, thus inhibiting the passage of microorganisms into the middle ear. If this nonspecific protective mechanism fails, bacteria may migrate up the tube and incite a purulent middle ear infection (see **C**).

9.4   Middle Ear: Auditory Ossicles and Tympanic Cavity

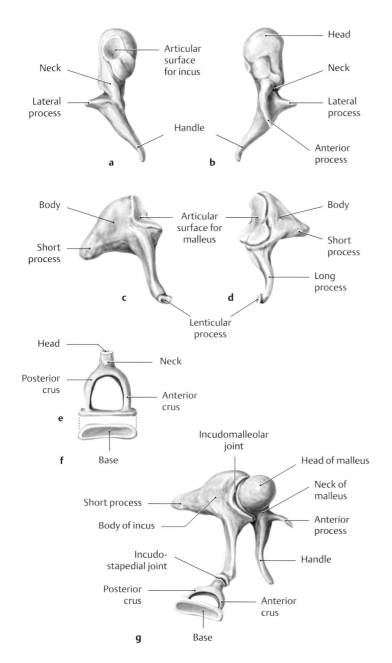

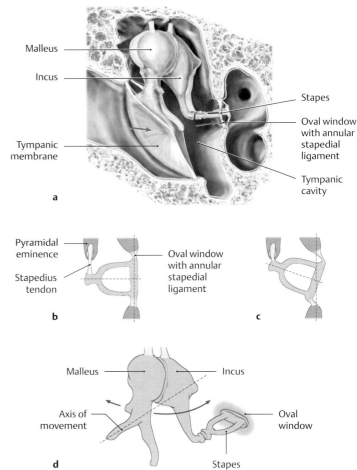

A Auditory ossicles

The auditory ossicles of the left ear. The ossicular chain consists of three small bones in the middle ear (chain function is described in **B**). It establishes an articular connection from the tympanic membrane to the oval window and consists of the following bones:

- Malleus ("hammer")
- Incus ("anvil")
- Stapes ("stirrup")

a, b Malleus: posterior view and anterior view
c, d Incus: medial view and anterolateral view
e, f Stapes: superior view and medial view
   g Medial view of the ossicular chain

Note the articulations between the malleus and incus (incudomalleolar joint) and between the incus and stapes (incudostapedial joint).

B Function of the ossicular chain

Anterior view.

a Sound waves (periodic pressure fluctuations in the air) set the tympanic membrane into vibration. The ossicular chain transmits the vibrations of the tympanic membrane (and thus the sound waves) to the oval window, which in turn communicates them to an aqueous medium, the perilymph. While sound waves encounter very little resistance in air, they encounter considerably higher impedance when they reach the fluid interface of the inner ear (perilymph). The sound waves must therefore be amplified ("impedance matching"). The difference in surface area between the tympanic membrane and oval window increases the sound pressure by a factor of 17, and this is augmented by the 1.3-fold mechanical advantage of the lever action of the ossicular chain. Thus, in passing from the tympanic membrane to the inner ear, the sound pressure is amplified by a factor of 22. If the ossicular chain fails to transform the sound pressure between the tympanic membrane and stapes base (footplate), the patient will experience conductive hearing loss of magnitude approximately 20 dB.

b, c Sound waves impinging on the tympanic membrane induce motion in the ossicular chain, causing a tilting movement of the stapes (**b** normal position, **c** tilted position). The movements of the stapes base against the membrane of the oval window (stapedial membrane) induce corresponding waves in the fluid column in the inner ear.

d The movements of the ossicular chain are essentially rocking movements (the dashed line indicates the axis of the movements, the arrows indicate their direction). Two muscles affect the mobility of the ossicular chain: the tensor tympani and the stapedius (see **C**).

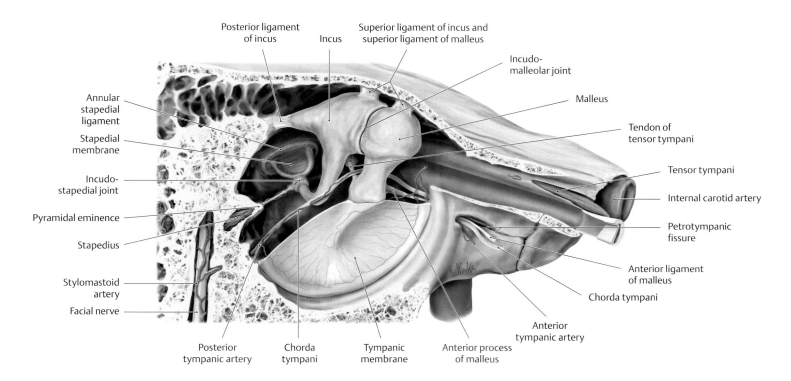

C Ossicular chain in the tympanic cavity

Lateral view of the right ear. The joints and their stabilizing ligaments can be seen. The two muscles of the middle ear—the stapedius and tensor tympani—can also be identified. The *stapedius* (innervated by the stapedial branch of the facial nerve) inserts on the stapes. When it contracts, it stiffens the sound conduction apparatus and decreases sound transmission to the inner ear. This filtering function is believed to be particularly important at high sound frequencies ("high-pass filter"). When sound is transmitted into the middle ear through a probe placed in the external ear canal, one can measure the action of the stapedius (stape-

dius reflex test) by measuring the change in acoustic impedance (i.e., the amplification of the sound waves). Contraction of the *tensor tympani* (innervated by the trigeminal nerve via the medial pterygoid nerve) stiffens the tympanic membrane, thereby reducing the transmission of sound. Both muscles undergo a reflex contraction in response to loud acoustic stimuli.

Note: The chorda tympani, which contains gustatory fibers for the anterior two-thirds of the tongue, passes through the middle ear without a bony covering (making it susceptible to injury during otological surgery).

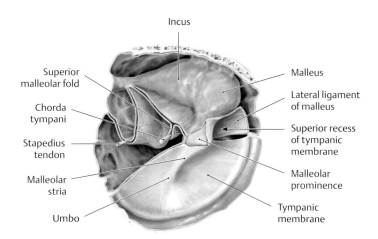

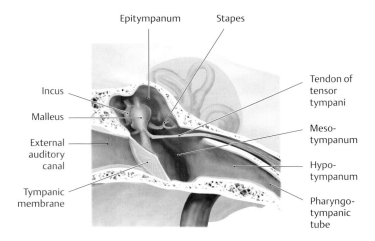

D Mucosal lining of the tympanic cavity

Posterolateral view with the tympanic membrane partially removed. The tympanic cavity and the structures it contains (ossicular chain, tendons, nerves) are covered with mucosa that is raised into folds and deepened into depressions conforming to the covered surfaces. The epithelium consists mainly of a simple squamous type, with areas of ciliated columnar cells and goblet cells. Because the tympanic cavity communicates directly with the respiratory tract through the pharyngotympanic tube, it can also be interpreted as a specialized paranasal sinus. Like the sinuses, it is susceptible to frequent infections (otitis media).

E Clinically important levels of the tympanic cavity

The tympanic cavity is divided into three levels in relation to the tympanic membrane:

- The epitympanum (epitympanic recess, attic) above the tympanic membrane
- The mesotympanum medial to the tympanic membrane
- The hypotympanum (hypotympanic recess) below the tympanic membrane

The epitympanum communicates with the mastoid air cells, and the hypotympanum communicates with the pharyngotympanic tube.

147

9.5 Inner Ear, Overview

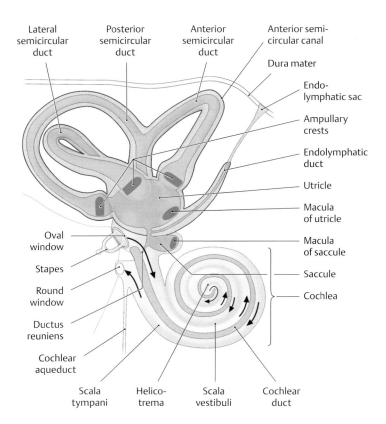

Lateral semicircular duct
Posterior semicircular duct
Anterior semicircular duct
Anterior semicircular canal
Dura mater
Endo-lymphatic sac
Ampullary crests
Endolymphatic duct
Utricle
Macula of utricle
Macula of saccule
Saccule
Cochlea
Oval window
Stapes
Round window
Ductus reuniens
Cochlear aqueduct
Scala tympani
Helico-trema
Scala vestibuli
Cochlear duct

A Schematic diagram of the inner ear

The inner ear is embedded within the petrous part of the temporal bone (see **B**) and contains the auditory and vestibular apparatus for hearing and balance (see p. 150 ff). It comprises a *membranous labyrinth* contained within a similarly shaped *bony labyrinth*. The **auditory apparatus** consists of the cochlear labyrinth with the membranous *cochlear duct*. The membranous duct and its bony shell make up the *cochlea*, which contains the sensory epithelium of the auditory apparatus (*organ of Corti*). The **vestibular apparatus** includes the vestibular labyrinth with three *semicircular canals* (semicircular ducts), a *saccule*, and a *utricle*, each of which contains sensory epithelium. While each of the membranous semicircular ducts is encased in its own bony shell (semicircular canal), the utricle and saccule are contained in a common bony capsule, the *vestibule*. The cavity of the *bony labyrinth* is filled with perilymph (*perilymphatic space*, beige), whose composition reflects its being an ultrafiltrate of blood. The perilymphatic space is connected to the subarachnoid space by the cochlear aqueduct (= perilymphatic duct). It ends at the posterior surface of the petrous part of the temporal bone below the internal acoustic meatus. The *membranous labyrinth* "floats" in the bony labyrinth, being loosely attached to it by connective-tissue fibers. It is filled with endolymph (*endolymphatic space*, blue-green), whose ionic composition corresponds to that of intracellular fluid. The endolymphatic spaces of the auditory and vestibular apparatus communicate with each other through the *ductus reuniens* and are connected by the *endolymphatic duct* to the endolymphatic sac, an epidural pouch on the posterior surface of the petrous bone in which the endolymph is reabsorbed.

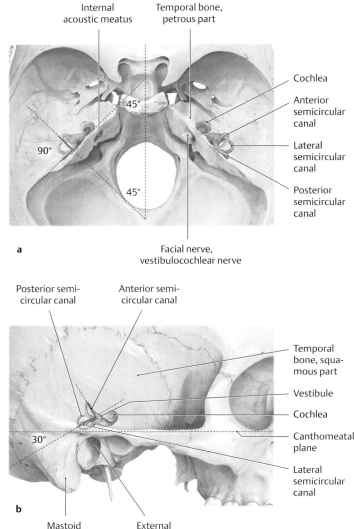

Internal acoustic meatus
Temporal bone, petrous part
Cochlea
Anterior semicircular canal
Lateral semicircular canal
Posterior semicircular canal
45°
90°
45°

a   Facial nerve, vestibulocochlear nerve

Posterior semicircular canal
Anterior semicircular canal
Temporal bone, squamous part
Vestibule
Cochlea
Canthomeatal plane
Lateral semicircular canal
30°

b   Mastoid process   External acoustic meatus

B Projection of the inner ear onto the bony skull

a Superior view of the petrous part of the temporal bone. **b** Right lateral view of the squamous part of the temporal bone.

The apex of the cochlea is directed anteriorly and laterally—not upward as one might intuitively expect. The bony semicircular canals are oriented at an approximately 45° angle to the cardinal body planes (coronal, transverse, and sagittal). It is important to know this arrangement when interpreting thin-slice CT scans of the petrous bone.

Note: The location of the semicircular canals is of clinical importance in thermal function tests of the vestibular apparatus. The lateral (horizontal) semicircular canal is directed 30° forward and upward (see **b**). If the head of the *supine* patient is elevated by 30°, the horizontal semicircular canal will assume a vertical alignment. Since warm fluids tend to rise, irrigating the auditory canal with warm (44°C) or cool (30°C) water (relative to the normal body temperature) can induce a thermal current in the endolymph of the semicircular canal, causing the patient to manifest vestibular nystagmus (jerky eye movements, vestibulo-ocular reflex). Because head movements always stimulate both vestibular apparatuses, caloric testing is the only method of *separately* testing the function of each vestibular apparatus (important in the diagnosis of unexplained vertigo).

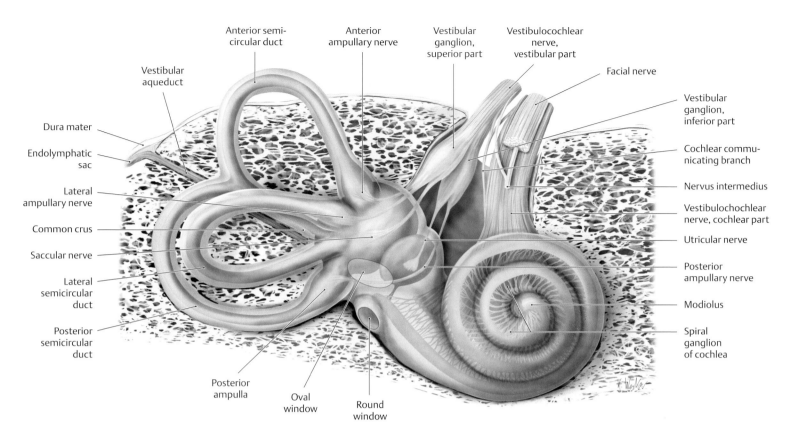

C Innervation of the membranous labyrinth

Right ear, anterior view. **Afferent impulses** from the receptor organs of the utricle, saccule, and semicircular canals (i.e., the **vestibular apparatus**) are first relayed by dendritic (peripheral) processes to the two-part *vestibular ganglion* (superior and inferior parts), which contains the cell bodies (perikarya) of the afferent neurons (bipolar ganglion cells). Their central processes form the *vestibular part* of the *vestibulocochlear nerve* through the internal acoustic meatus and the cerebellopontine angle to the brainstem.

Afferent impulses from the receptor organs of the cochlea (i.e., the **auditory apparatus**) are first transmitted by dendritic (peripheral) processes to the *spiral ganglia,* which contain the cell bodies of the bipolar ganglion cells. They are located in the central bony core of the cochlea (modiolus). Their central processes form the *cochlear part* of the *vestibulocochlear nerve.*

Note: also the section of the facial nerve with its parasympathetic fibers (nervus intermedius) within the internal auditory canal (see **D**).

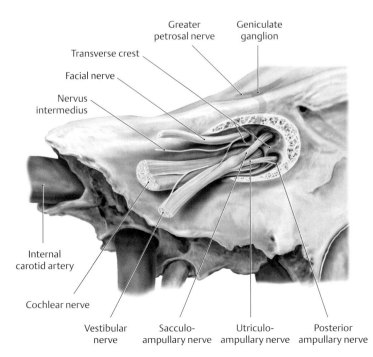

D Passage of cranial nerves through the right internal acoustic meatus

Posterior oblique view of the fundus of the internal acoustic meatus. The approximately 1-cm-long internal auditory canal begins at the internal acoustic meatus on the posterior wall of the petrous bone. It contains:

- the vestibulocochlear nerve with its cochlear and vestibular parts,
- the markedly thinner facial nerve with its parasympathetic fibers (nervus intermedius), and
- the labyrinthine artery and vein (not shown).

Given the close proximity of the vestibulocochlear nerve and facial nerve in the bony canal, a tumor of the vestibulocochlear nerve (*acoustic neuroma*) may exert pressure on the facial nerve, leading to peripheral facial paralysis (see also p. 79). Acoustic neuroma is a benign tumor that originates from the Schwann cells of vestibular fibers, and so it would be more accurate to call it a *vestibular schwannoma* (see also p. 82). Tumor growth always begins in the internal auditory canal; as the tumor enlarges it may grow into the cerebellopontine angle. Acute, unilateral inner ear dysfunction with hearing loss (sudden sensorineural hearing loss), often accompanied by tinnitus, typically reflects an underlying vascular disturbance (vasospasm of the labyrinthine artery causing decreased blood flow).

9.6   Ear: Auditory Apparatus

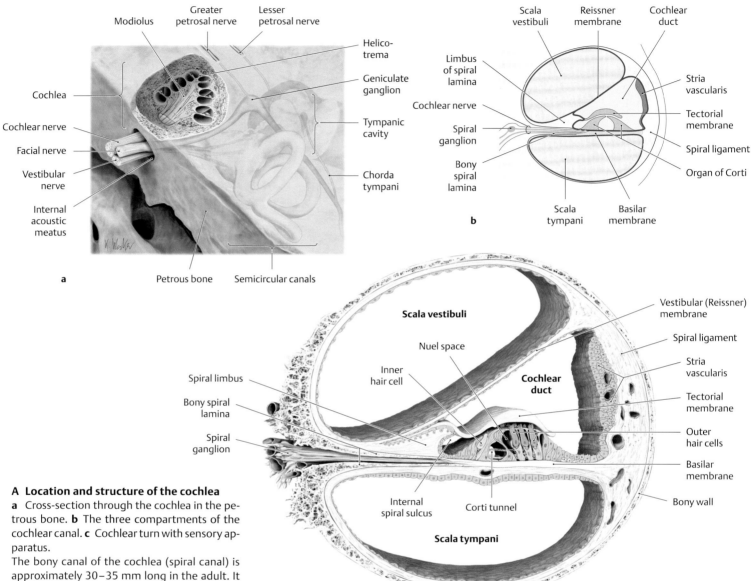

A Location and structure of the cochlea

a Cross-section through the cochlea in the petrous bone. **b** The three compartments of the cochlear canal. **c** Cochlear turn with sensory apparatus.

The bony canal of the cochlea (spiral canal) is approximately 30–35 mm long in the adult. It makes 2 ½ turns around its bony axis, the *modiolus,* which is permeated by branched cavities and contains the spiral ganglion (perikarya of the afferent neurons). The base of the cochlea is directed toward the internal acoustic meatus (**a**). A cross-section through the cochlear canal displays three membranous compartments arranged in three levels (**b**). The upper and lower compartments, the *scala vestibuli* and *scala tympani,* each contain perilymph, while the middle level, the *cochlear duct* (scala media), contains endolymph. The perilymphatic spaces are interconnected at the apex by the *helicotrema,* while the endolymphatic space ends blindly at the apex. The cochlear duct, which is triangular in cross-section, is separated from the scala vestibuli by the *vestibular Reissner membrane* and from the scala tympani by the *basilar membrane.* The basilar membrane represents a bony projection of the modiolus (*spiral lamina*) and widens

steadily from the base of the cochlea to the apex. High frequencies (up to 20,000 Hz) are perceived by the narrow portions of the basilar membrane while low frequencies (down to about 200 Hz) are perceived by its broader portions (*tonotopic organization*). The basilar membrane and bony spiral lamina thus form the floor of the cochlear duct, upon which the actual organ of hearing, the organ of Corti, is located. This organ consists of a system of sensory cells and supporting cells covered by an acellular gelatinous flap, the *tectorial membrane.* The sensory cells (inner and outer hair cells) are the receptors of the organ of Corti (**c**). These cells bear approximately 50–100 stereocilia, and on their apical surface synapse on their basal side with the endings of afferent and efferent neurons. They have the ability to

transform mechanical energy into electrochemical potentials (see below). A magnified cross-sectional view of a cochlear turn (**c**) also reveals the *stria vascularis,* a layer of vascularized epithelium in which the endolymph is formed. This endolymph fills the membranous labyrinth (appearing here as the cochlear duct, which is part of the labyrinth). The organ of Corti is located on the basilar membrane. It transforms the energy of the acoustic traveling wave into electrical impulses, which are then carried to the brain by the cochlear nerve. The principal cell of signal transduction is the inner hair cell. The function of the basilar membrane is to transmit acoustic waves to the inner hair cell, which transforms them into impulses that are received and relayed by the cochlear ganglion.

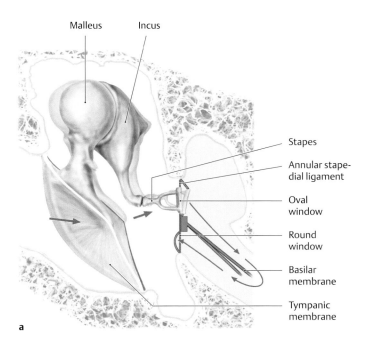

a

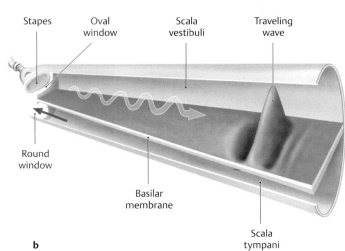

b

B Sound conduction during hearing

a Sound conduction from the middle ear to the inner ear: Sound waves in the air deflect the tympanic membrane, whose vibrations are conducted by the ossicular chain to the oval window. The sound pressure induces motion of the oval window membrane, whose vibrations are, in turn, transmitted through the perilymph to the basilar membrane of the inner ear (see **b**). The round window equalizes pressures between the middle and inner ear.

b Formation of a traveling wave in the cochlea: The sound wave begins at the oval window and travels up the scala vestibuli to the apex of the cochlea ("traveling wave"). The amplitude of the traveling wave gradually increases as a function of the sound frequency and reaches a maximum value at particular sites (shown greatly exaggerated in the drawing). These are the sites where the receptors of the organ of Corti are stimulated and signal transduction occurs. To understand this process, one must first grasp the structure of the organ of Corti (the actual organ of hearing), which is depicted in **C**.

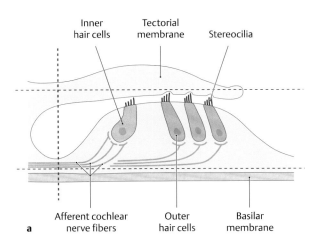

a

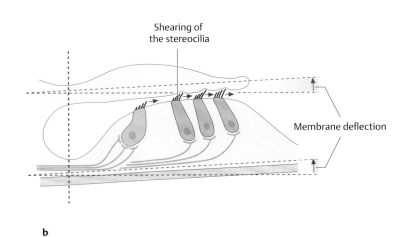

b

C Organ of Corti at rest (a) and deflected by a traveling wave (b)
The traveling wave is generated by vibrations of the oval window membrane (see **Bb**). At each site that is associated with a particular sound frequency, the traveling wave causes a maximum deflection of the basilar membrane and thus of the tectorial membrane, setting up shearing movements between the two membranes. These shearing move-

ments cause the stereocilia on the *outer* hair cells to bend. In response, the hair cells actively change their length, thereby increasing the local amplitude of the traveling wave. This additionally bends the stereocilia of the *inner* hair cells, stimulating the release of glutamate at their basal pole. The release of this substance generates an excitatory potential on the afferent nerve fibers, which is transmitted to the brain.

151

9.7 Inner Ear: Vestibular Apparatus

A Structure of the vestibular apparatus

The vestibular apparatus is the organ of balance. It consists of the membranous semicircular ducts, which contain sensory ridges (ampullary crests) in their dilated portions (ampullae), and of the saccule and utricle with their macular organs (their location in the petrous bone is shown in **B**, p. 148). The sensory organs in the semicircular ducts respond to angular acceleration while the macular organs, which have an approximately vertical and horizontal orientation, respond to horizontal (utricular macula) and vertical (saccular macula) linear acceleration, as well as to gravitational forces.

B Structure of the ampulla and ampullary crest

Cross-section through the ampulla of a semicircular canal. Each canal has a bulbous expansion at one end (ampulla) that is traversed by a connective-tissue ridge with sensory epithelium (ampullary crest). Extending above the ampullary crest is a gelatinous cupula, which is attached to the roof of the ampulla. Each of the sensory cells of the ampullary crest (approximately 7000 in all) bears on its apical pole one long kinocilium and approximately 80 shorter stereocilia, which project into the cupula. When the head is rotated in the plane of a particular semicircular canal, the inertial lag of the endolymph causes a deflection of the cupula, which in turn causes a bowing of the stereocilia. The sensory cells are either depolarized (excitation) or hyperpolarized (inhibition), depending on the direction of ciliary displacement (see details in **E**).

C Structure of the utricular and saccular maculae

The maculae are thickened oval areas in the epithelial lining of the utricle and saccule, each averaging 2 mm in diameter and containing arrays of sensory and supporting cells. Like the sensory cells of the ampullary crest, the sensory cells of the macular organs bear specialized stereocilia, which project into an otolithic membrane. The latter consists of a gelatinous layer, similar to the cupula, but it has calcium carbonate crystals or otoliths (*statoliths*) embedded in its surface. With their high specific gravity, these crystals exert traction on the gelatinous mass in response to linear acceleration, and this induces shearing movements of the cilia. The sensory cells are either depolarized or hyperpolarized by the movement, depending on the orientation of the cilia. There are two distinct categories of vestibular hair cells (type I and type II); type I cells (light red) are goldet shaped.

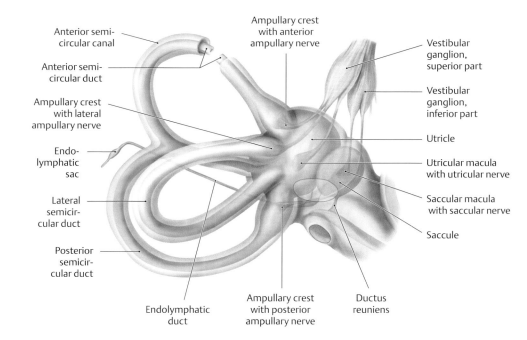

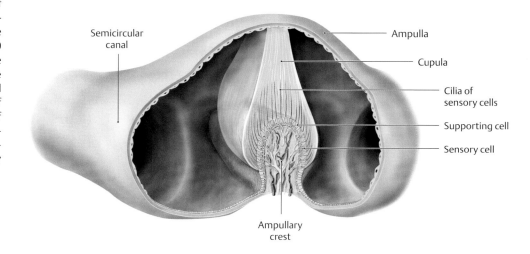

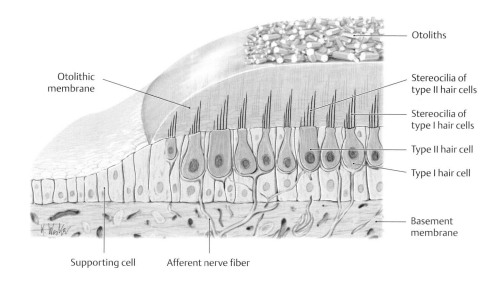

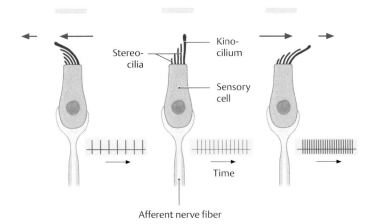

D Stimulus transduction in the vestibular sensory cells

Each of the sensory cells of the maculae and ampullary crest bears on its apical surface one long kinocilium and approximately 80 stereocilia of graduated lengths, forming an array that resembles a pipe organ. This arrangement results in a polar differentiation of the sensory cells. The cilia are straight while in a resting state. When the stereocilia are deflected toward the kinocilium, the sensory cell depolarizes and the frequency of action potentials (discharge rate of impulses) is increased (right side of diagram). When the stereocilia are deflected away from the kinocilium, the cell hyperpolarizes and the discharge rate is decreased (left side of diagram). This mechanism regulates the release of the transmitter glutamate at the basal pole of the sensory cell, thereby controlling the activation of the afferent nerve fiber (depolarization stimulates glutamate release, and hyperpolarization inhibits it). In this way the brain receives information on the magnitude and direction of movements and changes of position.

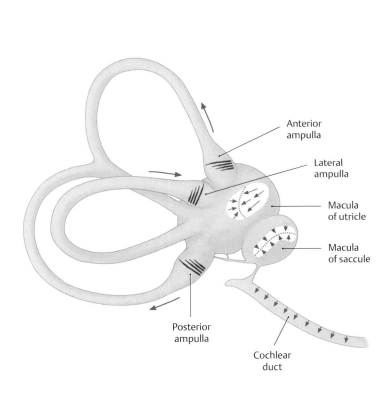

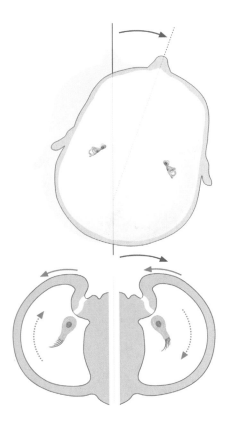

E Specialized orientations of the stereocilia in the vestibular apparatus (ampullary crest and maculae)

Because the stimulation of the sensory cells by deflection of the stereocilia *away from* or *toward* the kinocilium is what initiates signal transduction, the spatial orientation of the cilia must be specialized to ensure that every position in space and every movement of the head stimulates or inhibits certain receptors. The ciliary arrangement shown here ensures that every direction in space will correlate with the maximum sensitivity of a particular receptor field. The arrows indicate the polarity of the cilia, i.e., each of the arrowheads points in the direction of the kinocilium in that particular field.

Note that the sensory cells show an opposite, reciprocal arrangement in the sensory fields of the utricle and saccule.

F Interaction of contralateral semicircular canals during head rotation

When the head rotates to the right (red arrow), the endolymph flows to the left because of its inertial mass (solid blue arrow, taking the head as the reference point). Owing to the alignment of the stereocilia, the left and right semicircular canals are stimulated in opposite fashion. On the right side, the stereocilia are deflected toward the kinocilium (dotted arrow; the discharge rate increases). On the left side, the stereocilia are deflected away from the kinocilium (dotted arrow; the discharge rate decreases). This arrangement heightens the sensitivity to stimuli by increasing the stimulus contrast between the two sides. In other words, the difference between the decreased firing rate on one side and the increased firing rate on the other side enhances the perception of the kinetic stimulus.

9.8 Ear: Blood Supply

A Origin of the principal arteries of the tympanic cavity

Except for the caroticotympanic arteries, which arise from the petrous part of the internal carotid artery, all of the vessels that supply blood to the tympanic cavity arise from the external carotid artery. The vessels have many anastomoses with one another and reach the auditory ossicles, for example, through folds of mucosa. The ossicles are also traversed by intraosseous vessels.

Artery	Origin	Distribution
Caroticotympanic arteries	Internal carotid artery	Pharyngotympanic (auditory) tube and anterior wall of the tympanic cavity
Stylomastoid artery	Posterior auricular artery	Posterior wall of the tympanic cavity, mastoid air cells, stapedius muscle, stapes
Inferior tympanic artery	Ascending pharyngeal artery	Floor of the tympanic cavity, promontory
Deep auricular artery	Maxillary artery	Tympanic membrane, floor of the tympanic cavity
Posterior tympanic artery	Stylomastoid artery	Chorda tympani, tympanic membrane, malleus
Superior tympanic artery	Middle meningeal artery	Tensor tympani, roof of the tympanic cavity, stapes
Anterior tympanic artery	Maxillary artery	Tympanic membrane, mastoid antrum, malleus, incus

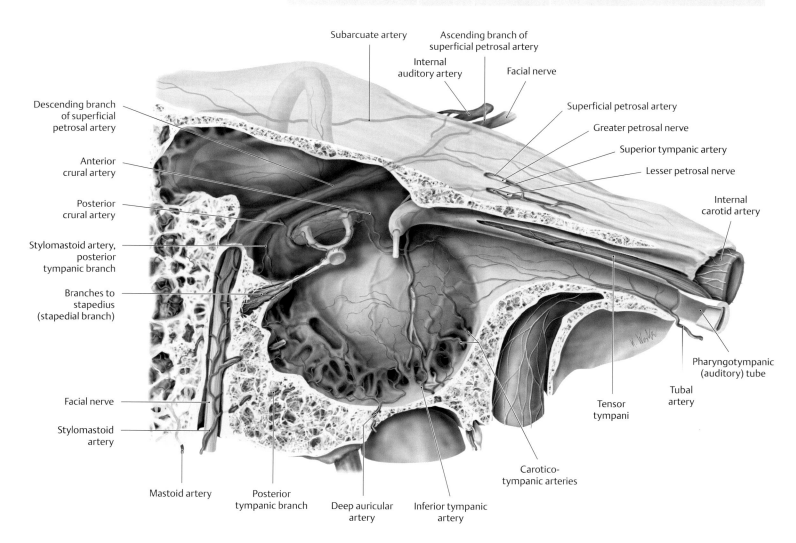

B Arteries of the tympanic cavity and mastoid air cells

Right petrous bone, anterior view. The malleus, incus, portions of the chorda tympani, and the anterior tympanic artery have been removed.

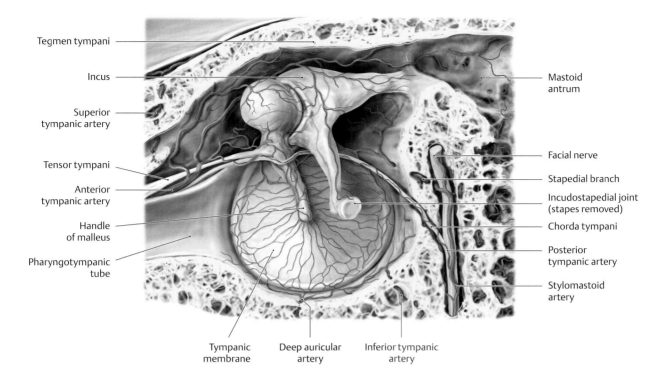

Tegmen tympani

Incus

Superior
tympanic artery

Tensor tympani

Anterior
tympanic artery

Handle
of malleus

Pharyngotympanic
tube

Tympanic
membrane

Deep auricular
artery

Inferior tympanic
artery

Mastoid
antrum

Facial nerve

Stapedial branch

Incudostapedial joint
(stapes removed)

Chorda tympani

Posterior
tympanic artery

Stylomastoid
artery

C Vascular supply of the ossicular chain and tympanic membrane
Medial view of the right tympanic membrane. This region receives most of its blood supply from the anterior tympanic artery. With inflammation of the tympanic membrane, the arteries may become so dilated that their course in the tympanic membrane can be seen, as illustrated here.

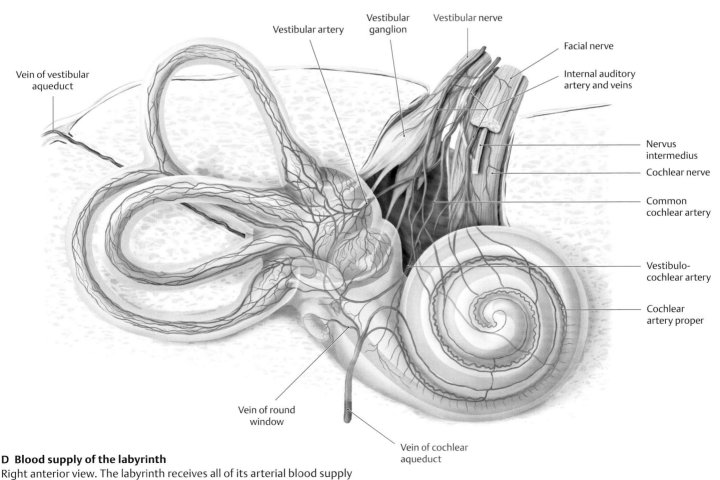

Vestibular artery

Vestibular
ganglion

Vestibular nerve

Facial nerve

Internal auditory
artery and veins

Vein of vestibular
aqueduct

Nervus
intermedius

Cochlear nerve

Common
cochlear artery

Vestibulo-
cochlear artery

Cochlear
artery proper

Vein of round
window

Vein of cochlear
aqueduct

D Blood supply of the labyrinth
Right anterior view. The labyrinth receives all of its arterial blood supply from the internal auditory artery, a branch of the anterior inferior cerebellar artery. The labyrinthine artery occasionally arises directly from the basilar artery.

155

10.1 Coronal Sections, Anterior Orbital Margin and Retrobulbar Space

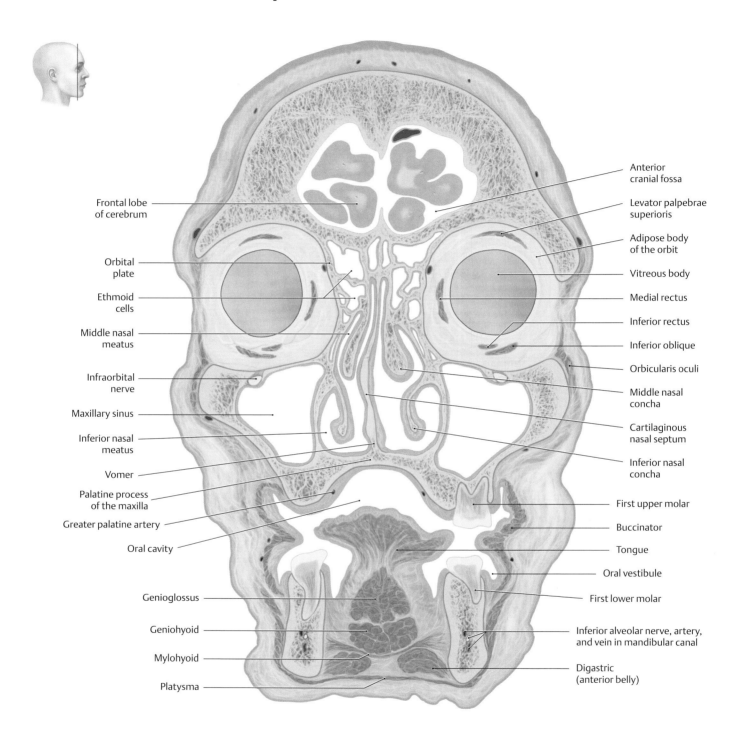

Frontal lobe of cerebrum

Orbital plate

Ethmoid cells

Middle nasal meatus

Infraorbital nerve

Maxillary sinus

Inferior nasal meatus

Vomer

Palatine process of the maxilla

Greater palatine artery

Oral cavity

Genioglossus

Geniohyoid

Mylohyoid

Platysma

Anterior cranial fossa

Levator palpebrae superioris

Adipose body of the orbit

Vitreous body

Medial rectus

Inferior rectus

Inferior oblique

Orbicularis oculi

Middle nasal concha

Cartilaginous nasal septum

Inferior nasal concha

First upper molar

Buccinator

Tongue

Oral vestibule

First lower molar

Inferior alveolar nerve, artery, and vein in mandibular canal

Digastric (anterior belly)

A Coronal section through the anterior orbital margin

Anterior view. This section of the skull can be roughly subdivided into four regions: the oral cavity, the nasal cavity and sinus, the orbit, and the anterior cranial fossa.

Inspecting the region in and around the **oral cavity**, we observe the muscles of the oral floor, the apex of the tongue, the neurovascular structures in the mandibular canal, and the first molar. The hard palate separates the oral cavity from the **nasal cavity**, which is divided into left and right halves by the nasal septum. The inferior and middle nasal conchae can be identified along with the laterally situated maxillary sinus. The structure bulging down into the roof of the sinus is the infraorbital canal, which transmits the infraorbital nerve (branch of the maxillary di-

vision of the trigeminal nerve, CN V$_2$). The plane of section is so far anterior that it does not cut the lateral bony walls of the **orbits** because of the lateral curvature of the skull. The section passes through the transparent vitreous body, and three of the six extraocular muscles can be identified in the retro-orbital fat. Two additional muscles can be seen in the next deeper plane of section (**B**). The space between the two orbits is occupied by the ethmoid cells.

Note: The bony orbital plate is very thin (lamina papyracea) and may be penetrated by infection, trauma, and neoplasms.

In the **anterior cranial fossa**, the section passes through both frontal lobes of the brain in the most anterior portions of the cerebral gray matter. Very little white matter is visible at this level.

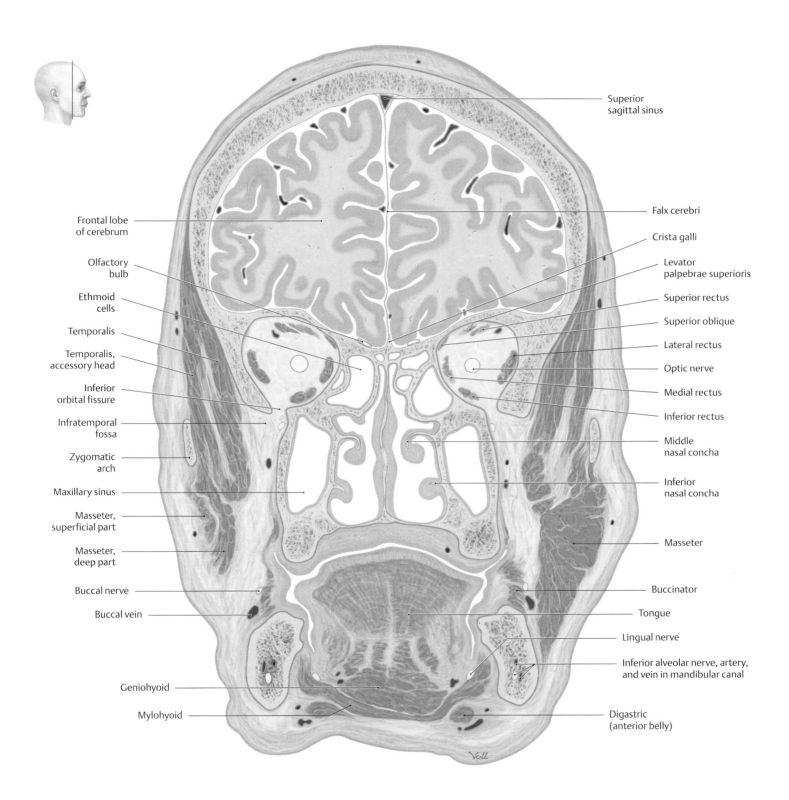

Frontal lobe of cerebrum

Olfactory bulb

Ethmoid cells

Temporalis

Temporalis, accessory head

Inferior orbital fissure

Infratemporal fossa

Zygomatic arch

Maxillary sinus

Masseter, superficial part

Masseter, deep part

Buccal nerve

Buccal vein

Geniohyoid

Mylohyoid

Superior sagittal sinus

Falx cerebri

Crista galli

Levator palpebrae superioris

Superior rectus

Superior oblique

Lateral rectus

Optic nerve

Medial rectus

Inferior rectus

Middle nasal concha

Inferior nasal concha

Masseter

Buccinator

Tongue

Lingual nerve

Inferior alveolar nerve, artery, and vein in mandibular canal

Digastric (anterior belly)

B Coronal section through the retrobulbar space
Anterior view. Here, the tongue is cut at a more posterior level than in **A** and therefore appears broader. In addition to the oral floor muscles, we see the muscles of mastication on the sides of the skull. In the orbital region we can identify the retrobulbar space with its fatty tissue, the extraocular muscles, and the optic nerve. The orbit communicates laterally with the infratemporal fossa through the inferior orbital fissure. This section cuts through both olfactory bulbs in the anterior cranial fossa, and the superior sagittal sinus can be recognized in the midline.

10.2 Coronal Sections, Orbital Apex and Pituitary

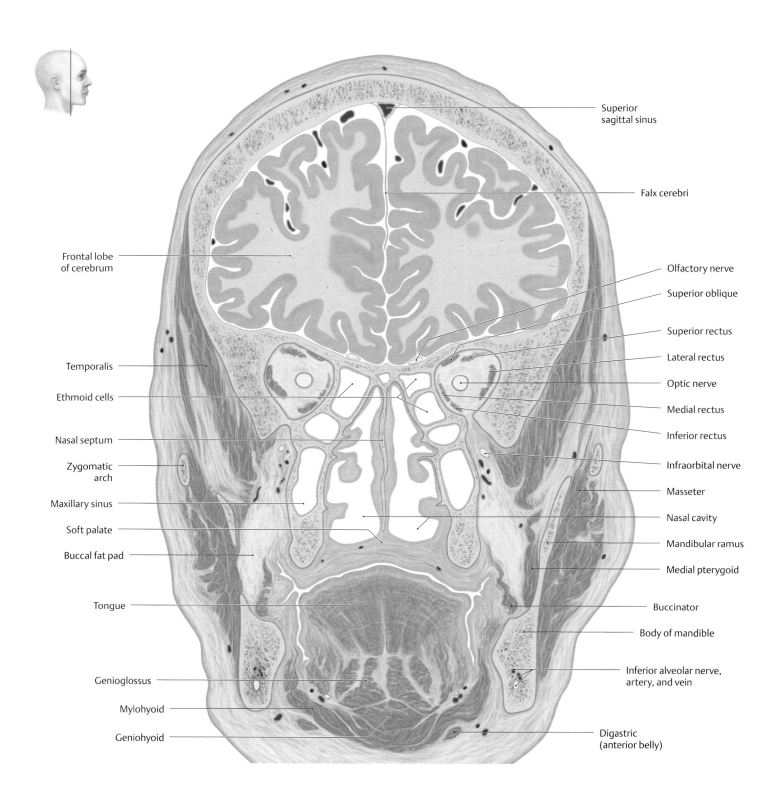

A Coronal section through the orbital apex

Anterior view. The soft palate replaces the hard palate in this plane of section, and the nasal septum becomes osseous at this level. The buccal fat pad is also visible in this plane. Because the buccal pad is composed of fat, it is attenuated in wasting diseases; this is why the cheeks are sunken in patients with end-stage cancer. This coronal section is slightly angled, producing an apparent discontinuity in the mandibular ramus on the left side of the figure (compare with the continuous ramus on the right side).

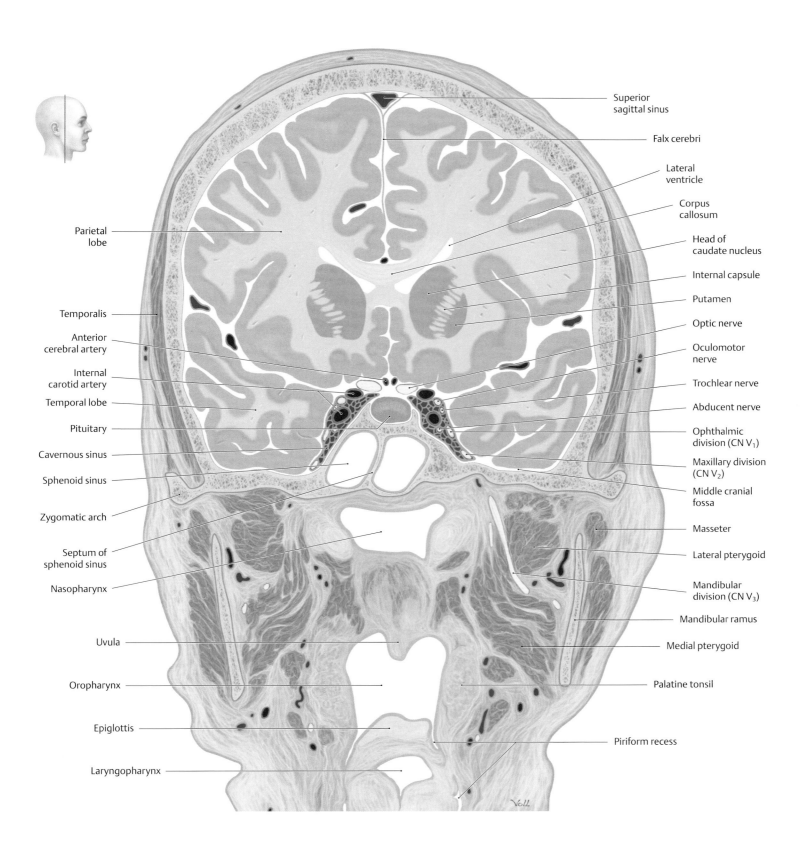

Parietal lobe

Temporalis

Anterior cerebral artery

Internal carotid artery

Temporal lobe

Pituitary

Cavernous sinus

Sphenoid sinus

Zygomatic arch

Septum of sphenoid sinus

Nasopharynx

Uvula

Oropharynx

Epiglottis

Laryngopharynx

Superior sagittal sinus

Falx cerebri

Lateral ventricle

Corpus callosum

Head of caudate nucleus

Internal capsule

Putamen

Optic nerve

Oculomotor nerve

Trochlear nerve

Abducent nerve

Ophthalmic division (CN V$_1$)

Maxillary division (CN V$_2$)

Middle cranial fossa

Masseter

Lateral pterygoid

Mandibular division (CN V$_3$)

Mandibular ramus

Medial pterygoid

Palatine tonsil

Piriform recess

B Coronal section through the pituitary

Anterior view. The nasopharynx, oropharynx, and laryngopharynx can now be identified. This section cuts the epiglottis, below which is the supraglottic space. The plane cuts the mandibular ramus on both sides, and a relatively long segment of the mandibular division (CN V$_3$) can be identified on the left side. The paired sphenoid sinuses are visible, separated by a median septum. Above the roof of the sphenoid sinuses is the pituitary (hypophysis), which lies in the hypophyseal fossa. In the cranial cavity, the plane of section passes through the middle cranial fossa. Due to the presence of the carotid siphon (a 180° bend in the cavernous part of the internal carotid artery), the section cuts the internal carotid artery twice on each side. Cranial nerves can be seen passing through the cavernous sinus on their way from the middle cranial fossa to the orbit. The superior sagittal sinus appears in cross-section at the attachment of the falx cerebri. At the level of the cerebrum, the plane of section passes through the parietal and temporal lobes. Intracerebral structures appearing in this section include the caudate nucleus, the putamen, the internal capsule, and the anterior horn of each lateral ventricle.

159

10.3 Transverse Sections, Orbits and Optic Nerve

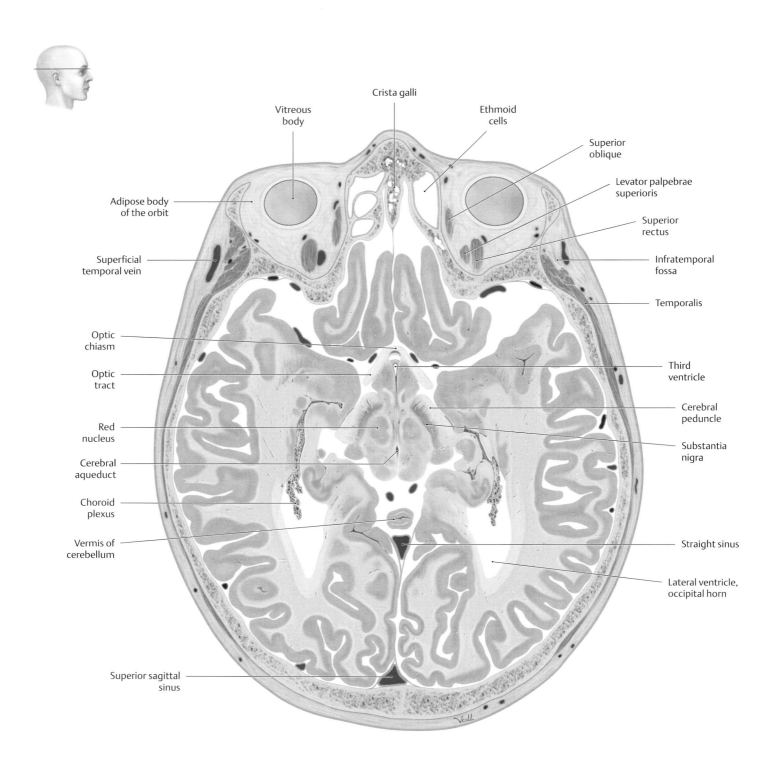

A Transverse section through the upper level of the orbits

Superior view. The highest section in this series displays the muscles in the upper level of the orbit (the orbital levels are described on p. 136 ff). The section cuts the bony crista galli in the anterior cranial fossa, flanked on each side by cells of the ethmoid sinus. The sections of the optic chiasm and adjacent optic tract are parts of the diencephalon, which surrounds the third ventricle at the center of the section. The red nucleus and substantia nigra are visible in the mesencephalon. The pyramidal tract descends in the cerebral peduncles. The section passes through the posterior (occipital) horns of the lateral ventricles and barely cuts the vermis of the cerebellum in the midline.

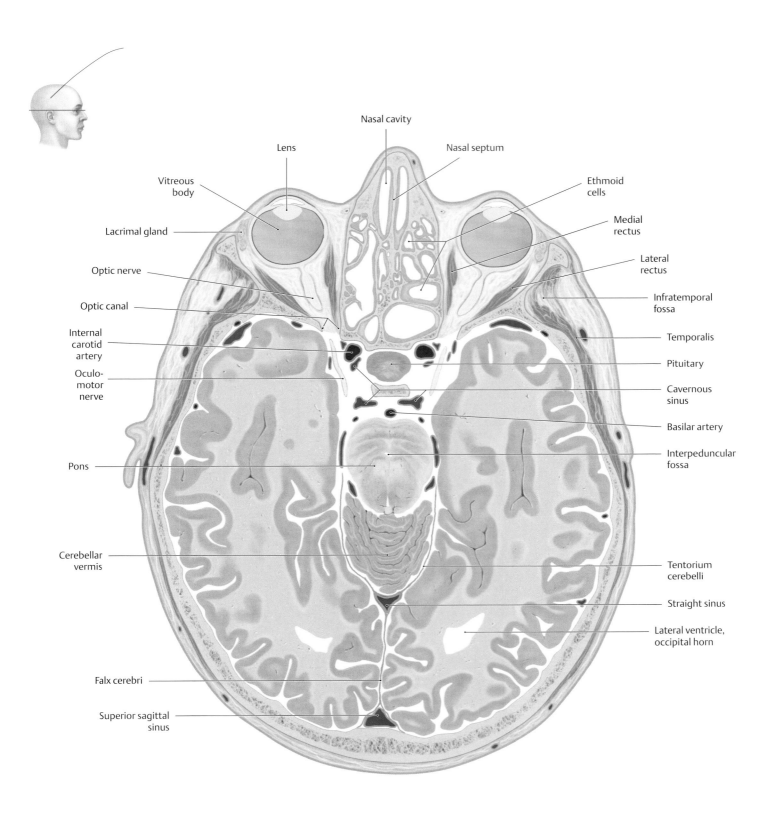

B Transverse section through the optic nerve and pituitary
Superior view. The optic nerve is seen just before its entry into the optic canal, indicating that the plane of section passes through the middle level of the orbit. Because the nerve completely fills the canal, growth disturbances of the bone at this level may cause pressure injury to the nerve. This plane cuts the ocular lenses and the cells of the ethmoid laby-rinth. The internal carotid artery can be identified in the middle cranial fossa, embedded in the cavernous sinus. The section cuts the oculomotor nerve on either side, which courses in the lateral wall of the cavernous sinus. The pons and cerebellar vermis are also seen. The falx cerebri and tentorium cerebelli appear as thin lines that come together at the straight sinus.

161

10.4 Transverse Sections, Sphenoid Sinus and Middle Nasal Concha

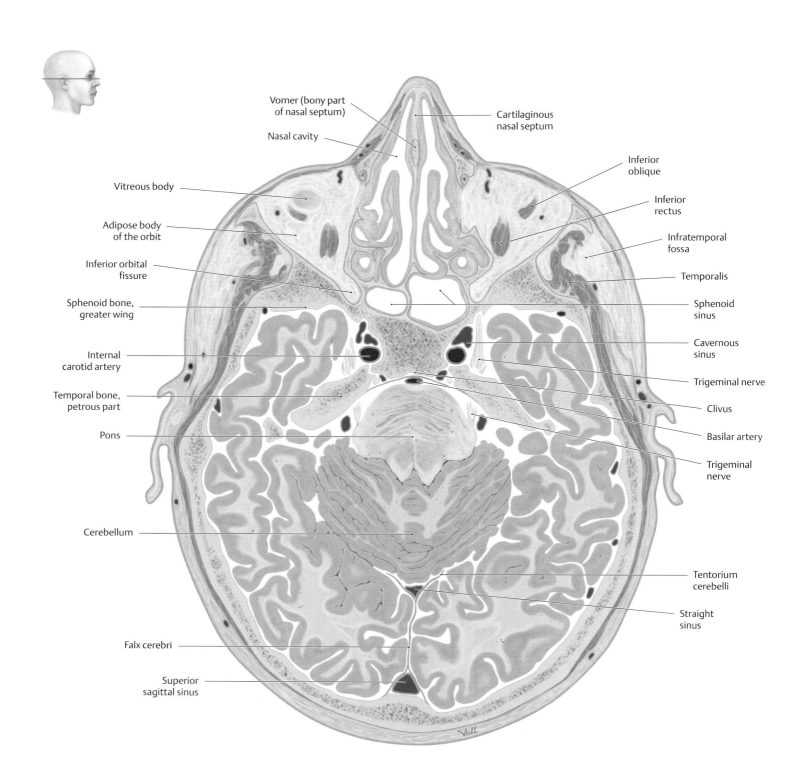

Vomer (bony part of nasal septum)
Cartilaginous nasal septum
Nasal cavity
Inferior oblique
Vitreous body
Inferior rectus
Adipose body of the orbit
Infratemporal fossa
Inferior orbital fissure
Temporalis
Sphenoid bone, greater wing
Sphenoid sinus
Internal carotid artery
Cavernous sinus
Temporal bone, petrous part
Trigeminal nerve
Pons
Clivus
Basilar artery
Trigeminal nerve
Cerebellum
Tentorium cerebelli
Straight sinus
Falx cerebri
Superior sagittal sinus

A Transverse section through the sphenoid sinus
Superior view. This section cuts the infratemporal fossa on the lateral aspect of the skull and the temporalis muscle that lies within it. The plane passes through the lower level of the orbit, and a small portion of the eyeball is visible on the left side. The orbit is continuous posteriorly with the inferior orbital fissure. This section displays the anterior extension of the two greater wings of the sphenoid bone and the posterior extension of the two "petrous bones" (petrous parts of the temporal bones), which mark the boundary between the middle and posterior cranial fossae (see p. 12 f). The clivus is part of the posterior cranial fossa and lies in contact with the basilar artery. The pontine origin of the trigeminal nerve and its intracranial course are clearly demonstrated.

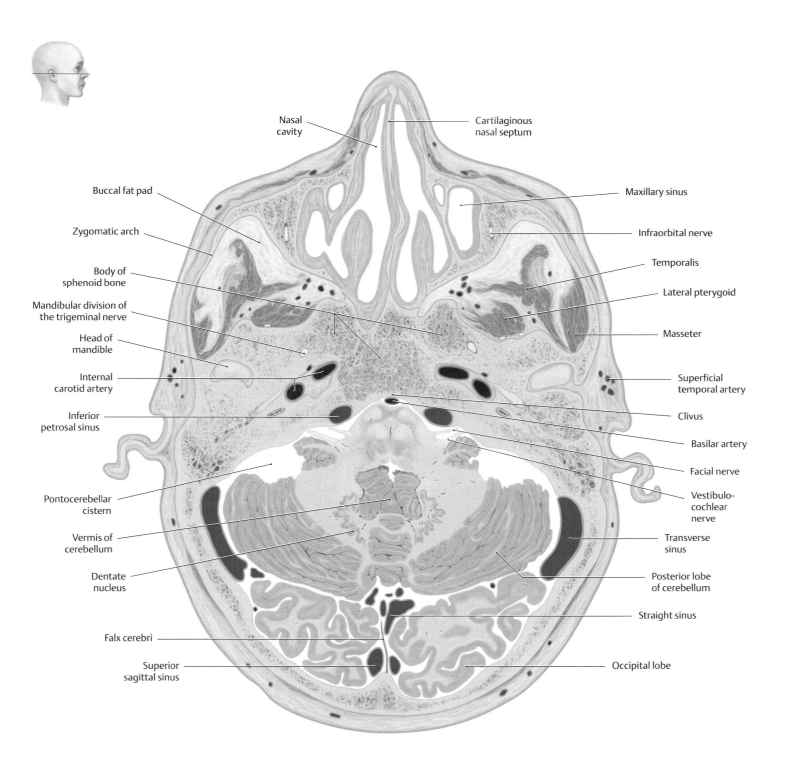

Nasal cavity

Cartilaginous nasal septum

Buccal fat pad

Maxillary sinus

Zygomatic arch

Infraorbital nerve

Body of sphenoid bone

Temporalis

Lateral pterygoid

Mandibular division of the trigeminal nerve

Masseter

Head of mandible

Internal carotid artery

Superficial temporal artery

Inferior petrosal sinus

Clivus

Basilar artery

Facial nerve

Vestibulo-cochlear nerve

Pontocerebellar cistern

Vermis of cerebellum

Transverse sinus

Dentate nucleus

Posterior lobe of cerebellum

Falx cerebri

Straight sinus

Superior sagittal sinus

Occipital lobe

B Transverse section through the middle nasal concha

Superior view. This section below the orbit passes through the infraorbital nerve in the accordingly named canal. Medial to the infraorbital nerve is the roof of the maxillary sinus. The zygomatic arch is visible in its entirety, and portions of the muscles of mastication medial to the zygomatic arch (masseter, temporalis, and lateral pterygoid) can be seen. The plane of section passes through the upper part of the head of the mandible. The mandibular division (CN V$_3$) appears in cross-section in its bony canal, the foramen ovale. It is evident that the body of the sphenoid bone forms the bony center of the base of the skull. The facial nerve and vestibulocochlear nerve emerge from the brainstem. The dentate nucleus lies within the white matter of the cerebellum. The space around the anterior part of the cerebellum, the pontocerebellar cistern, is filled with cerebrospinal fluid in the living individual. The transverse sinus is prominent among the dural sinuses of the brain.

10.5 Transverse Sections, Nasopharynx and Median Atlantoaxial Joint

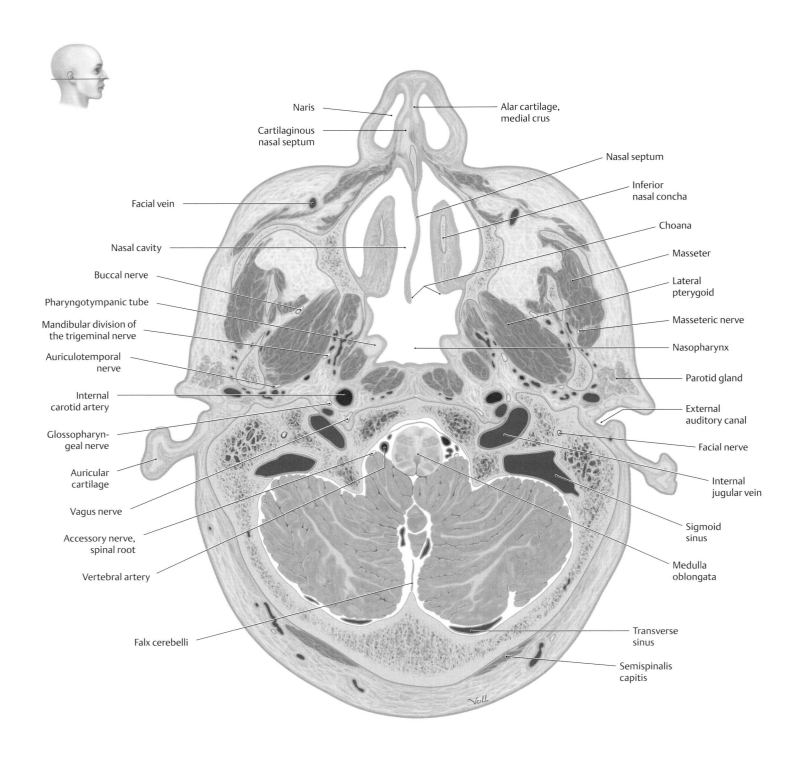

A Transverse section through the nasopharynx

Superior view. This section passes through the external nose and portions of the cartilaginous nasal skeleton. The nasal cavities communicate with the nasopharynx through the choanae. Cartilaginous portions of the pharyngotympanic tube project into the nasopharynx. The arterial blood vessels that supply the brain can also be seen: the internal carotid artery and vertebral artery.

Note the internal jugular vein and vagus nerve, which pass through the carotid sheath in company with the internal carotid artery.

A number of cranial nerves that emerge from the skull base are displayed in cross-section, such as the facial nerve coursing in the facial canal. This section also cuts the auricle and portions of the external auditory canal.

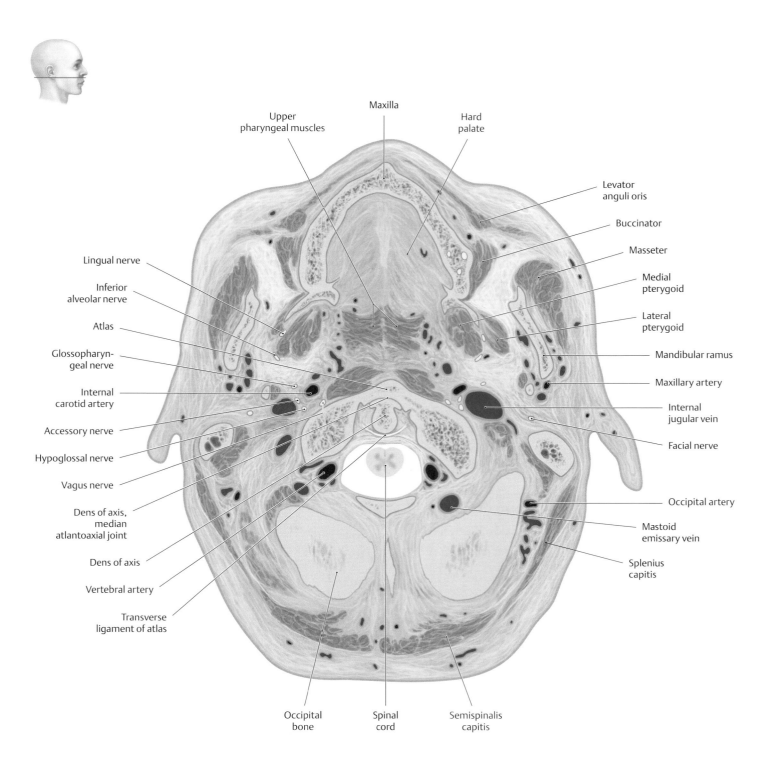

Maxilla

Upper pharyngeal muscles

Hard palate

Levator anguli oris

Buccinator

Masseter

Medial pterygoid

Lingual nerve

Lateral pterygoid

Inferior alveolar nerve

Mandibular ramus

Atlas

Maxillary artery

Glossopharyn- geal nerve

Internal carotid artery

Internal jugular vein

Accessory nerve

Facial nerve

Hypoglossal nerve

Vagus nerve

Occipital artery

Dens of axis, median atlantoaxial joint

Mastoid emissary vein

Dens of axis

Splenius capitis

Vertebral artery

Transverse ligament of atlas

Occipital bone

Spinal cord

Semispinalis capitis

B Transverse section through the median atlantoaxial joint
Superior view. The section at this level passes through the connective-tissue sheet that stretches over the bone of the hard palate. Portions of the upper pharyngeal muscles are sectioned close to their origin. The neurovascular structures in the carotid sheath are also well displayed. The dens of the axis articulates in the median atlantoaxial joint with the facet for the dens on the posterior surface of the anterior arch of the atlas. The transverse ligament of the atlas that helps to stabilize this joint can also be identified. The vertebral artery and its accompanying veins are displayed in cross-section, as is the spinal cord. In the occipital region, the section passes through the upper portion of the posterior neck muscles.

165

10.6 Midsagittal Section, Nasal Septum and Medial Orbital Wall

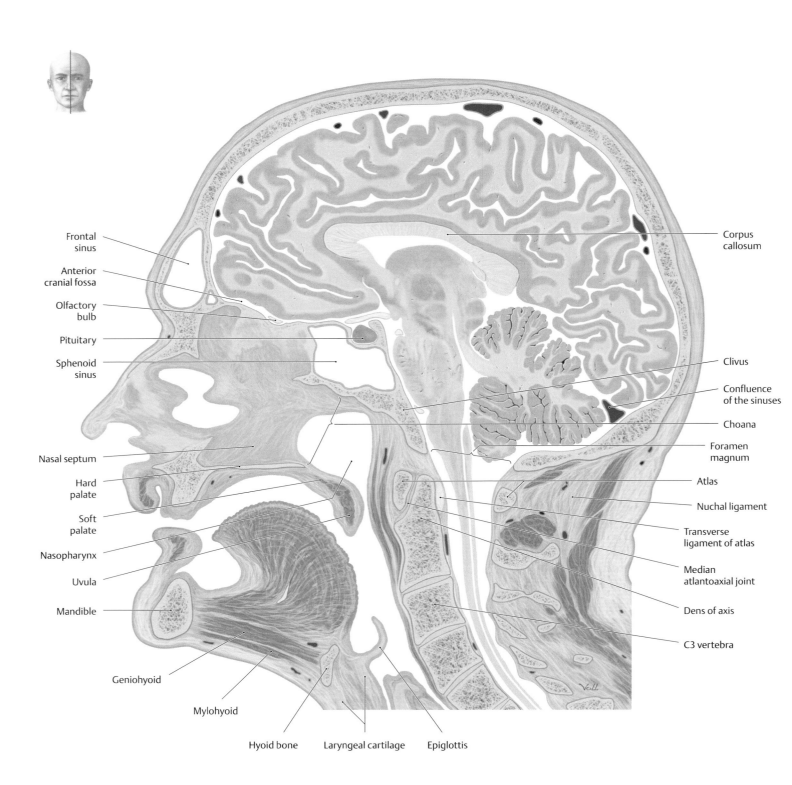

Frontal sinus

Anterior cranial fossa

Olfactory bulb

Pituitary

Sphenoid sinus

Nasal septum

Hard palate

Soft palate

Nasopharynx

Uvula

Mandible

Geniohyoid

Mylohyoid

Hyoid bone

Laryngeal cartilage

Epiglottis

Corpus callosum

Clivus

Confluence of the sinuses

Choana

Foramen magnum

Atlas

Nuchal ligament

Transverse ligament of atlas

Median atlantoaxial joint

Dens of axis

C3 vertebra

A Midsagittal section through the nasal septum

Left lateral view. The midline structures are particularly well displayed in this plane of section, and the anatomical structures at this level can be roughly assigned to the **facial skeleton** or neurocranium (cranial vault). The lowest level of the facial skeleton is formed by the oral floor muscles between the hyoid bone and mandible and the overlying skin. This section also passes through the epiglottis and the larynx below it, which are considered part of the cervical viscera. The hard and soft palate with the uvula define the boundary between the oral and nasal cavities. Posterior to the uvula is the oropharynx. The section includes the nasal septum, which divides the nasal cavity into two cavities (sectioned above and in front of the septum) that communicate with the nasopharynx through the choanae. Posterior to the frontal sinus is the anterior cranial fossa, which is part of the **neurocranium**. This section passes through the medial surface of the brain (the falx cerebri has been removed). The cut edge of the corpus callosum, the olfactory bulb, and the pituitary are also shown.

Note the median atlantoaxial joint (whose stability must be evalvuated after trauma to the cervical spine).

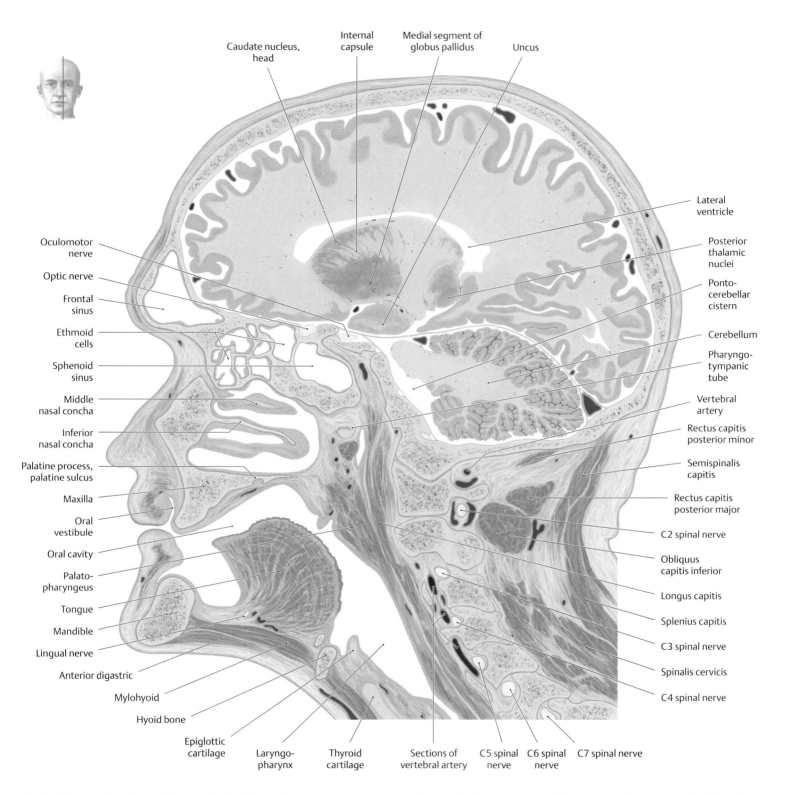

Caudate nucleus, head

Internal capsule

Medial segment of globus pallidus

Uncus

Lateral ventricle

Oculomotor nerve

Optic nerve

Frontal sinus

Ethmoid cells

Sphenoid sinus

Middle nasal concha

Inferior nasal concha

Palatine process, palatine sulcus

Maxilla

Oral vestibule

Oral cavity

Palato-pharyngeus

Tongue

Mandible

Lingual nerve

Anterior digastric

Mylohyoid

Hyoid bone

Epiglottic cartilage

Laryngo-pharynx

Thyroid cartilage

Sections of vertebral artery

C5 spinal nerve

C6 spinal nerve

C7 spinal nerve

Posterior thalamic nuclei

Ponto-cerebellar cistern

Cerebellum

Pharyngo-tympanic tube

Vertebral artery

Rectus capitis posterior minor

Semispinalis capitis

Rectus capitis posterior major

C2 spinal nerve

Obliquus capitis inferior

Longus capitis

Splenius capitis

C3 spinal nerve

Spinalis cervicis

C4 spinal nerve

B Sagittal section through the medial orbital wall
Left lateral view. This section passes through the inferior and middle nasal conchae within the nasal cavity. Above the middle nasal concha are the ethmoid cells. The only parts of the nasopharynx visible in this section are a small luminal area and the lateral wall, which bears a section of the cartilaginous portion of the pharyngothympanic tube. The sphenoid sinus is also displayed. In the region of the cervical spine, the section cuts the vertebral artery at multiple levels. The lateral sites where the spinal nerves emerge from the intervertebral foramina are clearly displayed.

10.7 Sagittal Sections, Inner Third and Center of the Orbit

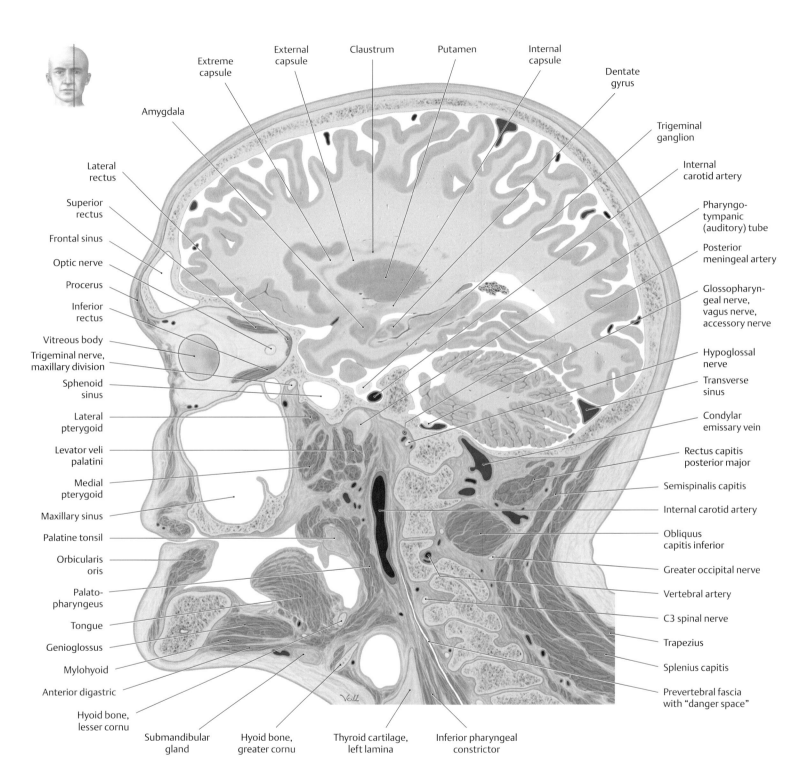

A Sagittal section through the inner third of the orbit
Left lateral view. This section passes through the maxillary and frontal sinuses while displaying one ethmoid cell and the peripheral part of the sphenoid sinus. It passes through the medial portion of the internal carotid artery and submandibular gland. The pharyngeal and masticatory muscles are grouped about the cartilaginous part of the pharyngotym-panic tube. The eyeball and optic nerve are cut peripherally by the section, which displays relatively long segments of the superior and inferior rectus muscles. Sectioned brain structures include the external and internal capsules and the intervening putamen. The amygdala and hippocampus can be identified near the base of the brain. A section of the trigeminal ganglion appears below the cerebrum.

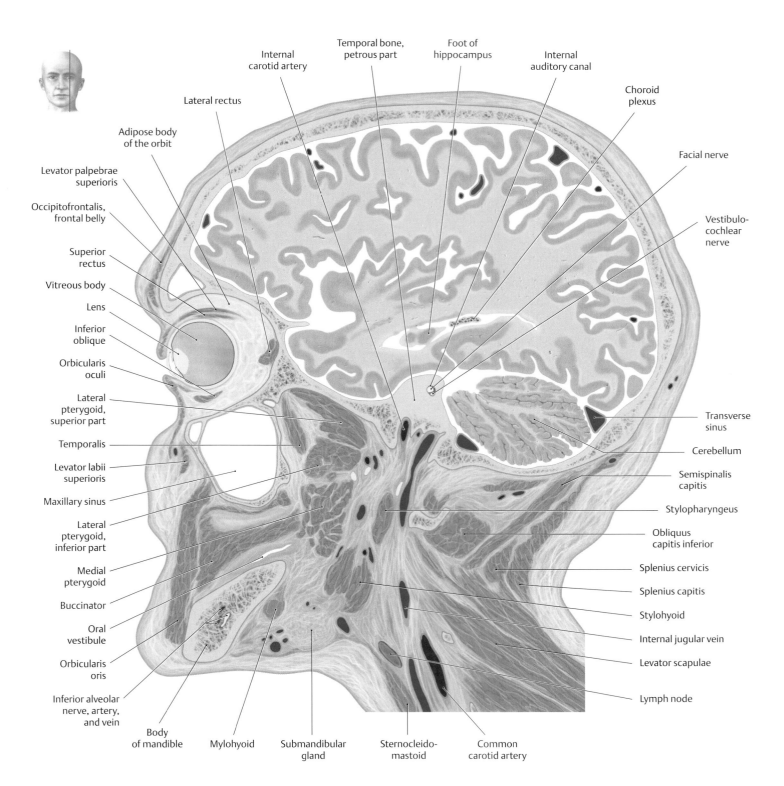

Temporal bone,
petrous part

Internal
carotid artery

Foot of
hippocampus

Internal
auditory canal

Lateral rectus

Choroid
plexus

Adipose body
of the orbit

Facial nerve

Levator palpebrae
superioris

Vestibulo-
cochlear
nerve

Occipitofrontalis,
frontal belly

Superior
rectus

Vitreous body

Lens

Inferior
oblique

Orbicularis
oculi

Lateral
pterygoid,
superior part

Transverse
sinus

Temporalis

Cerebellum

Levator labii
superioris

Semispinalis
capitis

Maxillary sinus

Stylopharyngeus

Lateral
pterygoid,
inferior part

Obliquus
capitis inferior

Medial
pterygoid

Splenius cervicis

Buccinator

Splenius capitis

Oral
vestibule

Stylohyoid

Orbicularis
oris

Internal jugular vein

Levator scapulae

Inferior alveolar
nerve, artery,
and vein

Lymph node

Body
of mandible

Mylohyoid

Submandibular
gland

Sternocleido-
mastoid

Common
carotid artery

B Sagittal section through the approximate center of the orbit
Left lateral view. Due to the obliquity of this section, the dominant
structure in the oral floor region is the mandible while the oral vestibule
appears as a narrow slit. The buccal and masticatory muscles are prominently displayed in this plane. Much of the orbit is occupied by the eyeball, which appears in longitudinal section. Aside from a few sections of

the extraocular muscles, the orbit in this plane is filled with fatty tissue.
Both the internal carotid artery and the internal jugular vein are demonstrated. Except for the foot of the hippocampus, the only visible cerebral
structures are the white matter and cortex. The facial nerve and vestibulocochlear nerve can be identified in the internal auditory canal.

169

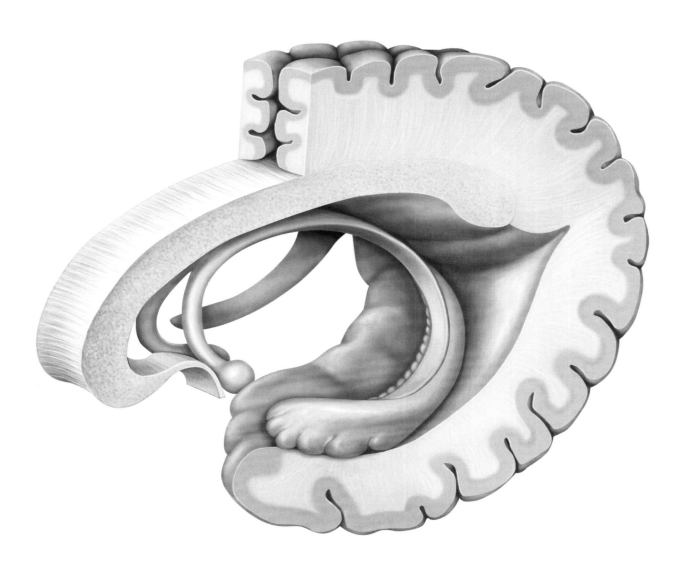

Neuroanatomy

1.1 Central Nervous System (CNS)

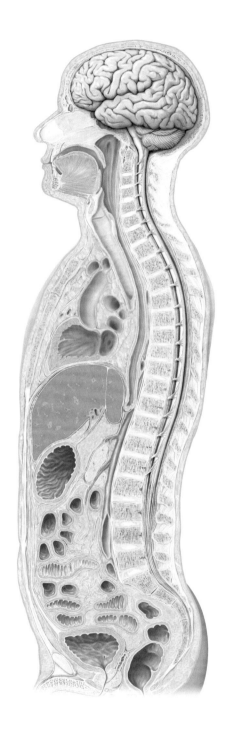

a

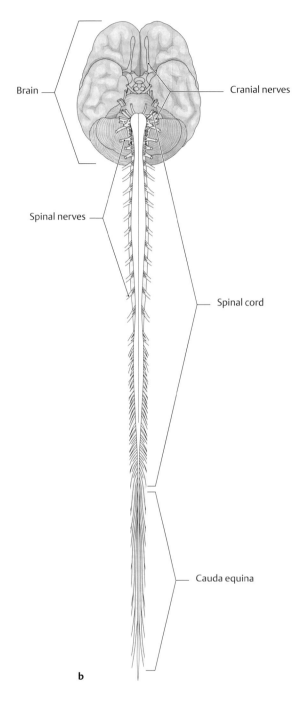

b

A Central nervous system, in situ and in isolation

a Central nervous system in situ, left lateral view. **b** Isolated central nervous system, anterior view.

The nervous system is concerned with the perception of processes that take place inside (enteroception) or outside the body (exteroception) and with internal and external communication. Given the diversity of these interrelated tasks, the body is endowed with a complex nervous system that can be subdivided in various ways. One basic principle of classification is to divide the nervous system morphologically into a peripheral nervous system (PNS) and a central nervous system (CNS). The central nervous system consists of the brain and spinal cord, which are seamlessly interconnected and comprise a functional unit. The *peripheral nervous system* is formed by the nerves that emerge from the brain and spinal cord (cranial nerves and spinal nerves) and ramify in the pe-

riphery of the body. Macroscopically, the brain and spinal cord consist of gray matter and white matter (see **B**). The surface of the brain is gray because of the presence of nerve cell bodies. The surface of the spinal cord is white because of the presence of nerve cell processes (axons) and their insulating myelin sheaths (= axons, see **C**). The CNS communicates with the rest of the body through the cranial nerves and spinal nerves, whose sites of emergence are shown in **b**. To shield the CNS from external injury, the brain and spinal cord are encased by bone (cranial bones and vertebrae). Situated between the bones and CNS are the coverings (meninges) of the brain and spinal cord, which are the first structures encountered when the overlying bone is removed. Having already described the bony anatomy in an earlier chapter, we now proceed to a description of the brain and spinal cord.

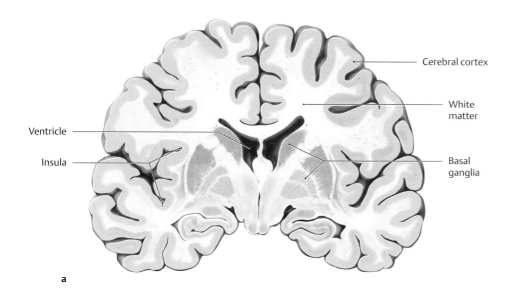
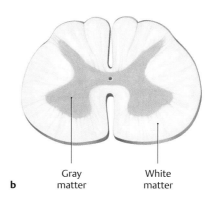

a

b

Cerebral cortex

White matter

Ventricle

Insula

Basal ganglia

Gray matter

White matter

B Distribution of gray and white matter in the CNS
a Coronal section through the cerebrum (telencephalon, see p. 198 ff).
b Cross-section through the spinal cord.
Even on gross inspection, sections of the brain and spinal cord differ markedly in their appearance due to differences in the distribution of gray and white matter. In the **cerebrum** (**a**), most of the *gray matter* is concentrated superficially in the cerebral cortex. The cerebrum also contains more deeply situated islands of gray matter (e.g., the basal

ganglia) in addition to other gray-matter structures that are not specifically addressed in this overview. The *white matter* of the cerebrum lies directly beneath the cortex and also surrounds more deeply placed groups of gray matter. Section **a** additionally shows part of the internal cavity system of the brain, the ventricles (see p. 192 ff). The gray/white matter arrangement is reversed in the **spinal cord** (**b**), in which the gray matter is placed centrally, forming a butterfly-shaped figure, while the white matter is external to it.

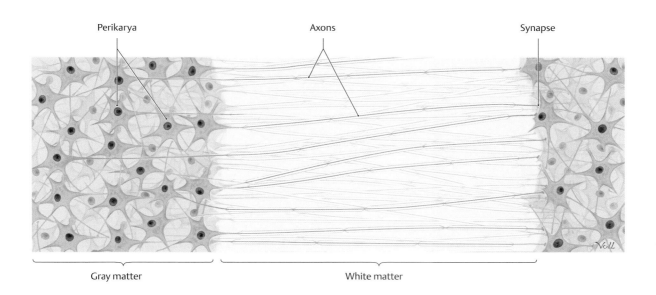

Perikarya

Axons

Synapse

Gray matter

White matter

C Histological appearance of the gray and white matter
The *gray* matter is made up of the cell bodies (*perikarya* or *somata*) of neurons, which are interconnected to form neuronal networks (neuron histology is described on p. 174 ff). The *white* matter, on the other hand, contains the processes (*axons*) of neurons that interconnect different areas of the brain and spinal cord. It derives its white color from the lipid content of the myelin sheaths. Many axons running in the same direction are collected to form fiber pathways or *tracts*. Because the processing of neural information begins in the perikaryon (soma) and ends at the synapse of the axon, these tracts are often named for their sites of origin and termination, e.g. the *corticospinal tract*. The perikarya of this

tract are located in the cerebral cortex, and its axons terminate in the spinal cord. This flow of information is also described macroscopically as a "projection," i.e., the corticospinal tract *projects* from the cortex to the spinal cord. The brain does not function as a "hard-wired computer," however. Learning processes like those that occur during puberty can alter the patterns of impulse transmission within the brain. An example is the physical awkwardness that is common during puberty, such as overturning a water glass at the dinner table. As the individual matures, these accidents become less frequent. Some time is needed for position sense to adapt to changes in body size and proportions.

173

1.2 Neurons

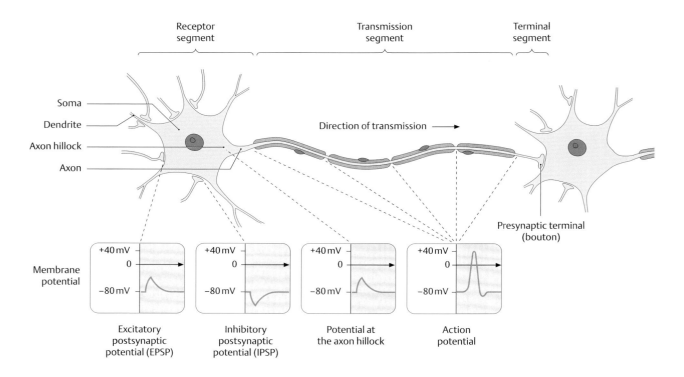

A The neuron (nerve cell)

The neuron is the smallest functional unit of the nervous system. It consists of a cell body, called the soma or perikaryon, from which two fundamentally different types of processes arise:

- Dendrites: Dendrites are called the *receptor segment* of the neuron because they conduct impulses to the cell body that they have received at synapses with other neurons. One neuron may have multiple dendrites, which may undergo very complex arborization to increase their surface area (see **C**). Dendrites, unlike axons, are not insulated by a myelin sheath.

- Axons or nerve fibers: The axon is the *projecting segment* of the neuron because it relays impulses to other neurons or other cells (e.g., skeletal muscle cells). Each neuron has only one axon. Axons in the CNS are generally covered by a myelin sheath (the axons plus their

myelin sheaths constitute the white matter). The myelin sheath may be absent in the peripheral nervous system (see details in **C**, p. 177).

Either excitatory or inhibitory neurotransmitters are released at synapses. These substances produce either an excitatory or inhibitory postsynaptic potential at the target neuron. In this way the transmitters released at synapses modulate the potential in the perikaryon of the neuron. The excitatory and inhibitory impulses are integrated in the axon hillock. When the potential exceeds the depolarization threshold of the neuron, the axon "fires," i.e., the hillock initiates an action potential that travels along the axon and triggers the release of a transmitter from its presynaptic knob (bouton). Although this simple characterization applies to most neurons, connections in the CNS can be much more complex than described here (see **C**, **D**, and **E**).

B Electron microscopy of the neuron

The organelles of neurons can be resolved with an electron microscope. Neurons are rich in rough endoplasmic reticulum (protein synthesis, active metabolism). This endoplasmic reticulum (called *Nissl substance* under a light microscope) is easily demonstrated by light microscopy when it is stained with cationic dyes (which bind to the anionic mRNA and nRNA of the ribosomes). The distribution pattern of the Nissl substance is used in neuropathology to evaluate the functional integrity of neurons. The neurotubules and neurofilaments that are visible by electron microscopy are referred to collectively in *light microscopy* as neurofibrils, as they are too fine to be resolved as separate structures under the light microscope. Neurofibrils can be demonstrated in light microscopy by impregnating the nerve tissue with silver salts. This is important in neuropathology, for example, because the clumping of neurofibrils is an important histological feature of Alzheimer's disease.

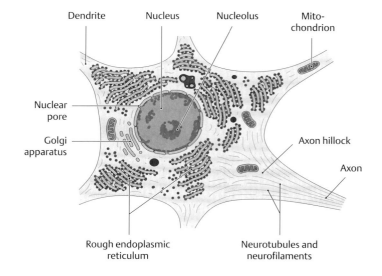

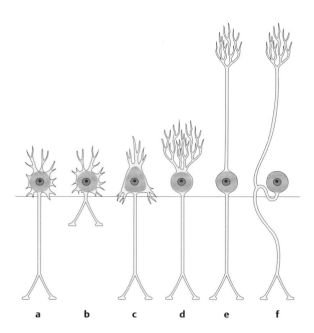

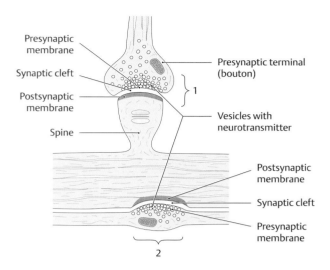

C Basic forms of the neuron and its functionally adapted variants

The horizontal line marks the region of the axon hillock, which represents the initial segment of the axon. (The structure of a peripheral nerve, which consists only of axons and sheath tissue, is shown on p. 180.)

a Multipolar neuron (multiple dendrites) with a long axon (= long transmission path). Examples are projection neurons such as alpha motor neurons in the spinal cord.

b Multipolar neuron with a short axon (= short transmission path). Examples are interneurons like those in the gray matter of the brain and spinal cord.

c Pyramidal cell: Dendrites are present only at the apex and base of the triangular cell body, and the axon is long. Examples are efferent neurons of the cerebral motor cortex (see pp. 180 and 200).

d Purkinje cell: An elaborately branched dendritic tree arises from one circumscribed site on the cell body. The Purkinje cell of the cerebellum has many synaptic contacts with other neurons (see p. 241).

e Bipolar neuron: The dendrite arborizes in the periphery. The bipolar cells of the retina are an example (see **C**, p. 131).

f Pseudounipolar neuron: The dendrite and axon are not separated by the cell body. An example is the primary afferent (sensory) neuron in the spinal (dorsal root) ganglion (see pp. 180, 272, and 274ff).

D Electron microscopic appearance of the two most common types of synapse in the CNS

Synapses are the functional connection between two neurons. They consist of a presynaptic membrane, a synaptic cleft, and a postsynaptic membrane. In a "spine synapse" (1), the presynaptic terminal (bouton) is in contact with a specialized protuberance (spine) of the target neuron. The side-by-side synapse of an axon with the flat surface of a target neuron is called a parallel contact or *bouton en passage* (2). The vesicles in the presynaptic expansions contain the neurotransmitters that are released into the synaptic cleft by exocytosis when the axon fires. From there the neurotransmitters diffuse to the postsynaptic membrane, where their receptors are located. A variety of drugs and toxins act upon synaptic transmission (antidepressants, muscle relaxants, nerve gases, botulinum toxin).

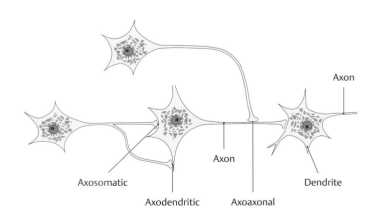

E Synaptic patterns in a small group of neurons

Axons may terminate at various sites on the target neuron and form synapses there. The synaptic patterns are described as axodendritic, axosomatic, or axoaxonal. Axodendritic synapses are the most common (see also **A**). The cerebral cortex consists of many small groups of neurons that are collected into functional units called columns (see p. 201 for details).

175

1.3 Neuroglia and Myelination

A Cells of the neuroglia in the CNS

Neuroglial cells surround the neurons, providing them with structural and functional support (see **D**). Various staining methods are used in light microscopy for more or less selectively defining specific portions of the neuroglial cells:

a Cell nuclei demonstrated with a basic stain.
b Cell body demonstrated by silver impregnation.

Neuroglial cells constitute the vast majority of cells in the CNS, outnumbering the neurons by approximately 10-to-1 (1 trillion neuroglial cells to 100 billion neurons by recent estimates). The neuroglia have an essential role in supporting the function of the neurons. For example, astrocytes absorb excess neurotransmitters from the extracellular milieu, helping to maintain a constant internal environment. While neurons are, almost without exception, permanently post-mitotic some neuroglial cells continue to divide throughout life. For this reason, most primary brain tumors originate from neuroglial cells and are named for their morphological similarity to normal neuroglial cells: astrocytoma, oligodendroglioma, and glioblastoma. Developmentally, most neuroglial cells arise from the same progenitor cells as neurons. This may not apply to microglial cells, which develop from precursor cells in the blood from the monocyte lineage.

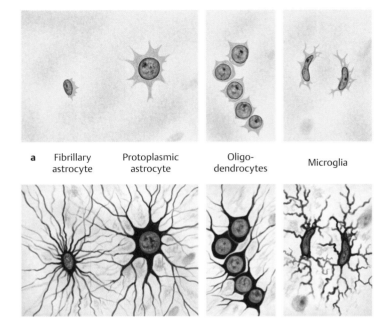

a Fibrillary astrocyte   Protoplasmic astrocyte   Oligodendrocytes   Microglia

b

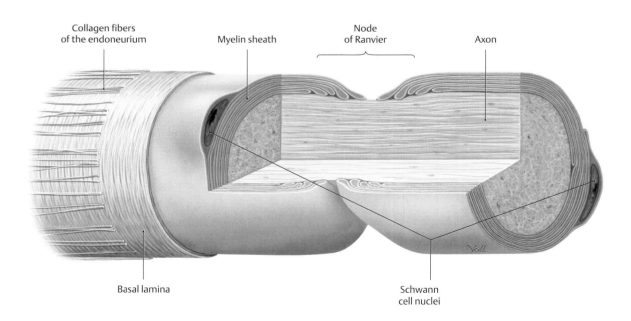

Collagen fibers of the endoneurium   Myelin sheath   Node of Ranvier   Axon

Basal lamina   Schwann cell nuclei

B Myelinated axon in the PNS

Most axons in the peripheral nervous system are insulated by a myelin sheath, although unmyelinated axons are also found in the PNS (see **C**).

The myelin sheath enables impulses to travel faster along the axon as they "jump" from one node of Ranvier to the next (saltatory nerve conduction), rather than travel continuously as in an unmyelinated axon.

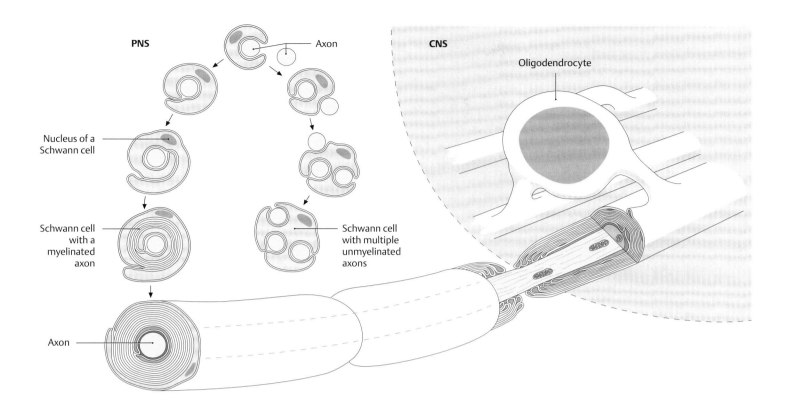

PNS

Axon

CNS

Oligodendrocyte

Nucleus of a
Schwann cell

Schwann cell
with a
myelinated
axon

Schwann cell
with multiple
unmyelinated
axons

Axon

C Myelination differences in the PNS and CNS

The purpose of myelination is to insulate the axons electrically. This significantly boosts the nerve conduction velocity as a result of saltatory conduction. While almost all axons in the CNS are myelinated, this is not the case in the PNS. The axons of the PNS are myelinated in regions where fast reaction speeds are needed (e.g., skeletal muscle contraction) and unmyelinated in regions that do not require rapid information transfer (e.g., the transmission of muscle spindle and tendon tension sensation). The very lipid-rich membranes of myelinating cells are wrapped around the axons to insulate them. There are differences between the myelinating cells of the central and peripheral nervous systems. Schwann cells (left) myelinate the axons in the PNS, whereas oligodendrocytes (right) form the myelin sheaths in the CNS.

Note: In the CNS, one oligodendrocyte always wraps around multiple axons; however, Schwann cells ensheath either one myelinated axon or multiple unmyelinated axons.

This difference in myelination has important clinical implications. In multiple sclerosis, the oligodendrocytes are damaged but the Schwann cells are not. As a result, the peripheral myelin sheaths remain intact in MS while the central myelin sheaths degenerate.

D Summary: Cells of the central nervous system (CNS) and peripheral nervous system (PNS) and their functional importance

Cell type	Function
Neurons (CNS and PNS) (see p. 179)	1. Impulse formation 2. Impulse conduction 3. Information processing
Glial cells	
Astrocytes (CNS only) (also called *macroglia*)	1. Maintain a constant internal milieu in the CNS 2. Help to form the blood brain–barrier 3. Phagocytosis of nonfunctioning synapses 4. Scar formation in the CNS (e.g., after cerebral infarction or in multiple sclerosis) 5. Absorb excess neurotransmitters and K+
Microglial cells (CNS only)	Cells specialized for phagocytosis and antigen processing (brain macrophages, part of the mononuclear phagocyte system); secrete cytokines and growth factors
Oligodendrocytes (CNS only)	Form the myelin sheaths in the CNS
Ependymal cells (CNS only)	Line cavities in the CNS
Cells of the choroid plexus (CNS only)	Secrete cerebrospinal fluid
Schwann cells (PNS only)	Form the myelin sheaths in the PNS
Satellite cells (PNS only) (also called *mantle cells*)	Modified Schwann cells; surround the cell body of neurons in PNS ganglia

1.4   Sensory Input, Perception and Qualities

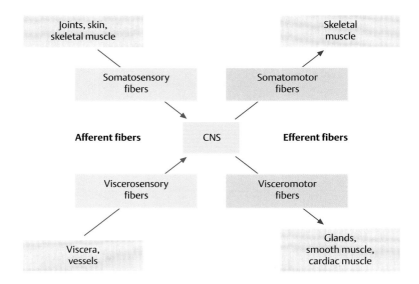

A Schematic diagram of information flow in the nervous system

We began this chapter (p. 172) by dividing the nervous system into the CNS and PNS. The nervous system can also be divided based the direction of information flow. Nerves that transmit impulses toward the brain or spinal cord are called *afferent* fibers (left), and nerves that transmit impulses away from the brain or spinal cord are called *efferent* fibers (right). The terms afferent and efferent are also used within the CNS to describe the connections between nuclei. The structure of the neuron is important in this scheme, because the dendritic tree and its processes are afferent while axons and their synapses are efferent. Another possible classification scheme shown here is to divide the nervous system into a somatic and autonomic (visceral, vegetative) nervous system (upper and lower parts of the diagram, respectively). The somatic nervous system is responsible for communication between the organism and its environment, and it coordinates locomotion. The autonomic (visceral) nervous system coordinates the function of the internal organs. Using the scheme pictured here, we can subdivide axons, as well as nerves and fiber tracts, into four different modalities: somatic afferent, somatic efferent, visceral afferent, and visceral efferent. Further subdivisions of the afferent and efferent fibers (e.g., special visceral afferent or secretomotor fibers) are omitted here in the interest of clarity.

B Special sensory qualities

The ability of the nervous and sensory system to perceive a great variety of stimuli is called *sensation*. This communication with the environment is mediated by specialized perceptual organs that are located at anatomically defined sites. The special sensory qualities include taste, smell, vision, hearing, and the sense of balance. All of these sensory perceptions are transmitted to the CNS by cranial nerves.

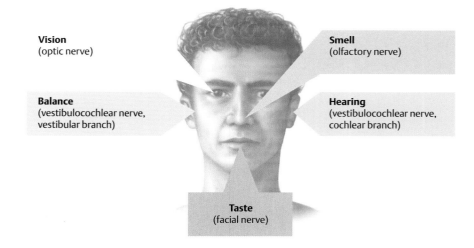

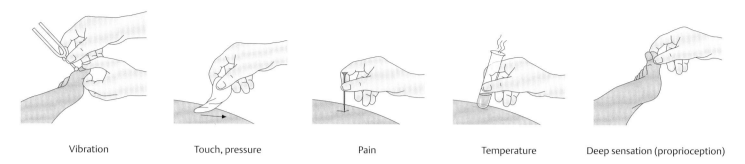

Vibration   Touch, pressure   Pain   Temperature   Deep sensation (proprioception)

C General sensory qualities

A basic distinction is drawn between *external perception (exteroception)* and *internal perception (proprioception)* depending on the source of the stimulus. Because the stimulus in exteroception comes from the external environment and is perceived by "exteroceptors" in the skin, this sense is also known as *superficial sensation*. In proprioception, the source of the stimulus lies "deep" within a muscle, tendon, or joint (information on the relative position of the body parts), and so this mode of perception is also called *deep sensation*. Moreover, two sensory qualities are distinguished in exteroception, which may both be perceived at the same location: (1) epicritic perception (light touch, vibration, two-point discrimination) and (2) protopathic perception (pain and temperature), which includes an emotional component (pain is distressing, for example). Exteroception, then, is largely a conscious mode of perception that is mediated by the gracile and cuneate fasciculi (epicritic) and the anterior and lateral spinalothalamic tracts (protopathic). Proprioception, on the other hand, is largely unconscious and is integrated chiefly by the cerebellum.

Testing superficial sensation:
- *Vibration sense:* tested with an alternately vibrating (64 or 128 Hz) and nonvibrating tuning fork, which may be placed on the shin, for example. The patient should be able to perceive the difference between the vibrating and nonvibrating states.
- *Pressure and touch sensation:* The skin is touched with a cotton swab.
- *Pain perception:* The skin is pricked with a sterile hypodermic needle. This test can also be used to test two-point discrimination.
- *Heat and cold sensation:* Test tubes containing warm or cold water are placed in contact with the skin.

Testing deep sensation (proprioception): With the patient's eyes closed, the examiner moves the distal phalanges of the toes, for example, and asks the patient to describe the position of the digits without looking at them.

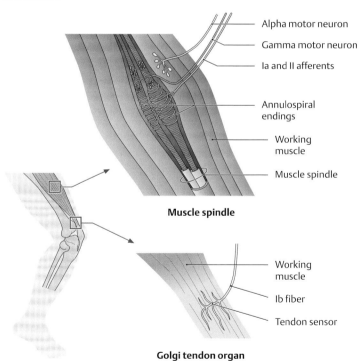

Alpha motor neuron
Gamma motor neuron
Ia and II afferents
Annulospiral endings
Working muscle
Muscle spindle

Muscle spindle

Working muscle
Ib fiber
Tendon sensor

Golgi tendon organ

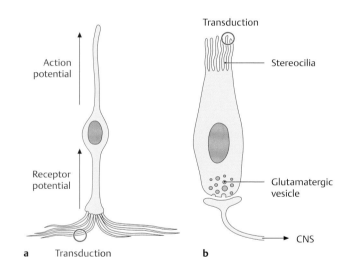

Action potential
Receptor potential
a Transduction

Transduction
Stereocilia
Glutamatergic vesicle
CNS
b

E Different types of sensory receptors

Proprioception as described above is mediated by specialized peripheral endings of primary sensory neurons whose cell bodies are in spinal (dorsal root) and cranial sensory ganglia. Other (exteroceptive) sensations involve receptor cells that are situated within special sense organs. These receptors can be neurons with axons that synapse onto secondary neurons (as in **a**, an olfactory receptor situated in the olfactory epithelium, which sends its axon into the olfactory bulb [CNS]). Other specialized receptor cells (**b**, vestibular hair cell) may have no axon, but instead participate in local synapses with neurons that, in turn, transmit the information to higher centers. The neurons that synapse with vestibular hair cells have cell bodies in the vestibular ganglion. The central processes of these ganglion cells travel in the vestibulocochlear nerve to the brainstem.

D Receptors in the muscles and tendons

The receptors in the muscles (muscle spindles), tendons (Golgi tendon organs), and joints (not shown) give the brain information about the position of joints, muscular force, and movements. This information is known collectively as *proprioception*. For example, we know when our hand is clenched into a fist even when it is behind our back. The brain receives additional information on the position of the head and limbs from the vestibular apparatus (sense of balance), the eyes, and mechanical sensors (mechanoreceptors) in the skin.

179

1.5 Peripheral and Central Nervous Systems

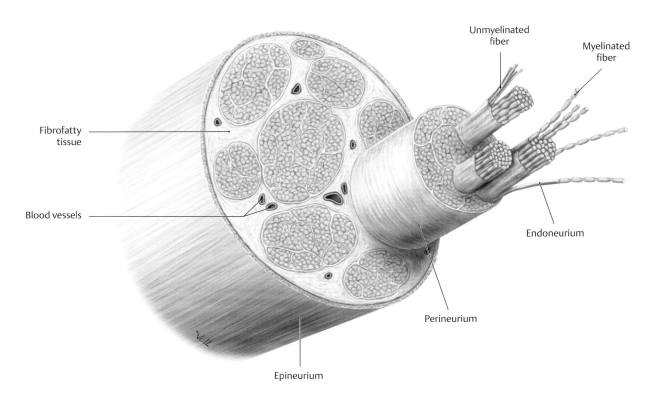

Unmyelinated fiber

Myelinated fiber

Fibrofatty tissue

Blood vessels

Endoneurium

Perineurium

Epineurium

A Peripheral nerve

Information travels in the PNS along nerves, which are the equivalent of tracts in the CNS. Like the tracts, the nerves consist of bundles of axons (neurites or nerve fibers). But whereas the axons in the CNS tracts are routed in an afferent or efferent direction (e.g., toward or away from the cortex), a typical peripheral nerve carries both afferent and efferent fibers and is therefore called a mixed nerve. Afferent and efferent fibers may be myelinated or unmyelinated (lacking a myelin sheath). It will be recalled that the peripheral nerves are myelinated by Schwann cells (see **C**, p. 177).

Note: The perikarya of neurons in the PNS are located in ganglia (see **B**).

B Ganglia

As noted above, the perikarya of neurons in the PNS are located in ganglia. Two main types of ganglion can be distinguished:

a **Spinal ganglia** are located at the dorsal root of spinal nerves and contain pseudounipolar neurons. These neurons convey *sensory information* from the periphery (e.g., pressure, temperature, pain) into the spinal cord, where the impulses are relayed to another neuron. The perikaryon has a T-shaped connection with the axon (see **C**, p. 175); thus, no synaptic relay in the spinal ganglion. Since the peripheral process receives sensory impulses, this neuron is called a *primary afferent neuron*. The sensory cranial-nerve ganglia also contain pseudounipolar neurons, which correspond functionally to the spinal ganglia.

b **Autonomic ganglia** are part of the autonomic nervous system. The efferent fibers to the (internal) organs are relayed in these ganglia (see p. 316).

Intramural ganglia in the intestinal wall (not shown) are part of the enteric nervous system (see p. 324).

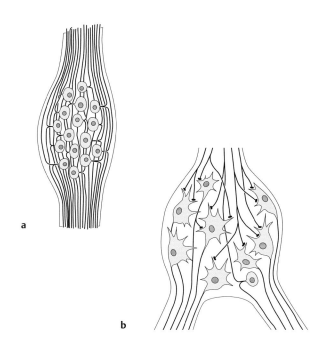

a

b

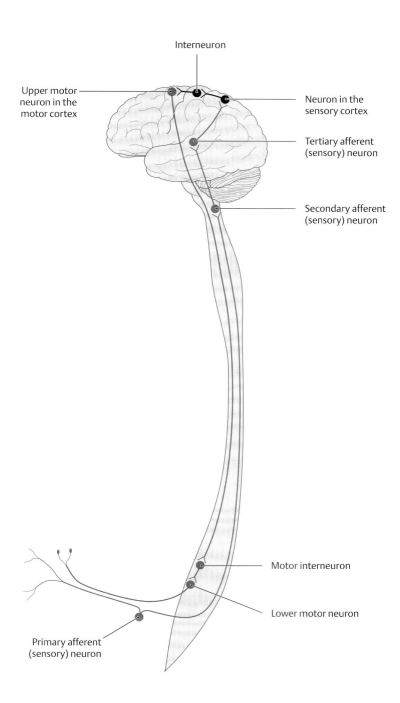

Interneuron

Upper motor neuron in the motor cortex

Neuron in the sensory cortex

Tertiary afferent (sensory) neuron

Secondary afferent (sensory) neuron

Motor interneuron

Lower motor neuron

Primary afferent (sensory) neuron

C Somatomotor integration

This greatly simplified circuit diagram shows how the sensory and motor systems work together during ordinary activities. An example: Placing the foot tentatively on the lower rung of a ladder to see if the ladder is stable initiates a flow of signals through a chain of neurons (the *sensory neurons* are shown in blue, the *motor neurons* in red). The sensation of the foot touching the rung is conveyed by the primary sensory neuron to the spinal cord. This neuron synapses with a secondary sensory neuron at the upper end of the spinal cord (dorsal column nuclei), which synapses with a third neuron in a specialized nucleus in the diencephalon. From there the information is relayed to the sensory cortex. Inter-

neurons in the brain then give rise to flow of impulses from the sensory cortex to the upper motor neuron in the motor cortex, which relays the motor command down to a motor interneuron. Finally this interneuron activates the lower motor neuron, which causes the muscle to contract and enables the individual to start climbing the ladder.

Note: Most diagrams omit the interneurons and show only the first and second motor neurons, which are called the "upper motor neuron" in the cortex and the "lower motor neuron" in the spinal cord. The distinction between these two neurons is very important clinically: A lesion of the upper motor neuron causes spastic paralysis, whereas a lesion of the lower motor neuron causes flaccid paralysis (see p. 343 for details).

1.6 Nervous System, Development

A Neural tube and neural crest (after Wolpert)

The tissues of the nervous system originate embryonically from the dorsal surface ectoderm. The notochord in the midline of the body induces the formation of the neural plate, which lies above the notochord, and of the neural crests, which are lateral to the notochord. With further development, the neural plate deepens at the center to form the neural groove, which is flanked on each side by the neural folds. Later the groove deepens and closes to form the neural tube, which sinks beneath the ectoderm. The *neural tube* is the structure from which the central nervous system (CNS)—the brain and spinal cord—develops (further development of the spinal cord is shown in **B**, further brain development in **D**). Failure of the neural groove to close completely will leave an anomalous cleft in the vertebral column, known as *spina bifida*. The administration of folic acid to potential mothers around the time of conception can reduce the incidence of spina bifida by 70 %. Cells that migrate from the *neural crest* develop into various structures, including cells of the peripheral nervous system (PNS) such as Schwann cells and the pseudounipolar cells of the spinal ganglion (see **C**).

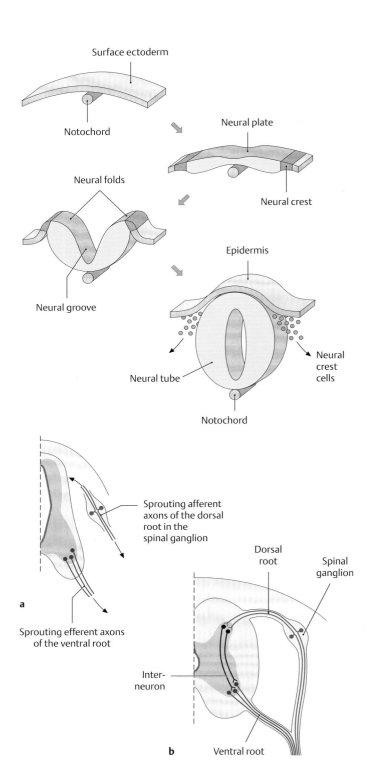

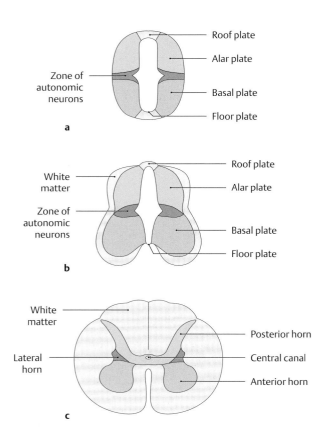

B Differentiation of the neural tube in the spinal cord during development

Cross-section, superior view.

a Early neural tube, **b** intermediate stage, **c** adult spinal cord.

The neurons that form in the basal plate are efferent (*motor neurons*), while the neurons that form in the alar plate are afferent (*sensory neurons*). In the future thoracic, lumbar, and sacral spinal cord, there is another zone between them that gives rise to sympathetic (autonomic) efferent neurons. The roof plate and floor plate do not form neurons.

C Development of a peripheral nerve

Afferent axons (blue) and efferent axons (red) sprout separately from the neuronal cell bodies during early embryonic development.

a Primary afferent neurons develop in the spinal ganglion, and alpha motor neurons develop from the basal plate of the spinal cord.

b The interneurons (black), which functionally interconnect the sensory and motor neurons, develop at a later stage.

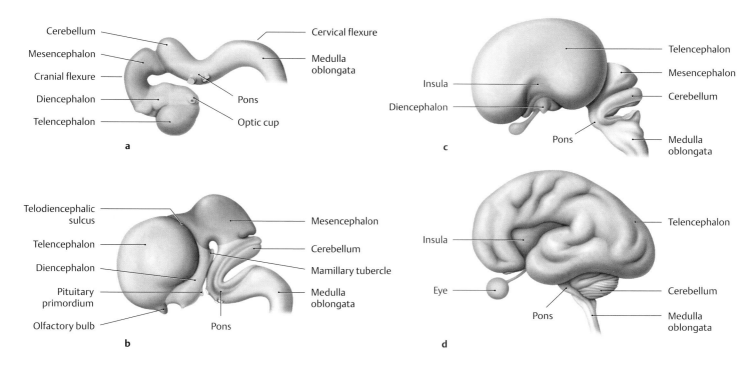

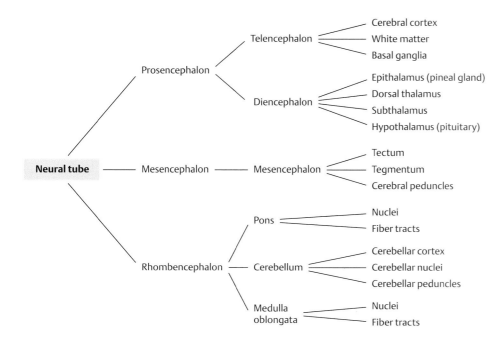

D Development of the brain

a Embryo with a greatest length (GL) of 10 mm at the beginning of the second month of development. Even at this stage we can see the differentation of the neural tube into segments that will generate various brain regions.

- Red: telencephalon (cerebrum)
- Yellow: diencephalon
- Dark blue: mesencephalon (midbrain)
- Light blue: cerebellum
- Gray: pons and medulla oblongata

Note: The telencephalon outgrows all the other brain structures as development proceeds.

b Embryo with a GL of 27 mm near the end of the second month of development (end of the embryonic period). The telencephalon and diencephalon have enlarged. The olfactory bulb is developing from the telencephalon, and the primordium of the pituitary gland is developing from the diencephalon.

c Fetus with a GL of 53 mm in approximately the third month of development. By this stage the telencephalon has begun to cover the other brain areas. The insula is still on the brain surface but will subsequently be covered by the hemispheres (compare with **d**).

d Fetus with a GL of 27 cm (270 mm) in approximately the seventh month of development. The cerebrum (telencephalon) has begun to develop well-defined gyri and sulci.

E Brain vesicles and their derivatives

The cranial end of the neural tube expands to form three primary brain vesicles for the

- forebrain (prosencephalon),
- midbrain (mesencephalon), and
- hindbrain (rhombencephalon).

The telencephalon and diencephalon develop from the prosencephalon. The mesencephalon gives rise to the superior and inferior colliculi and related structures. The rhombencephalon differentiates into the pons, cerebellum, and medulla oblongata. The pons and cerebellum are also known collectively as the *metencephalon*. Some important structures of the adult brain are listed in the diagram at left to illustrate the derivates of the brain vesicles. They can be traced back in the diagram to their developmental precursors..

1.7 Brain, Macroscopic Organization

A Left lateral view of the brain

The cerebrum is divided macroscopically into four lobes:

- Frontal lobe
- Parietal lobe
- Temporal lobe
- Occipital lobe

The surface contours of the cerebrum are defined by convolutions (gyri) and depressions (sulci). An example is the central sulcus, which separates the precentral gyrus from the postcentral gyrus. These two gyri are functionally important because the *precentral gyrus* is concerned with voluntary motor activity while the *postcentral gyrus* is concerned with the conscious perception of body sensation. Deep within the lateral sulcus is the *insular lobe*, often called simply the insula (see **B**, p. 173). The sulci are narrowed and compressed in *brain edema* (excessive fluid accumulation in the brain), but they are enlarged in *brain atrophy* (e.g., Alzheimer's disease) because of tissue loss from the gyri. The brains that are available for dissection in medical school courses frequently manifest signs of brain atrophy. Often the atrophy is predominantly frontal in males and predominantly occipital in females, but the reason for this disparity is unknown.

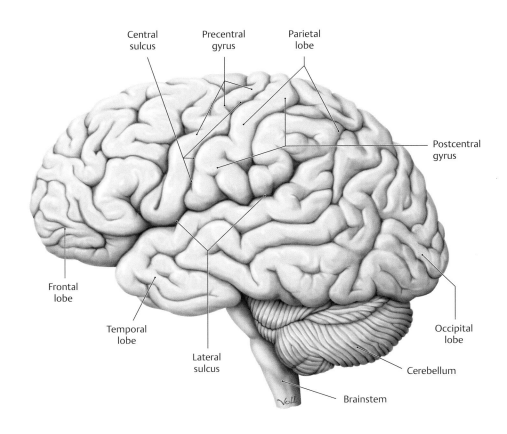

B Basal view of the brain

The spinal cord has been sectioned in its upper cervical portion. This view demonstrates the sites of emergence of most of the cranial nerves (yellow) from the brainstem (see p. 66 ff). The frontal lobes, temporal lobes, pons, medulla oblongata, and cerebellum are the principal structures that can be identified on the base of the brain. This view clearly displays the two hemispheres and the *longitudinal cerebral fissure* between them. The gyri vary considerably in different individuals, and even the convolutions of a single brain may show marked side-to-side differences, presumably due to the specialization of the hemispheres.

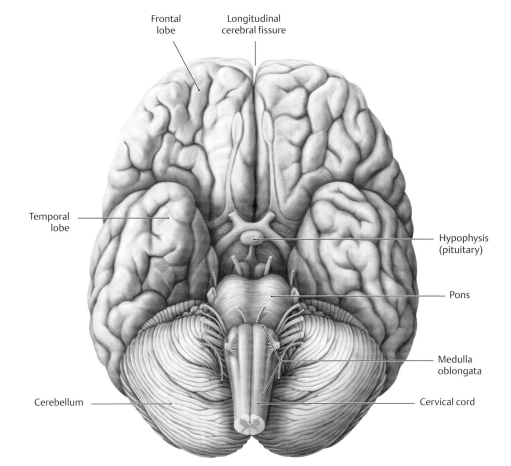

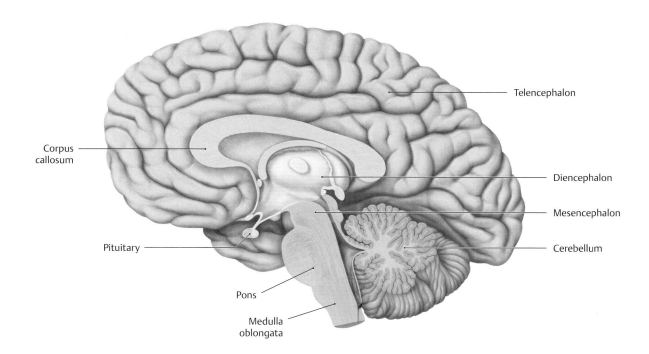

Corpus callosum

Pituitary

Pons

Medulla oblongata

Telencephalon

Diencephalon

Mesencephalon

Cerebellum

C Midsagittal section of the brain showing the medial surface of the right hemisphere

The brain has been split along the longitudinal cerebral fissure. Developmentally, the brain can be divided into several major parts (see p. 183), all of which are visible in this section:

- Telencephalon (cerebrum)
- Diencephalon
- Mesencephalon (midbrain)

- Pons
- Medulla oblongata
- Cerebellum

The medulla oblongata is continuous inferiorly with the spinal cord, with no definite anatomical boundary between them. The mesencephalon, pons, and medulla oblongata are collectively referred to as the *brainstem* based on their common embryological and functional features. The brainstem lies near the anterior surface of the cerebellum.

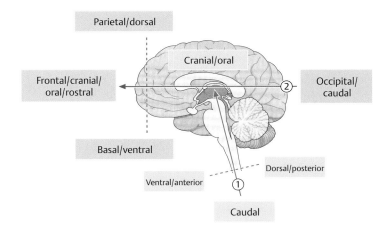

Parietal/dorsal

Cranial/oral

Frontal/cranial/ oral/rostral

Occipital/ caudal

Basal/ventral

Dorsal/posterior

Ventral/anterior

Caudal

D Terms of location and direction in the central nervous system

Midsagittal section viewed from the left side. Repeated references are made in subsequent units to two different axes of the brain: the *Meynert axis*, which is used to designate locations in the brainstem, and the *Forel axis*, which describes the topography of the diencephalon and telencephalon.

- The **Meynert axis** (1) passes through the brainstem and corresponds roughly to the longitudinal body axis.
- The **Forel axis** (2) runs horizontally through the diencephalon and telencephalon.

The following chapters on the CNS begin with the cerebrum and proceed downward to other brain structures and the spinal cord. Our approach to CNS topography also proceeds from outside to inside, following the order in which the structures are encountered in a dissection. Neuroanatomy is particularly challenging because we cannot directly infer the function of a structure from its appearance as we can with mus-

cle tissue, for example. Our presentation of the CNS therefore ends with a chapter on functional systems. In describing the functional systems, we will use a peripheral-to-central approach (i.e., from the simple to the complex) so that the reader may better understand the path followed by a stimulus from its source to its various relay stations in the CNS.

2.1 Brain and Menings in situ

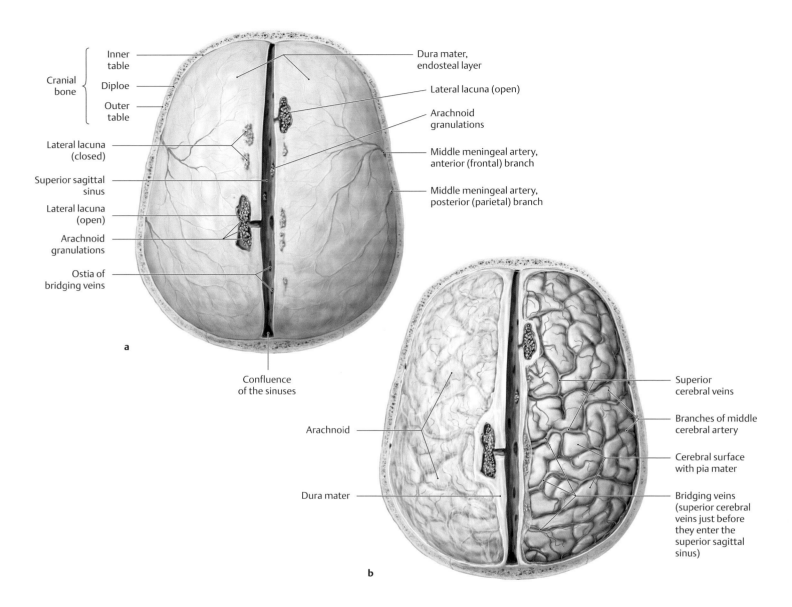

Inner table
Cranial bone { Diploe
Outer table
Lateral lacuna (closed)
Superior sagittal sinus
Lateral lacuna (open)
Arachnoid granulations
Ostia of bridging veins

Dura mater, endosteal layer
Lateral lacuna (open)
Arachnoid granulations
Middle meningeal artery, anterior (frontal) branch
Middle meningeal artery, posterior (parietal) branch

a

Confluence of the sinuses

Arachnoid

Dura mater

b

Superior cerebral veins
Branches of middle cerebral artery
Cerebral surface with pia mater
Bridging veins (superior cerebral veins just before they enter the superior sagittal sinus)

A Brain and menings in situ
Superior view. **a** The calvaria has been removed, and the superior sagittal sinus and its lateral lacunae have been opened; **b** The dura mater has been removed from the left hemisphere, and the dura and arachnoid have been removed from the right hemisphere.
The brain and spinal cord are covered by membranes called menings, which form a sac filled with cerebrospinal fluid. The menings are composed of the following three layers:

- Outer layer: The *dura mater* (often shortened to "dura") is a tough layer of collagenous connective tissue. It consists of two layers, an inner meningeal layer and an outer endosteal layer. The periosteal layer adheres firmly to the periosteum of the calvaria within the cranial cavity, but it is easy to separate the inner layer from the bone in this region, leaving it on the cerebrum as illustrated here (**a**).
- Middle layer: The *arachnoid* (arachnoid membrane) is a translucent membrane through which the cerebrum and the blood vessels in the subarachnoid space can be seen (**b**).
- Inner layer: The *pia mater* directly invests the cerebrum and lines its fissures (**b**).

The arachnoid and pia are collectively called the *leptomenings*. The space between them, called the subarachnoid space, is filled with cerebrospinal fluid and envelops the brain (see **C**, p. 191). It contains the major cerebral arteries and the superficial cerebral veins, which drain chiefly through "bridging veins" into the superior sagittal sinus. The dura mater in the midline forms a double fold between the periosteal and meningeal layers that encloses the endothelium-lined superior sagittal sinus (see **B**, p. 254), which has been opened in the illustration. Inspection of the opened sinus reveals the arachnoid granulations (Pacchionian granulations, arachnoid villi). These protrusions of the arachnoid are sites for the reabsorption of cerebrospinal fluid (see **A**, p. 194). Arachnoid granulations are particularly abundant in the lateral lacunae of the superior sagittal sinus. The dissection in **a** shows how the middle meningeal artery is situated between the dura and calvaria. Rupture of this vessel causes blood to accumulate between the bone and dura, forming an epidural hematoma (see p. 262).

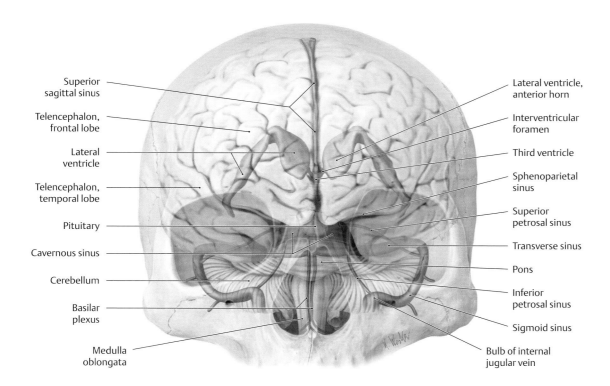

B Projection of important brain structures onto the skull
Anterior view. The largest structures of the cerebrum (telencephalon) are the frontal and temporal lobes. The falx cerebri separates the two cerebral hemispheres in the midline (not visible here). In the brainstem, we can identify the pons and medulla oblongata on both sides of the midline below the telencephalon. The superior sagittal sinus and the paired sigmoid sinuses can also be seen. The anterior horns of the two lateral ventricles are projected onto the forehead.

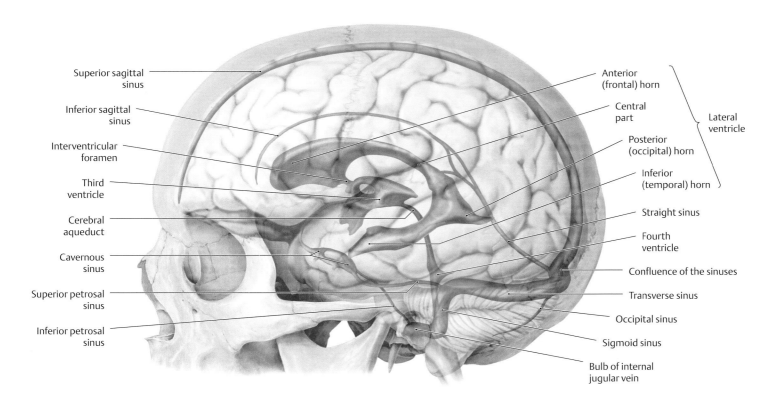

C Projection of important brain structures onto the skull
Left lateral view. The relationship of specific lobes of the cerebrum to the cranial fossae can be appreciated in this view. The frontal lobe lies in the anterior cranial fossa, the temporal lobe in the middle cranial fossa, and the cerebellum in the posterior cranial fossa. The following dural venous sinuses can be identified: the superior and inferior sagittal sinus, straight sinus, transverse sinus, sigmoid sinus, cavernous sinus, superior and inferior petrosal sinus, and occipital sinus.

187

2.2 Meninges and Dural Septa

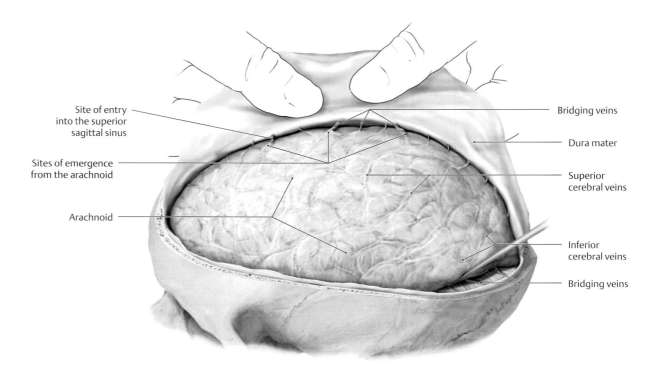

A Brain in situ with the dura partially dissected from the arachnoid
Viewed from upper left. The dura has been opened and reflected upward, leaving the underlying arachnoid and pia mater on the brain. Because the arachnoid is so thin, we can see the underlying subarachnoid space and the vessels that lie within it (see **C**). The subarachnoid space no longer contains cerebrospinal fluid at this stage of the dissection and is therefore collapsed. Before the superficial cerebral veins termi-

nate in the sinus, they leave the subarachnoid space for a short distance and course between the neurothelium of the arachnoid and the meningeal layer of the dura to the superior sagittal sinus. These segments of the cerebral veins are called *bridging veins* (see **C**). Some of the bridging veins, especially the inferior cerebral veins, open into the transverse sinus. Injury to the bridging veins leads to subdural hemorrhage (see pp. 191 and 262).

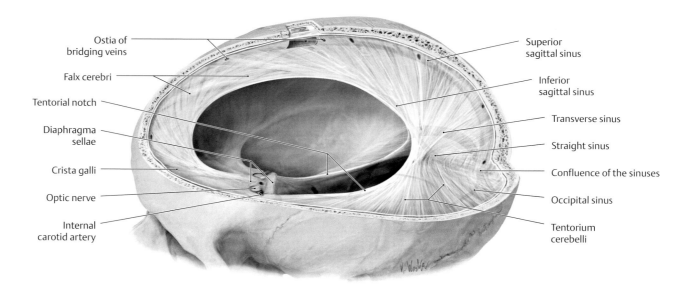

B Dural septa
Left anterior oblique view. The brain has been shelled out of its cavity to demonstrate the dural septa. The falx cerebri appears as a fibrous sheet that arises from the crista galli of the ethmoid bone and separates the two cerebral hemispheres. At its site of attachment to the calvaria, the falx cerebri expands to accommodate the superior sagittal sinus. Additional septa are the tentorium cerebelli and falx cerebelli (not shown

here). The tentorium cerebelli fans out into the groove between the cerebrum and cerebellum, while the falx cerebelli separates the two hemispheres of the cerebellum. Its root transmits the occipital sinus. Because the dural septa are rigid structures, portions of the brain may herniate beneath their free edges (see **D**). The brainstem passes through an opening in the tentorium cerebelli called the tentorial notch.

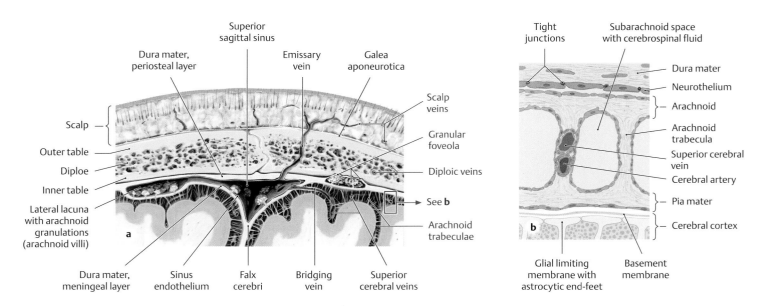

C Relationship of the meninges to the calvarium

a Coronal section through the vertex of the skull, anterior view. The endosteal layer of the dura mater and the periosteum of the skull are fused together (the periosteal layer of the dura mater), each layer consisting of a tough meshwork of fibrous tissue. At some sites the dura forms septa that dip into the fissures separating different brain regions. In the vertex region pictured here, the septum consists of the falx cerebri (other septa are shown in **B**). Located within the dura, between its endosteal and meningeal layers, are the principal venous channels of the brain, the dural venous sinuses (e.g., the superior sagittal sinus). Their walls are composed of dura and endothelium. Arachnoid granulations protrude from the subarachnoid space into the superior sagit-

tal sinus. These projections are channels through which cerebrospinal fluid from the subarachnoid space can be reabsorbed by the venous system (details on p. 194 f). They can produce pits in the inner table of the skull (granular foveolae, see p. 8). A schematic close-up (**b**) shows the relationship of the pia-arachnoid, which contains the slit-like subarachnoid space. This space is subdivided by arachnoid trabeculae that extend from the outer layer (arachnoid) to the inner layer (pia mater). At its boundary with the dura, the arachnoid is covered by flat cells which, unlike other meningeal cells, are joined together by "tight junctions" (neurothelium) to create a diffusion barrier between the blood and cerebrospinal fluid (see p. 196).

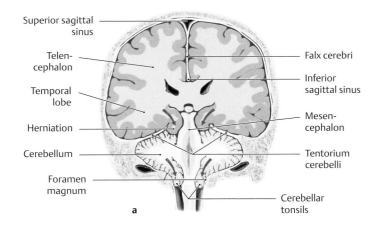

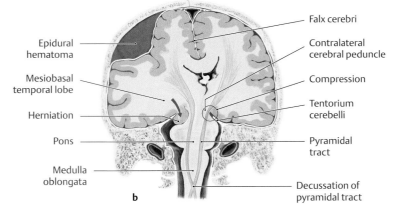

D Potential sites of brain herniation beneath the free edges of the meninges

Coronal section, anterior view. The tentorium cerebelli divides the cranial cavity into a supratentorial and an infratentorial space. The telencephalon is supratentorial, and the cerebellum is infratentorial (**a**). Because the dura is composed of tough, collagenous connective tissue, it creates a rigid intracranial framework. As a result, a mass lesion within the cranium may displace the cerebral tissue and cause portions of the cerebrum to become entrapped (herniate) beneath the rigid dural septa (= duplication of the meningeal layer of the dura).

a Axial herniation. This type of herniation is usually caused by generalized brain edema. It is a symmetrical herniation in which the middle and lower portions of both temporal lobes of the cerebrum herniate down through the tentorial notch, exerting pressure on the upper

portion of the midbrain (bilateral uncal herniation). If the pressure persists, it will force the cerebellar tonsils through the foramen magnum and also compress the lower part of the brainstem (tonsillar herniation). Because respiratory and circulatory centers are located in the brainstem, this type of herniation is life-threatening (see p. 231). Concomitant vascular compression may cause brainstem infarction.

b Lateral herniation. This type is caused by a unilateral mass effect (e.g., from a brain tumor or intracranial hematoma), as illustrated here on the right side. Compression of the ipsilateral cerebral peduncle usually produces contralateral hemiparesis. Sometimes, the herniating mesiobasal portions of the temporal lobe press the opposite cerebral peduncle against the sharp edge of the tentorium. This damages the pyramidal tract above the level of its decussation, causing hemiparesis to develop on the side opposite the injury.

2.3 Meninges of the Brain and Spinal Cord

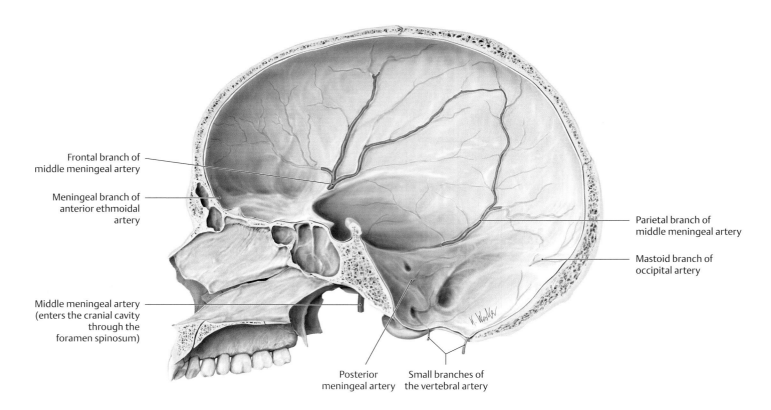

A Blood supply of the dura mater

Midsagittal section, left lateral view with branches of the middle meningeal artery exposed at several sites. Most of the dura mater in the cranial cavity receives its blood supply from the middle meningeal artery, a terminal branch of the maxillary artery. The other vessels shown here are of minor clinical importance. The essential function of the middle meningeal artery is, however, not to supply the meninges (as its name might suggest) but to supply the calvaria. Head injuries may cause the middle meningeal artery to rupture, leading to life-threatening complications (epidural hematoma; see **C** and pp. 189 and 262).

B Innervation of the dura mater in the cranial cavity (after von Lanz and Wachsmuth)

Superior view with the tentorium cerebelli removed on the right side. The intracranial meninges are supplied by meningeal branches from all three divisions of the trigeminal nerve and also by branches of the vagus nerve and the first two cervical nerves. Irritation of these sensory fibers due to meningitis is manifested clinically by headache and reflex nuchal stiffness (the neck is hyperextended in an attempt to relieve tension on the inflamed meninges). The brain itself is insensitive to pain.

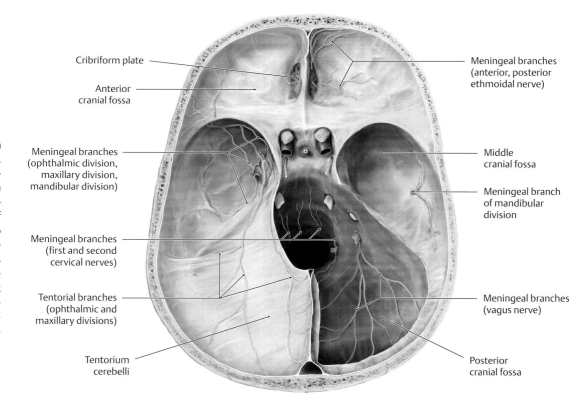

C Meninges and their spaces

Transverse section through the calvaria (schematic). The meninges have two spaces that do not exist under normal conditions, as well as one physiological space:

- Epidural space: This space is not normally present in the brain (contrast with **E**, which shows the physiological epidural space in the spinal canal). It develops in response to bleeding from the middle meningeal artery or one of its branches (arterial bleeding). The extravasated blood separates the dura mater from the bone, dissecting an epidural space between the inner table of the calvaria and the dura (epidural hematoma, see p. 262).
- Subdural space: Bleeding from the bridging veins artificially opens the subdural space between the meningeal layer of the dura mater and upper layer of the arachnoid membrane (subdural hematoma, see p. 262). The cells of the uppermost layer of

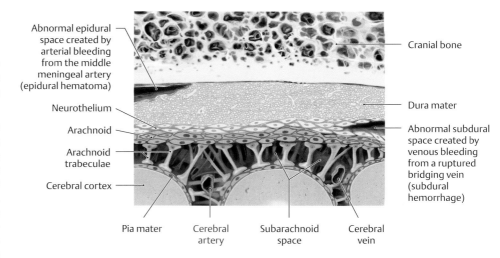

the arachnoid (neurothelium) are interconnected by a dense network of tight junctions, creating a tissue barrier (blood-cerebrospinal fluid barrier).
- Subarachnoid space: This physiologically normal space lies just beneath the arachnoid. It is filled with cerebrospinal fluid and is traversed by blood vessels. Bleeding into this space (subarachnoid hemorrhage) is usually arterial bleeding from an aneurysm (abnormal circumscribed dilation) of the basal cerebral arteries (see p. 262).

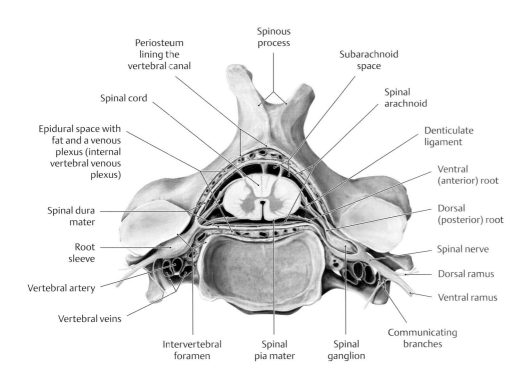

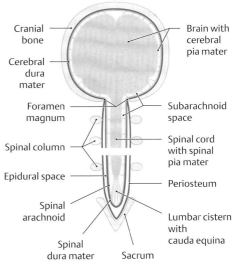

D Transverse section through the spinal cord and its meninges

Cervical vertebra viewed from above. Caudal to the foramen magnum, the dura mater separates from the periosteum; i.e., the meningeal and periosteal layers of the dura mater separate from each other to define a physiological space, the epidural space. This space is occupied by fatty tissue and venous plexuses. The dorsal and ventral roots of the spinal nerves course within the dural sac of the spinal cord and collectively form the cauda equina in the

lower part of the sac (not shown here). The dorsal and ventral roots unite within a dural sleeve at the intervertebral foramina to form the spinal nerves. After the two roots have fused lateral to the spinal ganglion, the spinal nerve emerges from the dural sac. The *pia mater* invests the surfaces of the brain and spinal cord in the same fashion. The denticulate ligaments are sheets of pial connective tissue that pass from the spinal cord to the dura and are oriented in the coronal plane.

E Meninges in the cranial cavity and spinal canal

The periosteum of the bones and the meningeal layer of the dura mater are fused together inside the cranial cavity. Caudal to the foramen magnum, however, these two layers of collagenous connective tissue separate from each other to form the epidural space. Due to the mobility of the spinal column, the periosteum of the vertebrae must be free to move relative to the dural sac. This is accomplished by the presence of the epidural space, which exists physiologically only within the spinal canal. It contains fat and venous plexuses (see **D**). This space has major clinical importance, as it is the compartment into which epidural anesthetics are injected.

3.1 Ventricular System, Overview

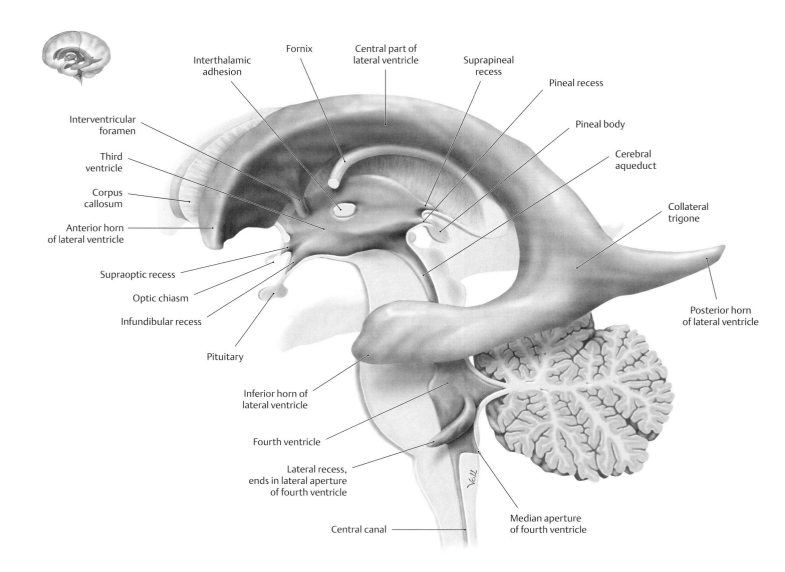

Fornix
Central part of
lateral ventricle
Interthalamic
adhesion
Suprapineal
recess
Pineal recess
Pineal body
Interventricular
foramen
Cerebral
aqueduct
Third
ventricle
Corpus
callosum
Collateral
trigone
Anterior horn
of lateral ventricle
Supraoptic recess
Optic chiasm
Posterior horn
of lateral ventricle
Infundibular recess
Pituitary
Inferior horn of
lateral ventricle
Fourth ventricle
Lateral recess,
ends in lateral aperture
of fourth ventricle
Central canal
Median aperture
of fourth ventricle

A Overview of the ventricular system and important neighboring structures

Left lateral view. The ventricular system is a greatly expanded and con-voluted tube that represents an upward prolongation of the central spi-nal canal into the brain. There are *four cerebral ventricles*, or cavities, filled with cerebrospinal fluid and lined by a specialized epithelium, the ependyma (see **D**, p. 197). The four ventricles are as follows:

- The *two* lateral ventricles, each of which communicates through an interventricular foramen with the
- third ventricle, which in turn communicates through the cerebral aq-ueduct with the
- fourth ventricle. This ventricle communicates with the subarachnoid space (see **B**).

The largest ventricles are the lateral ventricles, each of which consists of an anterior, inferior, and posterior horn and a central part. Certain por-tions of the ventricular system can be assigned to specific parts of the brain: the anterior (frontal) horn to the frontal lobe of the cerebrum, the inferior (temporal) horn to the temporal lobe, the posterior (occipital)

horn to the occipital lobe, the third ventricle to the diencephalon, the aqueduct to the midbrain (mesencephalon), and the fourth ventricle to the hindbrain (rhombencephalon). The anatomical relationships of the ventricular system can also be appreciated in coronal and transverse sections (see pp. 292 ff and 304 ff).

Cerebrospinal fluid is formed mainly by the choroid plexus, a network of vessels that is present to some degree in each of the four ventricles (see p. 195). Another site of cerebrospinal fluid production is the ependyma. Certain diseases (e.g., atrophy of brain tissue in Alzheimer's disease and internal hydrocephalus) are characterized by abnormal enlargement of the ventricular system and are diagnosed from the size of the ventricles in sectional images of the brain.

This unit deals with the ventricular system and neighboring structures. The next unit will trace the path of the cerebrospinal fluid from its pro-duction to its reabsorption. The last unit on the cerebrospinal fluid spaces will deal with the specialized functions of the ependyma, the circumventricular organs, and the physiological tissue barriers in the brain.

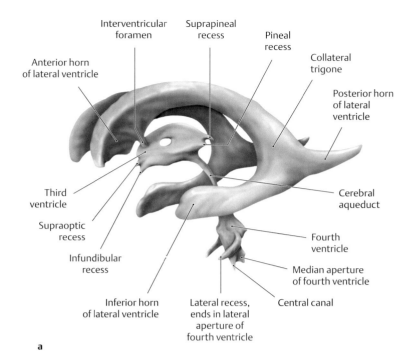

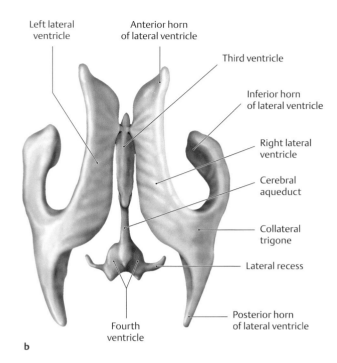

a

b

B Cast of the ventricular system

Left lateral view (**a**) and superior view (**b**). Cast specimens are used to demonstrate the connections between the ventricular cavities. Each lateral ventricle communicates with the third ventricle through an interventricular foramen. The third ventricle communicates through the cerebral aqueduct with the fourth ventricle in the rhombencephalon. The ventricular system has a fluid capacity of approximately 30 ml, while the subarachnoid space has a capacity of approximately 120 ml.

Note the three apertures (paired lateral apertures [foramina of Luschka] and an unpaired median aperture [foramen of Magendie]), through which cerebrospinal fluid flows from the deeper ventricular system into the more superficial subarachnoid space.

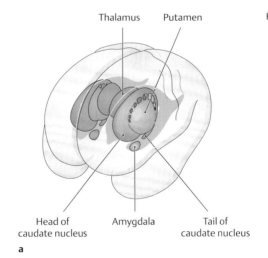

a

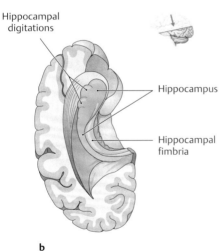

b

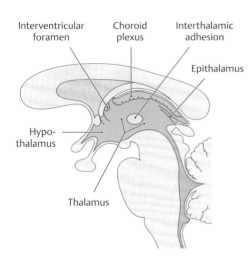

C Important structures neighboring the lateral ventricles

a View of the brain from upper left.

b View of the inferior horn of the left lateral ventricle in the opened temporal lobe.

a The following brain structures border on the lateral ventricles:
- The caudate nucleus (anterolateral wall of the anterior horn)
- The thalamus (posterolateral wall of the anterior horn)

- The putamen, which is lateral to the lateral ventricle and does not border it directly.

b The hippocampus (see p. 206) is visible in the anterior part of the floor of the inferior horn. Its anterior portions with the hippocampal digitations protrude into the ventricular cavity.

D Lateral wall of the third ventricle

Midsagittal section, left lateral view. The lateral wall of the third ventricle is formed by structures of the diencephalon (epithalamus, thalamus, hypothalamus). Protrusions of the thalami on both sides may touch each other (interthalamic adhesion) but are not functionally or anatomically connected and thus do not constitute a commissural tract.

193

3.2 Cerebrospinal Fluid, Circulation and Cisterns

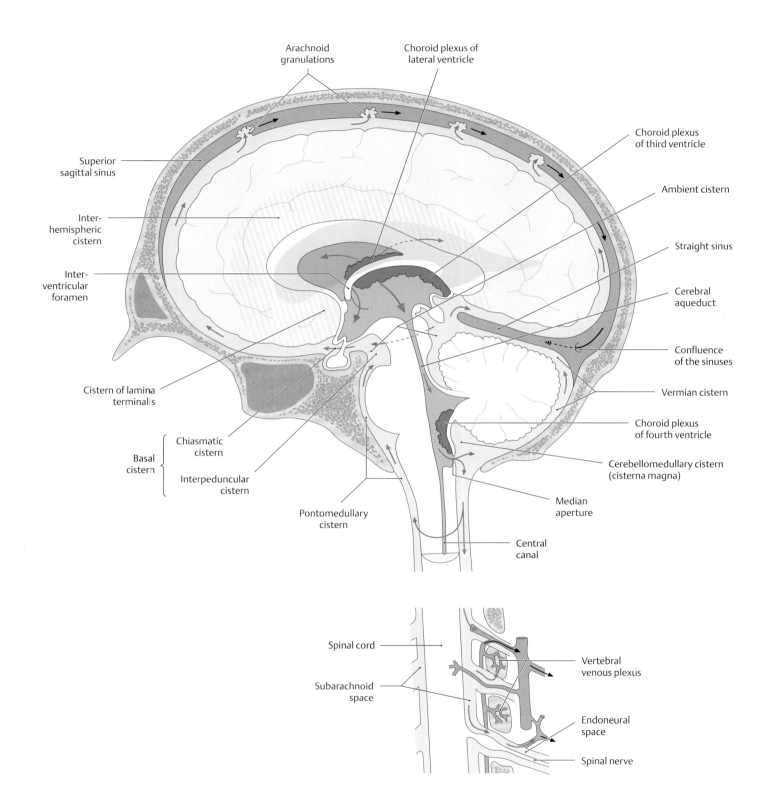

A Cerebrospinal fluid circulation and the cisterns

Cerebrospinal fluid (CSF) is produced in the choroid plexus, which is present to some extent in each of the four cerebral ventricles. It flows through the median aperture and paired lateral apertures (not shown; see p. 192 for location) into the subarachnoid space, which contains expansions called cisterns. Most of the CSF drains from the subarachnoid space through the arachnoid granulations, and smaller amounts drain along the proximal portions of the spinal nerves into venous plexuses or lymphatic pathways (see **F**). The cerebral ventricles and subarachnoid space have a combined capacity of approximately 150 ml of CSF (20 % in the ventricles and 80 % in the subarachnoid space). This volume is completely replaced two to four times daily, so that approximately 500 ml of CSF must be produced each day. Obstruction of CSF drainage will therefore cause a rise in intracranial pressure (see **E**, p. 197).

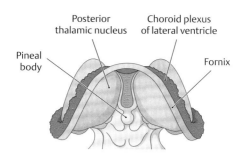

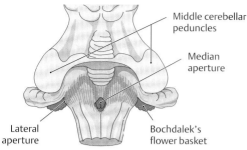

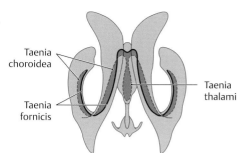

B Choroid plexus in the lateral ventricles

Rear view of the thalamus. Surrounding brain tissue has been removed down to the floor of the lateral ventricles, where the choroid plexus originates. The plexus is adherent to the ventricular wall at only one site (see **D**) and can thus float freely in the ventricular system.

C Choroid plexus in the fourth ventricle

Posterior view of the partially opened rhomboid fossa (with the cerebellum removed). Portions of the choroid plexus are attached to the roof of the fourth ventricle and run along the lateral aperture. Free ends of the choroid plexus may extend through the lateral apertures into the subarachnoid space on both sides ("Bochdalek's flower basket").

D Taeniae of the choroid plexus

Superior view of the ventricular system. The choroid plexus is formed by the ingrowth of vascular loops into the ependyma, which firmly attach it to the wall of the associated ventricle (see **F**). When the plexus tissue is removed with a forceps, its lines of attachment, called taeniae, can be seen.

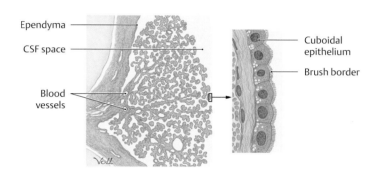

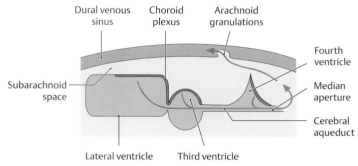

E Histological section of the choroid plexus, with a detail showing the structure of the plexus epithelium (after Kahle)

The choroid plexus is a protrusion of the ventricular wall. It is often likened to a cauliflower because of its extensive surface folds. The epithelium of the choroid plexus consists of a single layer of cuboidal cells and has a brush border on its apical surface (to increase the surface area further).

F Schematic diagram of cerebrospinal fluid circulation

As noted earlier, the choroid plexus is present to some extent in each of the four cerebral ventricles. It produces CSF, which flows through the two lateral apertures (not shown) and median aperture into the subarachnoid space. From there, most of the CSF drains through the arachnoid granulations into the dural venous sinuses.

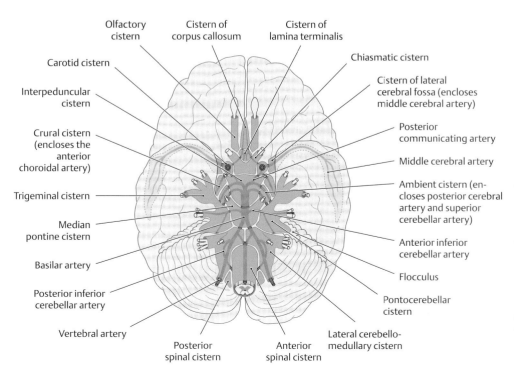

G Subarachnoid cisterns (after Rauber and Kopsch)

Basal view. The cisterns are CSF-filled expansions of the subarachnoid space. They contain the proximal portions of some cranial nerves and basal cerebral arteries (veins are not shown). When arterial bleeding occurs (as from a ruptured aneurysm), blood will slep into the subarachnoid space and enter the CSF. A ruptured intracranial aneurysm is a frequent cause of blood in the CSF (methods of sampling the CSF are described on p. 197).

3.3 Circumventricular Organs and Tissue Barriers in the Brain

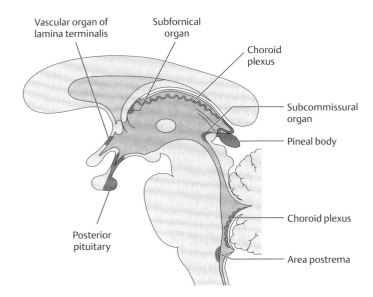

Vascular organ of lamina terminalis
Subfornical organ
Choroid plexus
Subcommissural organ
Pineal body
Choroid plexus
Area postrema
Posterior pituitary

B Summary of the smaller circumventricular organs

In addition to the four regions listed below, the circumventricular organs include the posterior pituitary, choroid plexus, and pineal body. The functional descriptions are based largely on experimental studies in animals.

Organ	Location	Function
Vascular organ of the lamina terminalis (VOLT)	Vascular loops in the rostral wall of the third ventricle (lamina terminalis); rudimentary in humans	Secretes the regulatory hormones somatostatin, luliberin, and motilin; contains cells sensitive to angiotensin II; is a neuroendocrine mediator
Subfornical organ (SFO)	Fenestrated capillaries between the interventricular foramina and below the fornices	Secretes somatostatin and luliberin from nerve endings; contains cells sensitive to angiotensin II; plays a central role in the regulation of fluid balance ("organ of thirst")
Subcommissural organ (SCO)	Borders on the pineal body; overlies the epithalamic commissure at the junction of the third ventricle and cerebral aqueduct	Secretes glycoproteins into the aqueduct that condense to form the Reissner fiber, which may extend into the central canal of the spinal cord; blood-brain barrier is intact; function is not completely understood
Area postrema (AP)	Paired organs in the floor of the caudal end of the rhomboid fossa, richly vascularized	Trigger zone for the emetic reflex (absence of the blood-brain barrier); atrophies in humans after middle age

A Location of the circumventricular organs

Midsagittal section, left lateral view. The circumventricular organs include the following:

- Posterior pituitary with the neurohemal region (see p. 222)
- Choroid plexus (see p. 195)
- Pineal body (see p. 224)
- Vascular organ of the lamina terminalis, subfornical organ, subcommissural organ, and area postrema (see **B**).

The circumventricular or ependymal organs all have several features in common. They are composed of modified ependyma, they usually border on the ventricular and subarachnoid CSF spaces, and they are located in the median plane (except the choroid plexus, though it does *develop* from an unpaired primordium in the median plane). The blood-brain barrier is usually absent in these organs (see **C** and **D**; except the subcommissural organ).

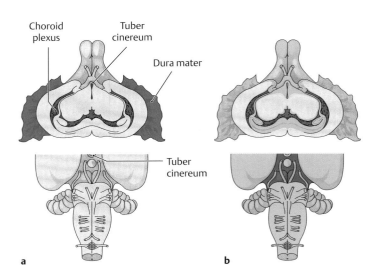

Choroid plexus
Tuber cinereum
Dura mater
Tuber cinereum
a
b

C Demonstration of tissue barriers in the brain (after Kahle)

a Blood-brain barrier, **b** blood-CSF barrier. The upper drawings show an inferior view of a transverse section through a rabbit brain, and the lower drawings show the brainstem from the basal aspect. The function of these barriers is to protect the brain from harmful substances in the bloodstream. These include macromolecular as well as small molecular pharmaceutical compounds.

a **Demonstration of the blood-brain barrier:** The *intravenous injection* of trypan blue dye (first Goldmann test) stains almost all organs blue except the brain and spinal cord. Even the dura and choroid plexus show heavy blue staining. Faint blue staining is noted in the tuber cinereum (neurohemal region of the posterior pituitary), area postrema, and spinal ganglia (absence of the blood-brain barrier in these regions). The same pattern of color distribution occurs naturally in *jaundice*, where bile pigment stains all organs but the brain and spinal cord, analogous to trypan blue in the first Goldmann test.

b **Demonstration of the blood-CSF barrier:** When the dye is injected *into the CSF* (second Goldmann test), the brain and spinal cord (CNS) show diffuse superficial staining while the rest of the body remains unstained. This shows that a barrier exists between the CSF and blood, but not between the CSF and the CNS.

D Blood-brain barrier and blood-CSF barrier
a Normal brain tissue with an intact blood-brain barrier;
b Blood-CSF barrier in the choroid plexus.

a The blood-brain barrier in normal brain tissue consists mainly of the tight junctions between capillary endothelial cells. It prevents the paracellular diffusion of hydrophilic substances from CNS capillaries into surrounding tissues and in the opposite direction as well. Essential hydrophilic substances that are needed by CNS must be channeled through the barrier with the aid of specific transport mechanisms (e.g., glucose by an insulin-dependent transporter).

b The blood-brain barrier is absent at fenestrated capillary endothelial cells in the choroid plexus and other circumventricular organs (see **A**), which allow substances to pass freely from the bloodstream into the brain tissue and vice versa. Tight junctions in the overlying ependyma (choroid plexus epithelium) do, however, create a two-way barrier between the brain tissue and ventricular CSF in these regions. In other words, the diffusion barrier is shifted from the vascular endothelium to the cells of the ependyma and choroid plexus.

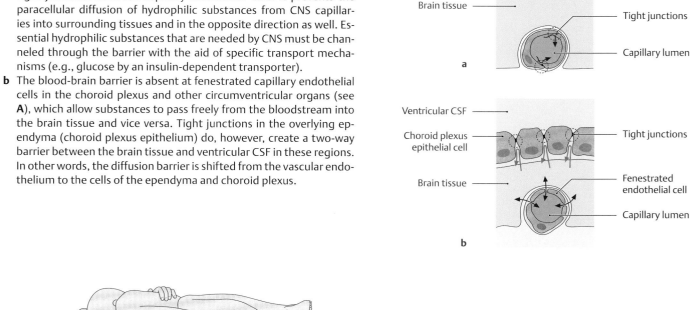

E Obtaining cerebrospinal fluid samples

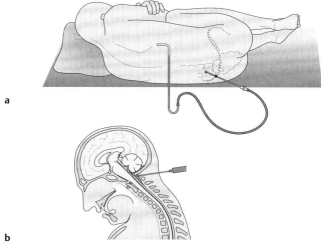

a Lumbar puncture: This is the *method of choice* for sampling the CSF. A needle is inserted precisely in the midline between the spinous processes of L 3 and L 4 and is advanced into the dural sac (lumbar cistern). At this time a fluid sample can be drawn and the CSF pressure can be measured for diagnostic purposes by connecting a manometer to the needle. Lumbar puncture is contraindicated if the intracranial pressure is markedly increased, as it may cause a precipitous cranial to spinal pressure gradient, causing the brainstem to herniate through the foramen magnum. This would exert pressure on vitally important centers in the medulla oblongata, with a potentially fatal outcome. Thus, the physician should always check for signs of increased intracranial pressure (e.g., papilledema, see p. 133) before performing a lumbar puncture.

b Suboccipital puncture: This technique should be used only in *exceptional cases* where a lumbar puncture is contraindicated (e.g., by a spinal cord tumor), because it may, rarely, produce a fatal complication. The mortality risk results from the need to pass a needle through the cerebellomedullary cistern (cisterna magna), which may endanger vital centers in the medulla oblongata.

F Comparison of cerebrospinal fluid and blood serum
Infection of the brain and its coverings (meningitis), subarachnoid hemorrhage, and tumor metastases can all be diagnosed by CSF examination. As the table indicates, CSF is more than a simple ultrafiltrate of blood serum. Its primary function is to impart buoyancy of the brain (the brain has an effective weight of only about 50 g despite a mass of 1300 g). Decreased CNS production therefore increases pressure on the spine and also renders the brain more susceptible to injury (less cushioning).

	CSF	Serum
Pressure	50–180 mm H$_2$O	
Volume	100–160 mL	
Osmolarity	292–297 mOsm/L	285–295 mOsm/L
Electrolytes		
Sodium	137–145 mM	136–145 mM
Potassium	2.7–3.9 mM	3.5–5.0 mM
Calcium	1–1.5 mM	2.2–2.6 mM
Chloride	116–122 mM	98–106 mM
pH	7.31–7.34	7.38–7.44
Glucose	2.2–3.9 mM	4.2–6.4 mM
CSF/serum glucose ratio	> 0.5–0.6	
Lactate	1–2 mM	0.6–1.7 mM
Total protein	0.2–0.5 g/L	55–80 g/L
Albumin	56–75 %	50–60 %
IgG	0.01–0.014 g/L	8–15 g/L
Leukocytes	< 4 cells/µL	
Lymphocytes	60–70 %	

4.1 Telencephalon, Development and External Structure

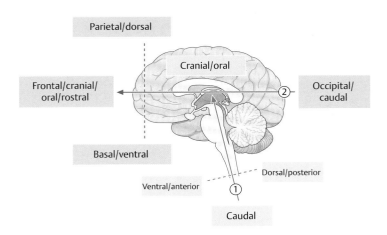

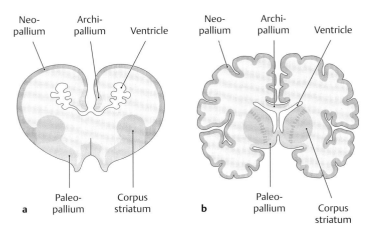

A Terms of location and direction
Midsagittal section viewed from the left side. Terms of location and direction in the telencephalon and diencephalon are based on the Forel axis (2), which runs horizontally through the forebrain. (1) Brainstem axis (Meynert axis).

B Development of the cerebral cortex
a Embryonic brain; **b** adult brain.
The cerebral hemispheres can be divided into phylogenetically ancient ("paleo"), old ("archi") and new ("neo") parts (see **D**). The cerebral cortex together with associated areas of underlying white matter is called the pallium, a term sometimes used interchangably with "cortex".

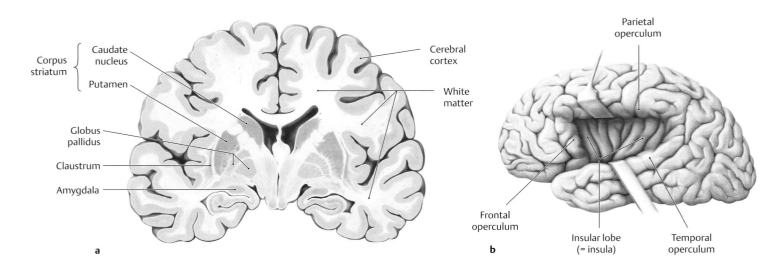

C Gray and white matter in the telencephalon
a Coronal section showing the distribution of gray and white matter in the brain.

Gray matter:
- Cerebral cortex: contains most of the gray matter of the telencephalon. It is divided on histological grounds into two parts:

  - Isocortex: corresponds to the neocortex (see **B**); largest part of the cerebral cortex, consisting of six layers (see p. 200).
  - Allocortex: corresponds to the paleo- and archicortexes (see **B**); consists of *three* or *four* layers (see p. 204).

- Subcortical nuclei: Basal ganglia: the caudate nucleus and putamen (collectively called the corpus striatum), and the globus pallidus.
  Note: The basal ganglia are often called the basal nuclei. Because they are located in the CNS, however, the term "ganglia" is more appropriate than "nuclei."

- Other white-matter nuclei that are not included among the basal ganlgia of the telencephalon:

  - Amygdala: often considered a transitional form between the two types of gray matter—cortex and basal ganglia—based on its location (see p. 207)
  - Claustrum

White matter: tissue below the cerebral cortex and surrounding the subcortical nuclei. *Note:* The white matter also contains nuclei of the diencephalon (see p. 215).

b Lateral view of the left hemisphere. Part of the cerebral cortex sinks below the surface during development, forming the insula. The portions of the cerebral cortex that overlie deeper cortical areas are called opercula ("little lids").

D Phylogenetic origins of major compoments of the telencephalon

Phylogenetic term	Structure in the embryonic brain	Structure(s) in the adult brain	Cortical structure
Paleopallium (oldest part)	Floor of the hemispheres	• Rhinencephalon (= olfactory bulb plus surrounding region)	Allocortex (see p. 204)
Archipallium (old part)	Medial portion of hemispheric wall	• Ammon's horn (largest part, not shown here) • Indusium griseum • Fornix	Allocortex
Neopallium (newest part)	Most of the brain surface plus the deeper corpus striatum	• Neocortex (= cortex), largest part of the cerebral cortex • Insula • Corpus striatum	Isocortex (see p. 200)

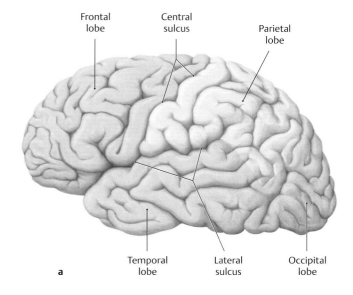

a

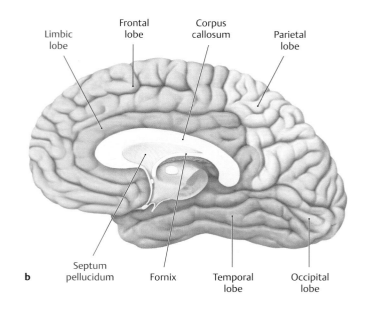

b

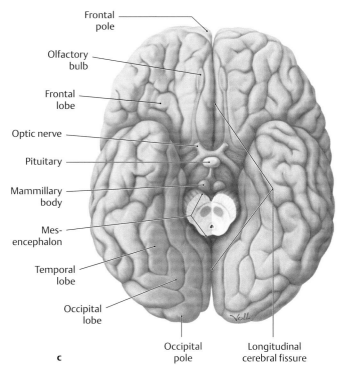

c

E Division of the cerebral hemispheres into lobes

a Left lateral view of the left hemisphere; **b** Left lateral view of the right hemisphere; **c** Basal view with the brainstem removed, showing the cut surface of the midbrain (mesencephalon).

The two cerebral hemispheres are the externally visible part of the telencephalon. They are separated from each other by the longitudinal cerebral fissure and are each subdivided into six lobes:

• Frontal lobe
• Parietal lobe
• Temporal lobe
• Occipital lobe
• Insular lobe (insula, see **Cb**)
• Limbic lobe (limbus)

The surface contours of the cerebral hemispheres are highly variable between individuals. A histological subdivision into cortical areas is more meaningful in terms of functional brain organization than a macroscopic subdivision into gyri and sulci (see p. 200).

199

4.2 Cerebral Cortex, Histological Structure and Functional Organization

A Histological structure of the cerebral cortex

A six-layered (laminar) structure is found throughout most of the neocortex. The silver impregnation (**a**) or Nissl staining of the cell bodies (**b**) allows for histological division of the neocortex according to the dominant structure of each layer:

I   Molecular layer: (outermost layer); relatively few neurons.
II   External granular layer: mostly stellate and scattered small pyramidal neurons.
III   External pyramidal layer: small pyramidal neurons.
IV   Internal granular layer: stellate an small pyramidal neurons.
V   Internal pyramidal layer: large pyramidal neurons.
VI   Multiform layer: (innermost layer); neurons of varied shape and size.

Cortical areas that are concerned primarily with information processing (e.g., primary somatosensory cortex) are rich in granule cells; the granular layers of these regions (*granular cortex*, see **Ba**) are also exceptionally thick. Areas in which information is transmitted out of the cortex (e.g. the prinary motor cortex) are distinguished by prominent layers of pyramidal cells and known as the *agranular cortex* (see **Bb**). Analysis of the distribution of nerve cells in the cerebral cortex allows for identification of functionally distinct areas (*cytoarchitectonics*, see **A,** p. 203).

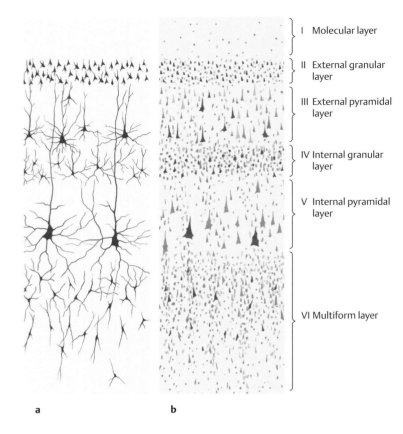

I   Molecular layer

II   External granular layer

III External pyramidal layer

IV Internal granular layer

V   Internal pyramidal layer

VI Multiform layer

a   b

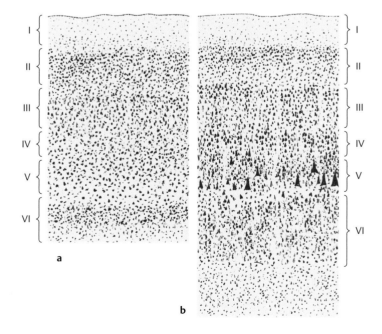

B Examples of granular and agranular cortex

a Granular cortex (koniocortex from the Greek konis = sand): The primary somatosensory cortex, in which the afferents from the thalamus terminate (at layer IV), is located in the postcentral gyrus. It is thinner overall than the primary somatomotor cortex (see **b**). A striking feature in the primary somatosensory cortex is that the external and internal granular layers (II and IV) where the large sensory tracts terminate are markedly widened. By contrast, the pyramidal cell layers (III and V) are thinned.

b Agranular cortex: The efferents fibers that project to the motor nuclei of the cranial nerves and motor columns of the spinal cord originate in the primary somatomotor cortex, located in the precentral gyrus. Its pyramidal layers (III and V) are greatly enlarged. Exceptionally large pyramidal neurons (Betz cells after the author who first described them) are found in the some areas of layer V. Their long axons extend into the sacral spinal cord (see p. 267).

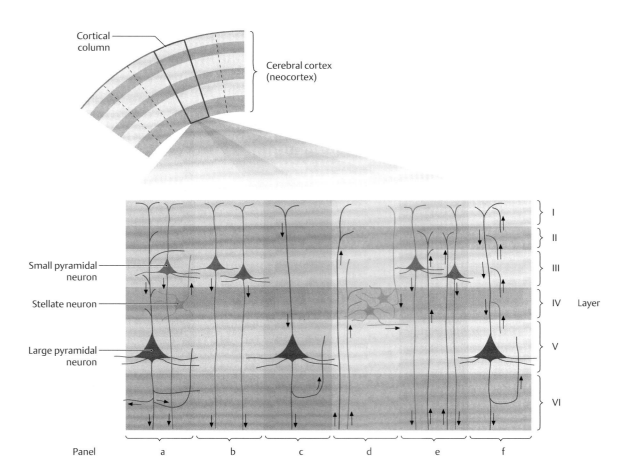

C Columnar organization of the cortex (after Klinke and Silbernagl)
While morphological considerations divide the cerebral cortex into horizontal layers (see **A**), functional considerations lead to its division into distinct units or modules (see **C**). Encompassing all six layers, these modules consist of vertically-arranged *cortical columns* of neurons that are interconnected a serve a common function, despite showing no distinct histological boundaries. In total, there are several million such modules in the cerebral cortex, with a variable width between 50 and 500 μm each. One cortical column has here been magnified to display its constituent neurons and connections in separate panels. Panels **a–c** show the principal types of cells participating in a cortical column: several thousand *stellate neurons* of various subtype and one hundred or so large and small pyramidal neurons (panel **a**). Panel **b** isolates the small pyramidal cells whose axons tend to terminate within the cortex

itself. In contrast, the deeper, large pyramidal neurons (panel **c**) have axons that generally project to subcortical structures. Large pyramidal cells are responsible for tracts of corticobulbar and corticospinal motor axons, which project to the brainstem and spinal cord, respectively. They may also send recurrent collateral fibers which end in the local cortex. Panels **d–f** contain axons projecting *into* the cerebral cortex. Panel **d** isolates thalamocortical projections that enter from the thalamus and synapse mostly on the stellate neurons of layer IV. Incoming association fibers of the nearby cortex and commissural fibers of the contralateral hemisphere frequently terminate on the dendrites of the small pyramidal neurons (panel **e**). Panel **f** shows the large pyramidal neurons whose apical dendrites reach from layer V to layer I. These large pyramidal neurons integrate inputs from various other local neurons and incoming fibers.

D Types of neuron in the cerebral cortex (simplified)

Neuron	Definition	Properties
Stellate neuron (layers II and IV)	Cell with short axon for local information processing; various types: basket, candelabra, double-bouquet cells	Inhibitory interneuron in most cortical areas; primary information-processing neuron (in layer II), especially in primary sensory areas
Small pyramidal neuron (layer III)	Cell with long axon that often ends within the cortex, either as: • Association fiber: axon ends in same hemisphere but different cortical area, or as • Commissural fiber: axon ends in opposite hemisphere but cortical area of similar function	Projection neuron whose axons end within the cortex
Large pyramidal neuron (layer V)	Cell with very long axon that projects outside the cortex, sometimes reaching distant structures	Excitatory projection neuron whose axons end outside the cortex
Granule cell (layers II and IV)	Generic term for small neuron, most often with stellate morphology	Depends on the cell type (see entries for stellate and small pyramidal neurons)

4.3 Neocortex, Cortical Areas

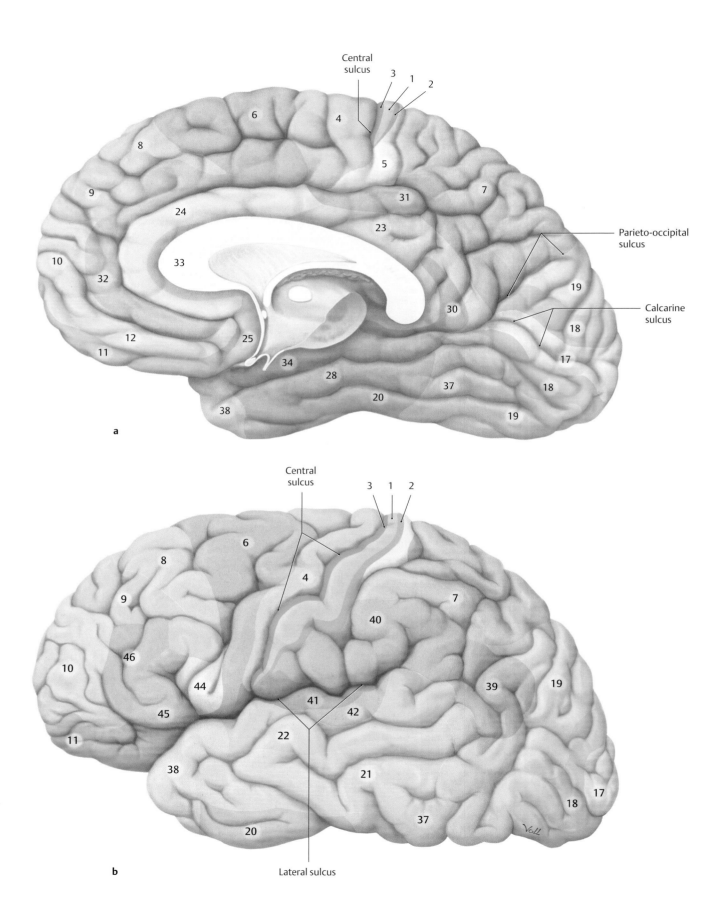

A Brodmann areas in the neocortex

a Midsagittal section of the right cerebral hemisphere, viewed from the left side; **b** Lateral view of the left cerebral hemisphere.

As noted earlier, the surface of the brain consists macroscopically of lobes, gyri, and sulci. Microscopically, however, subtle differences can be found in the distribution of the cortical neurons, and some of these differences do not conform to the gross surface anatomy of the brain. Portions of the cerebral cortex that have the same basic microscopic features are called *cortical areas* or *cortical fields*. This organization into cortical areas is based on the distribution of neurons in the different layers of the cortex (*cytoarchitectonics,* see **A**, p. 200). In the brain map shown at left, these areas are indicated by different colors. Although the size of the cortical areas may vary between individuals, the brain map pictured here is still used today as a standard reference chart. It was developed

in the early 20th century by the anatomist Korbinian Brodmann (1868–1918), who spent years painstakingly examining the cellular architecture of the cortex in a single brain. It has long been thought that the map created by Brodmann accurately reflects the functional organization of the cortex, and indeed, modern imaging techniques have shown that many of the cytologically defined areas are associated with specific functions. There is no need, of course, to memorize the location of all the cortical areas, but the following areas are of special interest:

- Areas 1, 2, and 3: primary somatosensory cortex
- Area 4 primary motor cortex
- Area 17: primary visual cortex (striate area, the extent of which is best appreciated in the midsagittal section)
- Areas 41 and 42: auditory cortex

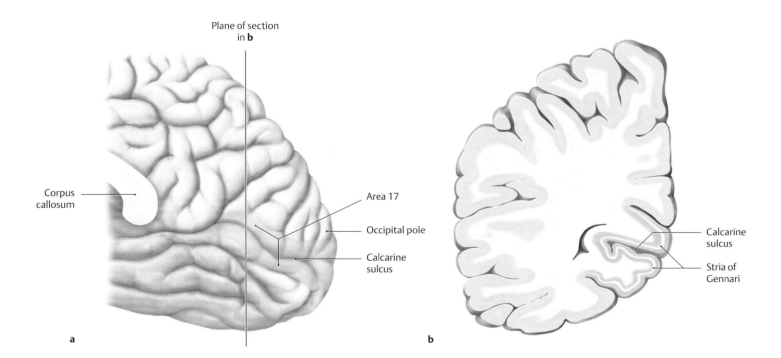

Plane of section in **b**

Corpus callosum

Area 17

Occipital pole

Calcarine sulcus

Calcarine sulcus

Stria of Gennari

a

b

B Visual cortex (striate area)

a Right hemisphere viewed from the left side; **b** Coronal section (plane of section shown in **a**), anterior view.

The primary visual cortex (striate area, shaded yellow) is the only cortical area that can be clearly recognized by its macroscopic appearance. It extends along both sides of the calcarine sulcus at the occipital pole. In

an unstained coronal section (**b**), the *stria of Gennari* can be identified as a prominent white stripe within the gray cortical area. This stripe contains cortical association fibers that synapse with the neurons of the internal granular layer (IV, see p. 201). The pyramidal cell layers (efferent fibers) are attenuated in the visual cortex, while the granular cell layers where the afferent fibers from the lateral geniculate nucleus terminate are markedly enlarged.

4.4 Allocortex, Overview

A Overview of the allocortex

View of the base of the brain (**a**) and the median surface of the right hemisphere (**b**). Structures belonging to the allocortex are indicated by colored shading (see listing of allocortical structures in **D**, p. 199).

The allocortex consists of the phylogenetically old part of the cerebral cortex. It is very small in relation to the cortex as a whole. Unlike the isocortex, which has a six-layered structure, the allocortex (*allo* = "other") usually consists of *three* layers that encompass the paleo- and archicortexes. Additionally, there exist *four*-layered transitional areas between the allocortex and isocortex: the *peri*paleocortex (not indicated separately in the drawing) and the *peri*archicortex (indicated by pink shading). An important part of the allocortex is the *rhinencephalon* ("olfactory brain"). Olfactory impulses that are perceived by the olfactory bulb are the only sensory afferent impulses that do not reach the cerebral cortex by way of the dorsal thalamus. Another important part of the allocortex is the hippocampus and its associated nuclei (see p. 206). As in the isocortex, the gyral patterns of the allocortex do not always conform to its histological organization.

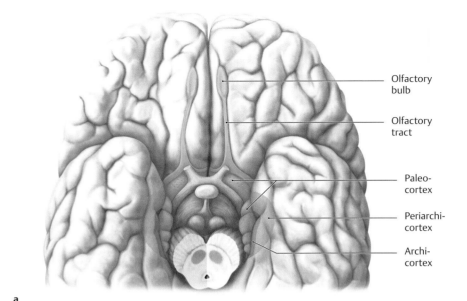

Olfactory bulb

Olfactory tract

Paleo-cortex

Periarchi-cortex

Archi-cortex

a

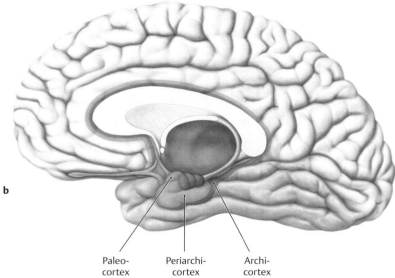

b

Paleo-cortex   Periarchi-cortex   Archi-cortex

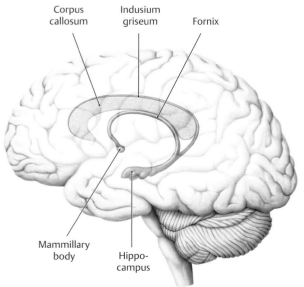

Corpus callosum   Indusium griseum   Fornix

Mammillary body   Hippo-campus

B Organization of the archipallium: deeper parts

Lateral view of the left hemisphere. The archicortex described in **A** is the *only* part of the archipallium that is located on the brain surface. The deeper parts of the archipallium, which lie within the white matter, are the hippocampus ("sea horse"), indusium griseum ("gray covering"), and fornix ("arch"). All three structures are part of the *limbic system* (see p. 374), and together form a border ("limbus") around the corpus callosum as a result of their migration during development.

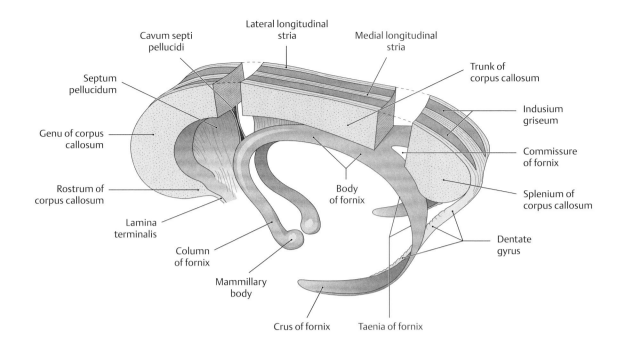

C Topography of the fornix, corpus callosum, and septum pellucidum (after Feneis)

Occipital view from upper left. The fornix is a tract of the archicortex that is closely apposed but functionally unrelated to the corpus callosum. The corpus callosum is the largest neocortical commissural tract between the hemispheres, serving to interconnect cortical areas of similer function in the two hemispheres (see also p. 376). The septum pellucidum is a thin plate that stretches between the corpus callosum and fornix, forming the medial boundary of the lateral ventricles. Between the two septa is a cavity of variable size, the *cavum septi pellucidi*. The cholinergic nuclei in the septa, which are involved in the organization of memory, are connected to the hippocampus by the fornix (see p. 206).

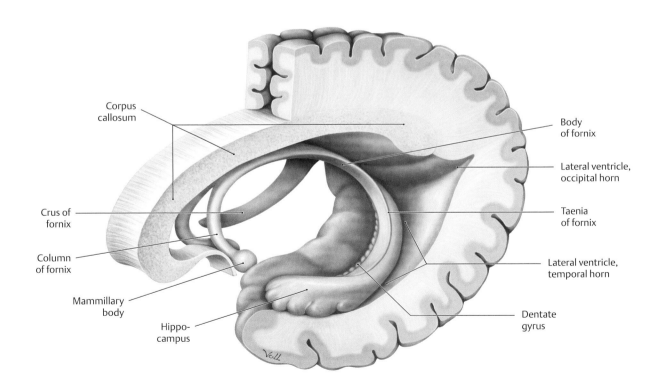

D Topography of the hippocampus, fornix, and corpus callosum

Viewed from the upper left and oral aspect. This drawing shows the hippocampus on the floor of the inferior horn of the lateral ventricle. The left and right *crura of the fornix* unite to form the *commissure of the fornix* (see **C**) and the *body of the fornix*, which divides anteriorly into left and right bundles, the *columns of the fornix*. The fornix is a white-matter tract connecting the hippocampus to the mammillary bodies in the diencephalon. Contained within the fornix are hippocampal neurons whose axons project to the septum, mammillary bodies, contralateral hippocamous, and other structures. This important pathway is part of the *limbic system* (see p. 374).

205

4.5 Allocortex: Hippocampus and Amygdala

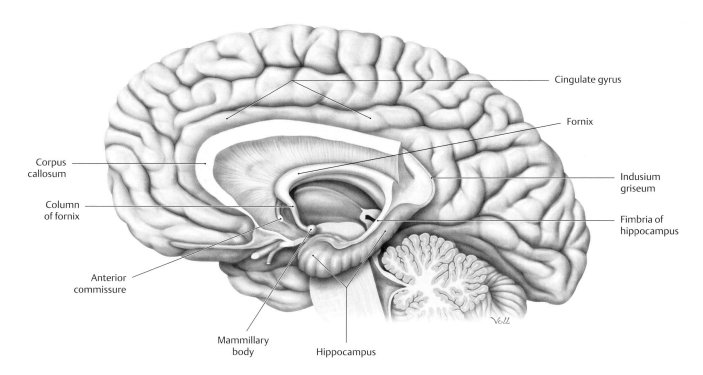

A Left hippocampal formation
Lateral view. Most of the left hemisphere has been dissected away, leaving only the corpus callosum, fornix, and hippocampus. The intact right hemisphere is visible in the background.
The hippocampal formation is an important component of the *limbic system* (see p. 374). It consists of three parts:

- Subiculum (see **Cb**)
- Hippocampus proper (Ammon's horn)
- Dentate gyrus (fascia dentata)

The fiber tract of the fornix connects the hippocampus to the mammillary body. The hippocampus integrates information from various brain areas and influences endocrine, visceral, and emotional processes via its efferent output. It is particulary associated with the establishment of short-term memory. Lesions of the hippocampus can therefore cause specific defects in memory formation.
Besides the hippocampus, which is the largest part of the archicortex, we can recognize another component of the archicortex, the indusium griseum.

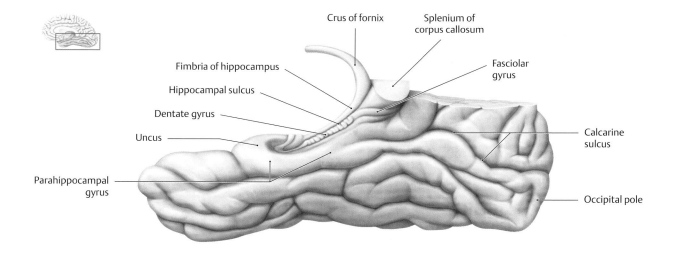

B Right hippocampal formation and the caudal part of the fornix
Left medial view. Compare this medial view of the right hippocampal formation with the lateral view in **A** above. A useful landmark is the calcarine sulcus, which leads to the occipital pole. The cortical areas that border the hippocampus (e.g., the parahippocampal gyrus) are particulary apparent in this view.

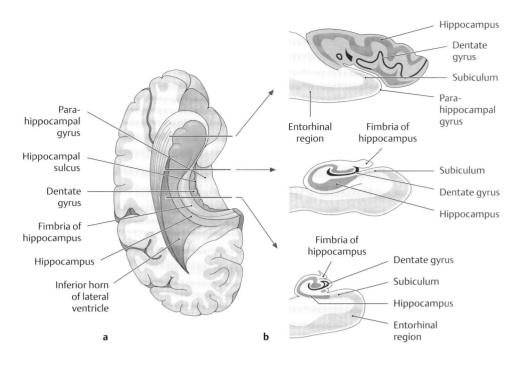

a   **b**

C Left temporal lobe with the inferior horn of the lateral ventricle exposed

a Transverse section, posterior view of the hippocampus on the floor of the inferior (temporal) horn. The following structures can be identified from lateral to medial: hippocampus, fimbria, dentate gyrus, hippocampal sulcus, and parahippocampal gyrus.

b Coronal sections of the left hippocampus. The hippocampus appears here as a curled band (Ammon's horn = the hippocampus proper), which shows considerable structural diversity in its different portions. The junction between the entorhinal cortex (entorhinal region) in the parahippocampal gyrus and Ammon's horn is formed by a transitional area, the subiculum. The entorhinal region is the "gateway" to the hippocampus, through which the hippocampus receives most of its afferent fibers.

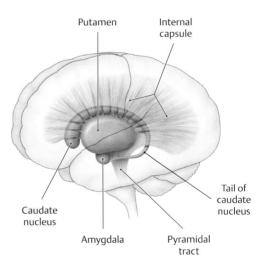

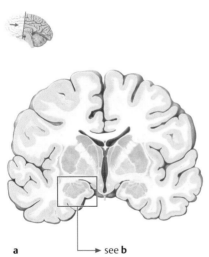

a   → see **b**

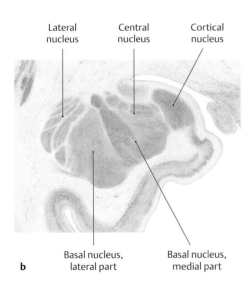

b

D Relationship of the amygdala to internal brain structures

Lateral view of the left hemisphere. The amygdala (amygdaloid body) is located below the putamen and anterior to the tail of the caudate nucleus. The fibers of the pyramidal tract run posterior and medial to the amygdala.

E Amygdala

a Coronal section at the level of the interventricular foramen. The amygdala extends medially to the inferior surface of the cortex of the temporal lobe. For this reason, it is considered to be part of the cortex as well as a nuclear complex that has migrated into the white matter. Stimulation of the amygdala in humans leads to changes in mood, ranging from rage and fear to rest and relaxation depending on the emotional state of the patient immediately prior to stimulation. Since the amygdala functions as an "emotional amplifier," lesions affect the patient's evaluation of events' emotional significance. The surrounding periamygdaline cortex and the corticomedial half of the amygdala are part of the primary olfactory

cortex. Hence these portions of the amygdala are considered part of the paleocortex, while the deeper portion is characterized as "nuclear."

b Detail from **a** showing the two main groups of nuclei in the amygdala:

- Phylogenetically old corticomedial group:
  – Cortical nucleus
  – Central nucleus
- Phylogenetically new basolateral group:
  – Basal nucleus
  – Lateral nucleus

The basal nucleus can be subdivided into a parvocellular medial part and a macrocellular lateral part.

207

4.6 Telencephalon: White Matter and Basal Ganglia

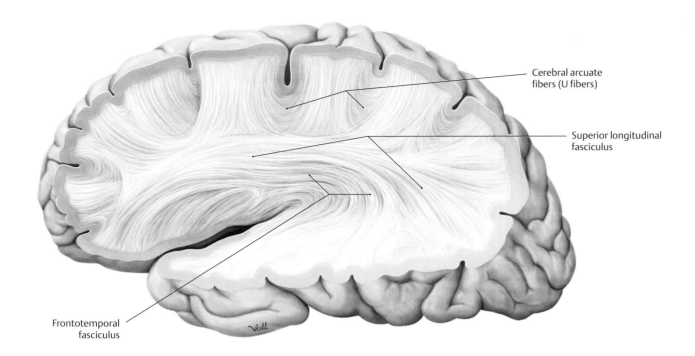

Cerebral arcuate fibers (U fibers)

Superior longitudinal fasciculus

Frontotemporal fasciculus

A Teased fiber preparation of the white matter of the telencephalon
Lateral view of the left hemisphere. This dissection shows the superficial layer of white matter located between the basal ganglia and the gray matter of the cerebral cortex. A special preparation technique was used to display the fiber structure of the white matter, which normally has a uniform white appearance. The fiber structure is defined by the tracts (bundles of myelinated axons) that interconnect different areas of the gray matter. For example, we can identify the short cerebral arcuate fibers (U fibers) that run between two adjacent gyri as well as the association fibers that span multiple gyri (e.g., the superior longitudinal and frontotemporal fasciculi). When these tracts are damaged (in multiple sclerosis, for example) the communication pathways within the brain cease to function normally. This may lead to central paralysis, visual disturbances (optic nerve damage), and behavioral changes (damage to the frontal cortex).

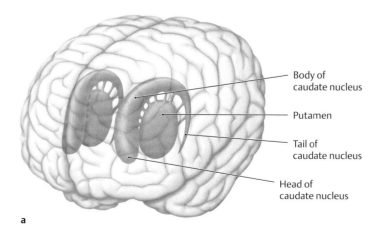

Body of caudate nucleus

Putamen

Tail of caudate nucleus

Head of caudate nucleus

a

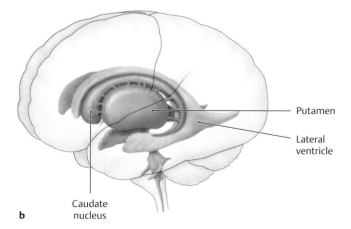

Putamen

Lateral ventricle

Caudate nucleus

b

B Projection of the basal ganglia onto the brain surface and ventricular system

a View from the upper left anterior aspect. The basal ganglia are masses of gray matter deep within the brain that contain the cell bodies of neurons. Further details on the basal ganglia are shown in **C**.

b Left lateral view. The caudate nucleus is closely applied to the concave lateral wall of the lateral ventricle. It is connected to the putamen by numerous streak-like bands of gray matter (corpus striatum, see **C**).

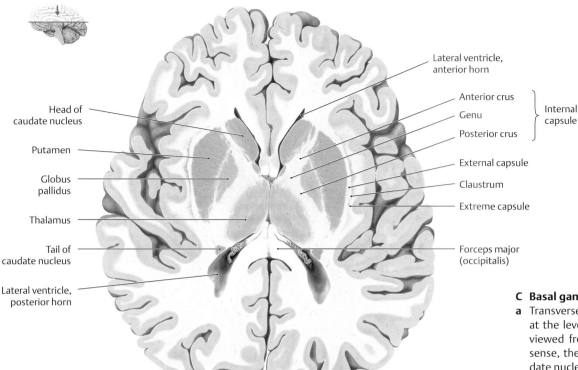

Head of caudate nucleus

Putamen

Globus pallidus

Thalamus

Tail of caudate nucleus

Lateral ventricle, posterior horn

Lateral ventricle, anterior horn

Anterior crus ⎫
Genu   ⎬ Internal capsule
Posterior crus ⎭

External capsule

Claustrum

Extreme capsule

Forceps major (occipitalis)

a

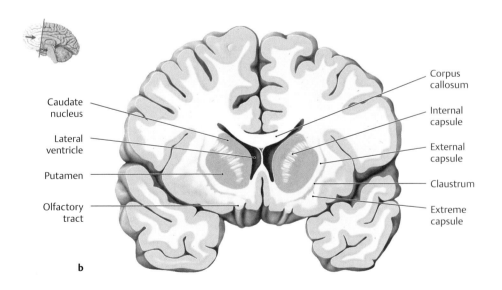

Caudate nucleus

Lateral ventricle

Putamen

Olfactory tract

Corpus callosum

Internal capsule

External capsule

Claustrum

Extreme capsule

b

C Basal ganglia

a Transverse section through the cerebrum at the level of the corpus striatum (see **D**), viewed from above. In a strict anatomical sense, the basal ganglia consist of the caudate nucleus, putamen, and globus pallidus. Developmentally, the globus pallidus is a part of the diencephalon (see **D**, p. 211) that has migrated into the telencephalon, but it is still counted among the basal ganglia. The basal ganglia are an essential component of the extrapyramidal motor system (its functional significance is described on p. 340). The claustrum ("barrier") is a strip of gray matter lateral to the putamen. It is not part of the basal ganglia but instead has reciprocal connections with sensory areas of the cerebral cortex.

b Coronal section through the cerebrum at the level of the olfactory tract, anterior view. This section demonstrates how the caudate nucleus and putamen are separated from each other by the fibrous white matter of the internal capsule. The caudate nucleus and putamen together constitute the corpus striatum (often shortened to "striatum"; see **D**). The globus pallidus is not visible because it is occipital to this plane of section.

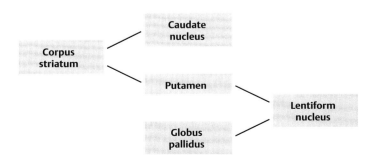

D Relationship between the corpus striatum and lentiform nucleus
The caudate nucleus and putamen together constitute the corpus striatum, while the putamen and globus pallidus make up the lentiform ("lens-shaped") nucleus. Although the globus pallidus and the putamen are anatomically juxtaposed, the putamen is functionally associated instead with the caudate nucleus. Developmentally, the putamen is part of the telencephalon and the globus pallidus is part of the diencephalon.

209

5.1   Diencephalon, Overview and Development

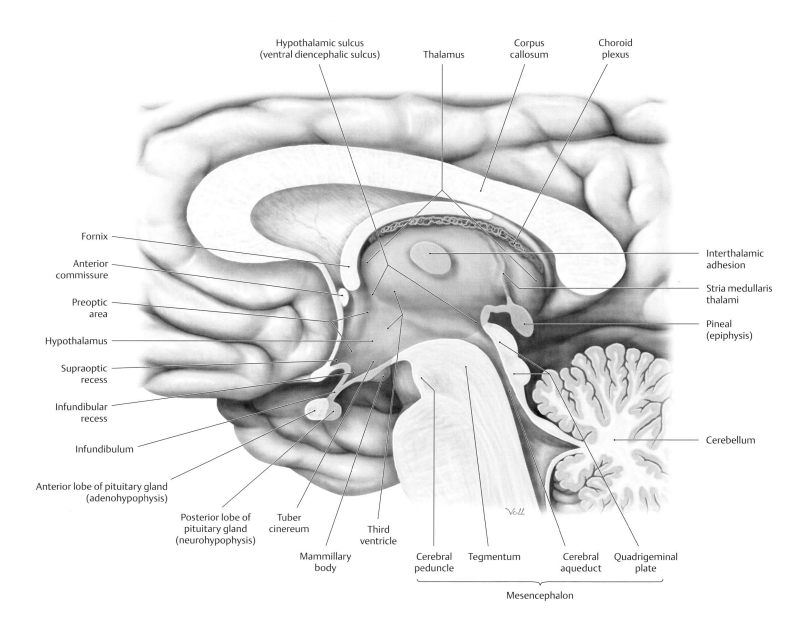

A The diencephalon in situ

Midsagittal section of the right hemisphere viewed from the medial side. The diencephalon is located below the corpus callosum, part of the telencephalon, and above the mesencephalon (midbrain). The lateral wall of the third ventricle, visible here, forms the medial boundary of the diencephalon. The *thalamus* makes up four-fifths of the entire diencephalon, but the only parts of the diencephalon that can be seen externally are the hypothalamus (visible from the basal aspect) and portions of the epithalamus (pineal, visible from the occipital aspect). The differentiation of these structures from the embryonic diencephalon is shown

in **D**, and their functions are listed on page 214 (**A**). In the adult brain, the diencephalon is involved in endocrine functioning and autonomic coordination of the pineal, posterior pituitary lobe and hypothalamus. It also acts as a relay station for sensory information and somatic motor control (via the thalamus). Units 5.2 and 5.3 deal with the external and internal structure of the diencephalon as a whole. Later units examine the individual parts of the diencephalon, devoting the most attention to the clinically important thalamus (5.4, 5.5) and hypothalamus (5.6, 5.7). The final unit covers the epithalamus and subthalamus (5.8).

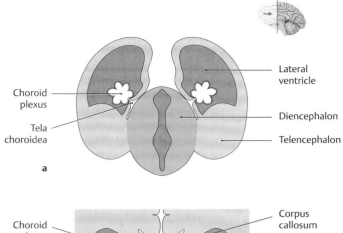

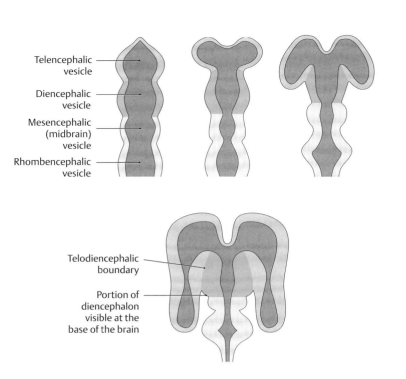

Telencephalic vesicle

Diencephalic vesicle

Mesencephalic (midbrain) vesicle

Rhombencephalic vesicle

Telodiencephalic boundary

Portion of diencephalon visible at the base of the brain

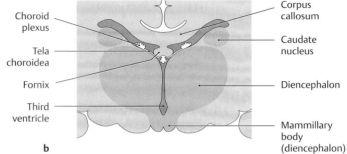

Choroid plexus

Tela choroidea

Lateral ventricle

Diencephalon

Telencephalon

a

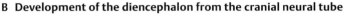

Choroid plexus

Tela choroidea

Fornix

Third ventricle

Corpus callosum

Caudate nucleus

Diencephalon

Mammillary body (diencephalon)

b

B Development of the diencephalon from the cranial neural tube
Anterior view. To understand the location and extent of the diencephalon in the adult brain, it is necessary to know how it develops from the neural tube. The diencephalon and telencephalon both develop from the prosencephalon, or telencephalic vesicle (see p. 183). As development proceeds, the two hemispheres of the telencephalic vesicle (red) expand, overgrowing the diencephalic vesicle (blue). This process shifts the boundary between the telencephalon and diencephalon until only a small area of the diencephalon can be seen at the base of the adult brain (see **A**).

C Posterior telodiencephalic boundary
Coronal sections.

a Embryonic brain. The development of the telencephalon (red) has progressed considerably in relation to **B**. The lateral ventricles containing the choroid plexus have already completely overgrown the diencephalon (blue) from behind. The medial wall of the lateral ventricles is very thin and has not yet fused to the diencephalon. Between the telencephalon and diencephalon is a vascularized sheet of connective tissue, the tela choroidea.

b Adult brain. By the adult stage, the tela choroidea and the medial wall of the lateral ventricle have become fused to the diencephalon. Removing the choroid plexus and the thin tela choroidea affords a direct view of the posteromedial boundary of the diencephalon (see **B**, p. 212).

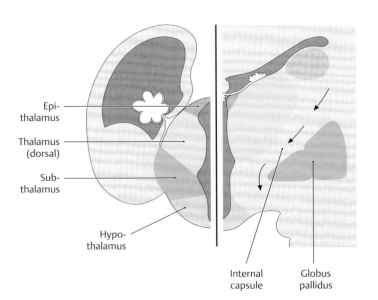

Epi-thalamus

Thalamus (dorsal)

Sub-thalamus

Hypo-thalamus

Internal capsule

Globus pallidus

D Organization of the diencephalon during embryonic development
Coronal section of an embryonic brain (left) and an adult brain (right) demonstrating the parts of the diencephalon.
Because the diencephalon of the adult brain lies between the telencephalon and mesencephalon, the ascending and descending axons must penetrate this part of the brain during development, forming the internal capsule. As development proceeds, the axon bundles that form the internal capsule migrate through the subthalamus (black arrows), displacing the greater portion of it laterally. This laterally displaced part of the subthalamus is called the *globus pallidus*. Although the globus pallidus is displaced anatomically into the telencephalon and is considered part of the telencephalon in a topographical sense, it still retains close functional ties with the subthalamus, as both are part of the extrapyramidal motor system. The *medial* part of the subthalamus remains in the diencephalon as the *true subthalamus* (not visible in this plane of section). As a result, the internal capsule of the telencephalon forms the lateral boundary of the diencephalon. The different parts of the diencephalon grow to reach different definitive sizes. The thalamus grows disproportionately and eventually occupies four-fifths of the mature diencephalon.

211

5.2 Diencephalon, External Structure

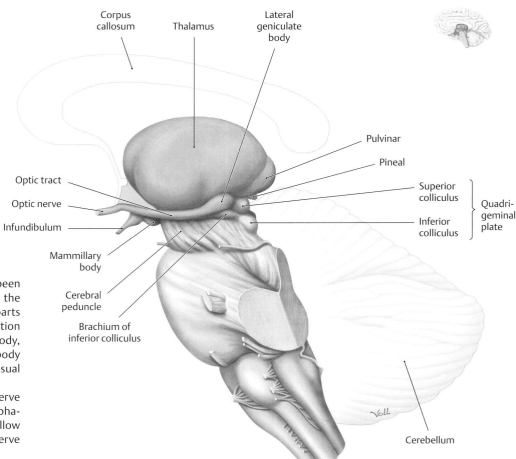

A The diencephalon and brainstem

Left lateral view. The telencephalon has been removed from around the thalamus, and the cerebellum has also been removed. The parts of the diencephalon visible in this dissection are the thalamus, the lateral geniculate body, and the optic tract. The lateral geniculate body and optic tract are components of the visual pathway.

Note: the retina and associated optic nerve form an anterior extension of the diencephalon. Departing from the convention of yellow for nerves, we have colored the optic nerve blue to emphasize this relationship.

B Arrangement of the diencephalon around the third ventricle

Posterior view of an oblique transverse section through the telencephalon with the corpus callosum, fornix, and choroid plexus removed. Removal of the choroid plexus leaves behind its line of attachment, the *taenia choroidea*. The thin wall of the third ventricle has been removed with the choroid plexus to expose the thalamic surface medial to the boundary line of the taenia choroidea. The thin ventricular wall has been left on the thalamus lateral to the taenia choroidea. This thin layer of telencephalon, called the *lamina affixa*, is colored brown in the drawing and covers the thalamus (part of the diencephalon), shown in blue. Because the thalamostriate vein marks this boundary between the diencephalon and telencephalon, it is featured prominently in the drawing. Lateral to the vein is the caudate nucleus, which is part of the telencephalon (compare with **C**, p. 211).

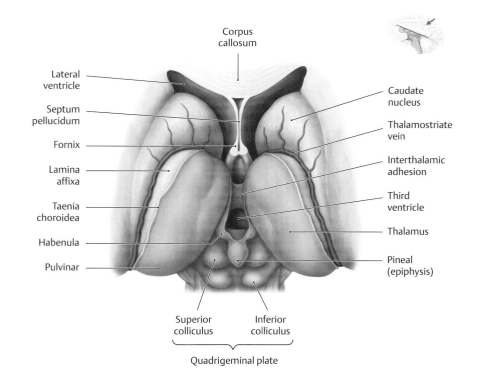

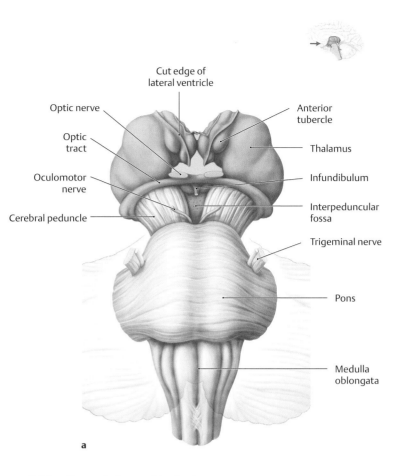

a

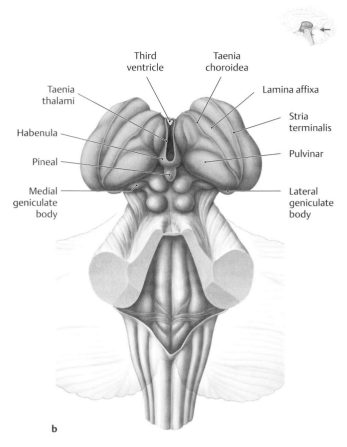

b

C The diencephalon and brainstem

a Anterior view, **b** posterior view with the cerebellum and telencephalon removed.

a The optic tract marks the lateral boundary of the diencephalon. It winds around the cerebral peduncles (crura cerebri), which are part of the adjacent midbrain (mesencephalon).

b The epithalamus, which is formed by the pineal and the two habenulae ("reins"), is well displayed in this posterior view. The lateral ge-

niculate body is an important relay station in the visual pathway, just as the medial geniculate body is an important relay station in the auditory pathway. Both are counted among the thalamic nuclei, and together they constitute the *metathalamus*, an extension of the thalamus proper. The pulvinar ("pillow"), which encompasses the posterior thalamic nuclei, is seen particularly well in this section.

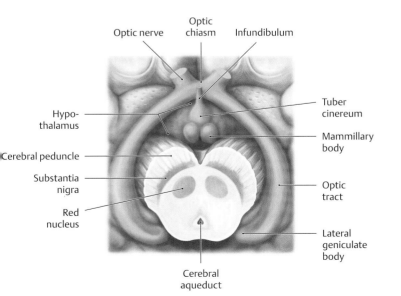

D Location of the diencephalon in the adult brain

Basal view of the brain (the brainstem has been sectioned at the level of the mesencephalon). The structures that can be identified in this view represent the parts of the diencephalon situated on the basal surface of the brain. This view also demonstrates how the optic tract, which is part of the diencephalon, winds around the cerebral peduncles of the mesencephalon (see **Ca**). Due to the expansion of the telencephalon, only a few structures of the diencephalon can be seen on the undersurface of the brain:

- Optic nerve
- Optic chiasm
- Optic tract
- Tuber cinereum with the infundibulum
- Mammillary bodies
- Medial geniculate body (see **Cb**)
- Lateral geniculate body
- Posterior lobe of the pituitary gland (neurohypophysis, see p. 222)

213

5.3 Diencephalon, Internal Structure

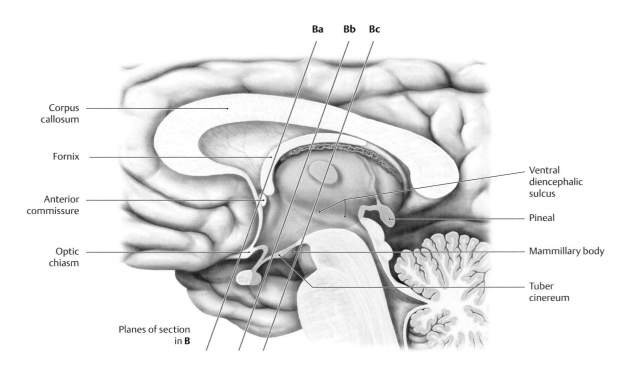

Ba Bb Bc

Corpus callosum

Fornix

Anterior commissure

Optic chiasm

Planes of section in **B**

Ventral diencephalic sulcus

Pineal

Mammillary body

Tuber cinereum

A The four parts of the diencephalon

Part	Boundary line	Structure	Function
Epithalamus		• Pineal gland • Habenulae	Regulation of circadian rhythms; linking of olfactory system to brainstem
	Dorsal diencephalic sulcus		
Thalamus		• Thalamus	Relay of sensory information; assistance in regulation of motor function
	Middle diencephalic sulcus		
Subthalamus		• Subthalamic nucleus • Zona incerta • Globus pallidus (see **E,** p. 225)	Relay of sensory information (somatomotor zone of diencephalon)
	Ventral diencephalic sulcus (= hypothalamic sulcus) *		
Hypothalamus		• Optic chiasm, optic tract • Tuber cinereum, neurohypophysis • Mammillary bodies	Coordination of autonomic nervous system with endocrine system; participation in visual pathway

* This is the only sulcus shown in **A**.

B Coronal sections through the diencephalon at three different levels

a Level of the optic chiasm: Portions of the diencephalon and telencephalon appear in this section, which clearly shows the position of the diencephalon on both sides of the third ventricle. An outpouching of the third ventricle, the preoptic recess, is located above the optic chiasm. Its connection to the third ventricle lies outside this plane of section.

b Level of the tuber cinereum, just behind the interventricular foramen: The boundary between the diencephalon and telencephalon is clearly defined only in the region about the ventricles; the underlying nuclear areas blend together with no apparent boundary. Along the lateral ventricles, the boundary between the diencephalon and telencephalon is marked by the lamina affixa, a narrow strip of telencephalon that overlies the thalamus. It can be seen that layers of gray matter permeate the internal capsule in its dorsal portion.

c Level of the mammillary bodies: This section displays the thalamic nuclei. More than 120 separate nuclei may be counted, depending on the system of nomenclature used. Most of these nuclei cannot be grossly identified in anatomical specimens. Their classification is reviewed on p. 216 (after Kahle and Frotscher, quoted from Villinger and Ludwig).

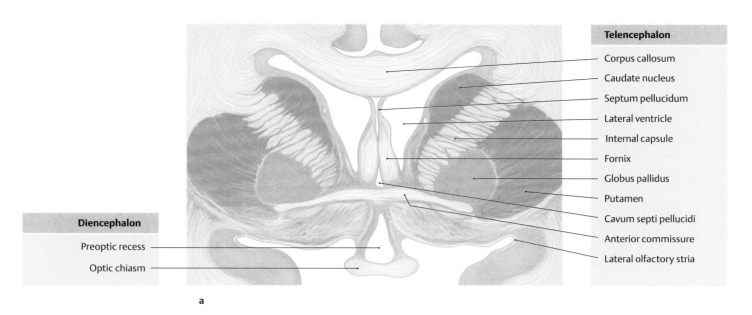

Telencephalon

- Corpus callosum
- Caudate nucleus
- Septum pellucidum
- Lateral ventricle
- Internal capsule
- Fornix
- Globus pallidus
- Putamen
- Cavum septi pellucidi
- Anterior commissure
- Lateral olfactory stria

Diencephalon

- Preoptic recess
- Optic chiasm

a

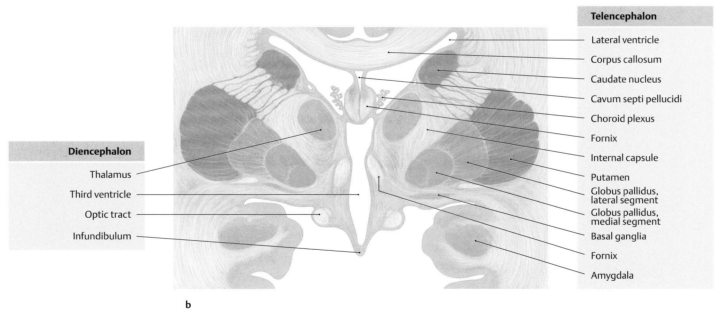

Telencephalon

- Lateral ventricle
- Corpus callosum
- Caudate nucleus
- Cavum septi pellucidi
- Choroid plexus
- Fornix
- Internal capsule
- Putamen
- Globus pallidus, lateral segment
- Globus pallidus, medial segment
- Basal ganglia
- Fornix
- Amygdala

Diencephalon

- Thalamus
- Third ventricle
- Optic tract
- Infundibulum

b

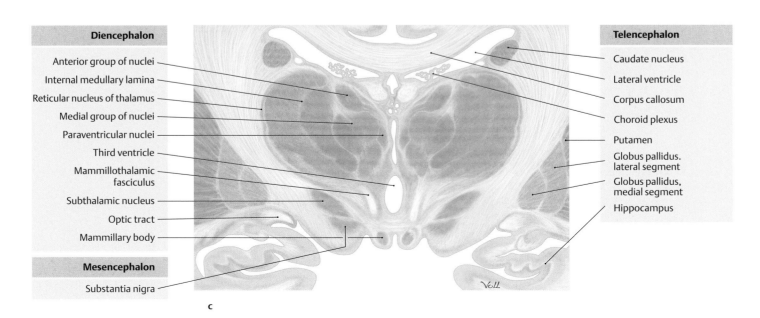

Diencephalon

- Anterior group of nuclei
- Internal medullary lamina
- Reticular nucleus of thalamus
- Medial group of nuclei
- Paraventricular nuclei
- Third ventricle
- Mammillothalamic fasciculus
- Subthalamic nucleus
- Optic tract
- Mammillary body

Mesencephalon

- Substantia nigra

Telencephalon

- Caudate nucleus
- Lateral ventricle
- Corpus callosum
- Choroid plexus
- Putamen
- Globus pallidus. lateral segment
- Globus pallidus, medial segment
- Hippocampus

c

5.4 Thalamus: Thalamic Nuclei

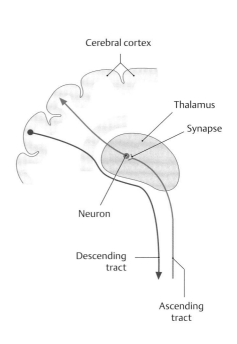

Cerebral cortex

Thalamus

Synapse

Neuron

Descending tract

Ascending tract

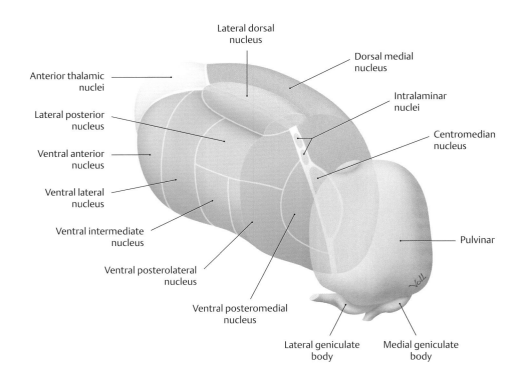

Lateral dorsal nucleus

Dorsal medial nucleus

Anterior thalamic nuclei

Intralaminar nuclei

Lateral posterior nucleus

Centromedian nucleus

Ventral anterior nucleus

Ventral lateral nucleus

Ventral intermediate nucleus

Pulvinar

Ventral posterolateral nucleus

Ventral posteromedial nucleus

Lateral geniculate body

Medial geniculate body

A Functional organization of the thalamus
Almost all of the sensory pathways are relayed via the thalamus and project to the cerebral cortex (see **G**, thalamic radiation). Consequently, a lesion of the thalamus or its cortical projection fibers caused by a stroke or other disease leads to sensory disturbances. Although a diffuse kind of sensory perception may take place at the thalamic level (especially pain perception), cortical processing (by the telencephalon) is necessary in order to transform unconscious perception into conscious perception. The olfactory system is an exception to this rule, although its olfactory bulb is still an extension of the telencephalon.
Note: Major descending motor tracts from the cerebral cortex generally bypass the thalamus.

B Spatial arrangement of the thalamic nuclear groups
Left thalamus viewed from the lateral and occipital aspect, slightly rotated relative to the views on p. 212. The thalamus is a collection of approximately 120 nuclei that process sensory information. They are broadly classified as specific or nonspecific:

- Specific nuclei and the fibers arising from them (thalamic radiation, see **G**) have direct connections with specific areas of the *cerebral cortex*. The specific thalamic nuclei are subdivided into four groups:

  - Anterior nuclei (yellow)
  - Medial nuclei (red)
  - Ventrolateral nuclei (green)
  - Dorsal nuclei (blue).

The dorsal nuclei are in contact with the the medial and lateral geniculate bodies. Located beneath the pulvinar, these two nuclear bodies contain the *nuclei of the medial and lateral geniculate bodies,* and are collectively called the *metathalamus.* Like the pulvinar, they belong to the category of specific thalamic nuclei.

- *Nonspecific nuclei* have no direct connections with the cerebral cortex. Part of a general arousal system, they are connected directly to the brainstem. The only nonspecific nuclei shown in this diagram (orange, see **F** for further details) are the centromedian nucleus and the intralaminar nuclei.

C Nomenclature of the thalamic nuclei

Name	Alternative name	Properties
Specific thalamic nuclei (cortically dependent)	Palliothalamus	Project to the cerebral cortex (pallium)
Nonspecific thalamic nuclei (cortically independent)	Truncothalamus	Project to the brainstem, diencephalon, and corpus striatum
Integration nuclei		Project to other nuclei within the thalamus (classified as nonspecific thalamic nuclei)
Intralaminar nuclei		Nuclei in the white matter of the internal medullary lamina (classified as nonspecific thalamic nuclei)

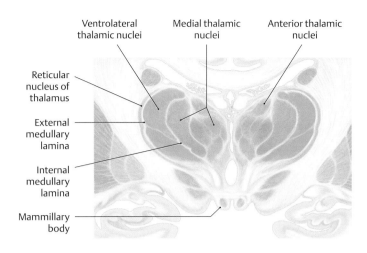

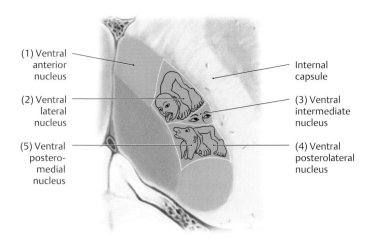

D Division of the thalamic nuclei by the medullary laminae

Coronal section at the level of the mammillary bodies. Several groups of thalamic nuclei are grossly separated into larger nuclear complexes by fibrous sheets called medullary laminae. The following laminae are shown in the diagram:

- Internal medullary lamina between the medial and ventrolateral thalamic nuclei
- External medullary lamina between the lateral nuclei and the reticular nucleus of the thalamus

E Somatotopic organization of the specific thalamic nuclei

Transverse section. The specific thalamic nuclei (defined in **B, C**) are topographically arranged according to their functional relation to specific regions of the body. Afferent fibers from the spinal cord, brainstem and cerebellum are localized to specific areas of the thalamus, where the corresponding thalamic nuclei are clustered. This pattern of somatotopic arrangement, a recurring theme in neural organization, is here illustrated for the ventrolateral thalamic nuclei (green in **B, D, E**). Axons from the crossed superior cerebral peduncle terminate in the ventral lateral nucleus of the thalamus (**2**); information on body position, coordination and muscle tone travels by this pathway to the motor cortex, which also shows a pattern of somatotopic organization (see p. 339). The *lateral* part of the ventral lateral nucleus relays impulses from the extremities, while the *medial* part relays impulses from the head. The ventral intermediate nucleus (**3**) receives afferent input from the vestibular nuclei concerning the coordination of gaze toward the ipsilateral side. The large sensory pathways of the spinal cord (the tracts of the posterior funiculus) are relayed to the nuclei cuneatus and gracilus, which send their axons through the medial lemniscus to terminate in the ventral posterolateral nucleus (**4**), while the trigeminal sensory pathways from the head terminate in the ventral posteromedial nucleus (**5**, trigeminal lemniscus, see p. 275). Topographical localization according to function is a basic principle of neural organization.

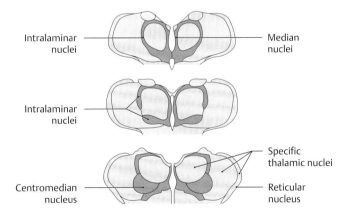

F Nonspecific thalamic nuclei

Coronal sections presented in an oral-to-caudal series. The nonspecific thalamic nuclei project to the brainstem, to other nuclei in the diencephalon (including other thalamic nuclei), and to the corpus striatum. They have no direct connections with the cerebral cortex, acting only indirectly on the cortex. The medial *nonspecific* thalamic nuclei are subdivided into two groups:

- Nuclei of the central thalamic gray matter (median nucleus): small groups of cells distributed along the wall of the third ventricle
- Intralaminar nuclei, located in the internal medullary lamina. The largest nucleus of this group is the centromedian nucleus.

The lateral *specific* thalamic nucleus shown in the diagram is the reticular nucleus of the thalamus, which is situated lateral to the other specific thalamic nuclei. The reticular nucleus is the source of the electrical impulses recorded in an electroencephalogram (EEG).

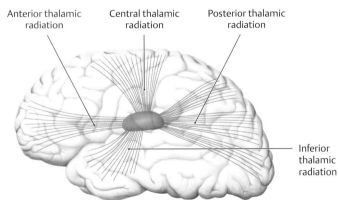

G Thalamic radiations

Lateral ventricle of the left hemisphere. The axons of the specific thalamic nuclei (so called because their fibers project to specific cortical areas) are collected into tracts that form the thalamic radiations. The arrangement of the fibers shows that the specific thalamic nuclei have connections with all areas of the cortex. The anterior thalamic radiation projects to the frontal lobe, the central thalamic radiation to the parietal lobe, the posterior thalamic radiation to the occipital lobe, and the inferior thalamic radiation to the temporal lobe.

5.5 Thalamus: Projections of the Thalamic Nuclei

A Ventrolateral thalamic nuclei: afferent and efferent connections

The ventral posterolateral nucleus (VPL) and ventral posteromedial nucleus (VPM) are the major thalamic relay centers for somatosensory information.

- The *medial lemniscus* ends in the *VPL*. It contains sensory fibers for position sense, vibration, pressure, discrimination, and touch that are relayed from the nucleus gracilis and nucleus cuneatus.
- Pain and temperature fibers from the trunk and limbs travel through the lateral *spinothalamic tract* to lateral portions of the *VPL*. These sensations are relayed from this nucleus to the somatosensory cortex.
- Pain and temperature information from the head region is conveyed by the *trigeminal system* (= trigeminothalamic tract) to the *VPM*. As in the VPL, they synapse with third-order thelamic neurons that project to the postcentral gyrus.

A *lesion of the VPL* leads to contralateral disturbances of superficial and deep sensation with dysesthesia and an abnormal feeling of heaviness in the limbs (lesion of the medial lemniscus). Because the pain fibers of the spinothalamic tract terminate in the basal portions of the VPL, lesions in that region may additionally cause severe pain ("thalamic pain"). The **ventral lateral nucleus** (VL) projects to somatomotor cortical areas (6aα and 6aβ). The VPL nuclei form a feedback loop with the motor areas of the cortex, and so lesions of these nuclei are characterized by motor deficits.

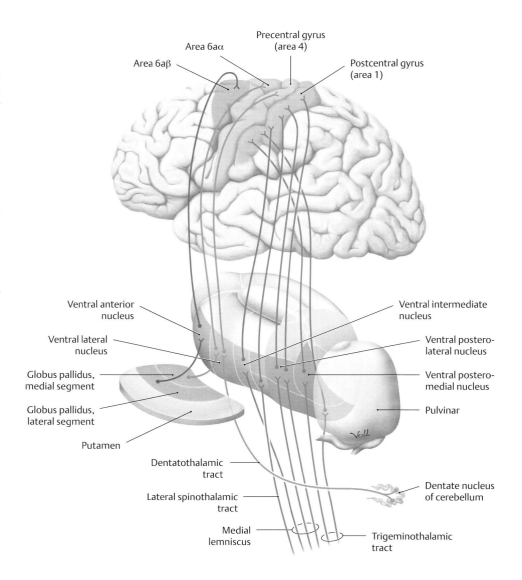

B Anterior nucleus and centromedian nucleus: afferent and efferent connections

The anterior nucleus receives *afferent fibers* from the mammillary body by way of the mammillothalamic fasciculus (bundle of Vicq-d'Azyr). The anterior nucleus establishes both afferent and efferent connections with the cingulate gyrus of the telencephalon. The largest nonspecific thalamic nucleus is the centromedian nucleus, which is one of the intralaminar nuclei. It receives *afferent fibers* from the cerebellum, reticular formation, and medial pallidus. Its *efferent fibers* project to the head of the caudate nucleus and the putamen. The centromedian nucleus is an important component of the **a**scending **r**eticular **a**ctivation **s**ystem (ARAS, arousal system). Essential for maintaining the waking state, the ARAS begins in the reticular formation of the brainstem and is relayed in the centromedian nucleus.

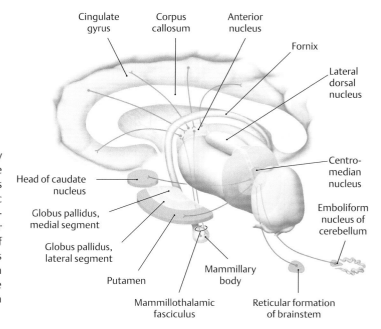

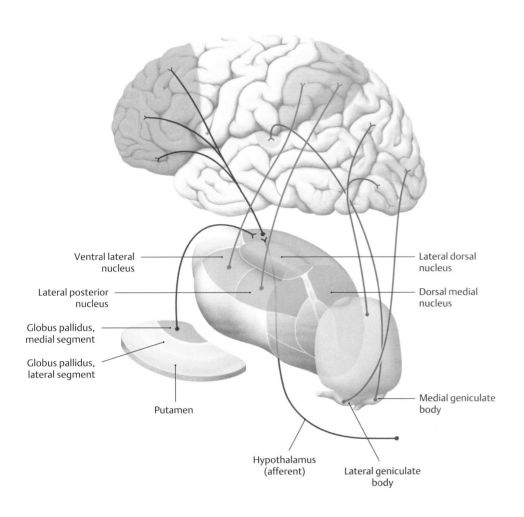

Ventral lateral nucleus

Lateral posterior nucleus

Globus pallidus, medial segment

Globus pallidus, lateral segment

Putamen

Lateral dorsal nucleus

Dorsal medial nucleus

Medial geniculate body

Hypothalamus (afferent)

Lateral geniculate body

C Medial, dorsal, and lateral thalamic nuclei: afferent and efferent connections

The **medial thalamic nuclei** receive their afferent input from ventral and intralaminar thalamic nuclei (not shown), the hypothalamus, the mesencephalon, and the globus/pallidus. Their efferent fibers project to the frontal lobe and premotor cortex, and afferent fibers from these regions return to the nuclei. The destruction of these tracts leads to *frontal lobe syndrome*, which is characterized by a loss of self-control (episodes of childish jocularity alternating with suspicion and petulance). The **dorsal nuclei** are formed by the pulvinar, which is the largest nuclear complex of the thalamus. The pulvinar receives afferent fibers from other thalamic nuclei, particularly the intralaminar nuclei (not shown). Its efferent fibers terminate in the association areas of the parietal and occipital lobes, which have reciprocal connections with the pulvinar. The lateral geniculate body (part of the visual pathway) projects to the visual cortex, while the medial geniculate body (part of the auditory pathway) projects to the auditory cortex. The **lateral nuclei** consists of the lateral dorsal nucleus and lateral posterior nucleus. They represent the dorsal portion of the ventrolateral group and receive their input from other thalamic nuclei (hence the term "integration nuclei," see p. 216). Their efferent fibers terminate in the parietal lobe of the brain.

D Synopsis of some clinically important connections of the specific thalamic nuclei

The specific thalamic nuclei project to the cerebral cortex. The table below lists the origins of the tracts that terminate in the nuclei, the nuclei themselves, and the sites to which their afferent fibers project.

Thalamic afferents (Structures that project *to the thalamus*)	Thalamic nucleus (abbreviation)	Thalamic efferents (Structure *to which* the thalamus projects)
Mammillary body (mammillothalamic fasciclus)	Anterior nucleus (NA)	Cingulate gyrus (limbic system)
Cerebellum, red nucleus	Ventral lateral nucleus (VL)	Premotor cortex (areas 6aα and 6aβ)
Posterior funiculus, lateral funiculus (somatosensory input, limbs, trunk)	Ventral posterolateral nucleus (VPL)	Postcentral gyrus (sensory cortex) = somatosensory cortex (see **A**)
Trigeminothalamic tract (somatosensory input, head)	Ventral posteromedial nucleus (VPM)	Postcentral gyrus (sensory cortex) = somatosensory cortex (see **A**)
Inferior brachium (part of the auditory pathway)	Medial geniculate nucleus (body) (MGB)	Transverse temporal gyri (auditory cortex)
Optic tract (part of the visual pathway)	Lateral geniculate nucleus (body) (LGB)	Striate area (visual cortex)

5.6 Hypothalamus

A Location of the hypothalamus

Coronal section. The hypothalamus is the lowest level of the diencephalon, situated below the thalamus. It is the only externally visible portion of the diencephalon (see **D**, p. 213). Located on either side of the third ventricle, its size is most clearly appreciated in a midsagittal section that bisects the third ventricle (see **Ba**).

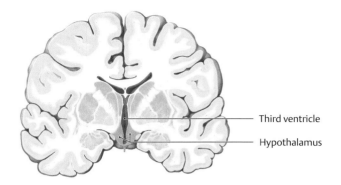

Third ventricle

Hypothalamus

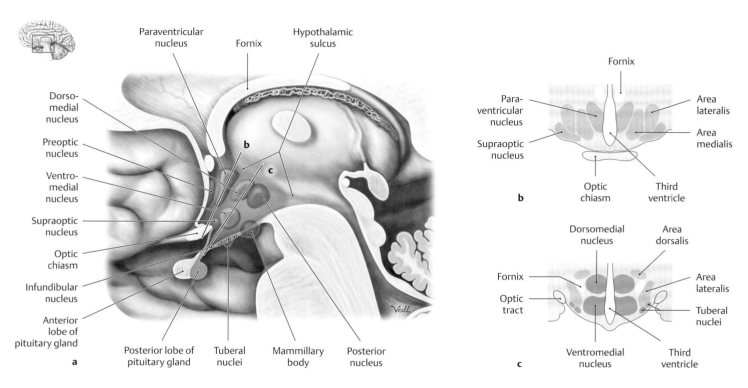

B Nuclei in the right hypothalamus

a Midsagittal section of the right hemisphere viewed from the medial side. **b, c** Coronal sections. The hypothalamus is a small nuclear complex located ventral to the thalamus and separated from it by the hypothalamic sulcus. Despite its small size, the hypothalamus is the command center for all autonomic functions in the body. The Terminologia Anatomica lists over 30 hypothalamic nuclei located in the lateral wall and floor of the third ventricle. Only a few of the larger, more clinically important nuclei are mentioned in this unit. Three groups of nuclei are listed below in an oral-to-caudal sequence, and their functions are briefly described:

- The anterior (rostral) group of nuclei (green) synthesizes the hormones released from the posterior lobe of the pituitary gland, and consists of the:
  - preoptic nucleus,
  - paraventricular nucleus, and
  - supraoptic nucleus.
- The middle (tuberal) group of nuclei (blue) controls hormone release from the anterior lobe of the pituitary gland, and consists of the:
  - dorsomedial nucleus,
  - ventromedial nucleus, and
  - tuberal nuclei.

- The posterior (mammillary) group of nuclei (red) activates the sympathetic nervous system when stimulated. It consists of the:
  - posterior nucleus and
  - mammillary nuclei located in the mammillary bodies.

The coronal section (**c**) shows the further subdivision of the hypothalamus by the fornix into lateral and medial zones. The three nuclear groups described above are part of the *medial* zone, whereas the nuclei in the *lateral* zone are not subdivided into specific groups (e.g., the area lateralis takes the place of a nucleus; the course of the fornix is described on p. 205). Bilateral lesions of the mammillary bodies and their nuclei are manifested by *Korsakoff syndrome*, which is frequently associated with alcoholism (cause: vitamin B_1 [thiamine] deficiency). The memory impairment that occurs in this syndrome mainly affects short-term memory, and the patient may fill in the memory gaps with fabricated information. A major neuropathological finding is the presence of hemorrhages in the mammillary bodies, which are sectioned at autopsy to confirm the diagnosis.

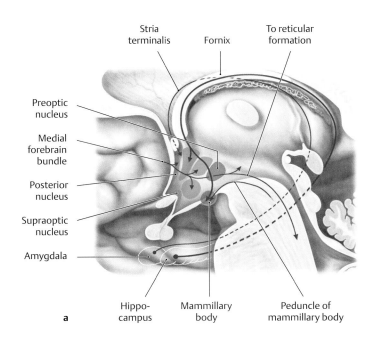

Stria terminalis   Fornix   To reticular formation

Preoptic nucleus
Medial forebrain bundle
Posterior nucleus
Supraoptic nucleus
Amygdala

a   Hippo-campus   Mammillary body   Peduncle of mammillary body

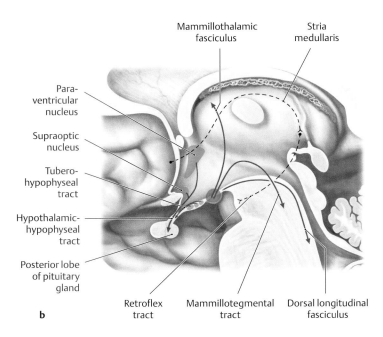

Mammillothalamic fasciculus   Stria medullaris

Para-ventricular nucleus
Supraoptic nucleus
Tubero-hypophyseal tract
Hypothalamic-hypophyseal tract
Posterior lobe of pituitary gland

b   Retroflex tract   Mammillotegmental tract   Dorsal longitudinal fasciculus

C Important afferent and efferent connections of the hypothalamus

Midsaggital section of the right hemisphere viewed from the medial side. Because the hypothalamus coordinates all the autonomic functions in the body, it establishes afferent (blue) and efferent (red) connections with many brain regions. The following are particularly important:

a Afferent connections (to the hypothalamus):
- The fornix conveys afferent fibers from the hippocampus; it is an important fiber tract of the limbic system.
- The medial forebrain bundle transmits afferent fibers from the olfactory areas to the preoptic nuclei.
- The stria terminalis conveys afferent fibers from the amygdala.
- The peduncle of the mammillary bodies transmits visceral afferent fibers and impulses from erogenous zones (nipples, genitalia).

b Efferent connections (from the hypothalamus):
- The dorsal longitudinal fasciculus passes to the brainstem where it is relayed several times before reaching the parasympathetic nuclei.
- The mammillotegmental tract distributes efferent fibers to the tegmentum of the midbrain; these are then relayed to the reticular formation. The fibers of this tract mediate the exchange of autonomic information between the hypothalamus, cranial nerve nuclei, and spinal cord.
- The mammillothalamic fasciculus (bundle of Vicq d'Azyr) conveys efferent fibers to the anterior thalamic nucleus, which is connected to the cingulated gyrus. This is part of the limbic system (see p. 374).
- The hypothalamic-hypophyseal and tuberohypophyseal tracts are efferent tracts to the pituitary gland (see p. 222).

D Functions of the hypothalamus
The hypothalamus is the coordinating center of the autonomic nervous system. There is no specific sympathetic or parasympathatic control center. Certain functions can be assigned to specific regions or nuclei in the hypothalamus, and these relationships are outlined in the table. Not all of the regions or nuclei listed in the table are shown in the drawings.

Region or nucleus	Function
Anterior preoptic region	Maintain constant body temperature; **Lesion:** central hypothermia
Posterior region	Respond to temperature changes, e.g., sweating; **Lesion:** hypothermia
Midanterior and posterior regions	Activate sympathetic nervous system
Paraventricular and anterior regions	Activate parasympathetic nervous system
Supraoptic and paraventricular nuclei	Regulate water balance; **Lesion:** Diabetes insipidus, also lack of thirst response resulting in hyponatremia
Anterior nuclei • Medial part • Lateral part	Regulate appetite and food intake • **Lesion:** Obesity • **Lesion:** Anorexia and emaciation

5.7   Pituitary Gland (Hypophysis)

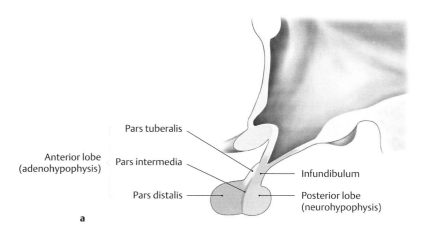

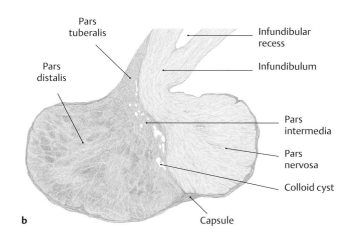

a

b

A Divisions of the pituitary gland

Midsagittal sections: **a** Schematic representation. **b** Histological appearance. The pituitary gland (hypophysis) consists of two lobes:

- Anterior lobe (adenohypophysis), the hormone-*producing* part (see **D** and **E**), and
- Posterior lobe (neurohypophysis), the hormone-*releasing* part (see **B**).

While the posterior pituitary lobe is an extension of the diencephalon, the anterior pituitary lobe is derived from the epithelium of the roof of the pharynx. The two lobes establish contact during embryonic development. The pituitary stalk (infundibulum) attaches both lobes of the gland to the hypothalamus, which contains the cell bodies of the neurosecretory neurons. The pituitary gland is surrounded by a fibrous capsule and lies in the *sella turcica* over the sphenoid sinus, which provides a route of surgical access to pituitary tumors.

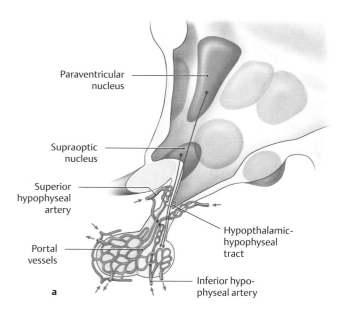

a

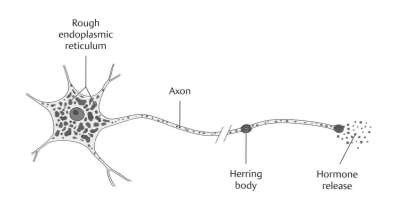

b

B Connections of the hypothalamic nuclei to the posterior lobe of the pituitary gland

a Hypothalamic-(neuro)pituitary axis. **b** Neurosecretory neuron in the hypothalamic nucleus.

Pituitary hormones are not synthesized in the *posterior pituitary lobe* (neurohypophysis) but in neurons located in the paraventricular nucleus and supraoptic nucleus of the hypothalamus. They are then transported by axons of the hypothalamic-hypophyseal tract to the neurohypophysis, where they are released as needed. Terminals of the paraventricular and supraoptic hypothalamic nuclei release two hormones in the posterior pituitary lobe :

- **Oxytocin** from the neurons of the paraventricular nucleus.
- **Antidiuretic hormone** (ADH) or **vasopressin** from the neurons of the supraoptic nucleus.

The axons from both nuclei pass through the pituitary stalk to the posterior lobe of the pituitary gland. The peptide hormones are stored in vesicles (aggregated into large "Herring bodies") in the cell bodies of the neurosecretory neurons and are carried to the posterior lobe by antegrade axoplasmic transport.

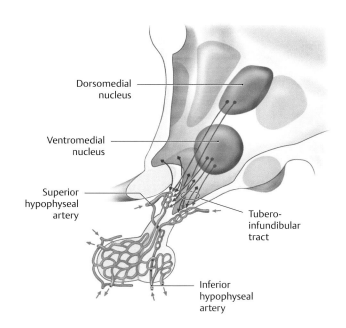

Dorsomedial nucleus

Ventromedial nucleus

Superior hypophyseal artery

Tubero-infundibular tract

Inferior hypophyseal artery

C Hypophyseal portal circulation and connections of the hypothalamic nuclei to the anterior pituitary lobe

The superior hypophyseal arteries from each side of the body form a vascular plexus around the infundibulum (pituitary stalk). The axons from neurons of the hypothalamic nuclei (dark red and dark blue arrows) terminate at this plexus and secrete hormones that have been produced in smaller (parvocellular) neurons of the hypothalamus. The secreted hypothalamic hormones are of two types:

- Releasing factors which stimulate hormone release from cells of the anterior pituitary lobe, and
- Release-inhibiting factors which inhibit release from these cells.

These hormones are carried by the hypophyseal portal venous system (named after the portal circulation of the liver) to capillaries in the anterior lobe, establishing communication between the hypothalamus and endocrine cells of the anterior pituitary.

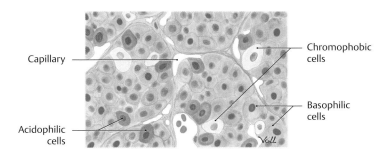

Capillary

Chromophobic cells

Basophilic cells

Acidophilic cells

D Histology of the anterior pituitary gland

Three types of cell can be distinguished in the anterior pituitary gland using classic histologic methods: acidophilic cells, basophilic cells, and chromophobic cells. The latter have already released their hormones, and are therefore negative in immunohistochemical tests that specifically detect peptide hormones; they are not listed in **E**. The acidophilic (a) cells secrete hormones that act directly on target cells (non-glandotropic hormones) while the basophilic (b) cells stimulate subordinate endocrine cells (glandotropic hormones).

E Hormones of the anterior pituitary lobe (adenohypophysis)

Hormones and synonyms	Cell designation*	Hormone actions
Somatotropin (STH) Growth hormone (GH) Somatotropic hormone	Somatotropic (a)	Stimulates longitudinal growth; acts on carbohydrate and lipid metabolism
Prolactin (PRL or LTH) Luteotropic hormone Mammotropic hormone	Mammotropic (a)	Stimulates lactation and proliferation of glandular breast tissue
Follitropin (FSH) Follicle-stimulating hormone	Gonadotropic (b)	Acts on the gonads; stimulates follicular maturation, spermatogenesis, estrogen production, expression of lutropin receptors and proliferation of granulosa cells
Lutropin (LH) Interstitial cell stimulating hormone - ICSH Luteinizing hormone	Gonadotropic (b)	Triggers ovulation; stimulates proliferation of follicular epithelial cells, production of testosterone in interstitial Leydig cells of the testis, and synthesis of progesterone; has general anabolic activity
Thyrotropin (TSH) Thyroid stimulating hormone Thyrotropic hormone	Thyrotropic (b)	Stimulates thyroid gland activity; increases O_2 consumption and protein synthesis; influences carbohydrate and lipid metabolism
Corticotropin (ACTH) Adrenocorticotropic hormone	Adrenotropic (b)	Stimulates hormone production in adrenal cortex; influences water and electrolyte balance; acts on carbohydrate formation in liver
Alpha/beta **Melanotropin (MSH)**	Melanotropic (b)	Aids in melanin formation and skin pigmentation; protects against UV radiation**

* Cells are classified as either acidophilic (a) or basophilic (b).

** In humans, melanotropin serves as a neurotransmitter in various brain regions.

5.8 Epithalamus and Subthalamus

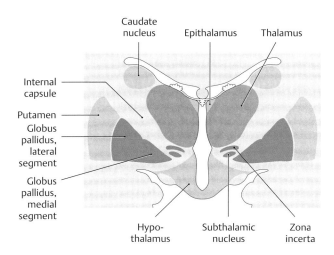

A Location of the epithalamus and subthalamus
Coronal section. The appropriateness of the term "epithalamus" can be appreciated in this plane of section, which shows the epithalamus riding upon the thalamus (*epi* = "upon"). The **epithalamus** (green) consists of the following structures:

- Pineal gland (epiphysis), see **B**.
- Habenulae with the habenular nuclei, see **D**.
- Habenular commissure, see **C**.
- Stria medullaris, see **D**.
- Epithalamic commissure (posterior), see **Ca**.

The region of the **subthalamus** (orange), formerly called the ventral thalamus, initially lies directly below the thalamus, but during embryonic development is displaced laterally into the telencephalon by fibers of the internal capsule, forming the *globus pallidus* (see **D**, p. 211). The subthalamus contains nuclei of the medial motor system (motor zones of the diencephalon), and has connections with the motor nuclei of the tegmentum. In fact, the subthalamus can be considered the cranial extension of the tegmentum.

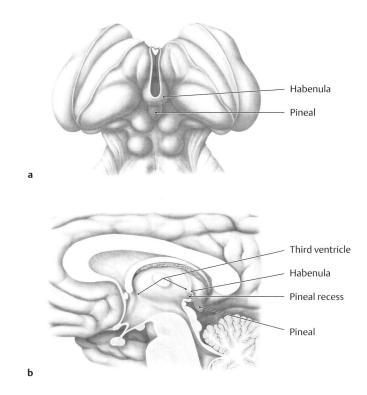

B Location of the pineal
a Posterior view. **b** Midsagittal section of the right hemisphere viewed from the medial side.
The pineal resembles a pine cone when viewed from behind. It is connected to the diencephalon by the habenula, which contains both afferent and efferent tracts. Its topographical relationship to the third ventricle is seen particularly well in midsagittal section (pineal recess). In reptiles, the calvaria over the pineal is thinned so that it is receptive to light stimuli. This is not the case in humans, although retinal afferents still communicate with the pineal through relay stations in the hypothalamus and the superior cervical (sympathetic) ganglion, helping to regulate circadian rhythms.

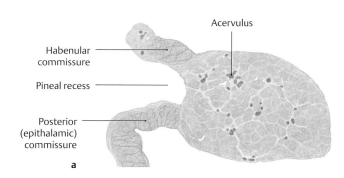

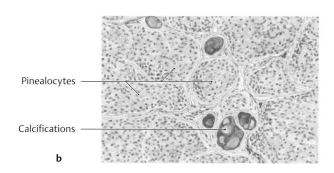

C Structure of the pineal gland
a Gross midsagittal tissue section. **b** Histological section.

a In the gross tissue section, the habenular commissure can be identified at the oral end of the pineal. Below it is the posterior (epithalamic) commissure. Between the two commissures is the CSF-filled pineal recess of the third ventricle. Calcifications (corpora arenacea, "brain sand") are frequently present and may be visible on radiographs; they have no pathological significance.

b The histological section demonstrates the specific cells of the pineal, the *pinealocytes*, which are embedded in a connective-tissue stroma and are surrounded by astrocytes. The pinealocytes produce *melatonin*, which plays a role in the regulation of circadian rhythms; it may be taken prophylactically, for example, to moderate the effects of jet lag. If the pineal ceases to function during childhood, the individual may undergo precocious puberty, as the pineal has significant, mostly inhibitory, effects on various endocrine systems.

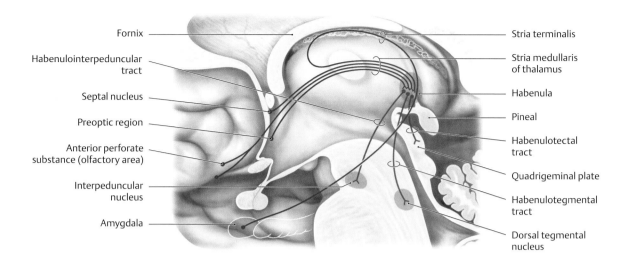

Fornix
Habenulointerpeduncular tract
Septal nucleus
Preoptic region
Anterior perforate substance (olfactory area)
Interpeduncular nucleus
Amygdala

Stria terminalis
Stria medullaris of thalamus
Habenula
Pineal
Habenulotectal tract
Quadrigeminal plate
Habenulotegmental tract
Dorsal tegmental nucleus

D Habenular nuclei and their fiber connections
Midsagittal section of the right hemisphere viewed from the medial side. The habenula ("reins") and their nuclei function as a relay station for afferent olfactory impulses. After their relay in the habenular nuclei, their efferent fibers are distributed to the salivatory and motor nuclei (mastication) in the brainstem.

Afferent connections (blue): Afferent impulses from the anterior perforate substance (olfactory area), septal nuclei, and preoptic region are transmitted by the stria medullaris to the habenular nuclei. These nuclei also receive impulses from the amygdala via the stria terminalis.

Efferent connections (red): Efferent fibers from the habenular nuclei are projected to the midbrain along three tracts:

- Habenulotectal tract: terminates in the roof of the mesencephalon, the quadrigeminal plate, supplying it with olfactory impulses.
- Habenulotegmental tract: terminates in the dorsal tegmental nucleus, establishing connections with the dorsal longitudinal fasciculus and with the salivatory and motor cranial nerve nuclei. (The smell of food stimulates salivation and gastric acid secretion: e.g., Pavlovian response).
- Habenulointerpeduncular tract: terminates in the interpeduncular nucleus, which then connects with the reticular formation.

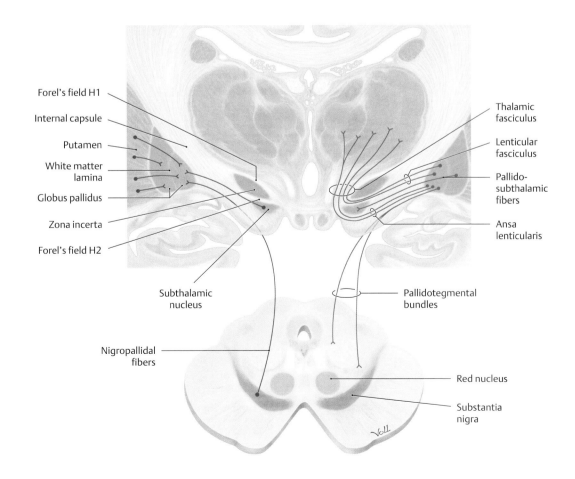

Forel's field H1
Internal capsule
Putamen
White matter lamina
Globus pallidus
Zona incerta
Forel's field H2
Subthalamic nucleus
Nigropallidal fibers

Thalamic fasciculus
Lenticular fasciculus
Pallido-subthalamic fibers
Ansa lenticularis
Pallidotegmental bundles
Red nucleus
Substantia nigra

E Subthalamic nuclei with their afferent (blue) and efferent (red) connections
The principal nucleus of the subthalamus is the *globus pallidus*, which is displaced laterally during development into the telencephalon by the internal capsule. A lamina of white matter subdivides the globus pallidus into a medial (internal) and lateral (external) segment. Certain small nuclei are exempt from this migration and remain near the midline: these are the *zona incerta* and *subthalamic nucleus.* The subthalamic nucleus, substantia nigra, and putamen send afferent fibers to the globus pallidus. The globus pallidus in turn distributes efferent fibers to these regions and also to the thalamus through a tract called the lenticular fasciculus. Functionally, these nuclei are classified as portions of the basal ganglia. Lesions of these nuclei lead to a movement disorder called contralateral hemiballism (the functional role of the subthalamus is described on p. 340).

225

6.1 Brainstem, Organization and External Structure

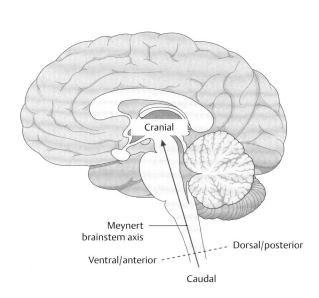

A Terms of location and direction in the brainstem

These terms are based on the nearly vertical *Meynert brainstem axis* (compare with the horizontal Forel axis, which was used as a reference line in previous units). Just dorsal to the brainstem is the cerebellum, which will be described in chapter 7.

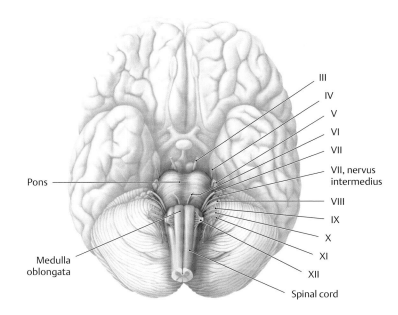

B Relationship of the brainstem to the cerebral and cerebellar hemispheres

Basal view. The brainstem is a midline structure flanked by the cerebrum and cerebellum. Its anatomical subdivisions are best appreciated in the midsagittal section (see **C**). The third through twelfth pairs of cranial nerves (CN III—XII) enter or emerge from the brainstem (see **Ea**).

D Overview of the brainstem

Topographical organization
- *Craniocaudal direction:*
  - Mesencephalon (midbrain)
  - Pons
  - Medulla oblongata
- *Anteroposterior direction:*
  - Base (mesencephalon: cerebral peduncles; pons: basal part; medulla oblongata: pyramids)
  - Tegmentum (present as such in all three parts)
  - Section of ventricular system (upper part: cerebral aqueduct, fourth ventricle, central canal)
  - Tectum ("roof"; present only in the mesencephalon; quadrigeminal plate)
- The cerebellum adjoins the brainstem dorsally.

Functional organization
- *Mediolaterally into four longitudinal nuclear columns:*
  - Somatic efferent (motor) column
  - Visceral efferent (motor) column
  - Visceral afferent (sensory) column
  - Somatic afferent (sensory) column
- *Organization into different structures:*
  - Nuclei of cranial nerves III—XII
  - Red nucleus, substantia nigra (motor coordination centers)
  - Reticular formation (diffuse nuclear aggregations for autonomic functions)
  - Ascending and descending tracts (see p. 232)
  - Dorsal column nuclei (nucleus gracilis and nucleus cuneatus)
  - Pontine nuclei

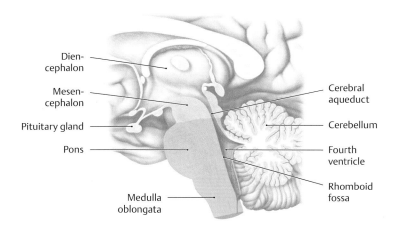

C Division of the brainstem into levels

Midsagittal section. The brainstem is divided macroscopically into three levels, with the bulge of the pons marking the boundary lines between the parts:

- Mesencephalon (midbrain)
- Pons
- Medulla oblongata

The location and contents of these parts are summarized in **D**. The three levels are easily distinguished from one another by gross visual inspection, although they are not differentiated in a functional sense. The *functional organization* of the brainstem (see **D**) is determined chiefly by the arrangement of the cranial nerve nuclei. Given the close proximity of nuclei and large fiber tracts in this region, even a small lesion of the brainstem (e.g., hemorrhage, tumor) may lead to extensive and complex alterations of sensorimotor function.

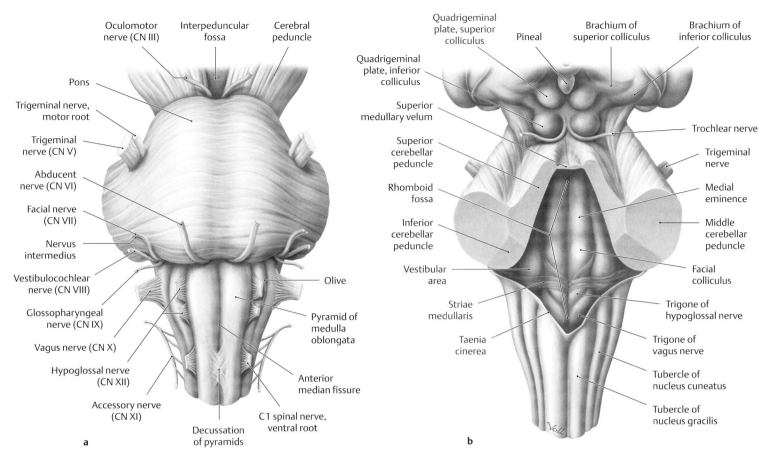

Oculomotor nerve (CN III)

Interpeduncular fossa

Cerebral peduncle

Pons

Trigeminal nerve, motor root

Trigeminal nerve (CN V)

Abducent nerve (CN VI)

Facial nerve (CN VII)

Nervus intermedius

Vestibulocochlear nerve (CN VIII)

Glossopharyngeal nerve (CN IX)

Vagus nerve (CN X)

Hypoglossal nerve (CN XII)

Accessory nerve (CN XI)

Olive

Pyramid of medulla oblongata

Anterior median fissure

Decussation of pyramids

C1 spinal nerve, ventral root

a

Quadrigeminal plate, superior colliculus

Pineal

Brachium of superior colliculus

Brachium of inferior colliculus

Quadrigeminal plate, inferior colliculus

Superior medullary velum

Superior cerebellar peduncle

Rhomboid fossa

Inferior cerebellar peduncle

Vestibular area

Striae medullaris

Taenia cinerea

Trochlear nerve

Trigeminal nerve

Medial eminence

Middle cerebellar peduncle

Facial colliculus

Trigone of hypoglossal nerve

Trigone of vagus nerve

Tubercle of nucleus cuneatus

Tubercle of nucleus gracilis

b

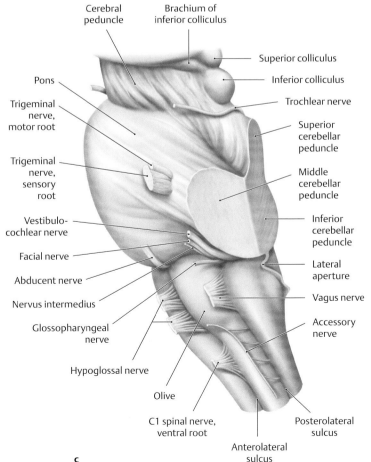

Cerebral peduncle

Brachium of inferior colliculus

Pons

Trigeminal nerve, motor root

Trigeminal nerve, sensory root

Vestibulo-cochlear nerve

Facial nerve

Abducent nerve

Nervus intermedius

Glossopharyngeal nerve

Hypoglossal nerve

Olive

C1 spinal nerve, ventral root

Anterolateral sulcus

Superior colliculus

Inferior colliculus

Trochlear nerve

Superior cerebellar peduncle

Middle cerebellar peduncle

Inferior cerebellar peduncle

Lateral aperture

Vagus nerve

Accessory nerve

Posterolateral sulcus

c

E Brainstem

a Anterior view. The sites of entry and emergence of the ten pairs of *true* cranial nerves (III–XII) are particularly well displayed in this view.
Note: Cranial nerve II (optic nerve) is a derivative of the diencephalon. Note also the site below the pyramids where the pyramidal fibers cross over the midline from each side (decussation of the pyramids). Most of the axons of the large motor pathway for the trunk and limbs cross to the opposite side at this level.

b Posterior view. Since the cerebellum has been removed, we can see the rhomboid fossa, which forms the floor of the fourth ventricle. The surface of the fossa is raised by several cranial nerve nuclei, which bulge into the fourth ventricle. The cerebellum is connected to the brainstem by three cerebellar peduncles on each side:

- Superior cerebellar peduncle
- Middle cerebellar peduncle
- Inferior cerebellar peduncle

The superior and inferior cerebellar peduncles border portions of the rhomboid fossa and thus contribute to the boundaries of the fourth ventricle.

c Left lateral view. In addition to the cerebellar peduncles, this view displays the superior and inferior colliculi. Together with their counterparts on the right side, the colliculi form the quadrigeminal plate (see **b**), which is a prominent structure of the mesencephalon. The two superior colliculi are part of the visual pathway, while the inferior colliculi are part of the auditory pathway. The trochlear nerve (CN IV) runs forward below the inferior colliculus, and is the only cranial nerve that emerges from the dorsal side of the brainstem. The olive appears as a prominence on the side of the medulla oblongata. The nuclei within the olive function as a relay station for the motor system (see p. 342).

6.2 Brainstem: Cranial Nerve Nuclei, Red Nucleus, and Substantia nigra

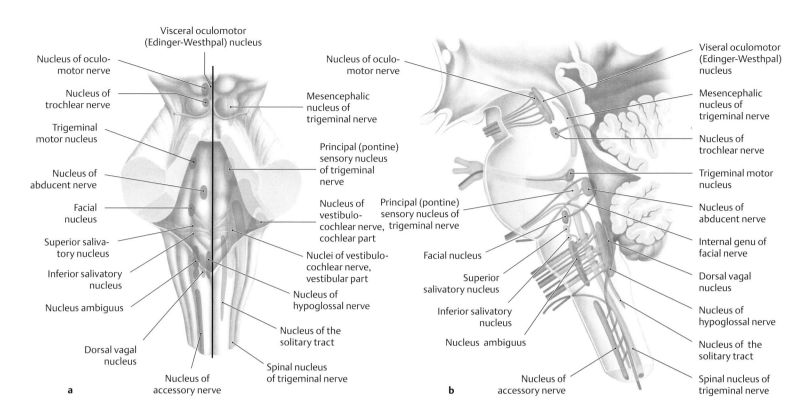

a

b

A Cranial nerve nuclei in the brainstem

a Posterior view with the cerebellum removed, exposing the rhomboid fossa; **b** Midsagittal section of the right half of the brainstem viewed from the left side.

The diagrams show the nuclei themselves and the course of the tracts leading to and away from them (to save space, the vestibular and cochlear nuclei are not shown).

The arrangement of the cranial nerve nuclei is easier to understand when we divide them into functional nuclear columns. The *motor nuclei*,

which give rise to the efferent fibers, are shown on the left side of diagram **a**, and the *sensory nuclei*, where the afferent fibers terminate, are shown in **b**. The arrangement of these nuclei can be derived from the arrangement of the nuclei in the spinal cord (see p. 68). The function and connections of some of these cranial nerves can be clinically evaluated by testing the *brainstem reflexes* (whose relay centers are located in the brainstem). These reflexes are important in the evaluation of comatose patients. A prime example is the pupillary reflexes, which are described more fully on p. 363.

B Overview of the nuclei of cranial nerves III—XII

Motor nuclei: give rise to efferent (motor) fibers, left in **Aa**	Sensory nuclei: where afferent (sensory) fibers terminate, right in **Aa**

Somatic efferent or somatic motor nuclei (red):
• Nucleus of oculomotor nerve (CN III)
• Nucleus of trochlear nerve (CN IV)
• Nucleus of abducent nerve (CN VI)
• Nucleus of accessory nerve (CN XI)
• Nucleus of hypoglossal nerve (CN XII)
 	
Visceral efferent (visceral motor) nuclei:
 	
Nuclei associated with the parasympathetic nervous system (light blue):
• Visceral oculomotor (Edinger-Westphal) nucleus (CN III)
• Superior salivatory nucleus (facial nerve, CN VII)
• Inferior salivatory nucleus (glossopharyngeal nerve, CN IX)
• Dorsal vagal nucleus (CN X)
 	
Nuclei of the branchial arch nerves (dark blue):
• Trigeminal motor nucleus (CN V)
• Facial nucleus (CN VII)
• Nucleus ambiguus (glossopharyngeal nerve, CN IX; vagus nerve, CN X; accessory nerve, CN XI, cranial root)
	Somatic afferent (somatic sensory) and vestibulocochlear nuclei (yellow):
	Sensory nuclei associated with the trigeminal nerve (CN V):
	• Mesencephalic nucleus of trigeminal nerve (special feature: pseudounipolar ganglion cells ("displaced sensory ganglion"), provide direct sensory innervation for muscles of mastication)
	• Principal (pontine) sensory nucleus of trigeminal nerve
	• Spinal nucleus of trigeminal nerve
	
	Nuclei of the vestibulocochlear nerve (CN VIII):
	o Vestibular part:
	  • Medial vestibular nucleus • Lateral vestibular nucleus
	  • Superior vestibular nucleus • Inferior vestibular nucleus
	o Cochlear part:
	  • Anterior cochlear nucleus • Posterior cochlear nucleus
	
	Visceral afferent (visceral sensory) nuclei (green):
	• Nucleus of the solitary tract (nuclear complex):
	o Superior part:
	  • Special visceral afferents (taste) from facial (CN VII), glossopharyngeal (CN IX), and vagus (CN X) nerves
	o Inferior part:
	  • General visceral afferents from glossopharyngeal (CN IX) and vagus (CN X) nerves

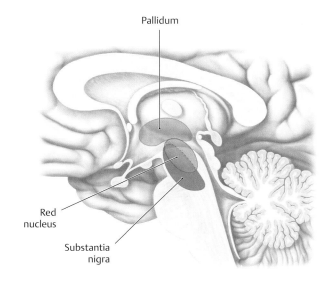

Pallidum

Red
nucleus

Substantia
nigra

C Location of the substantia nigra and red nucleus in the mesencephalon

Both of these nuclei, like the cranial nerve nuclei, are well-defined structures that belong functionally to the *extrapyramidal motor* system. Anatomically, the substantia nigra is part of the cerebral peduncles and therefore is not located in the tegmentum of the mesencephalon (see **A**, p. 234). Owing to their high respective contents of melanin and iron, the substantia nigra and red nucleus appear brown and red, respectively, in sections of fresh brain tissue. Both nuclei extend into the diencephalon and are connected to its nuclei by fiber tracts (see **E**).

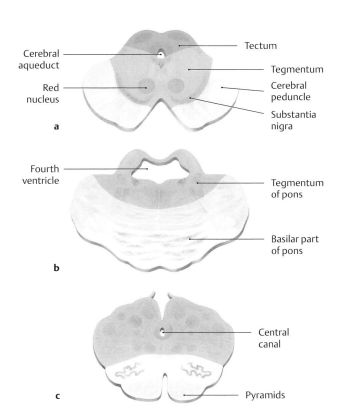

Cerebral
aqueduct — Tectum

Red
nucleus — Tegmentum

Cerebral
peduncle

Substantia
nigra

a

Fourth
ventricle

Tegmentum
of pons

Basilar part
of pons

b

Central
canal

Pyramids

c

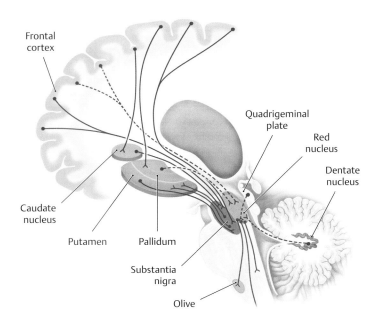

Frontal
cortex

Quadrigeminal
plate

Red
nucleus

Dentate
nucleus

Caudate
nucleus

Putamen   Pallidum

Substantia
nigra

Olive

D Cross-sectional structure of the brainstem at different levels

Transverse sections through the **a** mesencephalon, **b** pons, and **c** medulla oblongata, viewed from above.

A feature common to all three sections is the dorsally situated tegmentum ("hood," medium gray), the phylogenetically old part of the brainstem. The tegmentum of the adult brain contains the brainstem nuclei. Anterior to the tegmentum are the large ascending and descending tracts that run to and from the telencephalon. This region is called the cerebral peduncle (crus cerebri) in the mesencephalon, the basilar part (foot) of the pons at the pontine level, and the pyramids in the medulla oblongata. The tegmentum is covered dorsally by the tectum (= "roof") only in the region of the mesencephalon. In the mature brain pictured here, this structure forms the quadrigeminal plate containing the superior and inferior colliculi ("little hills"), shown faintly in **Da**. The brainstem is covered by the cerebellum at the level of the medulla oblongata and pons and therefore lacks a tectal covering at those levels.

E Afferent (blue) and efferent (red) connections of the red nucleus and substantia nigra

These two nuclei are important relay stations in the motor system. The *red nucleus* consists of a larger *neorubrum* and a smaller *paleorubrum*. It receives afferent axons from the dentate nucleus (dentatorubral tract), superior colliculi (tectorubral tract), inner pallidum (pallidorubral tract), and cerebral cortex (corticorubral tract). The red nucleus sends its axons to the olive (rubro-olivary fibers and reticulo-olivary fibers, part of the central tegmental tract) and to the spinal cord (rubrospinal tract). It coordinates muscle tone, body position, and gait. A lesion of the red nucleus produces resting tremor, abnormal muscle tone (tested as involuntary muscular resistance of the joints in the relaxed patient), and choreoathetosis (involuntary writhing movements, usually involving the distal parts of the limbs). The **substantia nigra** consists of a *compact part* (dark, contains melanin) and a *reticular part* (reddish, contains iron; for simplicity, the entire substantia nigra appears dark in the drawing). Most of its axons project diffusely to other brain areas and are not collected into tracts. Axons from the caudate nucleus (striatonigral fibers), anterior cerebral cortex (corticonigral fibers), putamen, and precentral cortex terminate in the substantia nigra.

229

6.3 Brainstem: Reticular Formation

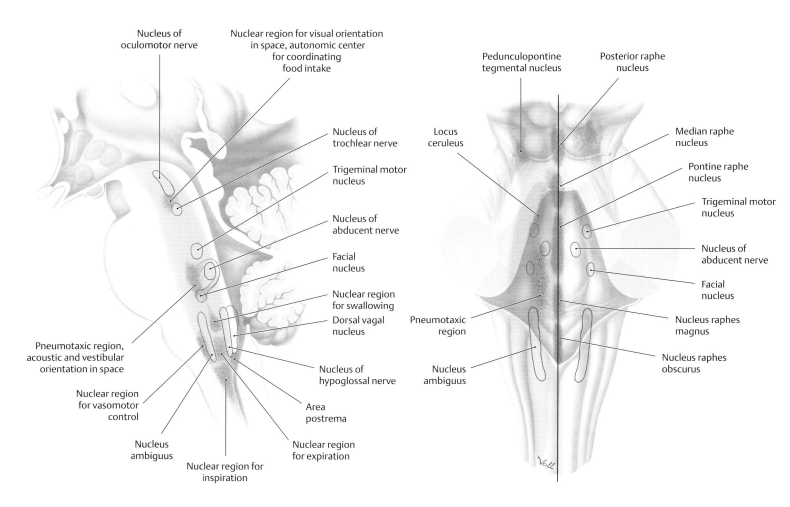

A Structural-functional relationships in the reticular formation

Midsagittal section of the brainstem viewed from the left side. While the cranial nerve nuclei, substantia nigra, and red nucleus have well-defined boundaries, as we have seen, the reticular formation (light green) is a relatively diffuse network of nerve cells and fibers in the brainstem, ocupying the areas between the cranial nerve nuclei described above. It can be roughly divided into two main *groups of nuclei:*

- *Medial group* (specific nuclei labeled in the diagram): nuclei containing *large neurons* whose axons form long ascending and descending tracts (see **E**).
- *Lateral group* (not individually labeled in the diagram): nuclei containing *small neurons* whose axons usually stay within the brainstem. They are therefore called "association areas."

Besides *respiratory and circulatory regulation*, the diffuse neuronal network of the reticular formation performs many other important autonomic functions that are mapped in the diagram neurotransmitters. Diagram **B** shows several nuclear regions and their neurotransmitters in some detail.

B Nuclear regions and neurotransmitters in the reticular formation

Posterior view of the brainstem (cerebellum removed). Reticular formation shown in green. Several nuclear regions and neurotransmitters are shown here. Left side: classification of the nuclear regions; right side: distribution of neurotransmitters in the nuclear regions. The nuclear regions of the reticular formation can be classified by their location (medial or lateral groups of nuclei, see **A**) or by the neurotransmitters they contain:

- Serotonergic (purple = serotonin)
- Cholinergic (red = acetylcholine)
- Noradrenergic (light blue = norepinephrine)
- Dopaminergic (orange = dopamine)
- Adrenergic (yellow = epinephrine)

The nuclei that flank the midline are called the *raphe nuclei* (shown in purple, raphe = "seam"). They contain the neurotransmitter seratonin, and their neurons project to the hypothaloamus, limbic system, and neocortex. The *locus ceruleus* (shown in blue, caeruleus = "blue") is a region that actually appears blue in the fresh brain. This nucleus contains noradrenergic neurons which send axons to the cerebellum, hypothalomus, and cerebral cortex.

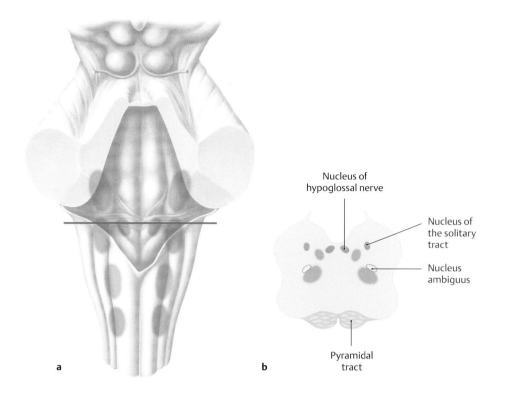

Nucleus of
hypoglossal nerve

Nucleus of
the solitary
tract

Nucleus
ambiguus

Pyramidal
tract

a   b

C Respiratory center in the reticular formation

a Posterior view with the cerebellum removed. **b** Transverse section at the level indicated, showing that the two nuclear groups in **a** do not lie in the same vertical plane.

An important autonomic function of the reticular formation is the regulation of breathing. The neurons controlling respiration are divided into an inspiratory group (red) and an expiratory group (blue). Their size is only approximate (as shown here) due to the extensive arborization of the axons and dendrites of these neurons. Respiratory rhythm is controlled by a group of cells in the ventral medulla called the pre-Bötzinger complex. When portions of the rhythmogenic neurons in this complex are destroyed in the rat, periods of apnea may be observed even during the day when activity normally peaks. It is believed that the loss of more than 60 % of these cells (which number in the thousands) is responsible for the development of sleep apnea in elderly patients.

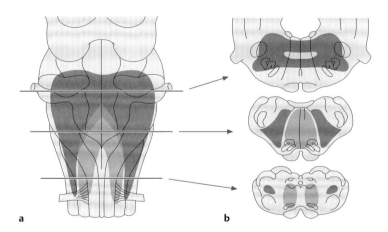

a   b

D Circulatory center in the reticular formation of the cat (after Kahle)

a Dorsal view, **b** transverse sections at the levels indicated.

Another important function of the reticular formation is circulatory regulation. The neurons responsible for this function have a diffuse arrangement similar to that of the respiratory neurons. Stimulating certain regions (dark red) via electrodes inserted into the reticular formation will cause the blood pressure to rise while stimulating other regions (pale red, depressor center) will cause it to fall.

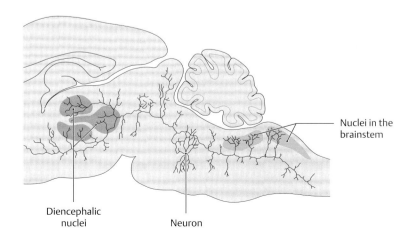

Nuclei in the
brainstem

Diencephalic
nuclei

Neuron

E Branching pattern of a neuron in the reticular formation of the rat brainstem (after Scheibel)

Midsagittal section viewed from the left side. Neurons can be selectively visualized by the silver-impregnation (Golgi) staining method. The axon of the neuron shown here divides into an ascending branch, which comes into contact with the diencephalic nuclei (shown in brown) and a descending branch, which establishes connections with cranial nerve nuclei (green) in the pons and medulla oblongata. This extensive arborization allows neurons of the reticular formation to have widespread effects on multiple brain regions.

231

6.4 Brainstem: Descending and Ascending Tracts

A Descending tracts in the brainstem
a Midsagittal section viewed from the left side. **b** Posterior view with the cerebellum removed.

The descending tracts shown here begin in the telencephalon and terminate partly in the brainstem but mostly in the spinal cord. The most prominent tract that descends through the brainstem, the *corticospinal tract*, terminates in the spinal cord. Its axons arise from large pyramidal neurons of the primary motor cortex and terminate on or near alpha motor neurons in the anterior horn of the spinal cord. Most of the axons cross to the opposite side (decussate) at the level of the pyramids. The fibers in this part of the pyramidal tract that descend through the brainstem are called *corticospinal fibers*. Those fibers in the pyramidal tract that terminate in the brainstem are called *corticonuclear fibers*. Corticonuclear axons connect the motor cortex to the brainstem motor nuclei of the cranial nerves.

Note: Direct cortical projections to the brainstem nuclei are predominantly:

- *bilateral* for:
    – the trigeminal motor nucleus (CN V)
    – neurons in the facial nucleus (CN VII) that innervate muscles in the forehead
    – nucleus ambiguus (CN X)
- *contralateral (crossed)* for:
    – the nucleus of the abducent nerve (CN VI)
    – neurons in the facial nucleus (CN VII) that innervate muscles in the lower face
    – the nucleus of the hypoglossal nerve (CN XII)
- *ipsilateral* for:
    – neurons in the nucleus of the accessory nerve (CN XI) that innervate the sternocleidomastoid muscle

The pattern of corticonuclear innervation is important in the diagnosis of different lesions, particularly involving the facial nerve (CN VII; see **D**, p. 79). Most cortical projections to the brainstem motor nuclei, however, are indirect, involving intermediate neurons, many of which are located in the surrounding reticular formation. Direct cortical control of brainstem motor neurons, specifically for the tongue and face, seems to be a recent evolutionary development, present in primates but not in other mammals. The nuclei of the oculomotor (CN III) and trochlear (CN IV) nerves, which do not receive direct cortical projections, are synaptically connected with the abducent nucleus through the *medial longitudinal fasciculus* (see **D**, p. 321), a brainstem tract that contains both ascending and descending fibers.

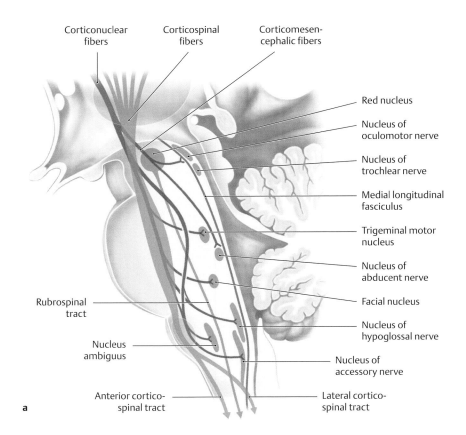

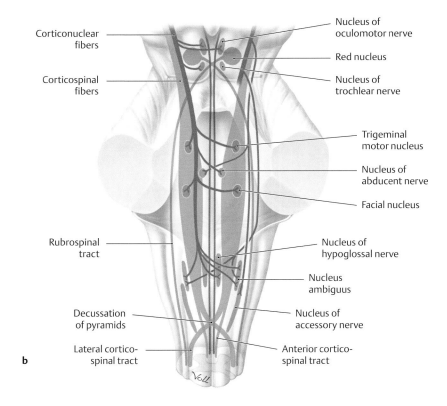

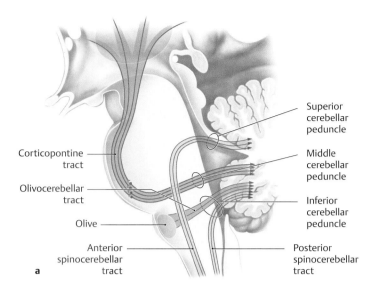

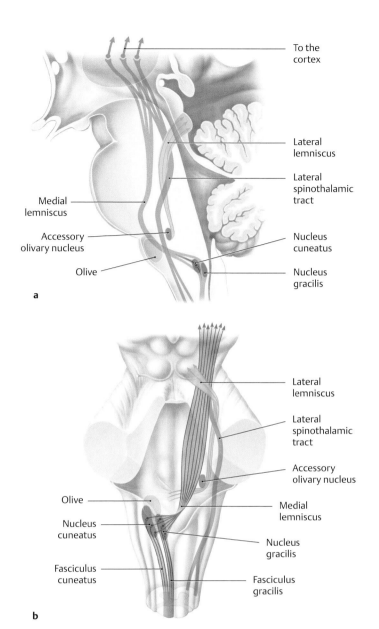

a

b

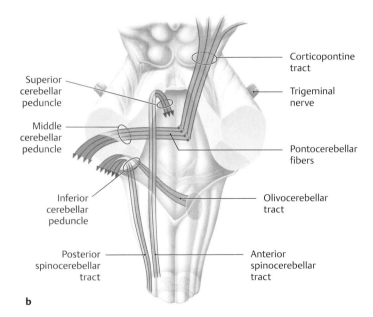

a

b

B Ascending tracts in the brainstem

a Left lateral view, **b** posterior view.

Two major ascending fiber bundles, the **posterior funiculus** (violet) and the **lateral spinothalamic tract** (dark blue), carry sensory information from the spinal cord to the brainstem. The posterior funiculus consists of the *medial fasciculus gracilis*, from the lower limb and trunk, and the *lateral fasciculus cuneatus*, from thoracic and cervical levels. Many of the fibers in these tracts are the central processes of dorsal root ganglion cells whose peripheral processes are in muscle spindles and tendon stretch receptors (proprioception) and cutaneous touch receptors. The first synapse in this ascending pathway is in the *nucleus gracilis or nucleus cuneatus*; the neurons from these nuclei send their axons in the *medial lemniscus* (lemniskos = "ribbon," Gr.) across the midline to the thalamus (see p. 216, 218). The lateral spinothalamic tract bears pain and temperature information from secondary neurons in the contralateral spinal cord, passing without an additional synaptic relay directly to the thalamus.

The other ribbon-like sensory tract in the brainstem – the *lateral lemniscus* – contains axons from the cochlear nuclei, some of which cross the midline in the trapezoid body, to synapse in the inferior colliculus of the quadrigeminal plate.

C Courses of the major cerebellar tracts through the brainstem

a Midsagittal section viewed from the left side. **b** Posterior view with the cerebellum removed.

The cerebellum is involved in the coordination of movement. Descending tracts (red) and ascending tracts (blue) enter the cerebellum through the superior, middle, and inferior cerebellar peduncles.

- **Superior cerebellar peduncle:** contains most of the *efferent* axons from the cerebellum (see p. 242). The only major *afferent* axon tract entering the cerebellum through the superior peduncle is the anterior spinocerebellar pathway.

- **Middle cerebellar peduncle:** largest of the three peduncles, occupied mostly by *afferent* fibers from contralateral basal pontine nuclei. These afferent fibers are the second step of a massive descending cortico-pontine to ponto-cerebellar projection.

- **Inferior cerebellar peduncle:** contains the *afferent* posterior spinocerebellar and olivocerebellar tracts. The posterior spinocerebellar tract enters ipsilaterally, the olivocerebellar tract from the contralateral (inferior) olivary nuclei.

233

6.5 Mesencephalon and Pons, Transverse Section

A Transverse section through the mesencephalon (midbrain)

Superior view.

Nuclei: The most rostral cranial nerve nucleus is the relatively small *nucleus of the oculomotor nerve* (see **B**, p. 226). In the same transverse plane is the *mesencephalic nucleus of the trigeminal nerve*; other trigeminal nuclei can be identified in sections at lower levels (see **C**). Unique in the CNS, the mesencephalic nucleus of the trigeminal nerve contains displaced pseudounipolar sensory neurons, closely related to the PNS neurons of the trigeminal ganglion (both populations are derived embryonically from the neural crest). The peripheral processes of these mesencephalic neurons are proprioceptors in the muscles of mastication. The *superior collicular nucleus* is part of the visual system. The *red nucleus* and *substantia nigra* are involved in coordination of motor activity. The red nucleus and all of the cranial nerve nuclei are located in the tegmentum of the mesencephalon, the superior colliculus is in the tectum (roof) of the mesencephalon, and the substantia nigra is in the cerebral peduncle (see **C**, p. 229). Different parts of the reticular formation, a diffuse aggregation of nuclear groups (see p. 230, 231), are visible here and in sections below.

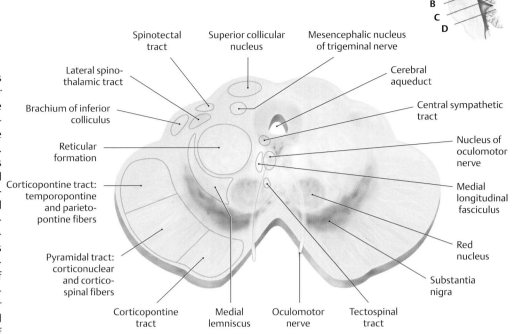

Tracts: The tracts at this level run anterior to the nuclear regions. Prominent descending tracts seen at this level include the pyramidal tract and the corticonuclear fibers that branch from it. Ascending tracts visible at this level include the lateral spinothalamic tract and the medial lemniscus, both of which terminate in the thalamus.

B Transverse section through the upper pons

Nuclei: The only cranial nerve nucleus appearing in this plane of section is the mesencephalic trigeminal nucleus. It can be seen that the fibers from the nucleus of the trochlear nerve (CN IV) cross to the opposite side (decussate) while still within the brainstem.

Tracts: The ascending and descending tract systems are the same as in **A** and **C**. The pyramidal tract appears less compact at this level compared with the previous section due to the presence of intermingled pontine nuclei. This section cuts the tracts (mostly efferent) that exit the cerebellum through the superior cerebellar peduncle. The lateral lemniscus at the dorsal surface of the section is part of the auditory pathway. The relatively large *medial longitudinal fasciculus* extends from the mesencephalon (see **A**) into the spinal cord. It interconnects the brainstem nuclei and contains a variety of fibers that enter and emerge at various levels (*"highway of the brainstem nuclei"*). The smaller *dorsal* longitudinal fasciculus connects hypothalamic nuclei with the parasym-

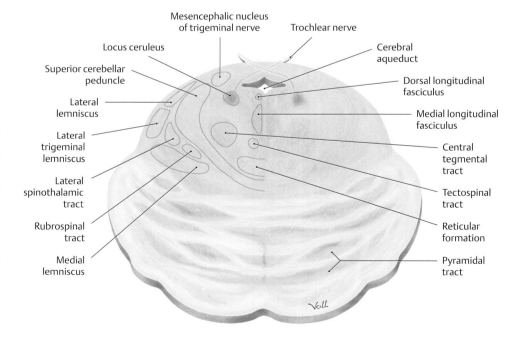

pathetic cranial nerve nuclei. The size and location of the nuclei of the reticular formation, which here are shown graphically within a compact area, vary with the plane of the section. This diagram indicates only the approximate location of the reticular formation, and other smaller nuclei and fibers may be found within these regions.

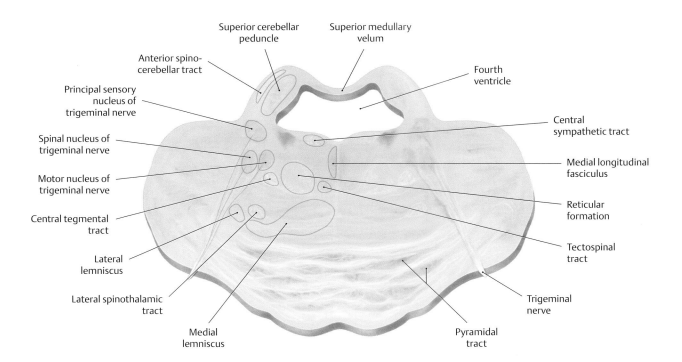

Superior cerebellar peduncle

Superior medullary velum

Anterior spino- cerebellar tract

Principal sensory nucleus of trigeminal nerve

Fourth ventricle

Central sympathetic tract

Spinal nucleus of trigeminal nerve

Medial longitudinal fasciculus

Motor nucleus of trigeminal nerve

Reticular formation

Central tegmental tract

Tectospinal tract

Lateral lemniscus

Trigeminal nerve

Lateral spinothalamic tract

Pyramidal tract

Medial lemniscus

C Transverse section through the midportion of the pons
Nuclei: The trigeminal nerve leaves the brainstem at the midlevel of the pons, its various nuclei dominating the pontine tegmentum. The *principal sensory nucleus* of the trigeminal nerve relays afferents for touch and discrimination, while its *spinal nucleus* relays pain and temperature fibers. The trigeminal motor nucleus contains the motor neurons for the muscles of mastication.

Tracts: This section cuts the anterior spinocerebellar tract, which passes to the cerebellum, immediately dorsal to the pons.
CSF space: At this level the cerebral aqueduct has given way to the fourth ventricle, which appears in cross section. It is covered dorsally by the medullary velum.

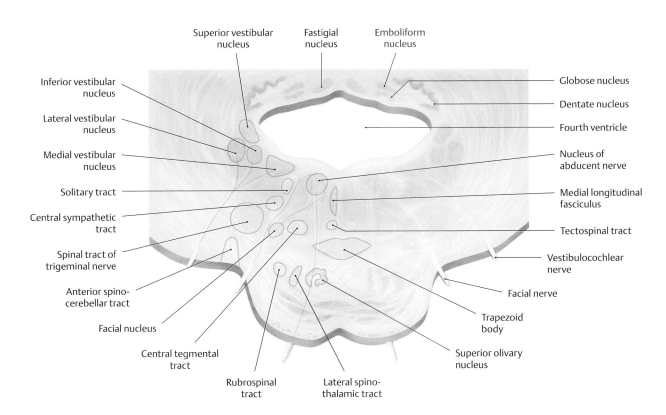

Superior vestibular nucleus

Fastigial nucleus

Emboliform nucleus

Inferior vestibular nucleus

Globose nucleus

Dentate nucleus

Lateral vestibular nucleus

Fourth ventricle

Medial vestibular nucleus

Nucleus of abducent nerve

Solitary tract

Medial longitudinal fasciculus

Central sympathetic tract

Tectospinal tract

Spinal tract of trigeminal nerve

Vestibulocochlear nerve

Anterior spino- cerebellar tract

Facial nerve

Facial nucleus

Trapezoid body

Central tegmental tract

Superior olivary nucleus

Rubrospinal tract

Lateral spino- thalamic tract

D Transverse section through the lower pons
Nuclei: The lower pons contains a number of cranial nerve nuclei including the nuclei of the vestibulocochlear and abducent nerves, and the facial (motor) nucleus. The rhomboid fossa is covered dorsally by the cerebellum, whose nuclei also appear in this section—the fastigial nucleus, emboliform nucleus, globose nucleus, and dentate nucleus.

Tracts: The trapezoid body with its subnuclei is an important relay station and crossing point in the auditory pathway (see p. 366). The central tegmental tract is an important pathway in the motor system.

6.6 Medulla oblongata, Transverse Section

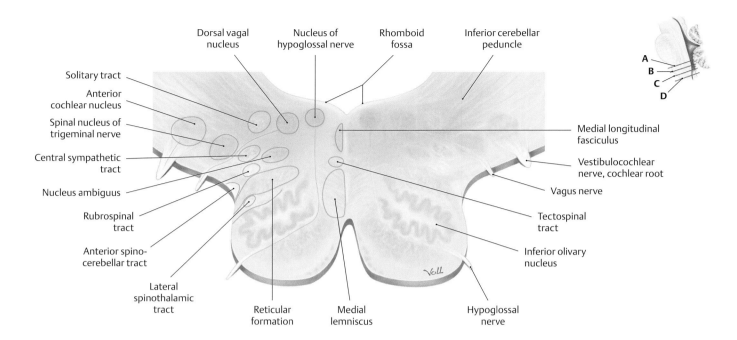

A Transverse section through the upper medulla oblongata

Nuclei: The nuclei of the hypoglossal nerve, vagus nerve, vestibulo-cochlear nerve, and the spinal nucleus of the trigeminal nerve appear in the *dorsal* part of the medulla oblongata. The inferior olivary nucleus, which belongs to the motor system, is located in the *ventral* part of the medulla oblongata. The reticular formation is interposed between the cranial nerve nuclei and the inferior olivary nucleus. It appears in all the transverse sections of this unit.

Tracts: Most of the ascending and descending tracts are the same as in the previous unit. A new structure appearing at this level is the *inferior cerebellar peduncle*, through which afferent tracts pass to the cerebellum (see p. 242).

CSF space: The floor of the fourth ventricle is the rhomboid fossa, which marks the dorsal boundary of this section.

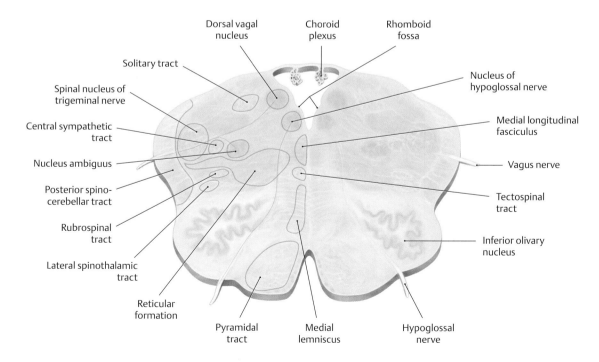

B Transverse section just above the middle of the medulla oblongata

Nuclei: The only cranial nerve nuclei visible at this level are those of the hypoglossal nerve, vagus nerve, and trigeminal nerve, appearing in the dorsal medulla. The lower portion of the inferior olivary nucleus appears in the ventral medulla.

Tracts: The ascending and descending tracts are the same as in the previous unit. Ascending sensory tracts (from nuclei gracilis and cuneatus, see p. 233, 326) decussate in the *medial lemniscus*. The solitary tract carries the gustatory fibers of cranial nerves V, VII, and X. Dorsolateral to it is the *nucleus of the solitary tract* (not shown). The *pyramidal tract* again appears as a compact structure at this level due to the absence of interspersed nuclei and decussating fibers.

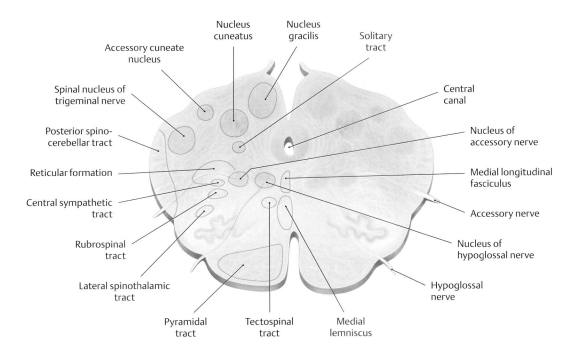

C Transverse section just below the middle of the medulla oblongata

Nuclei: The nuclei of the hypoglossal, vagus, and trigeminal nerves appear at this level. The irregular outline of the inferior olivary nucleus is still just visible in the ventral medulla. The nuclei that relay signals from the posterior funiculus—the nucleus cuneatus and nucleus gracilis—appear prominently in the dorsal part of the section. The tracts that arise from these nuclei decussate in the medial lemniscus (see above).

Tracts: The ascending and descending tracts correspond to those in the previous diagrams. The rhomboid fossa, which is the floor of the fourth ventricle, has narrowed substantially at this level to become the central canal.

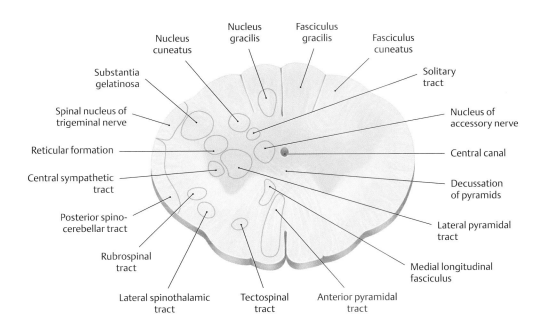

D Transverse section through the lower medulla oblongata

The medulla oblongata is continuous with the spinal cord at this level, showing no distinct transition.

Nuclei: The cranial nerve nuclei visible at this level are the spinal part of the trigeminal nerve and the nucleus of the accessory nerve. This section passes through the caudal ends of the nuclei in the relay station of the posterior funiculus—the nucleus cuneatus and nucleus gracilis.

Tracts: The ascending and descending tracts correspond to those in the previous diagrams of this unit. The section passes through the decussation of the pyramids, and we can now distinguish the anterior pyramidal tract (uncrossed) from the lateral pyramidal tract (crossed; see p. 338).

CSF space: This section passes through a portion of the central canal, which is markedly smaller at this level than in **C**. It may even be obliterated at some sites, but this has no clinical significance.

7.1 Cerebellum, External Structure

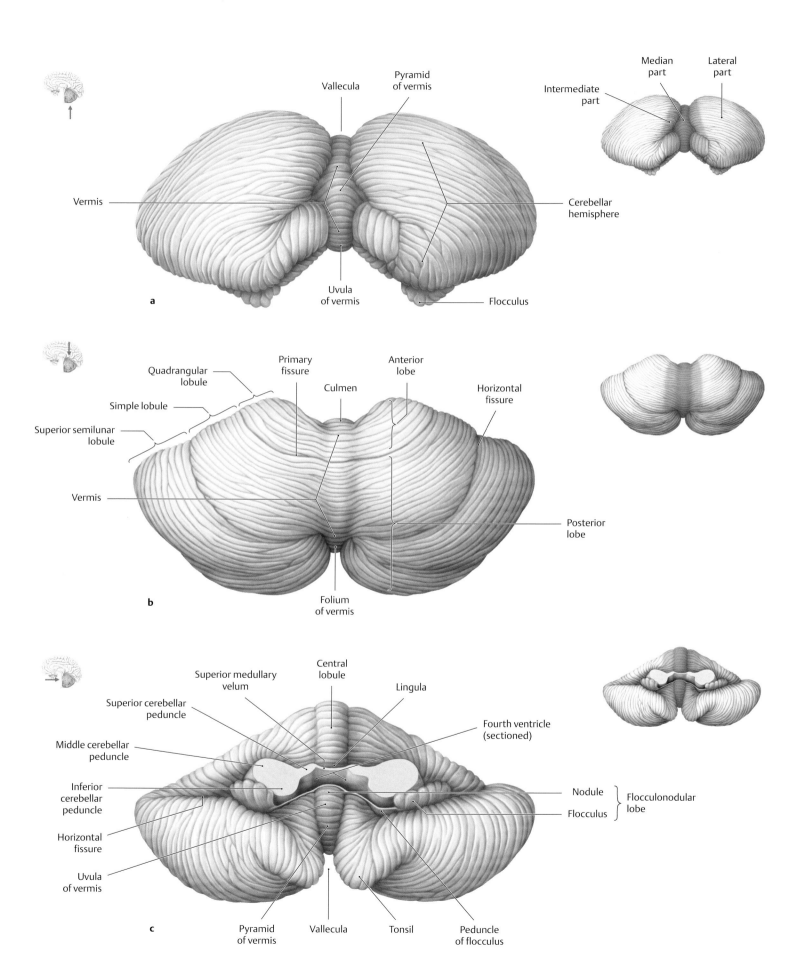

a

Median part · Lateral part · Intermediate part

Vallecula · Pyramid of vermis · Vermis · Cerebellar hemisphere · Uvula of vermis · Flocculus

b

Quadrangular lobule · Primary fissure · Anterior lobe · Culmen · Horizontal fissure · Simple lobule · Superior semilunar lobule · Vermis · Posterior lobe · Folium of vermis

c

Superior medullary velum · Central lobule · Lingula · Superior cerebellar peduncle · Fourth ventricle (sectioned) · Middle cerebellar peduncle · Inferior cerebellar peduncle · Nodule · Flocculonodular lobe · Flocculus · Horizontal fissure · Uvula of vermis · Pyramid of vermis · Vallecula · Tonsil · Peduncle of flocculus

A Isolated cerebellum

a Inferior view, **b** superior view, **c** anterior view. The cerebellum has been removed from the posterior cranial fossa and detached from the brainstem below the tentorium at the cerebellar peduncles (see also **B**).

The cerebellum is part of the motor system. It cannot initiate conscious movements by itself but is responsible for *unconscious* coordination and fine control of muscle actions (see **B**, p. 244). **Grossly**, the cerebellar surface presents a much finer arrangement of gyri and sulci than the cerebrum, providing an even greater expansion of its surface area. Externally the cerebellum consists of two large lateral masses, the *cerebellar hemispheres*, and a central part called the *vermis* (see **a**). *Cerebellar fissures* further subdivide the cerebellum into lobes. In particular:

- The primary fissure separates the anterior lobe of the cerebellum from the posterior lobe (see **b**).
- The posterolateral fissure separates the posterior lobe of the cerebellum from the flocculonodular lobe (see **B**).

Other, less important fissures have no clinical or functional significance and are not described here. Besides these anatomical divisions, the parts of the cerebellum can also be distinguished according to *phylogenetic* and *functional* criteria (see **C**; also **B**, p. 244). The cerebellum is connected to the brainstem by the three *cerebellar peduncles* (superior, middle, and inferior, see **c**), through which its afferent and efferent tracts enter and leave the cerebellum. The superior medullary velum stretches between the superior cerebellar peduncles and forms part of the roof of the fourth ventricle (see **c**). The cerebellar tonsils protrude downward near the midline on each side, almost to the foramen magnum at the base of the skull (not shown). Increased intracranial pressure may cause the cerebellar tonsils to herniate into the foramen magnum, impinging upon vital centers in the brainstem and posing a threat to life (see **D**, p. 189). **Functionally**, the *medial part* of the cerebellum (red) is distinguished from the *intermediate part* (pale red) and *lateral part* (gray). This functional classification does not conform to the anatomically defined lobar boundaries. Each of these parts projects to a specific cerebellar nucleus (see p. 240).

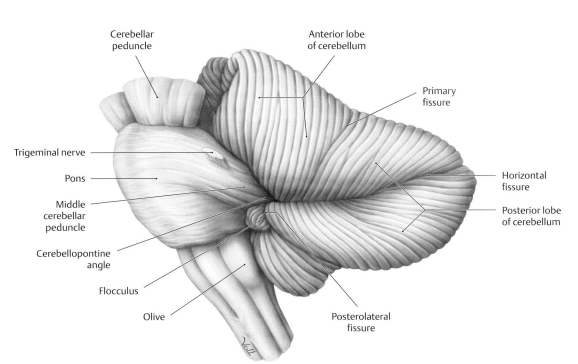

Cerebellar peduncle

Anterior lobe of cerebellum

Primary fissure

Trigeminal nerve

Pons

Middle cerebellar peduncle

Cerebellopontine angle

Flocculus

Olive

Horizontal fissure

Posterior lobe of cerebellum

Posterolateral fissure

B Relationship of the cerebellum to the brainstem

Left lateral view. The cerebellum overlies the dorsal aspect of the pons. Only the middle cerebellar peduncle can be identified in this external view. The *cerebellopontine angle* is clearly displayed. It has great clinical importance because it is the site where *cerebellopontine angle tumors* develop—most commonly acoustic neuromas (see **D**, p. 149).

C Synopsis of cerebellar classifications

Phylogenetic classification	Anatomical classification	Functional classification based on the origin of afferents
• Archicerebellum	• Flocculonodular lobe	• Vestibulocerebellum: maintenance of equilibrium
• Paleocerebellum	• Anterior lobe of cerebellum • Portions of the vermis • Medial portions of the posterior lobe	• Spinocerebellum: regulation of muscle tone
• Neocerebellum	• Lateral portions of the posterior lobe	• Pontocerebellum (= cerebrocerebellum): skilled movements

7.2 Cerebellum, Internal Structure

A The cerebellum, brainstem, and diencephalon

Midsagittal section viewed from the left side, displaying the internal structure of the cerebellum. The interior of the cerebellum is composed of *white matter* and its exterior of *gray matter* (cerebellar cortex, whose layers are shown in **D**). This section again shows how the cerebellum abuts the fourth ventricle, in which the choroid plexus can be seen. The superior medullary velum forms the *upper* portion of the roof of the fourth ventricle; the lingula is closely apposed to its dorsal surface. The *lower* portion of the roof of the fourth ventricle is in contact with the cerebellar nodule. This section demonstrates how the cerebellar cortex is deeply folded into *folia* (gyri, not individually labeled), producing a tree-like outline of the white matter called the *arbor vitae* ("tree of life").

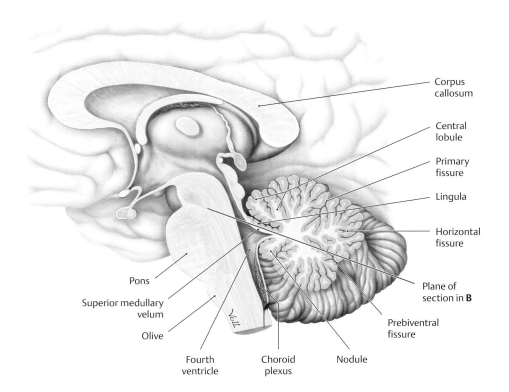

B Nuclei of the cerebellum

Section through the superior cerebellar peduncles (plane of section shown in **A**), viewed from behind. Deep within the cerebellar white matter are four pairs of nuclei that contain most of the *efferent* neurons of the cerebellum:

- Fastigial nucleus (green)
- Emboliform nucleus (blue)
- Globose nuclei (blue)
- Dentate nucleus (pink)

The cortical regions have been color-coded to match their target nuclei. The dentate nucleus is the largest of the cerebellar nuclei and extends into the cerebellar hemispheres. The cerebellar nuclei receive projections from Purkinje cells in the cerebellar cortex (see **D**). While the *efferent fibers* of the cerebellum can be assigned rather easily to anatomical structures, this is not true of the afferent fibers. Their sources are examined on p. 244.

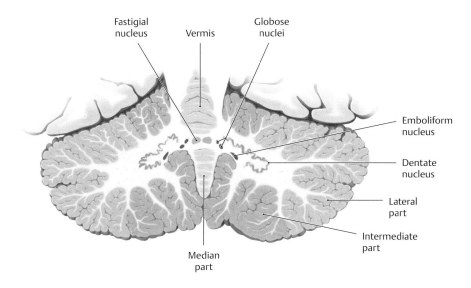

C Cerebellar nuclei and the regions of the cortex from which they receive projections (see also p. 238)

Cerebellar nucleus	Synonyms	Region of the cerebellar cortex that send axons to the nucleus
Dentate nucleus	Lateral cerebellar nucleus	Lateral part (lateral portions of the cerebellar hemispheres)
Emboliform nucleus	Anterior interpositus nucleus	Intermediate part (medial portions of the cerebellar hemispheres)
Globose nuclei	Posterior interpositus nucleus	Intermediate part (medial portions of the cerebellar hemispheres)
Fastigial nucleus	Medial cerebellar nucleus	Median part (cerebellar vermis)

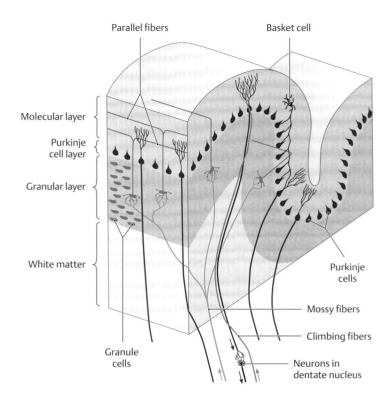

Molecular layer

Purkinje cell layer

Granular layer

White matter

Parallel fibers

Basket cell

Purkinje cells

Mossy fibers

Climbing fibers

Granule cells

Neurons in dentate nucleus

D Cerebellar cortex

The cerebellar cortex consists of three layers:

- Molecular layer: outer layer; contains *parallel fibers*, which are the axons of granule cells (blue) from the granular layer. They run parallel to the cerebellar folia and terminate in the molecular layer, where they synapse into the dendrites of the Purkinje cells. This layer also contains axons from the inferior olive and its accessory nuclei (*climbing fibers*) and a small number of inhibitory interneurons (*basket and stellate neurons*).
- Purkinje layer: contains the cell bodies of *Purkinje cells* (purple).
- Granular layer: contains mostly *granule cells* (blue), as well as *mossy* and *climbing fibers* (green and pink, respectively), and *Golgi cells* (not shown; the cell types are viewed in **F**).

The white matter of the cerebellum is located under the granular layer.

Note: The Purkinje cells are the only efferent cells of the cerebellar cortex. They project to the cerebellar nuclei.

E diagram

Glu — Granule cells — Glu

⊕

Glu — Inhibitory interneurons — GABA ⊖

⊕

Afferent connections

Axon collaterals

Purkinje cells

⊖ GABA

⊕

Asp

Axon collaterals

Neurons of cerebellar nuclei

Mossy fibers | Climbing fibers

Efferent connections

Pontine nuclei, spinal cord, nuclei of vestibular-cochlear nerve

Inferior olive

Thalamus, red nucleus, nuclei of vestibular-cochlear nerve, reticular formation

E Synaptic circuitry of the cerebellum

(after Bähr and Frotscher)

The cerebellum comprises 10% of the mass of the brain, but contains up to 50% of its neurons. This enormous population (cerebellar granule cells alone may number in excess of 100 billion) is composed of a few cell types arranged in a repetitive, highly ordered array. This repetition of simple elements has led to the description of the cerebellum as an intricate synaptic computer for motor coordination.

The basic cerebellar circuitry involves **afferents** including climbing and mossy fibers. *Climbing fibers* originate from the inferior olivary complex and form multiple excitatory synapses on the cell bodies and proximal dendritic tree of Purkinje cells (see **D**); collateral branches synapse in the (deep) cerebellar nuclei. *Mossy fibers* originate in the vestibular and pontine nuclei and the spinal cord to form excitatory contacts with granule cells in synaptic complexes called cerebellar glomeruli (see **D**); some branches excite local inhibitory neurons,

and collaterals also enter the cerebellar nuclei. The axons of granule cells form parallel fibers that form excitatory synapses on the dendritic trees of Purkinje cells. The Purkinje cells in turn send their axons mostly to the cerebellar nuclei (see **B**, above; also to vestibular nuclei), where they make inhibitory synapses. The identities of some neurotransmitters in this pathway have been established: local inhibitory neurons, and Purkinje cells themselves, use gamma-aminobutyric acid (GABA), while granule cells employ glutamate. Glutamate is probably also involved at mossy and climbing fiber synapses. The principal cerebellar **efferent** axons arise from the cerebellar nuclei. This circuitry combines direct activation (afferents to granule cells to Purkinje cells) and indirect inhibition (afferents to inhibitory interneurons to Purkinje cells), which may be integrated in a complex spatial pattern and temporal sequence in the cerebellar cortex and deep nuclei to provide indirect feedback control for motor coordination.

F Principal neurons and fiber types in the cerebellar cortex

Name	Definition
Climbing fibers	Axons of neurons of the inferior olive and its associated nuclei
Mossy fibers	Axons of neurons of the pontine nuclei, the spinal cord, and vestibular nuclei (pontocerebellar, spinocerebellar, and vestibular tracts)
Parallel fibers (see **D**)	Axons of granule cells
Granule cells	Interneurons of the cerebellar cortex
Purkinje cells	The only efferent cells of the cerebellar cortex; exert an inhibitory effect

241

7.3 Cerebellar Peduncles and Tracts

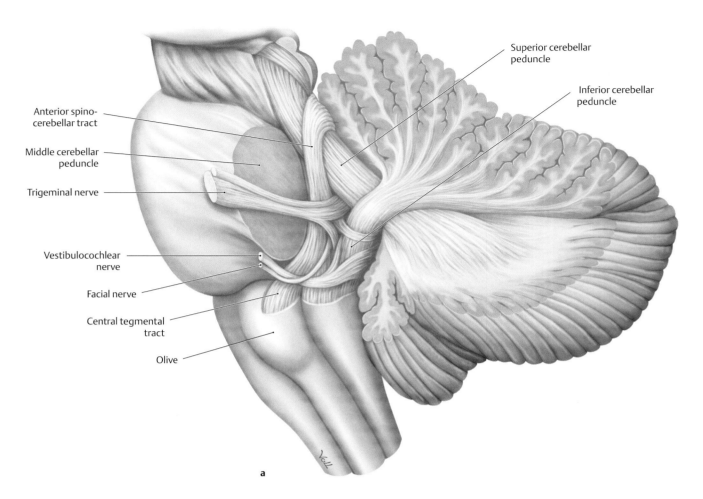

Superior cerebellar peduncle

Inferior cerebellar peduncle

Anterior spino-cerebellar tract

Middle cerebellar peduncle

Trigeminal nerve

Vestibulocochlear nerve

Facial nerve

Central tegmental tract

Olive

a

A Cerebellar peduncles

a Left lateral view with the upper portion of the cerebellum and lateral portions of the pons removed. This dissection, which has been prepared to show fiber structure, clearly shows the course of the cerebellar tracts. The size of the cerebellar peduncles, and thus the mass of entering and emerging axons, is substantial and reflects the extensive neural connections in the cerebellum (see p. 241). The cerebellum requires these numerous connections because it is an integrating center for the coordination of fine movements. In particular, it contains and processes vestibular and proprioceptive afferents and it modulates motor nuclei in other brain regions and in the spinal cord. The principal afferent and efferent connections of the cerebellum are reviewed in **B**.

b Left lateral view. Here the cerebellum has been sharply detached from its peduncles to demonstrate the complementary cut surface of the peduncles on the brainstem (compare with **Ac**, p. 238).

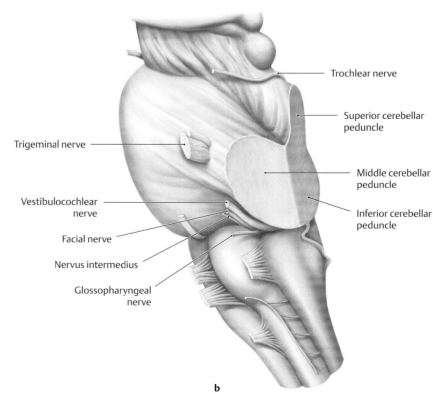

Trochlear nerve

Trigeminal nerve

Superior cerebellar peduncle

Vestibulocochlear nerve

Middle cerebellar peduncle

Facial nerve

Inferior cerebellar peduncle

Nervus intermedius

Glossopharyngeal nerve

b

B Synopsis of the cerebellar peduncles and their tracts

Tracts made up of afferent and efferent axons enter or leave the cerebellum through the cerebellar peduncles. The afferent axons originate in the spinal cord, vestibular organs, inferior olive and pons, while the efferent axons originate in the cerebellar nuclei (see p. 240). The representation of the body in the cerebellum, unlike in the cerebrum, is ipsilateral. Ascending cerebellar tracts thus cross (decussate) to the opposite side.

Cerebellar peduncle and constituent parts*	Origin**	Site of Termination
Superior cerebellar peduncle: contains mostly efferent tracts from the cerebellar nuclei. Some tracts cross in the decussation of the superior peduncle, then divide into a *descending* limb (to the pons) and an *ascending* limb (to the midbrain and thalamus).		
Descending parts (**e**)	Fastigial and globose nuclei	Reticular formation and vestibular nuclei (projection is mostly *contralateral*)
Ascending parts (**e**)	Dentate nucleus	Red nucleus and thalamus (both *contralateral*)
Anterior spinocerebellar tract (**a**)	Secondary neurons in intermediate gray matter, lumbosacral spinal cord. Relays proprioception (muscle spindles, tendon receptors, etc.) from dorsal root (spinal) ganglion cells, lower limb and trunk. Fibers cross locally and then re-cross in the pons to return to the ipsilateral side.	Vermis and intermediate part of anterior lobe of cerebellum (*ipsilateral*; terminates as mossy fibers)
Middle cerebellar peduncle: contains only afferent tracts.		
Pontocerebellar fibers (**a**)	Basal pontine nuclei. Relay cerebropontine to pontocerebellar projection (source of 90% of axons in middle peduncle)	Lateral regions of posterior and anterior lobes of cerebellum (*contralateral*; terminate as mossy fibers; branches to contralateral dentate nucleus)
Inferior cerebellar peduncle: contains both afferent and efferent tracts.		
Posterior spinocerebellar tract (**a**)	Posterior thoracic nucleus and thoracic spinal cord. Relays proprioception and cutaneous sensation from the lower limb. Contains large axons with high conduction velocity.	Vermis and nearby anterior lobe of cerebellum, pyramid and nearby posterior lobe of cerebellum. (*ipsilateral*; terminates as mossy fibers)
Cuneocerebellar tract (**a**)	Nucleus cuneatus and external cuneate nucleus. Relays proprioception (external cuneate nucleus) and cutaneous sensation (nucleus cuneatus) from the upper limb, with fast transmission, functionally corresponding to the posterior spinocerebellar tract.	Posterior part of anterior lobe of cerebellum (*ipsilateral*; terminates as mossy fibers).
Olivocerebellar tract (**a**)	Inferior olivary nuclear complex. Inferior olive receives numerous inputs from sensory and motor systems, including a large contralateral projection from the cerebellum itself (dentate nucleus, see below).	Molecular layer of cerebellar cortex (*contralateral*, terminates as *climbing* fibers)
Vestibulocerebellar tract (**a**)	Semicircular canal (vestibular ganglion) and vestibular nuclei. Transmits balance and body position/motion information either directly (vestibular axons via vestibulocochlear nerve [CN VIII], *ipsilateral*) or via synaptic relay in vestibular nuclei (*bilateral*).	Nodule, flocculus, anterior lobe, and vermis of cerebellum (*bilateral,* see left; terminates as *mossy* fibers)
Trigeminocerebellar fibers (**a**)	Trigeminal sensory nuclei in the brainstem. Relay proprioception and cutaneous sensation from the head.	Rostral part of posterior lobe of cerebellum (*ipsilateral*; terminate as mossy fibers)
Cerebello-olivary fibers (**e**)	Dentate nucleus	Inferior olive (*contralateral*)

*Subentries for constituent parts are classified as efferent (**e**) or afferent (**a**).
**In the case of afferents, the type of afferent is listed along with the site of origin.

7.4 Cerebellum, Simplified Functional Anatomy and Lesions

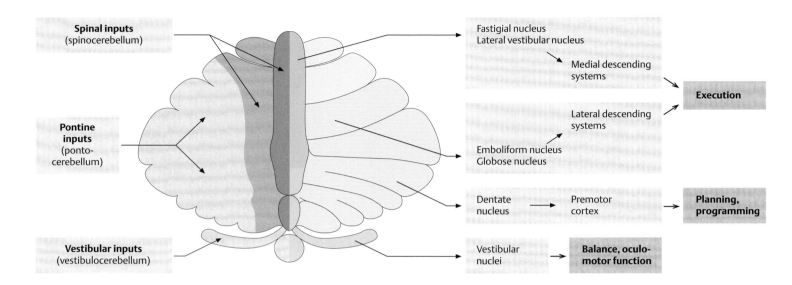

A Simplified functional anatomy of the cerebellum

(after Klinke and Silbernagl)

Two-dimensional representation of the cerebellum. Left: afferent inputs to the cerebellar cortex; Right: paths of cerebellar (efferent) output.

The coordination of motor activity by the cerebellum can be divided into three broad categories corresponding to the areas responsible for the coordination:

- Maintenance of posture and balance ("vestibulocerebellum")
- Dynamic control of muscle tone under various loads ("spinocerebellum")
- Integration of activity of various muscle groups during complex tasks ("pontocerebellum")

These categories of cerebellar function require different types of afferent information, and have different output (efferent) paths. Although afferent inputs and their corresponding tracts are not segregated by obvious anatomical boundaries in the cerebellum, there is a functional division that correlates with the evolution of the cerebellar structures (see **B**). The phylogenetically ancient part of the cerebellum (archicerebellum) receives vestibular input, projects to the fastigial nucleus and lateral vestibular nucleus, and controls trunk musculature through a "medial motor system" (see p. 282). Dynamic control of muscle tone requires feedback from muscle and tendon proprioceptors entering the cerebellum through spinocerebellar tracts. This "spinocerebellar" function utilizes more recently evolved paleocerebellar structures, the emboliform and globose cerebellar nuclei, and modulates muscle activity through a "lateral motor system" that involves muscles in the extremities. The most recent evolutionary developments in the cerebellum include the significant expansion of cerebral cortical projections via a relay in the pons, and a reciprocal massive cerebellar projection, through the dentate nucleus, back to the cerebral cortex via the thalamus. The neocerebellum thus sends information back to the cerebral cortex, which controls some musculature directly through corticonuclear projections to lower motor neurons controlling the tongue and face (see p. 232), and corticospinal projections to spinal motor neurons controlling the hands. This "pontocerebellar" pathway and function involves complex anticipatory activation of muscle groups to accept a load or limit a motion, and so can be characterized in part as a "planning" or "programming" function.

Note: this simplified outline of cerebellar function does not take into account the complexity of cerebellar contributions to a variety of other tasks. Visual inputs and oculomotor functions, specifically, have not been considered here.

B Synopsis of cerebellar classifications and their relationships to motor deficits

Some cerebellar lesions cause subtle cognitive deficits that cannot be explained simply as a loss of muscle coordination.

Functional classification	Phylogenetic classification	Anatomical classification	Deficit symptoms
Vestibulocerebellum	Archicerebellum	Flocculonodular lobe	<ul><li>Truncal, stance and gait ataxia</li><li>Vertigo</li><li>Nystagmus</li><li>Vomiting</li></ul>
Spinocerebellum	Paleocerebellum	Anterior lobe, parts of vermis; Posterior lobe, medial parts	<ul><li>Ataxia, chiefly affecting the lower limb</li><li>Oculomotor dysfunction</li><li>Speech disorder (asynergy of speech muscles)</li></ul>
Pontocerebellum (= cerebrocerebellum)	Neocerebellum	Posterior lobe, hemispheres	<ul><li>Dysmetria and hypermetria (positive rebound)</li><li>Intention tremor</li><li>Nystagmus</li><li>Decreased muscle tone</li></ul>

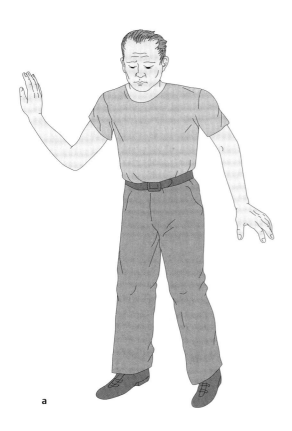

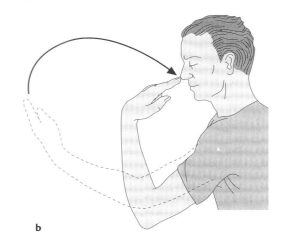

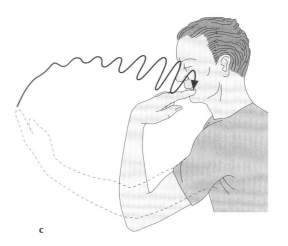

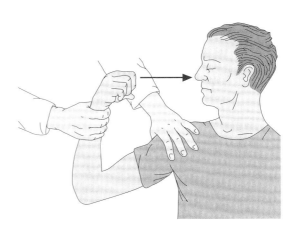

C Cerebellar lesions

Cerebellar lesions may remain clinically silent for some time because other brain regions can functionally compensate for them with reasonable effectiveness. Exceptions are direct lesions of the efferent cerebellar nuclei, which cannot be clinically compensated.

Cerebellar symptoms:

Asynergy	Lack of coordination among different muscle groups, especially in the performance of fine movements.
Ataxia	Uncoordinated sequence of movements. Truncal ataxia (patient cannot sit quietly upright) is distinguished from stance and gait ataxia (impaired limb movements, such as an unsteady gait in inebriation). The patient stands with the legs spread apart and places his hand on the wall for stability (**a**).
Decreased muscle tone	Ipsilateral muscle weakness and rapid fatigability (asthenia).
Intention tremor	Involuntary, rhythmical wavering movement of the hand when a purposeful movement is attempted, as in the finger-nose test: normal test (**b**), test indicating a cerebellar lesion (**c**).
Rebound phenomenon	The patient, with eyes closed, is told to move the arm against a resistance from the examiner (**d**). When the examiner suddenly releases the arm, it forcefully "rebounds" toward the patient (hypermetria).

8.1 Arteries of the Brain: Blood Supply and the Circle of Willis

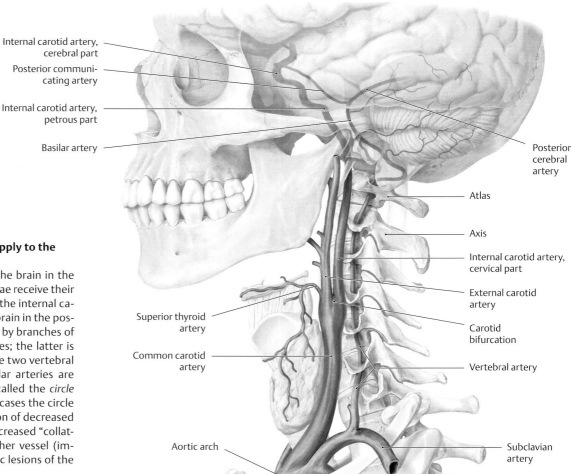

A Overview of the arterial supply to the brain

Left lateral view. The parts of the brain in the anterior and middle cranial fossae receive their blood supply from branches of the internal carotid artery, while parts of the brain in the posterior cranial fossa are supplied by branches of the vertebral and basilar arteries; the latter is formed by the confluence of the two vertebral arteries. The carotid and basilar arteries are connected by a vascular ring called the *circle of Willis* (see **C** and **D**). In many cases the circle of Willis allows for compensation of decreased blood flow in one vessel with increased "collateral" blood flow through another vessel (important in patients with stenotic lesions of the afferent arteries, see **E**).

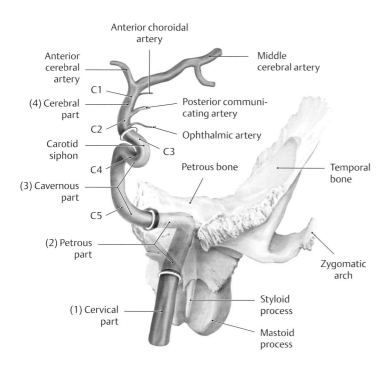

B The four anatomical divisions of the internal carotid artery

Anterior view of the left internal carotid artery. The internal carotid artery consists of four topographically distinct parts between the carotid bifurcation (see **A**) and the point where it divides into the anterior and middle cerebral arteries. The parts (separated in the figure by white disks) are:

(1) Cervical part (red): located in the lateral pharyngeal space.
(2) Petrous part (yellow): located in the carotid canal of the petrous bone.
(3) Cavernous part (green): follows an S-shaped curve in the cavernous sinus.
(4) Cerebral part (purple): located in the chiasmatic cistern of the subarachnoid space.

Except for the cervical part which generally does not give off branches, all the other parts of the internal carotid artery give off numerous branches (see p. 60). The *intracranial* parts of the internal carotid artery are subdivided into five segments (C1–C5) based on clinical criteria:

• C1–C2: the supraclinoid segments, located within the cerebral part. C1 and C2 lie above the anterior clinoid process of the lesser wing of the sphenoid bone.
• C3–C5: the infraclinoid segments, located within the cavernous sinus.

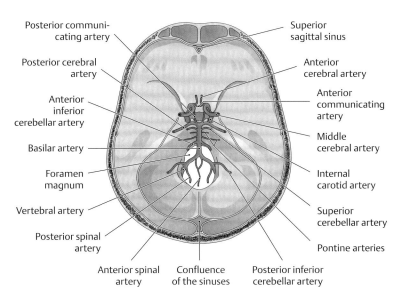

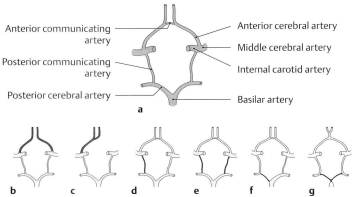

C Projection of the circle of Willis onto the base of the skull

Superior view. The two vertebral arteries enter the skull through the foramen magnum and unite behind the clivus to form the unpaired basilar artery. This vessel then divides into the two posterior cerebral arteries (additional vessels that normally contribute to the circle of Willis are shown in **D**).

Note: Each middle cerebral artery (MCA) is the direct continuation of the internal carotid artery on that side. Clots ejected by the left heart will frequently embolize to the MCA territory.

D Variants of the circle of Willis (after Lippert and Pabst)

The vascular connections within the circle of Willis are subject to considerable variation. As a rule, the segmental hypoplasias shown here do not significantly alter the normal functions of the arterial ring.

a In most cases, the circle of Willis is formed by the following arteries: the anterior, middle and posterior cerebral arteries; the anterior and posterior communicating arteries; the internal carotid arteries; and the basilar artery.

b Occasionally, the anterior communicating artery is absent.

c Both anterior cerebral arteries may arise from one internal carotid artery (10% of cases).

d The posterior communicating artery may be absent or hypoplastic on one side (10% of cases).

e Both posterior communicating arteries may be absent or hypoplastic (10% of cases).

f The posterior cerebral artery may be absent or hypoplastic on one side.

g Both posterior cerebral arteries may be absent or hypoplastic. In addition, the anterior cerebral arteries may arise from a common trunk (**g**).

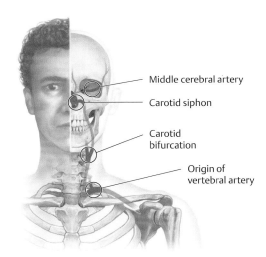

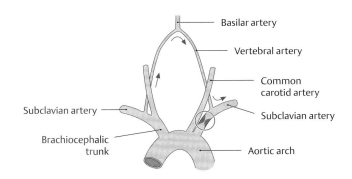

E Stenoses and occlusions of arteries supplying the brain

Atherosclerotic lesions in older patients may cause the narrowing (stenosis) or complete obstruction (occlusion) of arteries that supply the brain. Stenoses most commonly occur at arterial bifurcations, and the sites of predilection are shown. Isolated stenoses that develop gradually may be compensated for by collateral vessels. When stenoses occur simultaneously at multiple sites, the circle of Willis cannot compensate for the diminished blood supply, and cerebral blood flow becomes impaired (varying degrees of cerebral ischemia, see p. 264).

Note: The damage is manifested clinically in the brain, but the cause is located in the vessels that supply the brain. Because stenoses are treatable, their diagnosis has major therapeutic implications.

F Anatomical basis of subclavian steal syndrome

"Subclavian steal" usually results from stenosis of the left subclavian artery (red circle) located proximal to the origin of the vertebral artery. This syndrome involves a stealing of blood from the *vertebral artery* by the subclavian artery. When the left arm is exercised, as during yard work, insufficient blood may be supplied to the arm to accommodate the increased muscular effort (the patient complains of muscle weakness). As a result, blood is "stolen" from the vertebral artery circulation and there is a reversal of blood flow in the vertebral artery on the *affected* side (arrows). This leads to deficient blood flow in the basilar artery and may deprive the brain of blood, producing a feeling of lightheadedness.

247

8.2 Arteries of the Cerebrum

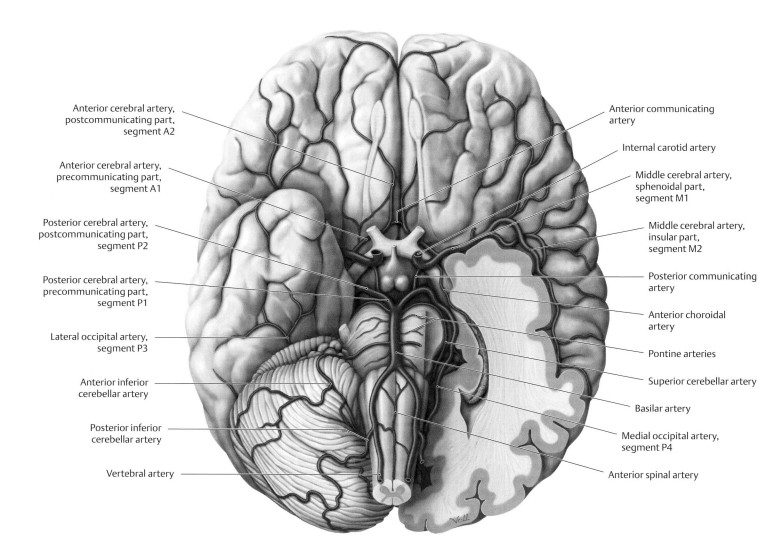

Anterior cerebral artery, postcommunicating part, segment A2

Anterior cerebral artery, precommunicating part, segment A1

Posterior cerebral artery, postcommunicating part, segment P2

Posterior cerebral artery, precommunicating part, segment P1

Lateral occipital artery, segment P3

Anterior inferior cerebellar artery

Posterior inferior cerebellar artery

Vertebral artery

Anterior communicating artery

Internal carotid artery

Middle cerebral artery, sphenoidal part, segment M1

Middle cerebral artery, insular part, segment M2

Posterior communicating artery

Anterior choroidal artery

Pontine arteries

Superior cerebellar artery

Basilar artery

Medial occipital artery, segment P4

Anterior spinal artery

A Arteries at the base of the brain
The cerebellum and temporal lobe have been removed on the left side to display the course of the posterior cerebral artery. This view was selected because most of the arteries that supply the brain enter the cerebrum from its basal aspect.
Note: the three principal arteries of the cerebrum, the anterior, middle and posterior cerebral arteries, arise from different sources. The ante-

rior and middle cerebral arteries are branches of the internal carotid artery, while the posterior cerebral arteries are terminal branches of the basiler artery (see p. 246 f). The vertebral arteries, which fuse to form the basilar artery, distribute branches to the spinal cord, brainstem, and cerebellum (anterior spinal artery, posterior spinal arteries, superior cerebellar artery, and anterior and posterior inferior cerebellar arteries).

B Segments of the anterior, middle, and posterior cerebral arteries

Artery	Parts	Segments
Anterior cerebral artery	• Precommunicating part • Postcommunicating part	• A1 = segment proximal to the anterior communicating artery • A2 = segment distal to the anterior communicating artery
Middle cerebral artery (MCA)	• Sphenoidal part • Insular part	• M1 = first horizontal segment of the artery (horizontal part) • M2 = segment on the insula
Posterior cerebral artery	• Precommunicating part • Postcommunicating part	• P1 = segment between the basilar artery bifurcation and posterior communicating artery • P2 = segment between the posterior communicating artery and anterior temporal branches • P3 = lateral occipital artery • P4 = medial occipital artery

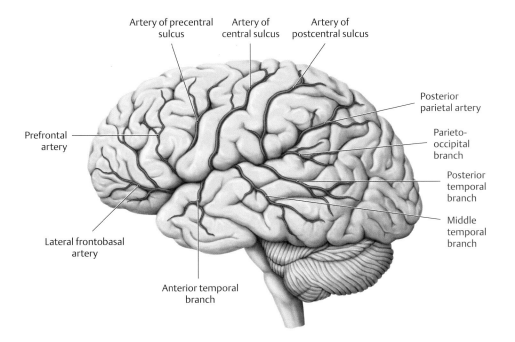

Artery of precentral sulcus

Artery of central sulcus

Artery of postcentral sulcus

Posterior parietal artery

Parieto-occipital branch

Posterior temporal branch

Middle temporal branch

Prefrontal artery

Lateral frontobasal artery

Anterior temporal branch

C Terminal branches of the middle cerebral artery on the lateral cerebral hemisphere

Left lateral view. Most of the blood vessels on the lateral surface of the brain are terminal branches of the middle cerebral artery (MCA). They can be subdivided into two main groups:

- Inferior terminal (cortical) branches: supply the temporal lobe cortex
- Superior terminal (cortical) branches: supply the frontal and parietal lobe cortex

Deeper structures supplied by these branches are not shown in the diagram (see p. 250 f).

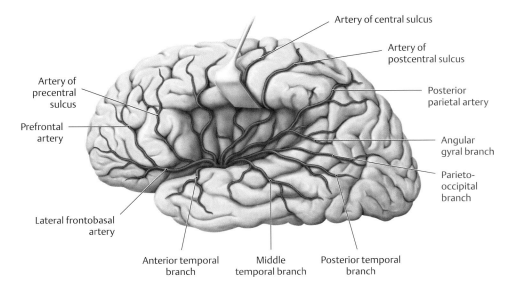

Artery of central sulcus

Artery of postcentral sulcus

Posterior parietal artery

Angular gyral branch

Parieto-occipital branch

Artery of precentral sulcus

Prefrontal artery

Lateral frontobasal artery

Anterior temporal branch

Middle temporal branch

Posterior temporal branch

D Course of the middle cerebral artery in the interior of the lateral sulcus

Left lateral view. On its way to the lateral surface of the cerebral hemisphere, the middle cerebral artery first courses on the base of the brain; this is the sphenoidal part of the MCA. It then continues through the lateral sulcus along the insula, which is the sunken portion of the cerebral cortex. When the temporal and parietal lobes are spread apart with a retractor, as shown here, we can see the arteries of the insula (which receive their blood from the insular part of the middle cerebral artery; see **A**). When viewed in an angiogram, the branches of the insular part of the MCA resemble the arms of a candelabrum, giving rise to the term "candelabrum artery" for that arterial segment.

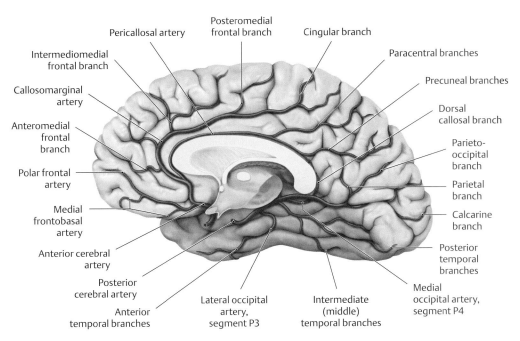

Posteromedial frontal branch

Pericallosal artery

Cingular branch

Paracentral branches

Intermediomedial frontal branch

Precuneal branches

Callosomarginal artery

Dorsal callosal branch

Anteromedial frontal branch

Parieto-occipital branch

Polar frontal artery

Parietal branch

Medial frontobasal artery

Calcarine branch

Anterior cerebral artery

Posterior temporal branches

Posterior cerebral artery

Anterior temporal branches

Lateral occipital artery, segment P3

Intermediate (middle) temporal branches

Medial occipital artery, segment P4

E Branches of the anterior and posterior cerebral arteries on the medial surface of the cerebrum

Right cerebral hemisphere viewed from the medial side, with the left cerebral hemisphere and brainstem removed. The medial surface of the brain is supplied by branches of the anterior and posterior cerebral arteries. While the *anterior cerebral artery* arises from the internal carotid artery, the *posterior cerebral artery* arises from the basilar artery (which is formed by the junction of the left and right vertebral arteries).

8.3 Arteries of the Cerebrum, Distribution

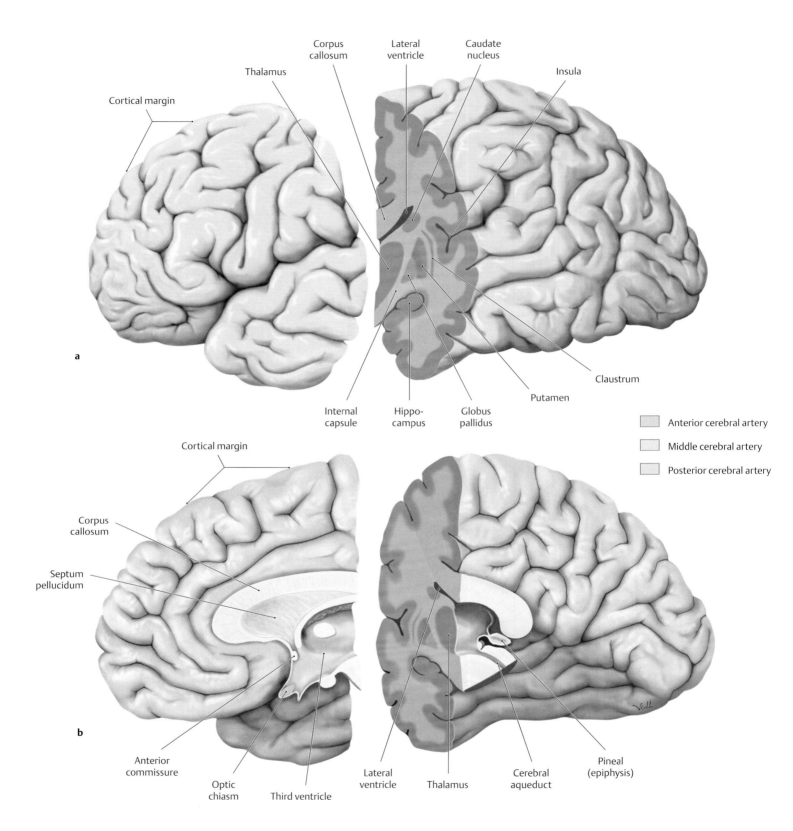

A Distribution areas of the main cerebral arteries

a Lateral view of the left cerebral hemisphere, **b** medial view of the right cerebral hemisphere. Most of the lateral surface of the brain is supplied by the *middle* cerebral artery (green), whose branches ascend to the cortex from the depths of the insula. The branches of the *anterior* cerebral artery supply the frontal pole of the brain and the cortical areas near the cortical margin (red and pink). The *posterior* cerebral artery supplies the occipital pole and lower portions of the temporal lobe (blue). The central gray and white matter have a complex blood supply (yellow) that includes the anterior choroidal artery. The anterior and posterior cerebral arteries supply most of the medial surface of the brain.

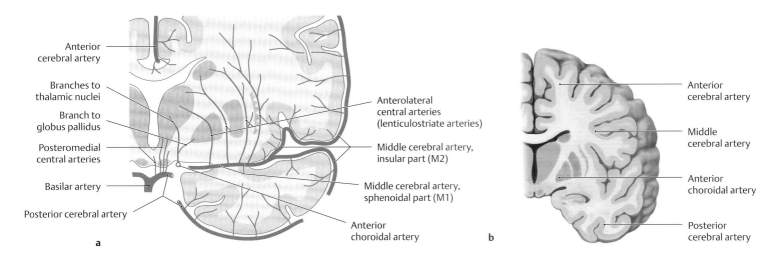

B Distribution of the three main cerebral arteries in transverse and coronal sections

a, b Coronal sections at the level of the mammillary bodies. **c** Transverse section at the level of the internal capsule.

The internal capsule, basal ganglia, and thalamus derive most of their blood supply from perforating branches of the following vessels at the base of the brain:

- Anterior choroidal artery (from the internal carotid artery)
- Anterolateral central arteries (lenticulostriate arteries and striate branches) with their terminal branches (from the middle cerebral artery)
- Posteromedial central arteries (from the posterior cerebral artery)
- Perforating branches (from the posterior communicating artery)

The internal capsule, which is traversed by the pyramidal tract and other structures, receives most of its blood supply from the middle cerebral artery (anterior crus and genu) and from the anterior choroidal artery (posterior crus). If these vessels become occluded, the pyramidal tract and other structures will be interrupted, causing paralysis on the contralateral side of the body (stroke: central paralysis, see **C** on p. 265).

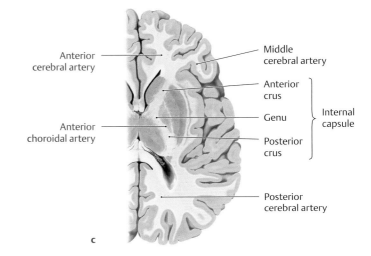

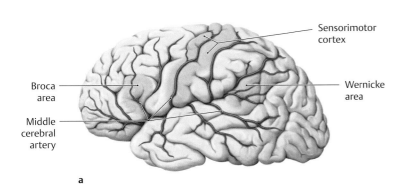

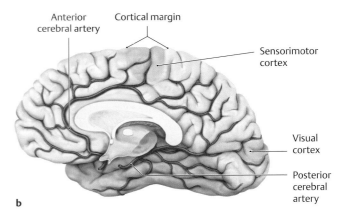

C Functional centers on the surface of the cerebrum

a Lateral view of the left cerebral hemisphere. Regions supplied by branches of the middle cerebral artery are shaded orange. Specific functions can be assigned to well-defined areas of the cerebrum. These areas are supplied by branches of the three main cerebral arteries. The sensorimotor cortex (pre- and postcentral gyrus) and the motor and sensory speech centers (Broca and Wernicke areas) are supplied by branches of the middle cerebral artery (see **b**). Therefore, a language deficit (aphasia) or the loss of motor or sensory function on one side of the body suggests an occlusion of the middle cerebral artery.

b Medial view of the right cerebral hemisphere. The "margin" of the sensorimotor cortex may be deprived of blood (clinically manifested by paralysis and sensory disturbances mainly affecting the lower limb) by an occlusion of the *anterior* cerebral artery. The visual cortex may lose its blood supply (causing blindness) through an occlusion of the *posterior* cerebral artery.

251

8.4 Arteries of the Brainstem and Cerebellum

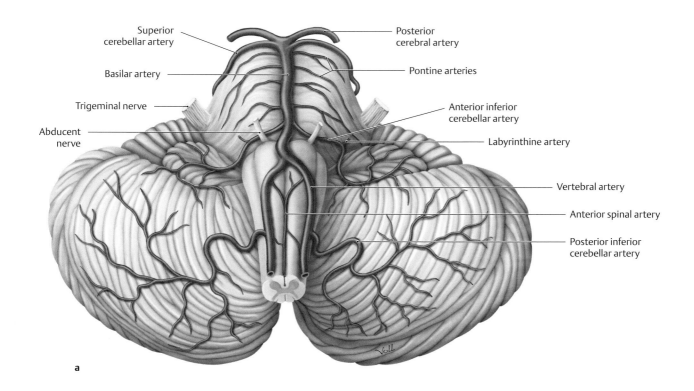

a

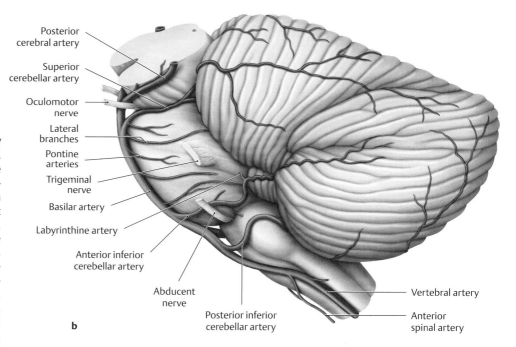

b

A Arteries of the brainstem and cerebellum

a Basal view, **b** left lateral view.

The brainstem and cerebellum are supplied by the basilar and cerebellar arteries (see below). Because the basilar artery is formed by the union of the two vertebral arteries, blood supplied by the basilar artery is said to come from the *vertebrobasilar complex*. The vessels that supply the **brainstem** (mesencephalon, pons, and medulla oblongata) arise either directly from the basilar artery (e.g., the pontine arteries) and vertebral arteries or from their branches. The branches are classified by their sites of entry and distribution as medial, mediolateral, or lateral (paramedian branches; short and long circumferential branches). Decreased perfusion in or occlusion of these vessels leads to transient or permanent impairment of blood flow (brainstem syndrome) and may produce a great variety of clinical symptoms, given the many nuclei and tract systems that exist in the brainstem. The **spinal cord**, receives a portion of its blood supply from the anterior spinal artery (see **b**), which arises from the vertebral artery (see p. 286). The **cerebellum** is supplied by three large arteries:

- Posterior inferior cerebellar artery (PICA), the largest branch of the vertebral artery. This vessel is usually referred to by its acronym, PICA.
- Anterior inferior cerebellar artery (AICA), the first major branch of the basilar artery.
- Superior cerebellar artery (SCA), the last major branch of the basilar artery before it divides into the posterior cerebral arteries.

Note: the labyrinthine artery which supplies the inner ear (see also **D**, p. 155) usually arises from the anterior inferior cerebellar artery, as pictured here, although it may also spring directly from the basilar artery. Impaired blood flow in the labyrinthine artery leads to an acute loss of hearing (sudden sensorineural hearing loss), frequently accompanied by tinnitus (see **D**, p. 149).

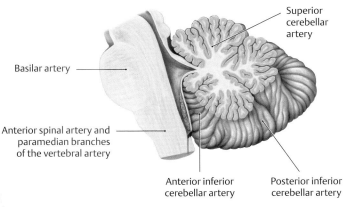

B Distribution of the arteries of the brainstem and cerebellum in midsagittal section (after Bähr and Frotscher)

All of the brain sections shown here and below are supplied by the vertebrobasilar complex. The transverse sections are presented in a caudal-to-cranial series corresponding to the direction of the vertebrobasilar blood supply.

Superior cerebellar artery

Basilar artery

Anterior spinal artery and paramedian branches of the vertebral artery

Anterior inferior cerebellar artery

Posterior inferior cerebellar artery

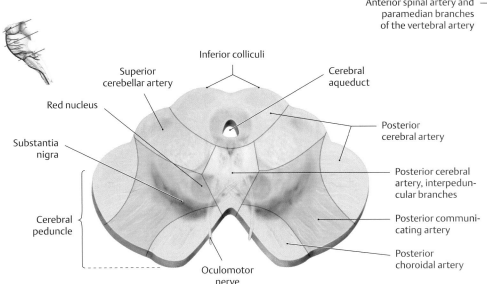

Inferior colliculi

Superior cerebellar artery

Red nucleus

Cerebral aqueduct

Substantia nigra

Posterior cerebral artery

Cerebral peduncle

Posterior cerebral artery, interpeduncular branches

Posterior communicating artery

Posterior choroidal artery

Oculomotor nerve

C Distribution of the arteries of the mesencephalon in transverse section

Besides branches from the superior cerebellar artery, the mesencephalon is supplied chiefly by branches of the posterior cerebral artery and posterior communicating artery.

Superior medullary velum

Superior cerebellar peduncle

Fourth ventricle

Basilar artery, long circumferential branches

Middle cerebellar peduncle

Basilar artery, short circumferential branches

Basilar artery, pontine and paramedian branches

Trigeminal nerve

D Distribution of the arteries of the pons in transverse section

The pons derives its blood supply from short and long branches of the basilar artery.

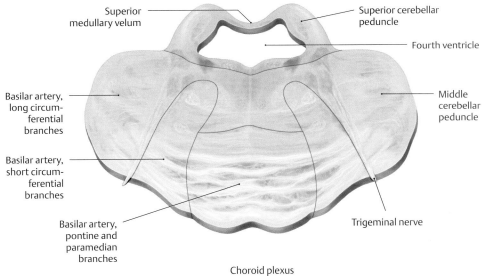

Choroid plexus

Fourth ventricle

Posterior inferior cerebellar artery

Vagus nerve

Anterior inferior cerebellar artery

Olive

Anterior spinal artery and paramedian branches of vertebral artery

Pyramidal tract

Hypoglossal nerve

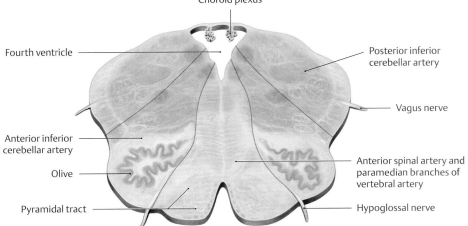

E Distribution of the arteries of the medulla oblongata in transverse section

The medulla oblongata is supplied by branches of the anterior spinal artery, and posterior inferior cerebellar artery (both arising from the vertebral artery), as well as the anterior inferior cerebellar artery (first large branch of the basilar artery).

253

8.5 Dural Sinuses, Overview

A Relationship of the principal dural sinuses to the skull
Oblique posterior view from the right side (brain removed and tentorium windowed on the right side). The dural sinuses are stiff-walled venous channels that receive blood from the internal and external cerebral veins, orbits, and calvaria, and convey it to the internal jugular veins on both sides. With few exceptions (inferior sagittal sinus, straight sinus), the walls of the dural sinuses are formed by both the periosteal and meningeal layers of the dura mater (see **C**, p. 189). The valveless dural sinuses are lined internally by endothelium and are expanded at some sites (particularly in the superior sagittal sinus) to form "lateral lacunae" (see **B**). These expansions contain the arachnoid villi through which cerebrospinal fluid (CSF) is absorbed into the venous blood (see p. 194f). The system of dural sinuses is divided into an upper group and a lower group:

- **Upper group:** superior and inferior sagittal sinuses, straight sinus, occipital sinus, transverse sinus, sigmoid sinus, and the confluence of the sinuses.
- **Lower group:** cavernous sinus with anterior and posterior intercavernous sinuses, sphenoparietal sinus, superior and inferior petrosal sinuses.

The upper and lower groups of dural sinuses communicate with the venous plexuses of the vertebral canal through the marginal sinus at the inlet to the foramen magnum and through the basilar plexus on the clivus (see **C**).

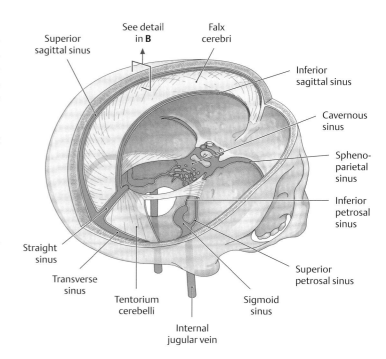

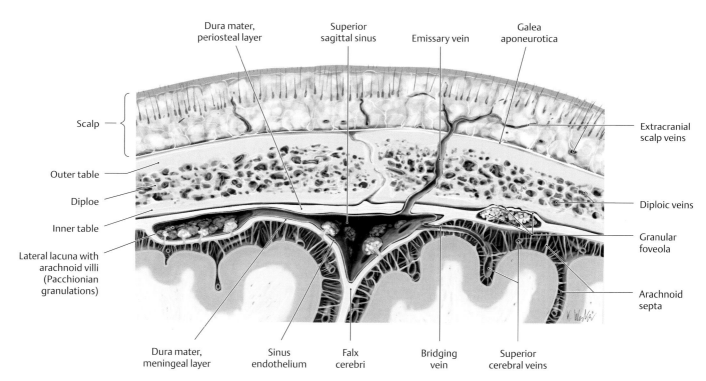

B Structure of a dural sinus, shown here for the superior sagittal sinus
Transverse section, occipital view (detail from **A**). The sinus wall is composed of endothelium and tough, collagenous dural connective tissue with a periosteal and meningeal layer. Between the two layers is the sinus lumen.

Note the lateral lacunae, where the arachnoid villi open into the venous system. Superficial cerebral veins (superior cerebral veins, bridging veins, see pp. 186 and 262) open into the sinus itself along with diploic veins from the adjacent cranial bone. The sinus also receives emissary veins—valveless veins that establish connections among the sinuses, the diploic veins, and the extracranial veins of the scalp.

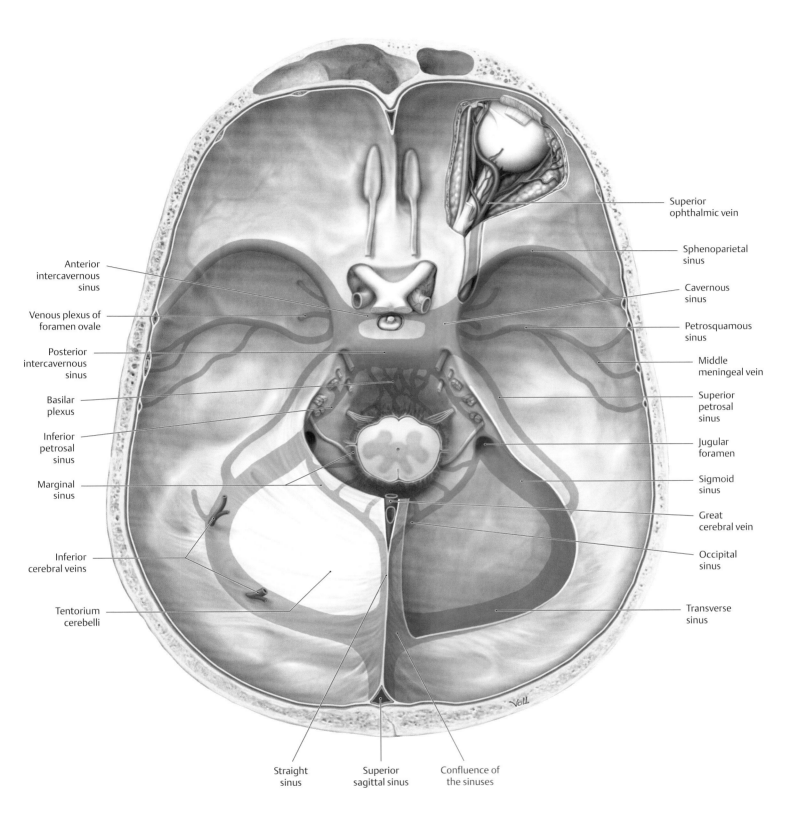

Superior
ophthalmic vein

Sphenoparietal
sinus

Cavernous
sinus

Petrosquamous
sinus

Middle
meningeal vein

Superior
petrosal
sinus

Jugular
foramen

Sigmoid
sinus

Great
cerebral vein

Occipital
sinus

Transverse
sinus

Anterior
intercavernous
sinus

Venous plexus of
foramen ovale

Posterior
intercavernous
sinus

Basilar
plexus

Inferior
petrosal
sinus

Marginal
sinus

Inferior
cerebral veins

Tentorium
cerebelli

Straight
sinus

Superior
sagittal sinus

Confluence of
the sinuses

C Dural sinuses at the skull base

Transverse section at the level of the tentorium cerebelli, viewed from above (brain removed, orbital roof and tentorium windowed on the right side). The cavernous sinus forms a ring around the sella turcica, its left and right parts being interconnected at the front and behind by an anterior and a posterior intercavernous sinus. Behind the posterior intercavernous sinus, on the clivus, is the basilar plexus. This plexus also contributes to the drainage of the cavernous sinus.

8.6 Dural Sinuses: Tributaries and Accessory Draining Vessels

A Dural sinus tributaries from the cerebral veins (after Rauber and Kopsch)

Right lateral view. Venous blood collected deep within the brain drains to the dural sinuses through *superficial* and deep cerebral veins (see p. 258). The red arrows in the diagram show the principal directions of venous blood flow in the major sinuses. Because of the numerous anastomoses, the isolated occlusion of even a complete sinus segment may produce no clinical symptoms.

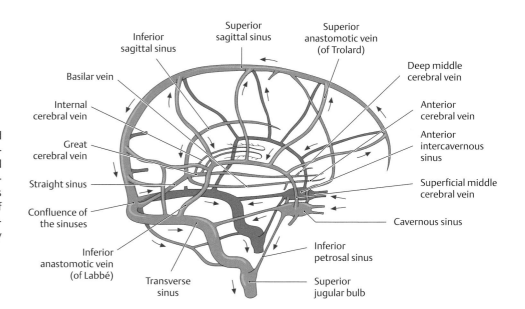

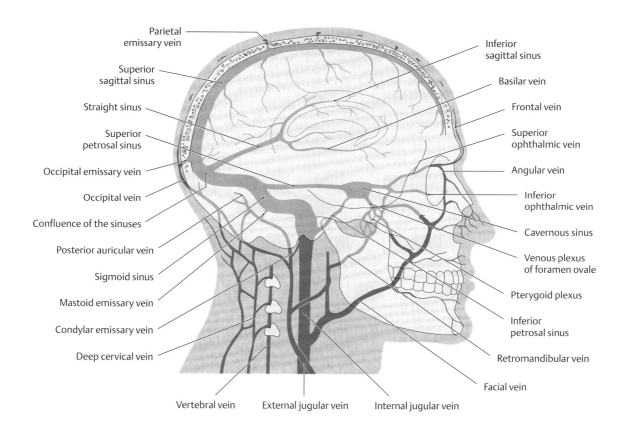

B Accessory drainage pathways of the dural sinuses

Right lateral view. The dural sinuses have many accessory drainage pathways besides their principal drainage into the two internal jugular veins. The connections between the dural sinuses and extracranial veins mainly serve to equalize pressure and regulate temperature. These anastomoses are of clinical interest because their normal direction of blood flow may reverse (no venous valves), allowing blood from extracranial veins to reflux into the dural sinuses. This mechanism may give rise to sinus infections that lead, in turn, to vascular occlusion (*venous sinus thrombosis*). The most important accessory drainage vessels include the following:

- Emissary veins (diploic and superior scalp veins), see **C**.
- Superior ophthalmic vein (angular and facial veins).
- Venous plexus of foramen ovale (pterygoid plexus, retromandibular vein).
- Marginal sinus and basilar plexus (internal and external vertebral venous plexus), see **C**.

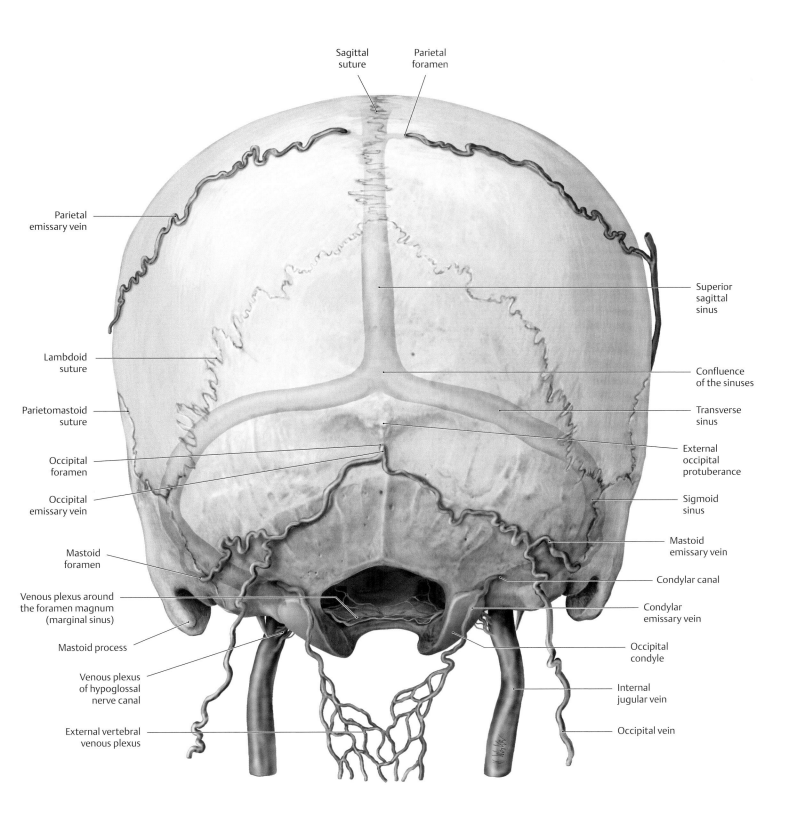

Sagittal suture

Parietal foramen

Parietal emissary vein

Superior sagittal sinus

Lambdoid suture

Confluence of the sinuses

Parietomastoid suture

Transverse sinus

Occipital foramen

External occipital protuberance

Occipital emissary vein

Sigmoid sinus

Mastoid foramen

Mastoid emissary vein

Venous plexus around the foramen magnum (marginal sinus)

Condylar canal

Mastoid process

Condylar emissary vein

Venous plexus of hypoglossal nerve canal

Occipital condyle

External vertebral venous plexus

Internal jugular vein

Occipital vein

C Occipital emissary veins

Emissary veins establish a direct connection between the intracranial dural sinuses and extracranial veins. They run through small cranial openings such as the parietal and mastoid foramina. Emissary veins are of clinical interest because they create a potential route by which bacteria from the scalp may spread to the dura mater and incite a purulent meningitis.

8.7 Veins of the Brain: Superficial and Deep Veins

Because the veins of the brain do not run parallel to the arteries, marked differences are noted between the regions of arterial supply and venous drainage. While all of the cerebral arteries enter the brain at its base, venous blood is drained from the entire surface of the brain, including the base, and also from the interior of the brain by two groups of veins: the *superficial cerebral veins* and the *deep cervical veins*. The superficial veins drain blood from the cerebral cortex (via cortical veins) and white matter (via medullary veins) directly into the dural sinuses. The deep veins drain blood from the deeper portions of the white matter, basal ganglia, corpus callosum, and diencephalon into the great cerebral vein, which enters the straight sinus. The two venous regions (those of the superficial and deep veins) are interconnected by numerous intracerebral anastomoses (see **D**).

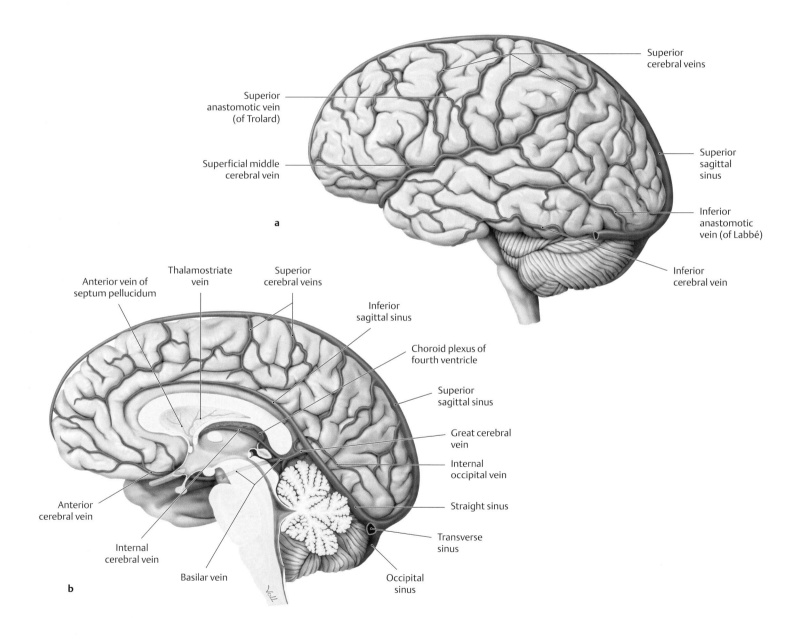

A Superficial veins of the brain (superficial cerebral veins)
Left lateral view (**a**) and medial view (**b**).
a, **b** The superficial cerebral veins drain blood from the short cortical veins and long medullary veins in the white matter (see **D**) into the dural sinuses. (The deep cerebral veins are described in **C**, p. 261.) Their course is extremely variable, and veins in the subarachnoid space do not follow arteries, gyri, or sulci. Consequently, only the most important of these vessels are named here.

Just before terminating in the dural sinuses, the veins leave the subarachnoid space and run a short subdural course between the dura mater and arachnoid. These short subdural venous segments are called *bridging veins*. The bridging veins have great clinical importance because they may be ruptured by head trauma, resulting in a subdural hematoma (see p. 262).

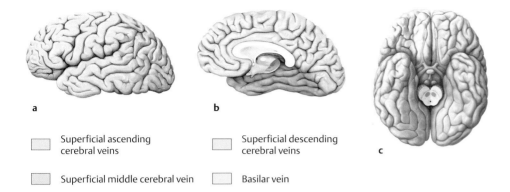

a

b

c

☐ Superficial ascending
cerebral veins

☐ Superficial descending
cerebral veins

☐ Superficial middle cerebral vein

☐ Basilar vein

B Regions drained by the superficial cerebral veins
a Left lateral view, **b** view of the medial surface of the right hemisphere, **c** basal view.
The veins on the lateral surface of the brain are classified by their direction of drainage as ascending (draining into the superior sagittal sinus) or descending (draining into the transverse sinus). The superficial middle cerebral vein drains into both the cavernous and transverse sinuses (see **A**, p. 254).

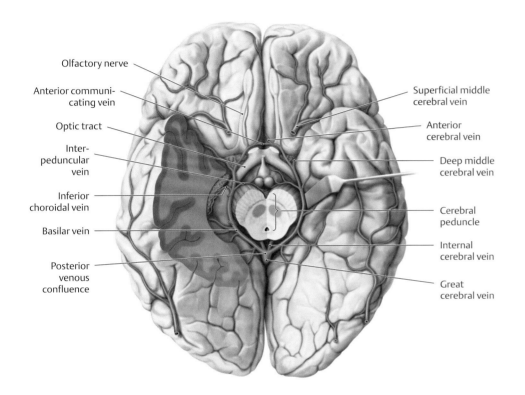

Olfactory nerve

Anterior communicating vein

Optic tract

Interpeduncular vein

Inferior choroidal vein

Basilar vein

Posterior venous confluence

Superficial middle cerebral vein

Anterior cerebral vein

Deep middle cerebral vein

Cerebral peduncle

Internal cerebral vein

Great cerebral vein

C Basal cerebral venous system
The basal cerebral venous system drains blood from both superficial and deep cerebral veins. A venous circle formed by the basilar veins (of Rosenthal, see below) exists at the base of the brain, analogous to the arterial circle of Willis. The basilar vein is formed in the anterior perforate substance by the union of the anterior cerebral and deep middle cerebral veins. Following the course of the optic tract, the basilar vein runs posteriorly around the cerebral peduncle and unites with the basilar vein from the opposite side on the dorsal aspect of the mesencephalon. The two internal cerebral veins also terminate at this venous junction, the posterior venous confluence. This junction gives rise to the midline great cerebral vein, which enters the straight sinus. The basilar vein receives tributaries from deep brain regions in its course (e.g., veins from the thalamus and hypothalamus, choroid plexus of the inferior horn, etc.). The two anterior cerebral veins are interconnected by the anterior communicating vein, creating a closed, ring-shaped drainage system.

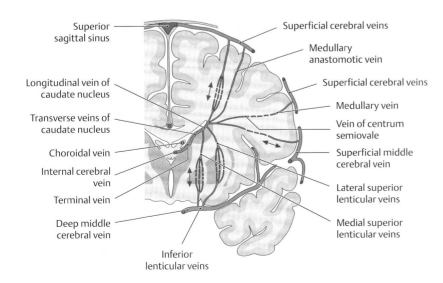

Superior sagittal sinus

Longitudinal vein of caudate nucleus

Transverse veins of caudate nucleus

Choroidal vein

Internal cerebral vein

Terminal vein

Deep middle cerebral vein

Inferior lenticular veins

Superficial cerebral veins

Medullary anastomotic vein

Superficial cerebral veins

Medullary vein

Vein of centrum semiovale

Superficial middle cerebral vein

Lateral superior lenticular veins

Medial superior lenticular veins

D Anastomoses between the superficial and deep cerebral veins
Transverse section through the left hemisphere, anterior view. The superficial cerebral veins communicate with the deep cerebral veins through the anastomoses shown here (see p. 260). Flow reversal (double arrows) may occur in the boundary zones between two territories.

8.8 Veins of the Brainstem and Cerebellum: Deep Veins

A Deep cerebral veins

Multiplanar transverse section (combining multiple transverse planes) with a superior view of the opened lateral ventricles. The temporal and occipital lobes and tentorium cerebelli have been removed on the left side to demonstrate the upper surface of the cerebellum and the superior cerebellar veins. On the lateral walls of the anterior horns of both lateral ventricles, the superior thalamostriate vein runs toward the interventricular foramen in the groove between the thalamus and caudate nucleus. After receiving the anterior vein of the septum pellucidum and the superior choroidal vein, it forms the internal cerebral vein and passes through the interventricular foramen along the roof of the diencephalon toward the quadrigeminal plate, which contains the superior and inferior colliculi. There it unites with the internal cerebral vein of the opposite side, and the basal veins to form the posterior venous confluence, which gives rise to the great cerebral vein.

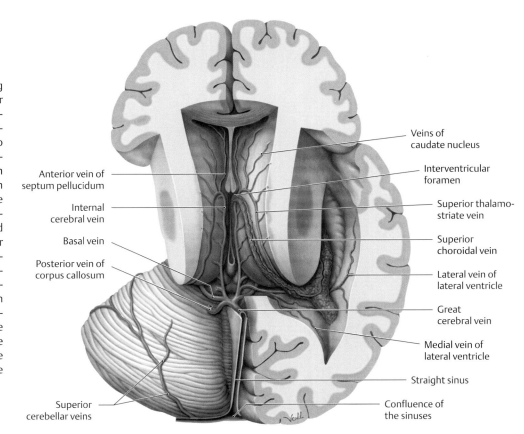

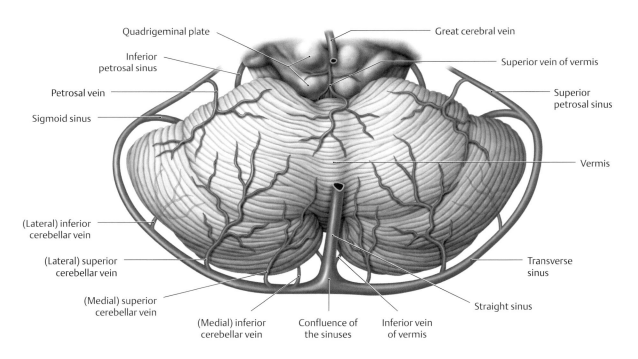

B Cerebellar veins

Posterior view. Like the other veins of the brain, the cerebellar veins are distributed independently of the cerebellar arteries. Larger trunks cross over gyri and sulci, running mainly in the sagittal direction. A *medial* and a *lateral* group can be distinguished based on their gross topographical anatomy. The medial group of cerebellar veins drains the vermis and adjacent portions of the cerebellar hemispheres (precentral vein, superior and inferior veins of the vermis) and the medial portions of the superior and inferior cerebellar veins. The *lateral group* (petrosal vein and lateral portions of the superior and inferior cerebellar veins) drains most of the two cerebellar hemispheres. All of the cerebellar veins anastomose with one another; their outflow is exclusively infratentorial (i.e., below the tentorium cerebelli).

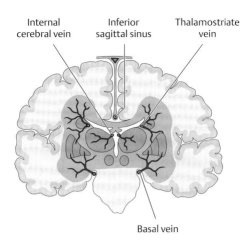

Internal cerebral vein — Inferior sagittal sinus — Thalamostriate vein

Basal vein

C Region drained by the deep cerebral veins

Coronal section. Three principal venous segments can be identified in each hemisphere:

- Thalamostriate vein
- Internal cerebral vein
- Basal vein

The region drained by the deep cerebral veins encompasses large portions of the base of the cerebrum, the basal ganglia, the internal capsule, the choroid plexuses of the lateral and third ventricles, the corpus callosum, and portions of the diencephalon and mesencephalon.

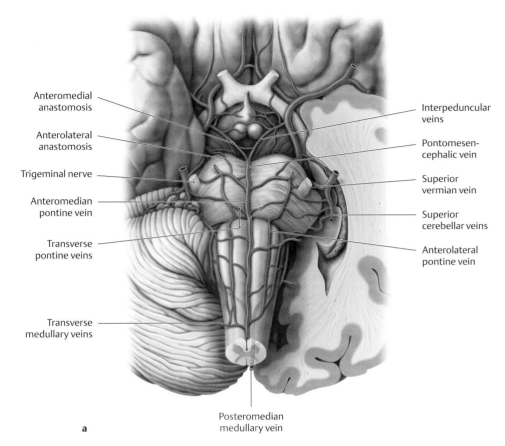

Anteromedial anastomosis — Anterolateral anastomosis — Trigeminal nerve — Anteromedian pontine vein — Transverse pontine veins — Transverse medullary veins

Interpeduncular veins — Pontomesencephalic vein — Superior vermian vein — Superior cerebellar veins — Anterolateral pontine vein

Posteromedian medullary vein

a

D Veins of the brainstem

a Anterior view of the brainstem in situ (the cerebellum and part of the occipital lobe have been removed on the left side). **b** Posterior view of the isolated brainstem with the cerebellum removed.

The veins of the brainstem are a continuation of the veins of the spinal cord and connect them with the basal veins of the brain. As on the spinal cord, the veins on the lower part of the brainstem form a venous plexus consisting of a powerfully developed *longitudinal* system and a more branched *transverse* system. The veins of the medulla oblongata, pons, and cerebellum make up the infratentorial venous system. Various anastomoses (e.g., anteromedial and lateral) exist at the boundary between the infra- and supratentorial systems.

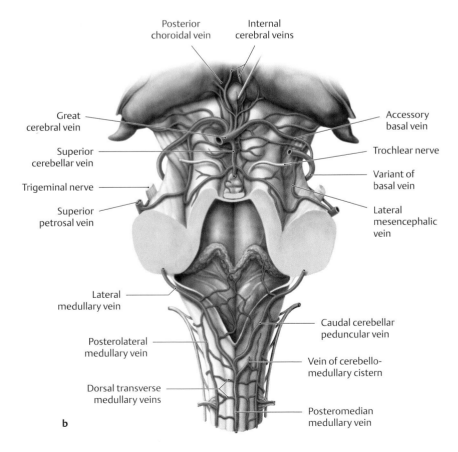

Posterior choroidal vein — Internal cerebral veins

Great cerebral vein — Superior cerebellar vein — Trigeminal nerve — Superior petrosal vein — Lateral medullary vein — Posterolateral medullary vein — Dorsal transverse medullary veins

Accessory basal vein — Trochlear nerve — Variant of basal vein — Lateral mesencephalic vein — Caudal cerebellar peduncular vein — Vein of cerebellomedullary cistern — Posteromedian medullary vein

b

8.9 Blood Vessels of the Brain: Intracranial Hemorrhage

Intracranial hemorrhages may be extracerebral (see **A**) or intracerebral (see **C**).

A Extracerebral hemorrhages

Extracerebral hemorrhages are defined as bleeding between the calvaria and brain. Because the bony calvaria is immobile, the developing hematoma exerts pressure on the soft brain. Depending on the source of the hemorrhage (arterial or venous), this may produce a rapidly or slowly developing incompressible mass with a rise of intracranial pressure that may damage not only the brain tissue at the bleeding site but also in more remote brain areas. Three types of intracranial hemorrhage can be distinguished based on their relationship to the dura mater:

a **Epidural hematoma** (epidural = above the dura). This type generally develops after a head injury involving a skull fracture. The bleeding most commonly occurs from a ruptured middle meningeal artery (due to the close proximity of the middle meningeal artery to the calvaria, a sharp bone fragment may lacerate the artery). The hematoma forms between the calvaria and the periosteal layer of the dura mater. Pressure from the hematoma separates the dura from the calvaria and displaces the brain. Typically there is an initial transient loss of consciousness caused by the impact, followed 1–5 hours later by a second decline in the level of consciousness, this time due to compression of the brain by the arterial hemorrhage. The interval between the first and second loss of consciousness is called the *lucid interval* (occurs in approximately 30–40 % of all epidural hematomas). Detection of the hemorrhage (CT scanning of the head) and prompt evacuation of the hematoma are life-saving.

b **Subdural hematoma** (subdural = below the dura). Trauma to the head causes the rupture of a *bridging vein* (see p. 254) that bleeds between the dura mater and arachnoid. The bleeding occurs into a potential "subdural space," which exists only when extravasated blood has dissected the arachnoid membrane from the dura (the spaces are described in **C**, p. 191). Because the bleeding source is venous, the increased intracranial pressure and mass effect develop more slowly than with an arterial epidural hemorrhage. Consequently, a subdural hematoma may develop *chronically* over a period of weeks, even after a relatively mild head injury.

c **Subarachnoid hemorrhage** is an arterial bleed caused by the rupture of an aneurysm (abnormal outpouching) of an artery at the base of the brain (see **B**). It is typically caused by a brief, sudden rise in blood pressure, like that produced by a sudden rise of intra-abdominal pressure (straining at stool or urine, lifting a heavy object, etc.). Because the hemorrhage is into the CSF-filled subarachnoid space, blood can be detected in the cerebrospinal fluid by means of lumbar puncture. The cardinal symptom of a subarachnoid hemorrhage is a sudden, excruciating headache accompanied by a stiff neck caused by meningeal irritation.

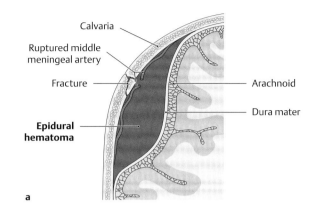

a

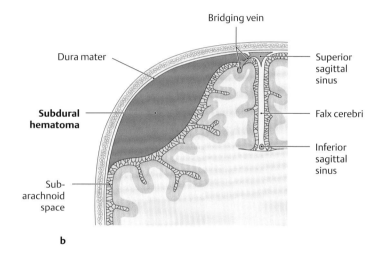

b

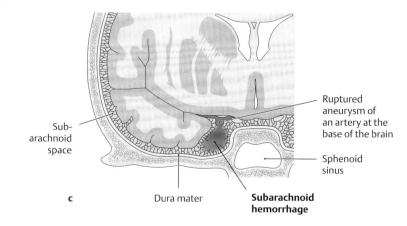

c

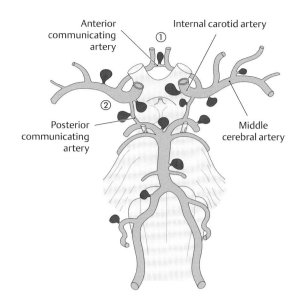

B Sites of berry aneurysms at the base of the brain

(after Bähr and Frotscher)

The rupture of congenital or acquired arterial aneurysms at the base of the brain is the most frequent cause of subarachnoid hemorrhage and accounts for approximately 5 % of all strokes. These are abnormal saccular dilations of the circle of Willis and are especially common at the site of branching. When one of these thin-walled aneurysms ruptures, arterial blood escapes into the subarachnoid space. The most common site is the junction between the anterior cerebral and anterior communicating arteries (1); the second most likely site is the branching of the posterior communicating artery from the internal carotid artery (2).

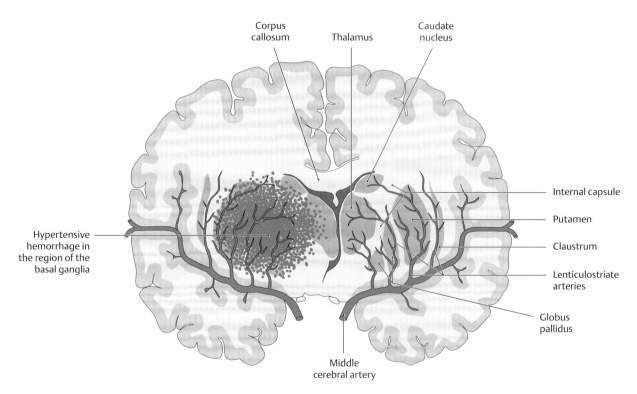

C Intracerebral hemorrhage

Coronal section at the level of the thalamus. Unlike the intracranial *extracerebral* hemorrhages described above, *intracerebral* hemorrhage occurs when damaged arteries bleed directly *into the substance of the brain*. This distinction is of very great clinical importance because extracerebral hemorrhages can be controlled by surgical hemostasis of the bleeding vessel, whereas intracerebral hemorrhages cannot. The most frequent cause of intracerebral hemorrhage (hemorrhagic stroke) is high blood pressure. Because the soft brain tissue offers very little resistance, a large hematoma may form within the brain. The most common sources of intracerebral bleeding are specific branches of the middle cerebral artery—the lenticulostriate arteries pictured here (known also as the "stroke arteries"). The hemorrhage causes a cerebral infarction in the region of the internal capsule, one effect of which is to disrupt the pyramidal tract, which passes through the capsule (see **E**, p. 377). The loss of pyramidal tract function below the lesion is manifested clinically by spastic paralysis of the limbs on the side of the body *opposite* to the injury (the pyramidal tracts cross below the level of the lesion). The hemorrhage is not always massive, and smaller bleeds may occur in the territories of the three main cerebral arteries, producing a typical clinical presentation.

8.10 Blood Vessels of the Brain: Cerebrovascular Disease

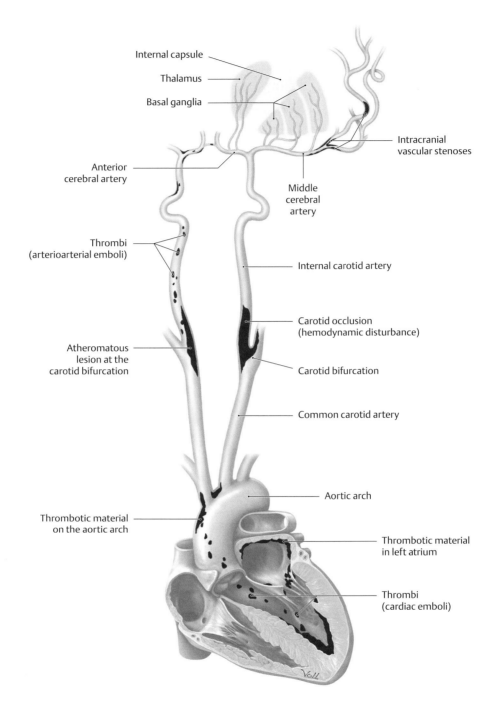

A Frequent causes of cerebrovascular disease (after Mumenthaler) Disturbances of cerebral blood flow that deprive the brain of oxygen (cerebral ischemia) are the most frequent cause of central neurological deficits. The most serious complication is stroke: the vast majority of all strokes are caused by cerebral *ischemic* disease. Stroke has become the third leading cause of death in western industrialized countries (approximately 700,000 strokes occur in the United States each year). Cerebral ischemia is caused by a prolonged diminution or interruption of blood flow and involves *the distribution area of the internal carotid artery* in up to 90% of cases. Much less commonly, cerebral ischemia is caused by an obstruction of venous outflow due to cerebral venous thrombosis (see

B). A decrease of arterial blood flow in the carotid system most commonly results from an embolic or local thrombotic occlusion. Most emboli originate from atheromatous lesions at the carotid bifurcation (arterioarterial emboli) or from the expulsion of thrombotic material from the left ventricle (cardiac emboli). Blood clots (thrombi) may be dislodged from the heart as a result of valvular disease or atrial fibrillation. This produces emboli that may be carried by the bloodstream to the brain, where they may cause the functional occlusion of an artery supplying the brain. The most common example of this involves all of the distribution region of the middle cerebral artery, which is a direct continuation of the internal carotid artery.

Right   Left

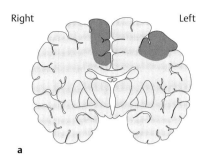

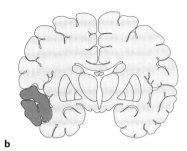

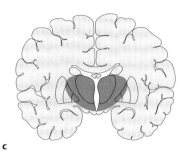

a   b   c

B Cerebral venous thrombosis

Coronal section, anterior view. The cerebral veins, like the cerebral arteries, serve specific territories (see pp. 258 and 260). Though much less common than decreased arterial flow, the obstruction of venous outflow is an important potential cause of ischemia and infarction. With a thrombotic occlusion, for example, the quantity of blood and thus the venous pressure are increased in the tributary region of the occluded vein. This causes a drop in the capillary pressure gradient, with an increased extravasation of fluid from the capillary bed into the brain tissue (edema). There is a concomitant reduction of arterial inflow into the affected region, depriving it of oxygen. The occlusion of specific cerebral veins (e.g., due to cerebral venous thrombosis) leads to brain infarctions at characteristic locations:

a **Superior cerebral veins:** Thrombosis and infarction in the areas drained by the:

- Medial superior cerebral veins (right, *symptoms*: contralateral lower limb weakness);
- Posterior superior cerebral veins (left, *symptoms*: contralateral hemiparesis).

Motor aphasia occurs if the infarction involves the motor speech center in the dominant hemisphere.

b **Inferior cerebral veins:** Thrombosis of the right inferior cerebral veins leads to infarction of the right temporal lobe (*symptoms*: sensory aphasia, contralateral hemianopia).

c **Internal cerebral veins:** Bilateral thrombosis leads to a symmetrical infarction affecting the thalamus and basal ganglia. This is characterized by a rapid deterioration of consciousness ranging to coma.

Because the dural sinuses have extensive anastomoses, a limited occlusion affecting part of a sinus often does not cause pronounced clinical symptoms, unlike the venous thromboses described here (see p. 256).

C Cardinal symptoms of occlusion of the three main cerebral arteries (after Masuhr and Neumann)

When the *anterior, middle* or *posterior cerebral artery* becomes occluded, characteristic functional deficits occur in the oxygen-deprived brain areas supplied by the occluded vessel (see p. 250). In many cases the affected artery can be identified based on the associated neurological deficit:

- Bladder weakness (cortical bladder center) and paralysis of the lower limb (hemiplegia with or without hemisensory deficit, predominantly affecting the leg) on the side opposite the occlusion (see motor and sensory homunculi, pp. 329 and 339) indicate an infarction in the territory of the **anterior cerebral artery**.
- Contralateral hemiplegia affecting the arm and face more than the leg indicates an infarction in the territory of the **middle cerebral artery**. If the dominant hemisphere is affected, aphasia also occurs (the patient cannot name objects, for example).
- Visual disturbances affecting the contralateral visual field (hemianopia) may signify an infarction in the territory of the **posterior cerebral artery**, because the structures supplied by this artery include the visual cortex in the calcarine sulcus of the occipital lobe. If branches to the thalamus are also affected, the patient may also exhibit a contralateral hemisensory deficit because the afferent sensory fibers have already crossed below the thalamus.

The extent of the infarction depends partly on whether the occlusion is proximal or distal. Generally a proximal occlusion will cause a much more extensive infarction than a distal occlusion. MCA infarctions are the most common because the middle cerebral artery is essentially a direct continuation of the internal carotid artery.

Vascular territory	Neurological symptoms	
Anterior cerebral artery	Hemiparesis (with or without hemisensory deficit)	Bladder dysfunction
Middle cerebral artery	Hemiparesis (with or without hemisensory deficit) mainly affecting the arm and face (Wernicke-Mann type)	Aphasia
Posterior cerebral artery	Hemisensory losses	Hemianopia

9.1 Spinal Cord, Segmental Organization

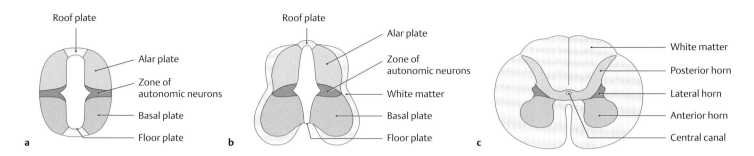

a | **b** | **c**

Roof plate — Alar plate — Zone of autonomic neurons — Basal plate — Floor plate

Roof plate — Alar plate — Zone of autonomic neurons — White matter — Basal plate — Floor plate

White matter — Posterior horn — Lateral horn — Anterior horn — Central canal

A Development of the spinal cord
Transverse section, superior view.
a Early neural tube, **b** intermediate stage, **c** adult spinal cord. The spinal cord develops from the neural tube:

- **Posterior horn:** develops from the posterior part of the neural tube (the *alar plate*). It contains the afferent (sensory) neurons.
- **Anterior horn:** develops from the anterior part of the neural tube (the *basal plate*). It contains the efferent (motor) neurons.
- **Lateral column:** develops from the intervening zone. Present only in the thoracic, lumbar, and sacral regions of the cord, it contains the autonomic (sympathetic and parasympathetic) neurons. (Its longitudinal distribution is shown in **C**, p. 283.)

Neurons do not develop from the roof or floor plates. Viewing the spinal cord in transverse section, we see that it consists of gray matter that is arranged about the central canal and is surrounded by white matter. The **gray matter** contains the cell bodies of neurons while the **white matter** consists of nerve fibers (axons).
Note: axons that have the same function are collected into bundles called *tracts*. Tracts that terminate in the brain are called *ascending, afferent* or *sensory* tracts, while tracts that pass from the brain into the spinal cord are called *descending, efferent* or *motor* tracts.

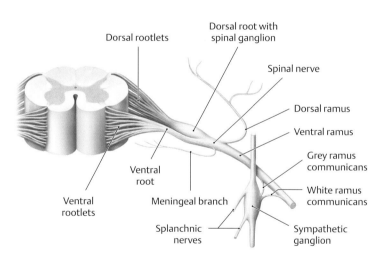

Dorsal rootlets — Dorsal root with spinal ganglion — Spinal nerve — Dorsal ramus — Ventral ramus — Grey ramus communicans — White ramus communicans — Sympathetic ganglion — Splanchnic nerves — Meningeal branch — Ventral root — Ventral rootlets

B Structure of a spinal cord segment
Two main organizational principles are observed in the spinal cord:

1. **Functional organization within a segment** (viewed in a transverse section of the spinal cord). In each spinal cord segment, the *afferent* dorsal rootlets enter the back of the cord while the *efferent* ventral rootlets emerge from the front of the cord. The rootlets in each set combine to form the dorsal (posterior) and ventral (anterior) roots. Each dorsal and ventral root fuses to form a mixed *spinal nerve*, which carries both sensory and motor fibers. Shortly after the fusion of its two roots, the spinal nerve divides into various branches.
2. **Topographical organization of the segments** (viewed in a longitudinal section of the spinal cord). The spinal cord consists of a vertical series of 31 segments (see **C**), each of which innervates a specific area in the trunk and limbs.

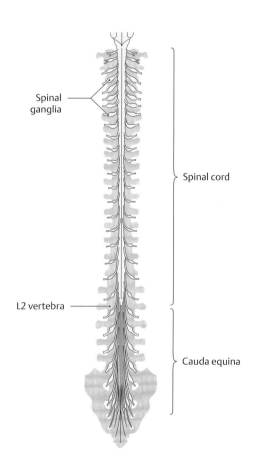

Spinal ganglia — Spinal cord — L2 vertebra — Cauda equina

C Spinal cord and spinal ganglia in situ
Posterior view with the laminar arches of the vertebral bodies removed. The longitudinal growth of the spinal cord lags behind that of the bony vertebral column. As a result, the lower end of the spinal cord in the adult lies at approximately the level of the first lumbar vertebral body (L1, see **D**). Below L1, the spinal nerve roots descend from the end of the cord to the intervertebral foramina, where they join to form the spinal nerves. The collection of these spinal roots is called the *cauda equina* ("horse's tail").

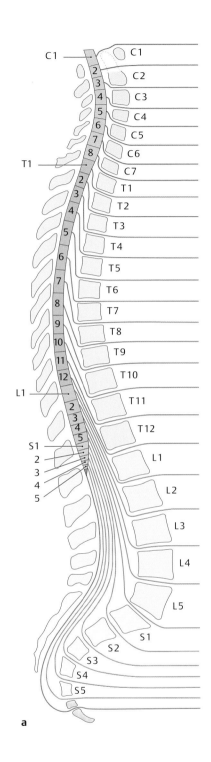

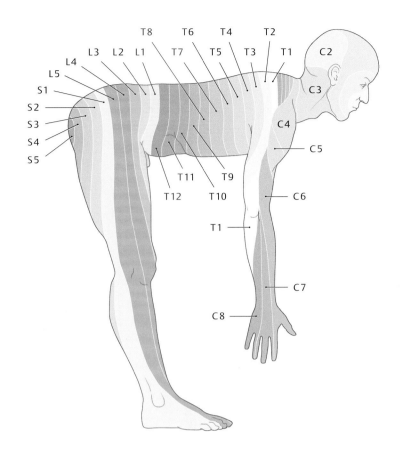

E Simplified schematic representation of the segmental innervation of the skin
(after Mumenthaler)

Distribution of the dermatomes on the body. Sensory innervation of the skin correlates with the sensory roots of the spinal nerves in **D**. Every spinal cord segment (except for C 1, see below) innervates a particular skin area (= dermatome). From a clinical standpoint, it is important to know the precise correlation of dermatomes with spinal cord segments so that the level of a spinal cord lesion can be determined based on the location of the affected dermatome. For example, a lesion of the C 8 spinal nerve root is characterized by a loss of sensation on the ulnar (small-finger) side of the hand.

Note: There is no C 1 dermatome because the first spinal nerve is purely motor.

Spinal cord segment	Vertebral body	Spinous process
C 8	Inferior margin of C 6, superior margin of C 7	C 6
T 6	T 5	T 4
T 12	T 10	T 9
L 3	T 11	T 11
S 1	T 12	T 12

D Spinal cord segments and vertebral bodies in the adult

a Midsagittal section, viewed from the right side. The spinal cord can be divided into four major regions: cervical cord (C, pink); thoracic cord (T, blue); lumbar cord (L, green); and sacral cord (S, yellow). The spinal cord segments are numbered according to the exit point of their associated nerves and do not necessarily correlate numerically with the nearest skeletal element (see **b**). The spinal cord generally terminates at the level of the L 1 vertebral body, and the region below this is known as the *cauda equina*. The cauda equina consists of dorsal (sensory) and ventral (motor) spinal nerve roots, and provides safe access for introducing a spinal needle to sample CSF (lumbar puncture).

b Differential growth of the spinal cord and vertebral column may separate spinal cord segments from their associated skeletal elements, with progressively greater "mismatch" occurring at more caudal levels. It is important to know the relationship of the spinal cord segments to the associated vertebral bodies when assessing injuries to the vertebral column (e.g., spinal fracture and cord lesions, see p. 357). The parts in the table are only approximations and may differ slightly in individual cases.

Note: there are only seven cervical vertebra (C1–C7), but eight pairs of cervical nerves (C1–C8).

9.2　Spinal Cord, Organization of Spinal Cord Segments

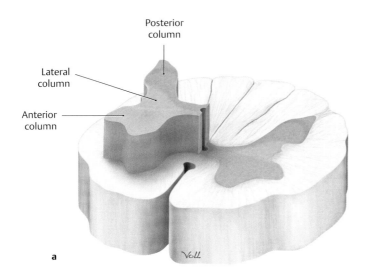

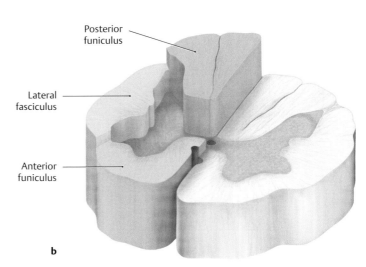

A Gray and white matter of the spinal cord
Three-dimensional representation, oblique anterior view from upper left.
a Gray matter, **b** white matter.
This three-dimensional view shows how the gray matter is divided into three columns:
- **Anterior column** (anterior horn): contains motor neurons.
- **Lateral column** (lateral horn): contains sympathetic or parasym-

pathetic (visceromotor) neurons.
- **Posterior column** (posterior horn): contains sensory neurons.
The gray matter partitions the white matter analogously into anterior, lateral and posterior funiculi. When the spinal cord is viewed in cross-section, the gray-matter columns are traditionally referred to as "horns."

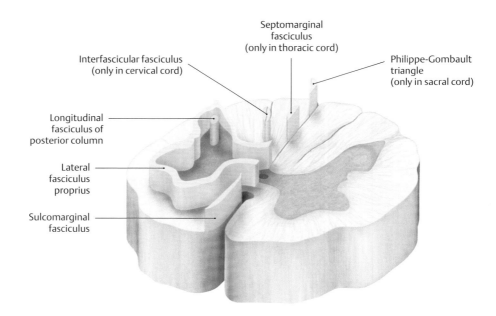

B Principal intrinsic fascicles of the spinal cord (shaded yellow)
Three-dimensional representation, oblique anterior view from upper left. Because most of the muscles have a plurisegmental mode of innervation, axons must be able to ascend and descend for multiple segments within the spinal cord in order to coordinate spinal reflexes (see p. 272).

The neurons of these axons originate from *interneurons* (see p. 271 **E**) in the gray matter, which form the intrinsic reflex pathways of the spinal cord (see p. 273 **C**). These axons are collected into *intrinsic fascicles* known also as *fasciculi proprii*. Arranged chiefly around the gray matter, these bundles make up the "intrinsic circuits" of the spinal cord.

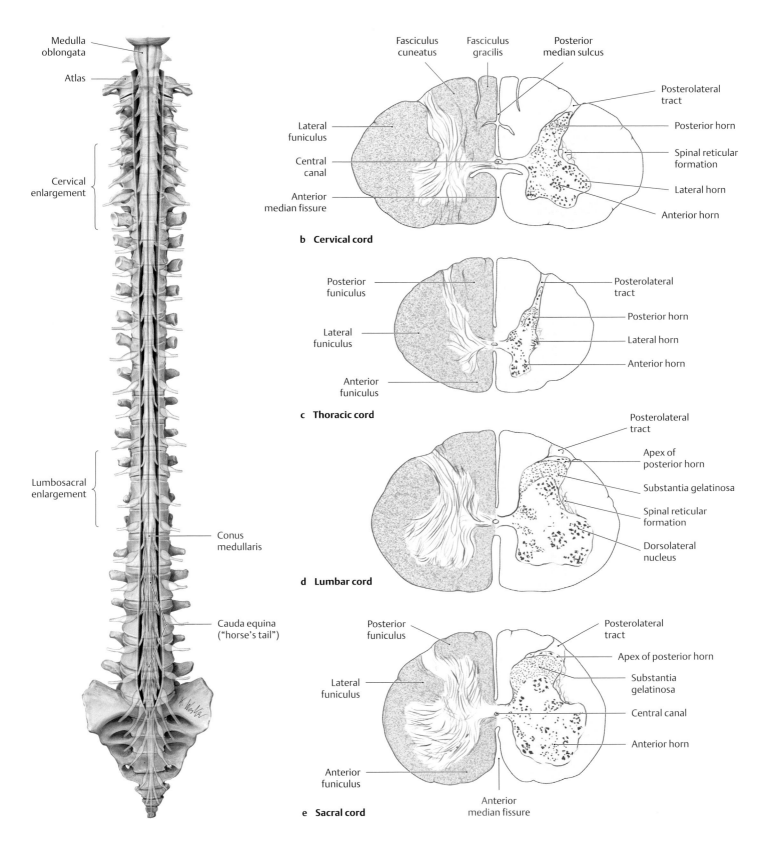

b Cervical cord

c Thoracic cord

d Lumbar cord

e Sacral cord

C Position of the spinal cord in the dural sac
a Anterior view with the vertebral bodies partially removed to display the anterior aspect of the spinal cord. The transverse sections (**b–e**) depict fiber tracts (left side, myelin stain) and neuron cell bodies (right side, Nissl stain) at different levels of the spinal cord. The areas of the cervical and lumbrosacral enlargements have been demarcated (**a**). In these areas, which provide innervation to the limbs, the gray matter is significantly expanded.

9.3 Spinal Cord: Internal Divisions of the Gray Matter

A Organizational principles of the anterior column of the spinal cord

Motor neurons that innervate specific muscles are arranged into vertical columns in the anterior (ventral) horn of the gray matter of the spinal cord. Analogous to the brainstem motor nuclei, these columns can themselves be called nuclei, and are arranged in a somatotopic fashion (see **B** for a mapping of these nuclei to their target muscles). The motor columns innervating the trunk have a relatively simple arrangement that follows the linear segmental organization of spinal nerves and dermatomes. The cervical and lumbrosacral enlargments, which innervate the limbs, have a more complex pattern of innervation than the trunk muscles: during the migratory processes of embryonic development, muscle precursors "carry" their original innervation with them, generating a motor column that sends its axons through multiple nerve roots from multiple spinal cord levels. The muscles innervated by such a column are accordingly called *multisegmental muscles* (see **B**, p. 272). Muscles whose motor neurons are situated entirely within one segment are referred to as *indicator muscles;* testing the function of indicator muscles is valuable in clinical assessment.

Note: although one muscle may be innervated by axons from multiple spinal segments, those axons arise from a *single* motor column.

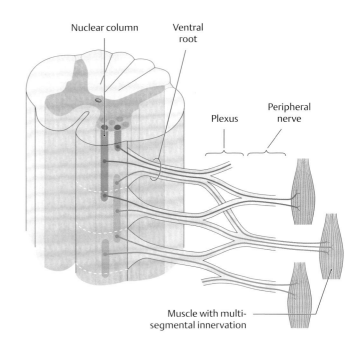

B Somatotopic organization of nuclear columns of the anterior horn (after Bossy)

a Common pattern of organization in the spinal cord. More medial nuclear columns of the anterior horn innervate muscles close to the midline, while more lateral nuclear columns tend to innervate muscles outside the trunk.

b Enlargement of cervical cord. The same pattern of medial-to-lateral organization exists (see **a**) with medial nuclei innervating axial mus-

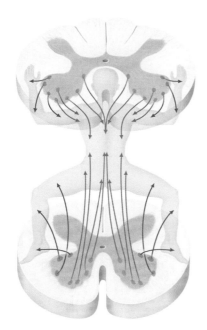

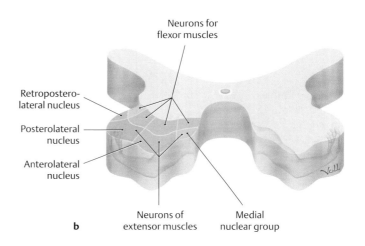

cles and lateral nuclei innervating muscles at the extremities. However, there is also an anterior-to-posterior segregation of motor columns. Neurons serving extensor muscles (shades of blue) are found in the most anterior parts of the anterior horn, while those serving flexor muscles (shades of pink) are found in the more posterior regions. These nuclei are further divided into:

- Medial nuclei: innervate nuchal, back, intercostal, and abdominal muscles
- Anterolateral nucleus: innervates shoulder girdle and upper arm muscles
- Posterolateral nucleus: innervates forearm muscles
- Retroposterolateral nucleus: innervates small muscles of the fingers

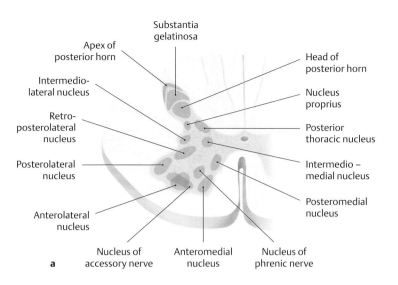

a Nucleus of accessory nerve | Anteromedial nucleus | Nucleus of phrenic nerve

b Anterolateral nucleus | Anteromedial nucleus | Central nucleus

C Cell groups in the gray matter of the spinal cord

a Cervical cord, **b** lumbar cord.

Besides the somatotopic organization of the anterior horn, the gray matter contains a particular pattern of neuron clustering. When the motor columns described in **A** and **B** are shown in red and the neurons participating in the sensory pathways are shown in blue, an obvious pattern of functional sequestration can be seen. The larger anterior (ventral) horn contains the motor nuclei, and is the source of the ventral (motor) root of the spinal nerve, whereas the more slender posterior (dorsal) horn contains the cell bodies of secondary sensory neurons and receives the dorsal (sensory) root. The sensory neurons of the posterior horn receive synapses from entering processes of spinal (dorsal root) ganglion cells, and in turn send their axons to other, mostly more cranial, levels. *Note:* some ganglion cell axons enter ascending tracts without synapsing locally.

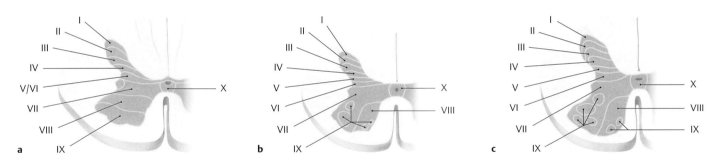

D Synaptic layers in the gray matter

a Cervical cord, **b** thoracic cord, **c** lumbar cord. Motor neurons are shown in red, sensory neurons in blue.

The gray matter can also be divided into layers of axon termination, based on cytological criteria. This was first done by the Swedish neuroanatomist Bror Rexed (1914–2002), who divided the gray matter into laminae I–X. This laminar architecture is especially well defined in the posterior (dorsal) horn, where primary sensory axons make synapses in specific layers.

E Gray matter neurons of the spinal cord

Motor neurons (neurons which send axons in the ventral root to the spinal nerve and periphery):
- *Somatic motor neurons* (including alpha and gamma motor neurons)
- *Visceral motor neurons:* preganglionic neurons which innervate ganglion cells. At thoracolumbar levels these are preganglionic sympathetic neurons; at mid-sacral levels, these are preganglionic parasympathetic motor neurons.

Intrinsic neurons (neurons which send axons to other CNS locations):
- *Secondary sensory neurons* (tract cells): neurons which send their axons in ascending tracts (white matter). These neurons receive synapses from primary sensory neurons whose cell bodies are in spinal (dorsal root) ganglia.
- *Local interneurons:* neurons distributed through the gray matter whose axons remain in the local spinal cord (see **C**, p.273). These include:
  – Intercalated cells: neurons whose axons remain at the same segmental level.

  – Commissural cells: neurons whose axons cross in the spinal white commissure to the contralateral side.
  – Association (intersegmental) cells: neurons whose axons interconnect different spinal segments.
  – Renshaw cells: a specific type of inhibitory interneuron that is excited by axon collaterals from alpha motor neurons. The excited Renshaw cell inhibits the motor neuron that stimulated it, and also neighboring motor neurons, creating a negative-feedback loop that modulates the firing rate of the group of neurons. The Renshaw cell also synapses on other local inhibitory neurons, and receives input from descending pathways.

Some of these distinctions are not exact. Tract cells, for instance, have collaterals that synapse locally. Specific intrinsic neuron types like the Renshaw cell have been identified not only by their pattern of connections but also by pharmacological and electrophysiological behavior.

9.4 Spinal Cord: Reflex Arcs and Intrinsic Circuits

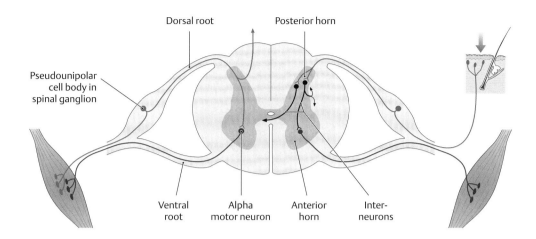

A **Integrative function of the gray matter of the spinal cord: reflexes**

Afferent nerves are shown in blue, efferent nerves in red. Black indicates neurons of the spinal reflex circuit.

The gray matter of the spinal cord supports muscular function at the unconscious (reflex) level, holding the body upright during stance and enabling us to walk and run without conscious control. To perform this coordinating function, the neurons of the gray matter must receive information from the muscles and their surroundings; this information enters the posterior horn of the spinal cord via the axons of neurons in the spinal ganglia (see p. 328). Two types of reflex exist:

- **Monosynaptic reflex** (left): intrinsic reflex in which information from the periphery (e.g., on muscle length and stretch) comes from the muscle itself. Receptors in the muscle transmit signals to

alpha motor neurons via neurons whose cell bodies are in the spinal ganglia. These afferent neurons release excitatory transmitters which cause the alpha motor neurons to stimulate muscle contraction (see **D**).
- **Polysynaptic reflex** (right): reflex mediated by receptors in the skin or other sites *outside* the muscle. These receptors act via *interneurons* (see **C**) to stimulate muscular contraction

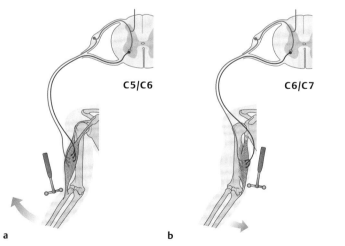

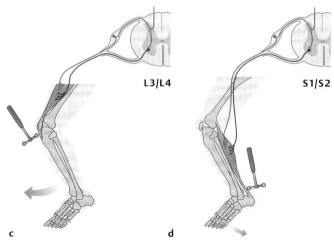

B Clinically important monosynaptic reflexes

a Biceps reflex, **b** triceps reflex, **c** patellar reflex (quadriceps reflex), **d** Achilles tendon reflex.

The drawings show the muscles, the trigger points for eliciting the reflexes, the nerves involved in the reflexes (afferent nerves in blue, efferent nerves in red), and the corresponding spinal cord segments.

The principal monosynaptic reflex es are should be tested in every physical examination. Each reflex is elicited by briskly tapping theappropriate

tendon with a reflex hammer to stretch the muscle. If the muscle contracts in response to this stretch, the reflex arc is intact. Although each test involves just one muscle and one nerve supplying the muscle, the innervation involves several spinal cord segments (= multisegmental muscles, see **A**, p. 270). The right and left sides should always be compared in clinical reflex testing, as this is the only way to recognize a *unilateral* increase, decrease, or other abnormality.

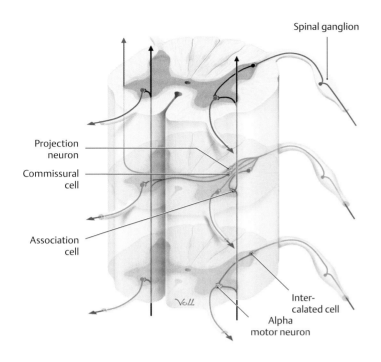

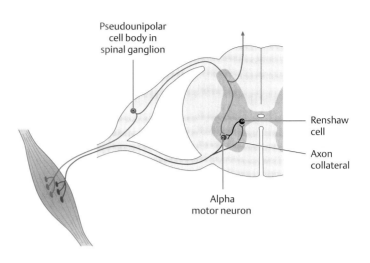

C Components of the intrinsic circuits of the spinal cord

Afferent neurons are shown in blue, efferent neurons in red. The neurons of the spinal reflex circuits are shown in black. Polysynaptic reflexes often must be coordinated at the spinal cord level by multiple segments. Interneurons, some of whose axons show a T-shaped branching pattern, convey the afferent signals to higher and lower segments along crossed and uncrossed pathways (types of interneurons are described in **E**, p. 271). These chains of interneurons, which are entirely contained within the spinal cord, make up the *intrinsic circuits* of the cord. The axons of the neurons in the intrinsic circuits pass to adjacent segments in intrinsic fascicles (fasciculi proprii) located as the edge of the gray matter (see **B**, p. 268). These fascicles are the conduction apparatus of the intrinsic circuits.

D Effects of the Renshaw cell on the alpha motor neuron

The afferent fibers in a monosynaptic reflex originate in neurons of the spinal ganglia. They terminate on the alpha motor neurons, where they release the excitatory transmitter acetylcholine. In response to this transmitter release, the alpha motor neuron transmits excitatory impulses to the neuromuscular synapse (the transmitter at the synapse is also acetylcholine). The excitatory alpha motor neuron has axon collaterals that enable it to exert a stimulatory effect on an inhibitory interneuron called a Renshaw cell. In response to this stimulation, the Renshaw cell releases the *inhibitory* transmitter glycine. This self-inhibiting mechanism serves to prevent overexcitation of the alpha motor neurons (recurrent inhibition). The clinical importance of the Renshaw cells is dramatically illustrated in patients with tetanus. The tetanus toxin inhibits the release of glycine from the Renshaw cells. Inhibition of the alpha motor neurons fails to occur, and so the patient experiences sustained (tetanic) muscle contractions.

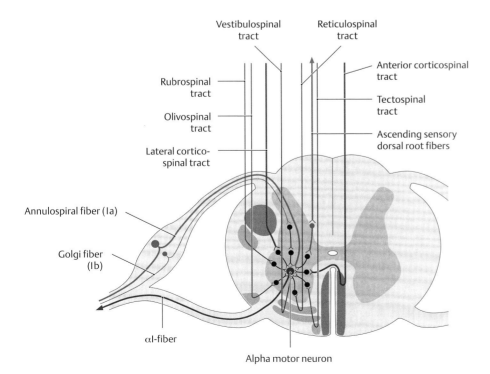

E Effects of long tracts on the alpha motor neuron

The alpha motor neuron not only receives efferent fibers from the spinal cord itself, but is also strongly modulated by efferent fibers from long tracts that originate in the brain. Most of these efferent fibers have an inhibitory effect on the alpha motor neuron. If these effects are abolished due to a complete cord lesion, for example, the disproportionately strong influence of the spinal intrinsic circuits will lead to spastic paralysis (see p. 343).

9.5 Ascending Tracts of the Spinal Cord: Spinothalamic Tracts

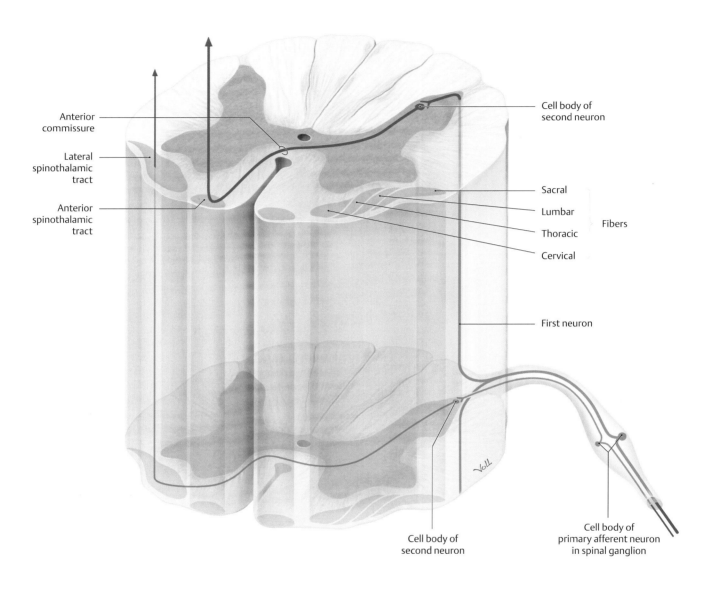

A Course of the anterior and lateral spinothalamic tracts in a transverse section of the spinal cord

See p. 284 for overview of ascending tracts. The axons of the anterior spinothalamic tract run in the anterior funiculus of the spinal cord, while those of the lateral spinothalamic tract run in both the anterior and lateral funiculi. (These two tracts are sometimes referred to collectively as the *anterolateral funicular tract.*) The anterior spinothalamic tract is the pathway for crude touch and pressure sensation, while the lateral spinothalamic tract conveys pain, temperature, tickle, itch, and sexual sensation. The cell bodies of the primary afferent neurons for both tracts are located in the spinal ganglia. Both tracts contain second neurons and cross in the anterior commissure. The somatotopic organization of the lateral spinothalamic tract is shown on the left side of the diagram. Starting dorsally and moving clockwise, we successively encounter the sacral, lumbar, thoracic, and cervical fibers. In older terminology a distinction is sometimes drawn between *epicritic* and *protopathic* sensation. According to this terminology, the anterior and lateral spinothalamic tracts are classified as *protopathic pathways* while the tracts of the posterior funiculus are classified as an *epicritic sensory pathway.* Today the original classification has been dropped because it does not correspond well to the assignment of sensory qualities to anatomically defined tracts.

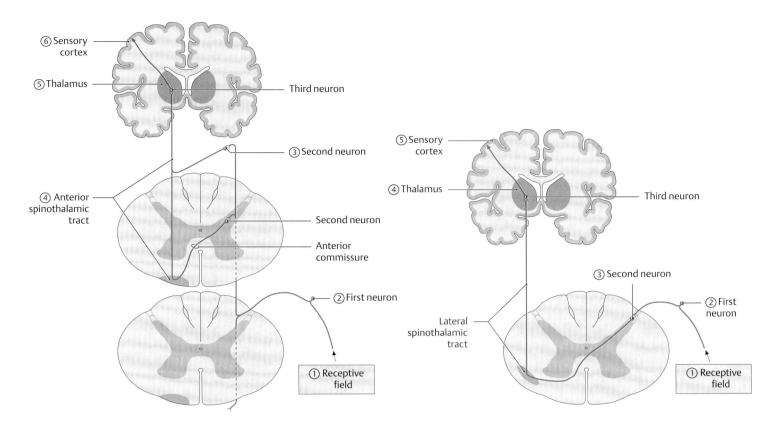

B Anterior spinothalamic tract and its central connections

1 Impulses from tactile corpuscles and from receptors about the hair follicles are carried to the anterior spinothalamic tract by moderately large-caliber myelinated axons (dendritic axons).

2 The cell bodies of these axons are located in the spinal ganglia (first neuron, primary afferent neuron).

3 The axons pass through the dorsal roots and enter the gray matter, where they branch in a T-shaped pattern. These branches descend for 1–2 segments and ascend for 2–15 segments. The synapses of these axons terminate on neurons in the posterior column (second neuron).

4 The axons of the second neuron form the anterior spinothalamic tract. They cross at the anterior commissure and ascend in the opposite anterior funiculus.

5 In the mesencephalon, the tract runs in the medial lemniscus as the spinal lemniscus (the lemnisci are described in **D**) and terminates in the posterolateral ventral nucleus of the thalamus (third neuron, see **A**, p. 218).

6 The axons of the third neurons terminate in the primary somatosensory cortex, which is located in the postcentral gyrus.

C Lateral spinothalamic tract and its central connections

1 Free nerve endings in the skin function as receptors for pain and temperature sensation.

2 The cell bodies of these free nerve endings are located in the spinal ganglia (first neuron).

3 The central processes of these neurons pass through the dorsal roots into the spinal cord, where they terminate on projection neurons in the substantia gelatinosa (second neuron).

4 The axons of the second neurons cross in the anterior commissure in the corresponding spinal cord segment and ascend in the anterolateral funiculus on the opposite side. They terminate in the thalamus (third neuron).

5 The axons of the third neurons terminate in the primary somatosensory cortex, which is located in the postcentral gyrus.

D Synopsis of the lemniscal tracts (lemnisci)

Cerain sensory pathways cross in the form of a lemniscal tract (*lemniskus* = "ribbon"). The characteristics of the four lemnisci are reviewed below.

Lemniscus	Connection	Functional importance
Lateral lemniscus	Trapezoid body/superior olive with inferior colliculus	Auditory pathway
Medial lemniscus	Dorsal column nuclei (gracilis and cuneatus) with thalamus	Touch, conscious proprioception (see p. 284) of the trunk and limbs
Spinal lemniscus* (borders the medial lemniscus)	Posterior horns (lateral and anterior spinothalamic tract) with thalamus	Pain pathway for the trunk and limbs
Trigeminal lemniscus (borders the medial lemniscus)	Sensory trigeminal nuclei with thalamus	Sensory pathway for the head

* The spinal lemniscus is the portion of the anterior spinothalamic tract located in the mesencephalon. The course of the anterior spinothalamic tract in the brainstem is not fully understood, and therefore cannot be clearly depicted in these diagrams.

9.6 Ascending Tracts of the Spinal Cord: Fasciculus gracilis and Fasciculus cuneatus

A Ascending axons in the fasciculus gracilis and fasciculus cuneatus

See p. 284 for overview of ascending tracts. The fasciculus gracilis ("slender fasciculus") and fasciculus cuneatus ("wedge-shaped fasciculus") are the two large ascending tracts in the posterior funiculus. Both tracts convey fibers for position sense (conscious proprioception, see p. 284) and fine cutaneous sensation (touch, vibration, fine pressure sense, two-point discrimination). The fasciculus gracilis carries fibers from the lower limbs, while the fasciculus cuneatus carries fibers only from the upper limbs and is therefore not present in the spinal cord below the T3 level. The cell bodies of the first neuron are located in the spinal ganglion. Their fibers are heavily myelinated and therefore conduct impulses rapidly. They pass uncrossed (the level of the decussation is shown in **C**) to the dorsal column nuclei (nucleus gracilis and cuneatus, see **C**). Both nuclei are located in the caudal portion of the medulla oblongata. Thus, the fasciculi are somatotopically organized.

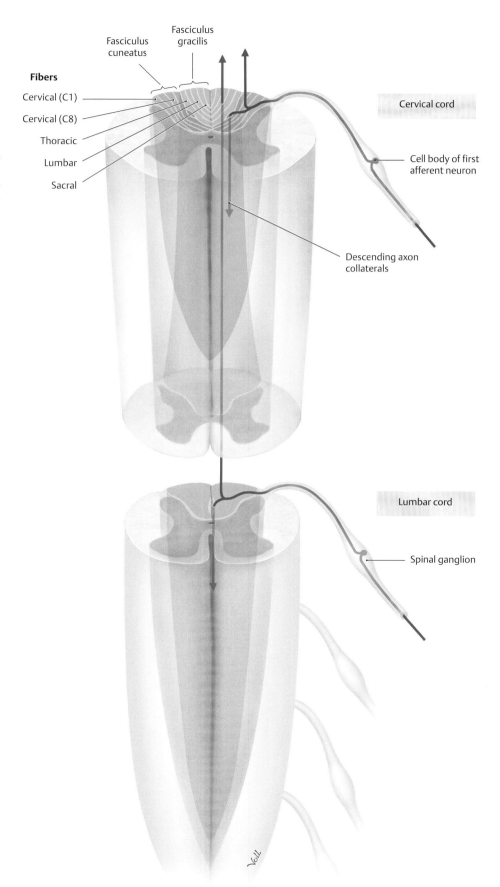

Fibers

Cervical (C1)
Cervical (C8)
Thoracic
Lumbar
Sacral

Fasciculus cuneatus
Fasciculus gracilis

Cervical cord

Cell body of first afferent neuron

Descending axon collaterals

Lumbar cord

Spinal ganglion

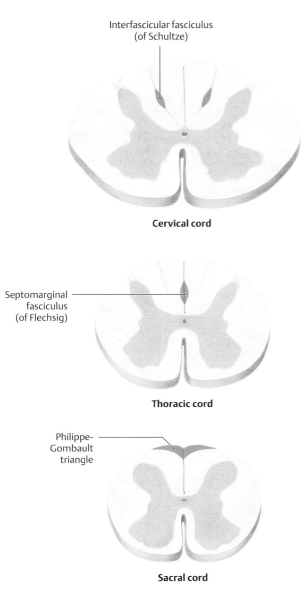

Cervical cord

Interfascicular fasciculus (of Schultze)

Septomarginal fasciculus (of Flechsig)

Thoracic cord

Philippe-Gombault triangle

Sacral cord

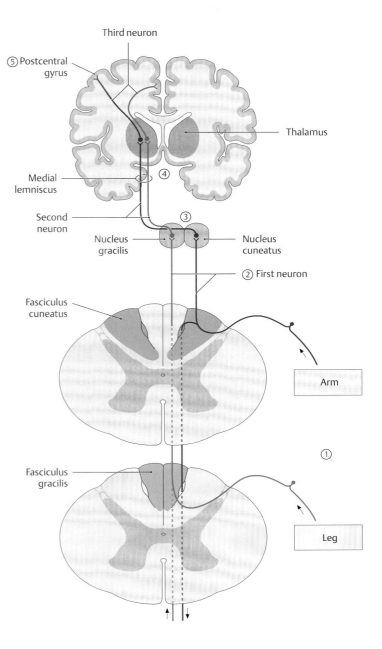

Third neuron

⑤ Postcentral gyrus

Thalamus

Medial lemniscus

Second neuron

③

Nucleus gracilis

Nucleus cuneatus

② First neuron

Fasciculus cuneatus

④

Fasciculus gracilis

Arm

①

Leg

B Descending axons

Besides the ascending axons contained in the fasciculus gracilis and fasciculus cuneatus (both shown in **A**), there are also descending axon collaterals that are distributed to lower segments. This pathway takes different shapes at different levels, appearing as the comma tract of Schultze (interfascicular fasciculus) in the cervical cord, the oval area of Flechsig (septomarginal fasciculus) in the thoracic cord, and the Philippe-Gombault triangle in the sacral cord. These tracts are concerned with sensorimotor innervation at the spinal cord level and are thus considered part of the intrinsic circuits of the spinal cord (see p. 273).

C Tracts of the posterior funiculus and their central connections

1 Muscle and tendon receptors, and Vater-Pacini corpuscles are receptors for conscious proprioception. Receptors about the hair follicles and additional receptors mediate the fine touch sensation of the skin.

2 The cell bodies of the neurons that relay this information are located in the spinal ganglia (first neuron).

3 The axons of these neurons ascend uncrossed in the posterior funiculi to the nucleus cuneatus and nucleus gracilis (second neuron) in the lower medulla oblongata.

4 The axons from the second neurons cross in the medial lemniscus (see **D**, p. 275) to the thalamus (third neuron).

5 The axons of the third neuron terminate in the primary somatosensory cortex, located in the postcentral gyrus.

9.7 Ascending Tracts of the Spinal Cord: Spinocerebellar Tracts

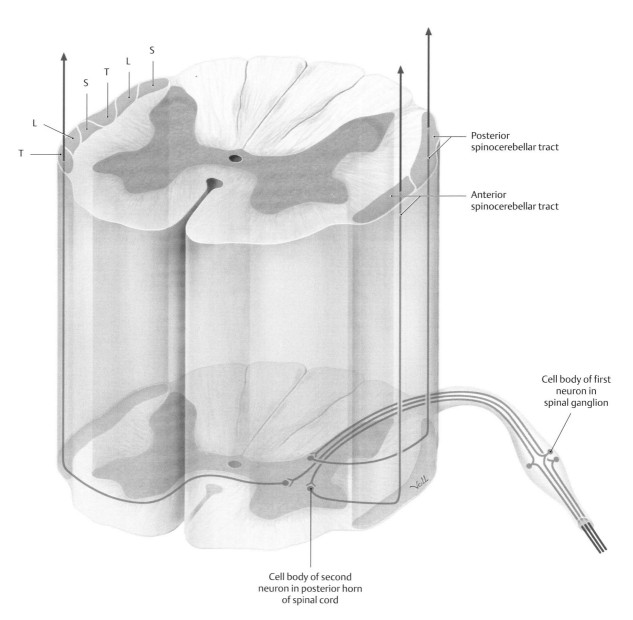

Posterior spinocerebellar tract

Anterior spinocerebellar tract

Cell body of first neuron in spinal ganglion

Cell body of second neuron in posterior horn of spinal cord

A Anterior and posterior spinocerebellar tracts

See p. 284 for overview of ascending tracts. Both the anterior and posterior spinocerebellar tracts are located in the lateral funiculus of the spinal cord. Their afferent fibers, which convey afferent impulses from muscles, tendons, and joints to the cerebellum, are involved in the unconscious coordination of motor activities (unconscious proprioception, automatic processes below the conscious level, such as jogging and riding a bicycle, see p. 284). The projection (second) neurons of both spinocerebellar tracts receive their proprioceptive signals from primary afferent fibers originating at the first neurons of the spinal ganglia. In the **anterior spinocerebellar tract,** the second neurons are located at the center of the posterior column. Their projection fibers ascend both ipsilaterally and contralaterally to the cerebellum via the superior cerebellar peduncle. The second neurons of the **posterior spinocerebellar tract** are located in the posterior thoracic nucleus of the posterior horn; this nuclear column spans segments C8–L2. The projection fibers from these second neurons ascend ipsilaterally to the cerebellum via the inferior cerebellar peduncle. Both the anterior and posterior spinocerebellar tracts have the same somatotopic organization from front to back: thoracic (T), lumbar (L), and sacral (S) fibers. Fibers of similar function from the cervical region pass through the fasciculus cuneatus to the accessory cuneate nucleus and continue as cuneocerebellar fibers to the cerebellum. However, these do not pass through the posterior spinocerebellar tract, which contains no fibers from the cervical cord.

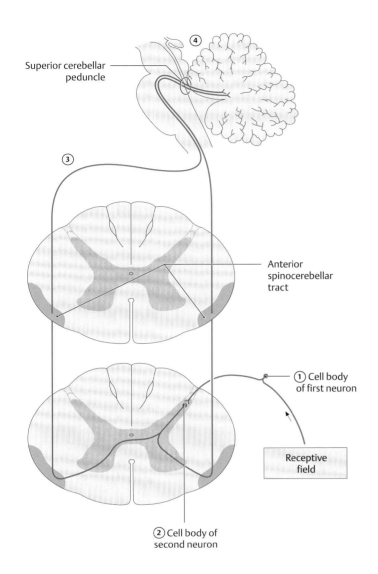

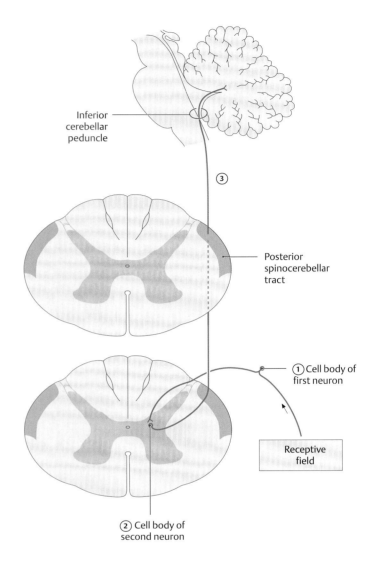

B Anterior spinocerebellar tract and its central connections

1 Proprioceptive signals from muscle spindles and tendon receptors are carried by fast-conducting myelinated axons (IA fibers) to pseudounipolar first neurons in the spinal ganglia.

2 The signals then proceed to the second neurons (projection neurons of the anterior spinocerebellar tract) at the center of the posterior column.

3 The axons of the second neurons ascend both *ipsilaterally* and *contralaterally* to the cerebellum and then pass through the floor of the rhomboid fossa to the midbrain.

4 Once in the midbrain, the axons change direction and pass through the superior cerebellar peduncle and superior medullary velum to the vermis of the cerebellum.

C Posterior spinocerebellar tract and its central connections

1 Muscle spindles and tendon receptors convey proprioceptive information via fast IA fibers that arise from pseudounipolar first neurons in the spinal ganglia.

2 The IA fibers proceed to the second neurons of the posterior column. The second neurons are contained in the thoracic nucleus, which spans spinal cord segments C8 to L2.

3 The axons of the second neurons (projection neurons of the spinocerebellar tract) ascend *ipsilaterally* to the cerebellum, entering through the inferior cerebellar peduncle.

9.8 Descending Tracts of the Spinal Cord: Pyramidal (Corticospinal) Tracts

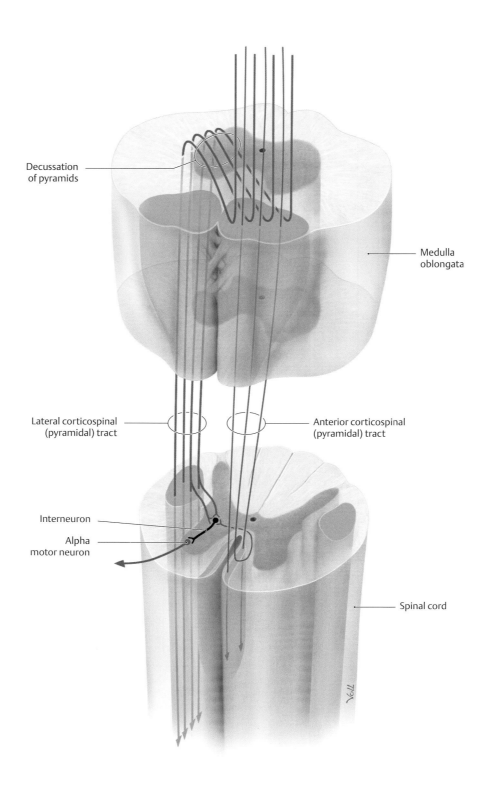

A Course of the anterior and lateral corticospinal tracts (pyramidal tract) in the lower medulla oblongata and spinal cord

The pyramidal tract, which begins in the motor cortex, is the most important pathway for voluntary motor function. See p. 285 for overview of descending tracts. Some of its axons, the *corticonuclear fibers*, termi-nate at the cranial nerve nuclei while others, the *corticospinal fibers*, terminate on the motor anterior horn cells of the spinal cord (see **B** for further details). A third group, the *corticoreticular fibers*, are distributed to nuclei of the reticular formation.

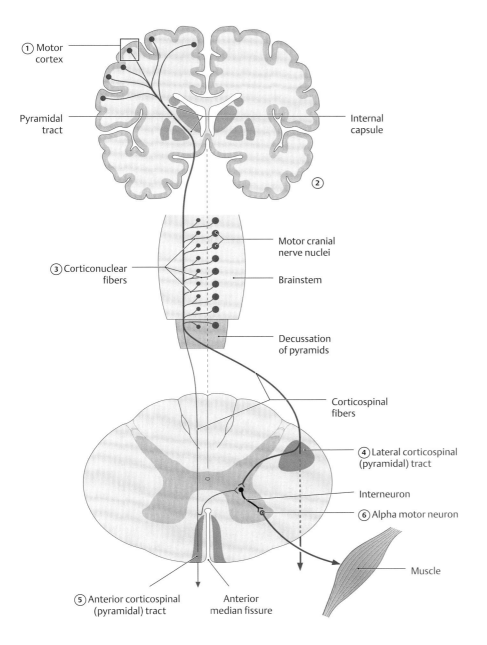

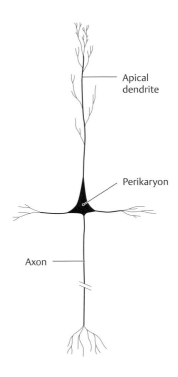

C Silver-impregnation (Golgi) method staining of pyramidal cell

This method produces a silhouette of the stained neurons. The axons of the pyramidal cells form the pyramidal tract. Approximately 40 % are located in the motor cortex (Brodmann area 4, see p. 202).

B Course of the pyramidal tract

1 The pyramidal tract originates in the motor cortex at the pyramidal cells (large afferent neurons with pyramid-shaped cell bodies, see **C**). The pyramidal tract has three components:
- *Corticonuclear fibers* for the cranial nerve nuclei
- *Corticospinal fibers* for the spinal cord
- *Corticoreticular fibers* to the reticular formation

2 All three components pass through the internal capsule from the telencephalon, continuing into the brainstem and spinal cord.

3 In the brainstem, the cortico*nuclear* fibers are distributed to the motor nuclei of the cranial nerves.

4 The cortico*spinal* fibers descend to the decussation of the pyramids in the lower medulla oblongata, where approximately 80 % of them cross to the opposite side. The fibers continue into the spinal cord, where they form the lateral corticospinal tract, which has a somatotopic organization: the fibers for the sacral cord are the most lateral, while the fibers for the cervical cord are the most medial.

5 The remaining 20 % of cortico*spinal* fibers continue to descend with-out crossing, forming the *anterior corticospinal tract,* which borders the anterior median fissure in a transverse section of the spinal cord. The anterior corticospinal tract is particularly well developed in the cervical cord, but is not present in the lower thoracic, lumbar, or sacral cords.

6 Most fibers of the *anterior corticospinal tract* cross at the segmental level to terminate on the same motor neurons as the *lateral corticospinal tract.* The axons of the pyramid cells terminate via intercalated cells on alpha and gamma motor neurons, Renshaw cells, and inhibitory interneurons (not shown, see p. 273, **C**).

Lesions of the pyramidal tract are discussed on p. 343. Other motor tracts are closely applied to the pyramidal tract in the region of the internal capsule and will be described in the next unit. While the pyramidal tract controls conscious movement (voluntary motor activity), *supplementary motor tracts* are essential for involuntary muscle processes (e.g., standing, walking, running; see p. 342).

281

9.9 Descending Tracts of the Spinal Cord: Extrapyramidal and Autonomic Tracts

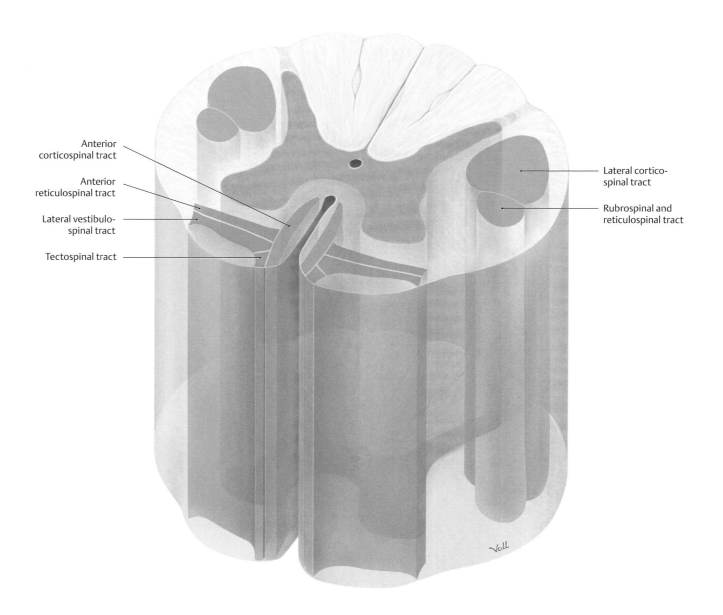

Anterior corticospinal tract

Anterior reticulospinal tract

Lateral vestibulospinal tract

Tectospinal tract

Lateral corticospinal tract

Rubrospinal and reticulospinal tract

A Tracts of the extrapyramidal motor system in the spinal cord
See p. 285 for overview of descending tracts. Unlike the pyramidal tract, which controls conscious, voluntary motor activities (e.g., raising a cup to the mouth), the *extra*pyramidal motor system (cerebellum, basal ganglia, and motor nuclei of the brainstem) is necessary for *automatic* and *learned* motor processes (e.g., walking, running, cycling). The division into a pyramidal and extrapyramidal system has proven useful in clinical practice. A recent alternative classification divides the descending tracts into a lateral and medial system. Under this classification, the *lateral system* includes:
- Lateral corticospinal tract (= pyramidal tract, see p. 280)
- Rubrospinal tract (extrapyramidal)

The lateral system projects predominantly to the distal muscles, particularly those of the upper limb, and thus critically influences fine, discriminating motor functions of the hand and arm. The *medial system* projects mainly to the neurons of the trunk and lower limb muscles and is thus concerned with the motor aspects of trunk position and stance. The *medial system* consists of three extrapyramidal tracts:
- Anterior reticulospinal tract
- Lateral vestibulospinal tract
- Tectospinal tract

The central connections of this system are illustrated in **B**. Because the pyramidal and extrapyramidal tracts are closely interconnected and run close to one other, lesions generally affect both tract systems simultaneously (see p. 343). Isolated lesions of either the pyramidal or extrapyramidal pathway at the spinal cord level are virtually unknown.

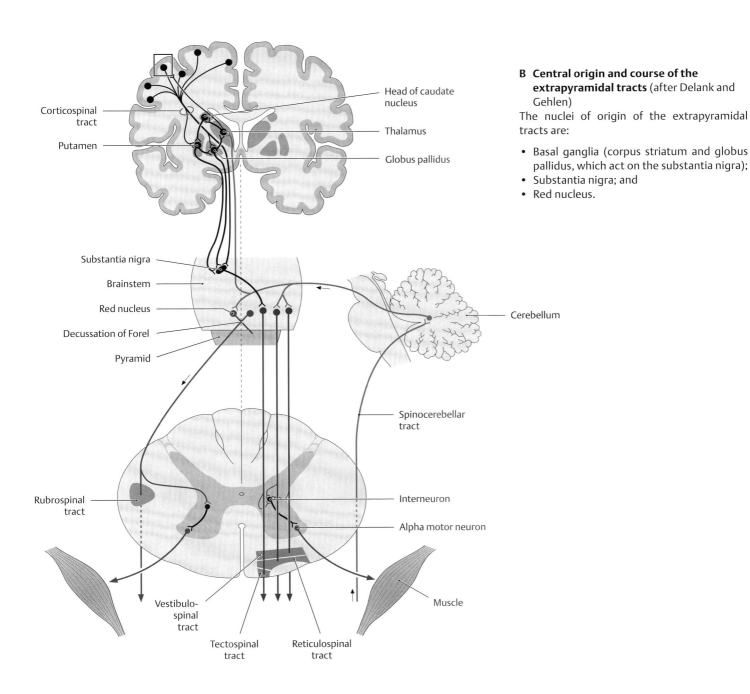

Corticospinal tract

Putamen

Head of caudate nucleus

Thalamus

Globus pallidus

Substantia nigra

Brainstem

Red nucleus

Decussation of Forel

Pyramid

Cerebellum

Spinocerebellar tract

Rubrospinal tract

Interneuron

Alpha motor neuron

Muscle

Vestibulo-spinal tract

Tectospinal tract

Reticulospinal tract

B Central origin and course of the extrapyramidal tracts (after Delank and Gehlen)

The nuclei of origin of the extrapyramidal tracts are:

- Basal ganglia (corpus striatum and globus pallidus, which act on the substantia nigra);
- Substantia nigra; and
- Red nucleus.

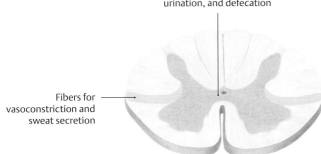

Fibers for genital function, urination, and defecation

Fibers for vasoconstriction and sweat secretion

C Autonomic pathways of the spinal cord

Autonomic pathways have a somewhat diffuse arrangement in the spinal cord and rarely form closed tract systems. There are two exceptions:

- The descending central sympathetic tract for vasoconstriction and sweat secretion borders the pyramidal tract anteriorly and shows the same somatotopic organization as the pyramidal tract.
- The parependymal tract runs on both sides of the central canal and contains both ascending and descending fibers. Passing from the spinal cord to the hypothalamus, this tract is concerned with urination, defecation, and genital functions.

9.10 Tracts of the Spinal Cord, Overview

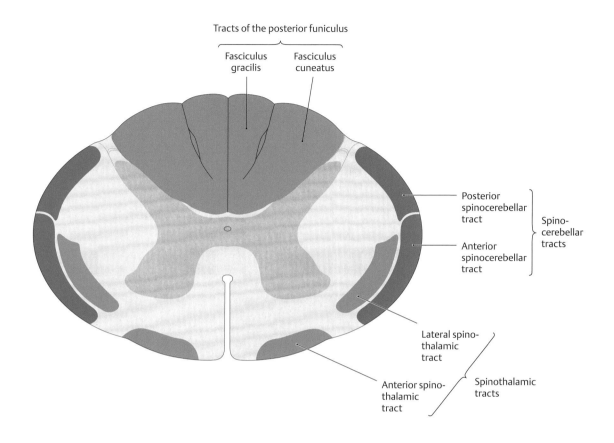

A Ascending tracts in the spinal cord

Transverse section through the spinal cord. Ascending tracts are afferent (= sensory) pathways that carry information from the trunk and limbs to the brain. The most important ascending tracts and their functions are listed below.

Spinothalamic tracts
– Anterior spinothalamic tract (coarse touch sensation)
– Lateral spinothalamic tract (pain and temperature sensation)

Tracts of the posterior funiculus
– Fasciculus gracilis (fine touch sensation, conscious proprioception of the *lower* limb)
– Fasciculus cuneatus (fine touch sensation, conscious proprioception of the *upper* limb).

Spinocerebellar tracts
– Anterior spinocerebellar tract (unconscious proprioception to the cerebellum)
– Posterior spinocerebellar tract (unconscious proprioception to the cerebellum)

Proprioception involves the perception of limb position in space ("position sense"). It lets us know, for example, that our arm is in front of or behind our chest even when our eyes are closed. The information involved in proprioception is complex. Thus, our position sense tells us where our joints are in relation to one another while our motion sense tells us the speed and direction of joint movements. We also have a "force sense" by which we can perceive the muscular force that is associated with joint movements. Moreover, proprioception takes place on both a conscious (I know that my hand is making a fist in my pants pocket without seeing it) and an unconscious level, enabling us to ride a bicycle and climb stairs without thinking about it. The table on p. 327 gives a comprehensive review of all the ascending tracts.

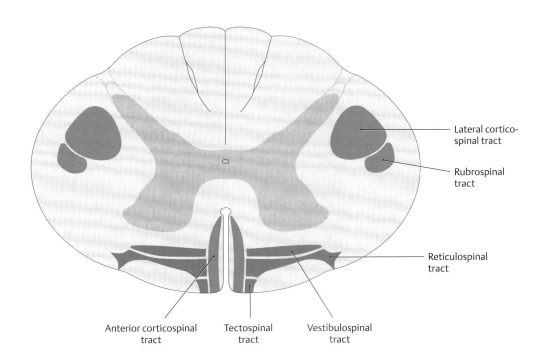

Lateral cortico-
spinal tract

Rubrospinal
tract

Reticulospinal
tract

Anterior corticospinal
tract

Tectospinal
tract

Vestibulospinal
tract

B Descending tracts in the spinal cord

Transverse section through the spinal cord. The descending tracts of the spinal cord are concerned with motor function. They convey information from higher motor centers to the motor neurons in the spinal cord. According to a relatively recent classification (not yet fully accepted in clinical medicine), the descending tracts of the spinal cord can be divided into two motor systems:

- **Lateral motor system** (concerned with fine, precise motor skills in the hands):
  - Pyramidal tract (anterior and lateral corticospinal tract)
  - Rubrospinal tract
- **Medial motor system** (innervates medially situated motor neurons controlling trunk movement and stance):
  - Reticulospinal tract
  - Tectospinal tract
  - Vestibulospinal tract

Except for the pyramidal tract, which may be represented as a monosynaptic pathway in a simplified scheme, it is difficult to offer a simple and direct classification of the motor system because sequences of movements are programmed and coordinated in multiple feedback mechanisms called "motor loops" (see p. 341). There is no point, then, in listing the various tracts in a simplified table. While the tracts can be distinguished rather clearly from one another at the level of the spinal cord, their fibers are so intermixed at the higher cortical levels that isolated motor disturbances (unlike sensory disturbances) essentially do not occur at the level of the spinal cord.

9.11   Blood Vessels of the Spinal Cord: Arteries

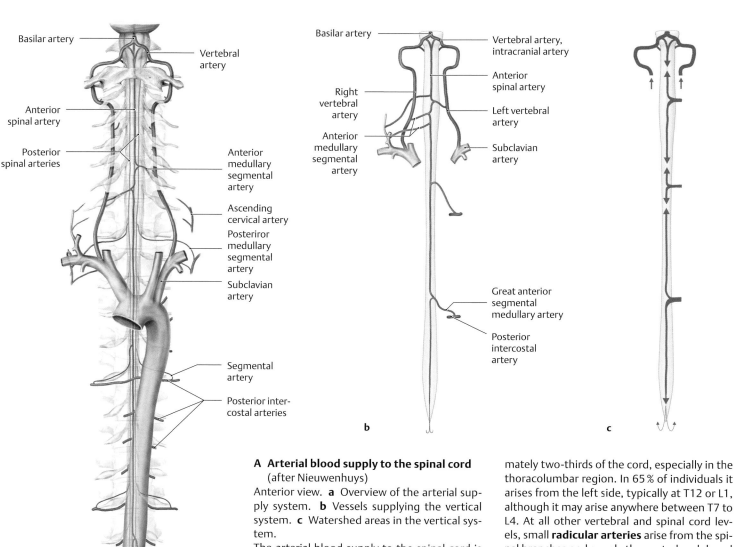

A Arterial blood supply to the spinal cord
(after Nieuwenhuys)

Anterior view. **a** Overview of the arterial supply system. **b** Vessels supplying the vertical system. **c** Watershed areas in the vertical system.

The arterial blood supply to the spinal cord is derived from both vertical and horizontal components. The *vertical system* consists of the unpaired *anterior spinal arteries* and the paired *posterior spinal arteries*. The **spinal arteries** typically arise intracranially from the vertebral arteries, though the posterior spinal arteries may arise from the posterior inferior cerebellar artery. The descending spinal arteries are small where they originate at the vertebral arteries, and would significantly decrease in caliber without reinforcing contributions from the anterior and posterior **segmental medullary arteries**. These segmental medullary vessels arise from spinal branches of the vertebral, ascending cervical, deep cervical, posterior intercostal, lumbar, and lateral sacral arteries, depending upon the level of the spinal cord. The segmental medullary vessels vary in both their level of origin and number (an average of 8 anterior, and 12 posterior arteries are seen). One of these arteries, the great anterior segmental medullary artery (of Adamkiewicz), is usually significantly larger than the others, and reinforces the blood supply to approxi-

mately two-thirds of the cord, especially in the thoracolumbar region. In 65 % of individuals it arises from the left side, typically at T12 or L1, although it may arise anywhere between T7 to L4. At all other vertebral and spinal cord levels, small **radicular arteries** arise from the spinal branches and supply the ventral and dorsal nerve roots, as well as the peripheral portions of the anterior and posterior horns. The radicular arteries do not reach or contribute to the spinal arteries. Since the spinal arteries receive variable reinforcement from segmental medullary arteries, certain regions of the spinal cord may receive their blood supply from multiple sources (see **c**). Restriction of blood supply at such a region may result in ischemic injury to the cord. The T1–T4 and the L1 cord segments are particularly vulnerable.

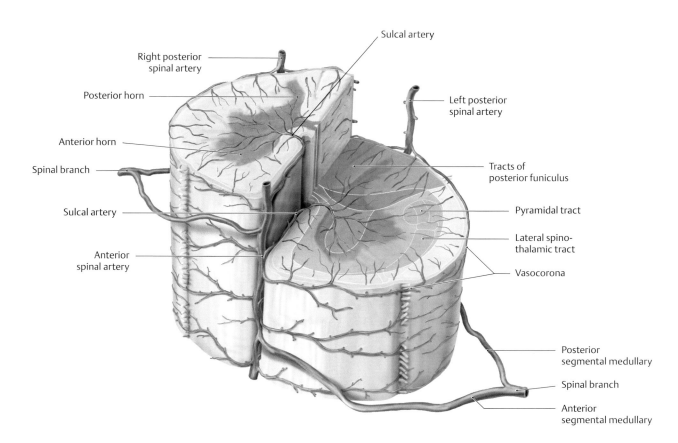

B Blood supply to the spinal cord segments

In each spinal cord segment, the *anterior spinal artery* gives off several (5–9) **sulcal arteries** which course posteriorly in the anterior median fissure. Typically, each sulcal artery enters one half of the spinal cord, supplying the anterior horn, base of the posterior horn, and the anterior and lateral funiculi (approximately two-thirds of the total area) in that half; the sulcal arteries tend to alternate direction (left or right) to supply both halves of the spinal cord segment. The paired *posterior spinal arteries* provide the blood supply to the posterior one-third of the cord, including the posterior horn and funiculus. All three spinal arteries contribute numerous delicate anastomosing **vasocorona** on the pial sur-

face of the spinal cord which in turn send branches into the periphery of the cord. The sulcal arteries are the only end-arteries within the spinal cord, and their occlusion may produce clinical symptoms. Occlusion of the anterior spinal artery at segmental levels may damage the anterior horn and ventral roots resulting in flaccid paralysis of the muscles supplied by these segments. If the pyramidal tract in the lateral funiculus is involved, spastic paralysis will develop below the lesion level. An occlusion of the posterior spinal arteries in one or more segments will affect the posterior horn and funiculus leading to disturbances of proprioception, vibration, and pressure sensation.

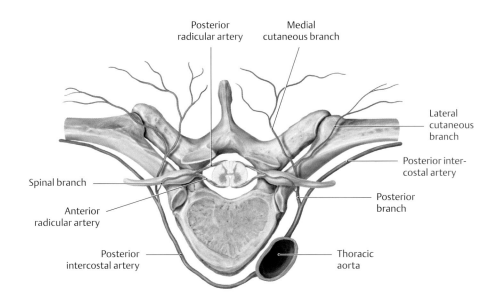

C Blood vessels supplying the spinal cord

Thoracic vertebra viewed from above. The spinal branches arise from the posterior branches of segmental arteries and divide into an anterior and a posterior radicular artery. The radicular arteries supply the dorsal and ventral roots, and peripheral portions of the dorsal and ventral horns; they also communicate with the vasocorona. These arteries have a better-developed connection with the anterior spinal artery at some levels and with the posterior spinal artery at other levels.

9.12 Blood Vessels of the Spinal Cord: Veins

A Venous drainage of the spinal cord
(after Nieuwenhuys)

Anterior view. Analogous to the arterial supply, the venous drainage of the spinal cord consists of a *horizontal system* (venous rings, see **B**) and a *vertical system* that drains the venous rings. The vertical system is illustrated here. While the arterial blood supply is based on three vessels, the interior of the spinal cord drains through venous plexuses into only two unpaired vessels: an anterior and a posterior spinal vein (see **B**). The *anterior* spinal vein communicates superiorly with veins of the brainstem. Its lower portion enters the filum terminale (a glial filament extending from the conus medullaris to the sacral end of the dural sac, where it is attached). The larger *posterior* spinal vein communicates with the radicular veins at the cervical level and ends at the conus medullaris. The **radicular veins** connect these veins, which lie within the pia mater, with the internal vertebral venous plexus (see **C**). Blood from the cord drains into the **vertebral veins**, which open into the superior vena cava. Blood from the thoracic cord drains into the **intercostal veins**, which drain into the superior vena cava via the azygos and hemiazygos system. Radicular veins are present at only certain segments, as shown. Their distribution varies among individuals.

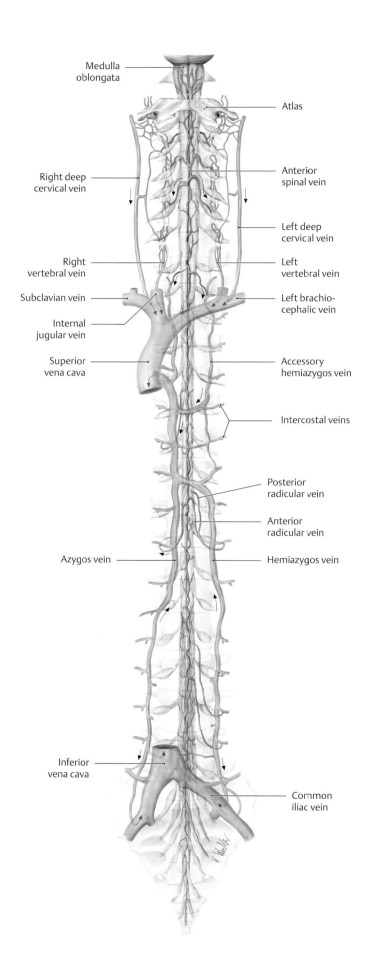

Medulla oblongata

Atlas

Right deep cervical vein

Anterior spinal vein

Left deep cervical vein

Right vertebral vein

Left vertebral vein

Subclavian vein

Left brachio-cephalic vein

Internal jugular vein

Superior vena cava

Accessory hemiazygos vein

Intercostal veins

Posterior radicular vein

Anterior radicular vein

Azygos vein

Hemiazygos vein

Inferior vena cava

Common iliac vein

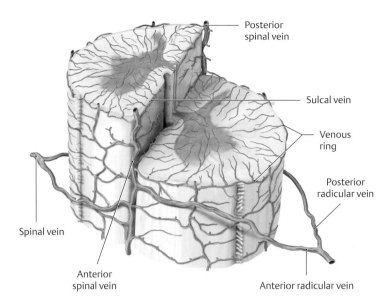

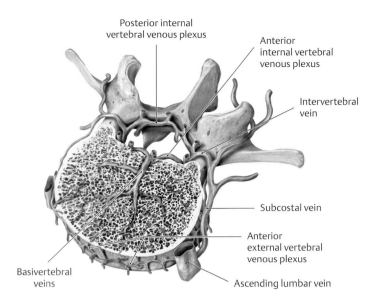

B Venous drainage of a spinal cord segment

Anterior view from upper left. A spinal cord segment is drained by the anterior and posterior spinal veins. These vessels are located within the pia mater and are interconnected by an anastomotic venous ring. Both veins channel blood through the radicular veins to the internal vertebral venous plexus (see **C**). Unlike the radicular veins, the veins *inside* the spinal cord have no valves. As a result, venous stasis may cause a hazardous rise of pressure in the spinal cord. A typical cause of increased intramedullary venous pressure is an arteriovenous fistula, which is an abnormal communication between an artery and vein in the spinal cord. Because the pressure in the arteries is higher than in the veins, arterial blood tends to enter the veins of the spinal cord through the fistulous connection. The fistula will remain asymptomatic as long as the intramedullary veins maintain an adequate drainage capacity. But if the flow across the fistula outstrips their drainage capacity, the functions of the spinal cord will be impaired by the increased pressure. This is manifested clinically by disturbances of gait, spastic paralysis, and sensory disturbances. Untreated, the decompensated fistula will eventually cause a complete functional transection of the spinal cord. The treatment of choice is surgical correction of the fistula.

C Vertebral venous plexus

Transverse section viewed obliquely from upper left. The veins of the spinal cord and its coverings are connected to the internal vertebral venous plexus via the radicular and spinal veins. Located in the fatty tissue of the epidural space, this plexus occupies the inner circumference of the vertebral canal. The internal plexus is connected to the external vertebral venous plexus by the *inter*vertebral and *basi*vertebral veins. Anastomoses exist between the tributary regions of the anterior and posterior spinal veins. Oblique anastomoses are located in the interior of the spinal cord and may extend over several segments (not shown). These connections are particularly important in maintaining a constant intramedullary venous pressure.

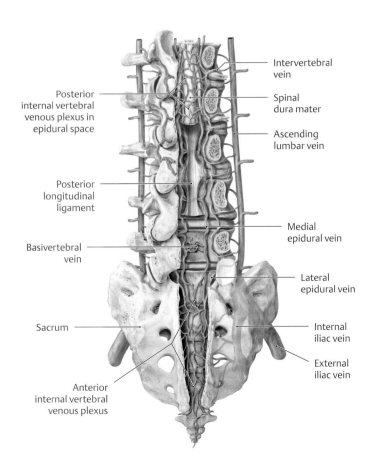

D Epidural veins in the sacral and lumbar vertebral canals
(after Nieuwenhuys)

Posterior view (vertebral canal windowed). The internal veins of the spinal cord are valveless up to the point at which they emerge from the spinal dura mater. The internal vertebral venous plexus is connected by other valveless veins (not shown here) to the venous plexus of the prostate. It is relatively easy for prostatic carcinoma cells to pass along the veins of the prostatic venous plexus to the sacral venous plexus and destroy the surrounding tissue. For this reason, prostatic carcinoma frequently metastasizes to this region and destroys the surrounding bone, resulting in severe pain.

289

9.13 Spinal Cord, Topography

A Spinal cord and spinal nerve in the vertebral canal at the level of the C 4 vertebra

Transverse section viewed from above. The spinal cord occupies the center of the vertebral foramen and is anchored within the subarachnoid space to the spinal dura mater by the denticulate ligament. The root sleeve, an outpouching of the dura mater in the intravertebral foramen, contains the spinal ganglion and the dorsal and ventral roots of the spinal nerve. The spinal dura mater is bounded externally by the epidural space, which contains venous plexuses, fat and connective tissue. The epidural space extends upwards as far as the foramen magnum, where the dura becomes fused to the cranial periosteum (see p. 191).

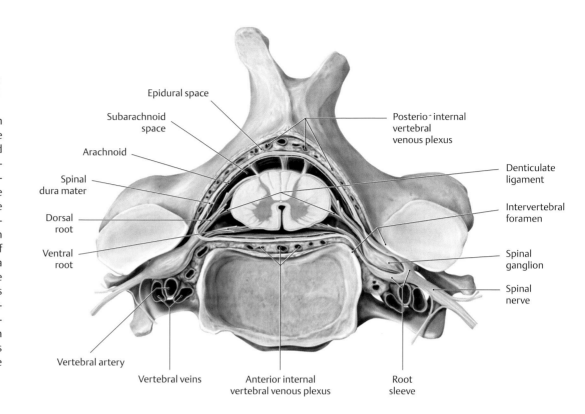

Epidural space

Subarachnoid space

Arachnoid

Spinal dura mater

Dorsal root

Ventral root

Vertebral artery

Vertebral veins

Anterior internal vertebral venous plexus

Root sleeve

Posterior internal vertebral venous plexus

Denticulate ligament

Intervertebral foramen

Spinal ganglion

Spinal nerve

B Cauda equina at the level of the L 2 vertebra

Transverse section viewed from below. The spinal cord usually ends at the level of the first lumbar vertebra (L1). The space below the lower end of the spinal cord is occupied by the cauda equina and filum terminale in the dural sac (lumbar cistern, see p. 191), which ends at the level of the S 2 vertebra (see **C** and p. 267 **D**). The epidural space expands at that level and contains extensive venous plexuses and fatty tissue.

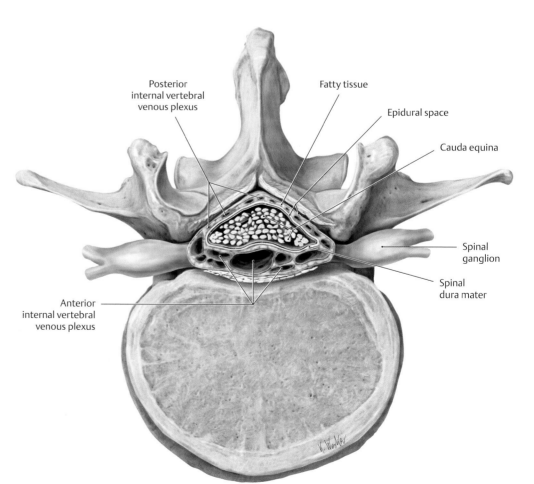

Posterior internal vertebral venous plexus

Anterior internal vertebral venous plexus

Fatty tissue

Epidural space

Cauda equina

Spinal ganglion

Spinal dura mater

290

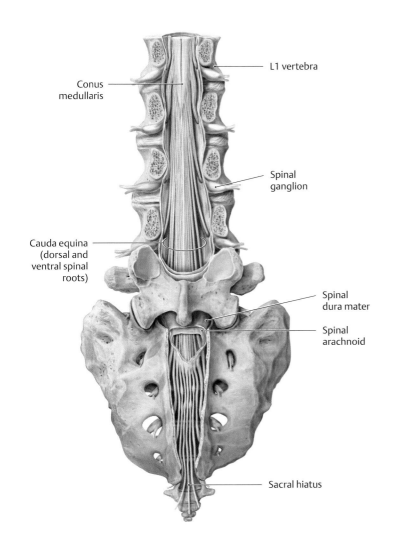

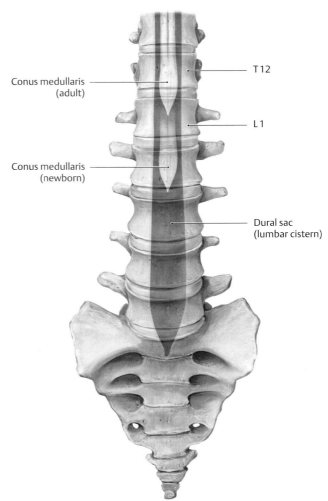

C Cauda equina in the vertebral canal
Posterior view. The laminae and the dorsal surface of the sacrum have been partially removed. The spinal cord in the adult terminates at approximately level of the first lumbar vertebra (L1). The dorsal and ventral spinal nerve roots extending from the lower end of the spinal cord (conus medullaris) are known collectively as the cauda equina. During lumbar puncture at this level, a needle introduced into the subarachnoid space (lumbar cistern) normally slips past the spinal nerve roots without injuring them.

D The spinal cord, dural sac, and vertebral column at different ages
Anterior view. As an individual grows, the longitudinal growth of the spinal cord increasingly lags behind that of the vertebral column. At birth the distal end of the spinal cord, the conus medullaris, is at the level of the L3 vertebral body (where lumbar puncture is contraindicated). The spinal cord of a tall adult ends at the T12/L1 level, while that of a short adult extends to the L2/L3 level. The dural sac always extends into the upper sacrum. It is important to consider these anatomical relationships during lumbar puncture. It is best to introduce the needle at the L3/L4 interspace (see **E**).

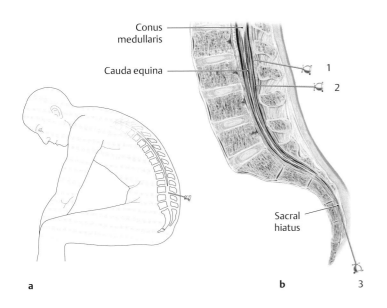

E Lumbar puncture, epidural anesthesia, and lumbar anesthesia
In preparation for a **lumbar puncture**, the patient bends far forward to separate the spinous processes of the lumbar spine. The spinal needle is usually introduced between the spinous processes of the L3 and L4 vertebrae. It is advanced through the skin and into the dural sac (lumbar cistern, see **D**) to obtain a cerebrospinal fluid sample. This procedure has numerous applications, including the diagnosis of meningitis. For **epidural anesthesia**, a catheter is placed in the epidural space without penetrating the dural sac (1). **Lumbar anesthesia** is induced by injecting a local anesthetic solution into the dural sac (2). Another option is to pass the needle into the epidural space through the sacral hiatus (3).

291

10.1   Coronal Sections: I and II (Frontal)

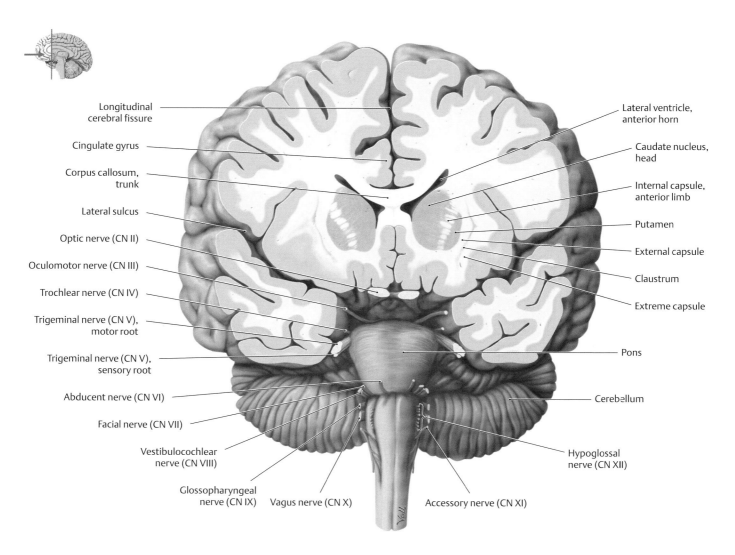

Longitudinal cerebral fissure

Cingulate gyrus

Corpus callosum, trunk

Lateral sulcus

Optic nerve (CN II)

Oculomotor nerve (CN III)

Trochlear nerve (CN IV)

Trigeminal nerve (CN V), motor root

Trigeminal nerve (CN V), sensory root

Abducent nerve (CN VI)

Facial nerve (CN VII)

Vestibulocochlear nerve (CN VIII)

Glossopharyngeal nerve (CN IX)   Vagus nerve (CN X)   Accessory nerve (CN XI)

Lateral ventricle, anterior horn

Caudate nucleus, head

Internal capsule, anterior limb

Putamen

External capsule

Claustrum

Extreme capsule

Pons

Cerebellum

Hypoglossal nerve (CN XII)

General remarks on sectional brain anatomy

The series of sections (coronal, transverse, and sagittal) in this chapter is intended to help the reader gain an appreciation of the three-dimensional anatomy of the brain. This is necessary for the correct interpretation of modern sectional imaging modalities (CT and MRI for the investigation of suspected stroke, brain tumors, meningitis, and trauma). In offering this synoptic perspective, we assume that the reader has read the previous chapters and has gained at least a general appreciation of the functional and descriptive anatomy of the brain. The legends and especially the small accompanying schematic diagrams are intended to facilitate a three-dimensional understanding of the two-dimensional sections (the plane of the section in each figure is indicated by a red line in the small, inset image).

The planes of section have been selected to display the structures of *greatest clinical importance* more clearly than can be done in actual tissue sections, which are not always optimally fixed and preserved. Because the sections were modeled on specimens taken from different individuals, some structures will not be found at the same location in every figure. The structures of the brain were assigned to specific ontogenetic regions in previous chapters, and these relationships are summarized in **B**, p. 315, at the end of this chapter.

Note the relationship of the sectional planes to the Forel axis in the anterior part of the brain and to the Meynert axis in the brainstem region (see **D**, p. 185).

A Coronal section I

The body (trunk) of the *corpus callosum*, which interconnects the two cerebral hemispheres, is prominently displayed in this coronal section. Superior to the corpus callosum is the *cingulate gyrus*, which also appears in subsequent sections. Inferior to the corpus callosum is the *caudate nucleus,* which appears particularly large because this section passes through the widest portion of its head (see **C**). The nucleus appears different in later sections because it tapers occipitally to a narrow tail (see the units that follow). The schematic lateral view (**C**) shows how the caudate nucleus is closely applied to the *lateral ventricle* and follows its concavity (shown in green). The caudate nucleus and the *putamen* together form the *corpus striatum,* whose "striation" is formed by the anterior limb of the internal capsule, a streak of white matter. The putamen still appears quite small at this level because the section passes only through its anterior tip. It becomes larger as the planes of section move further occipitally. The structures *anterior* to this plane consist of the cortex and white matter of the frontal lobe, both of which are easily identified. The temporal lobes, which still appear to be separate, detached structures, join the rest of the telencephalon in more occipital sectional planes (see **B**).

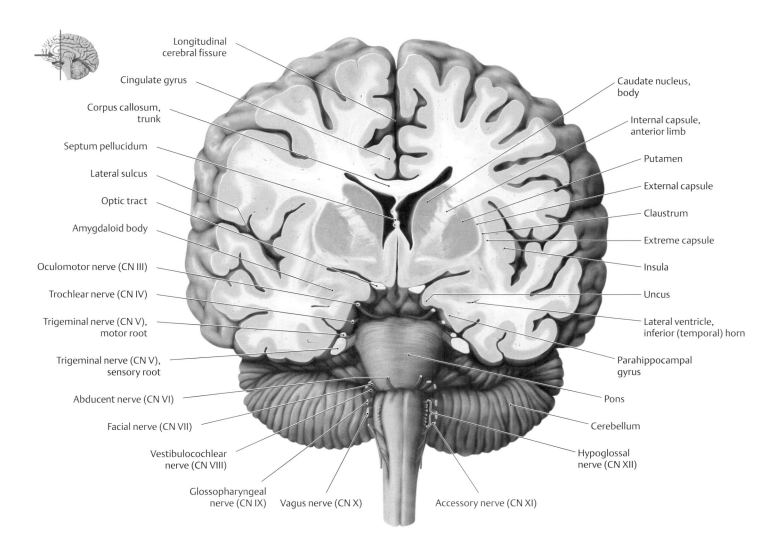

Longitudinal cerebral fissure

Cingulate gyrus

Corpus callosum, trunk

Septum pellucidum

Lateral sulcus

Optic tract

Amygdaloid body

Oculomotor nerve (CN III)

Trochlear nerve (CN IV)

Trigeminal nerve (CN V), motor root

Trigeminal nerve (CN V), sensory root

Abducent nerve (CN VI)

Facial nerve (CN VII)

Vestibulocochlear nerve (CN VIII)

Glossopharyngeal nerve (CN IX) Vagus nerve (CN X)

Accessory nerve (CN XI)

Caudate nucleus, body

Internal capsule, anterior limb

Putamen

External capsule

Claustrum

Extreme capsule

Insula

Uncus

Lateral ventricle, inferior (temporal) horn

Parahippocampal gyrus

Pons

Cerebellum

Hypoglossal nerve (CN XII)

B Coronal section II

This section contains essentially the same structures as in **A**. The plane no longer passes through the *head* of the candate nucleus, instead passing through its slender *body*. The *inferior horn* (temporal horn) of the lateral ventricle appears as a slitlike structure and also provides a useful landmark: ventral to the inferior horn is a portion of the *parahippocampal gyrus*. Superior and medial to the inferior horn are the *amygdalae* (amygdaloid bodies, visible here for the first time; compare with **D**). They are bordered by the *uncus*, which is the hook-shaped anterior end of the parahippocampal gyrus. The internal capsule, which pierces the corpus striatum, appears considerably thicker in this plane than in **A**. The temporal lobe has merged at this level with the rest of the telencephalon, and the *insular cortex* is clearly visible.

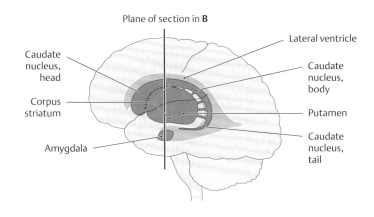

Plane of section in **B**

Caudate nucleus, head

Corpus striatum

Amygdala

Lateral ventricle

Caudate nucleus, body

Putamen

Caudate nucleus, tail

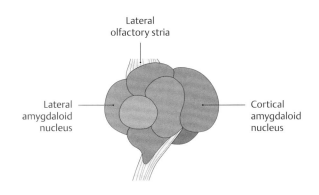

Lateral olfactory stria

Lateral amygdaloid nucleus

Cortical amygdaloid nucleus

C Relationship between the caudate nucleus and lateral ventricle.
Left lateral view.

D Amygdala
Right lateral view.

10.2   Coronal Sections: III and IV

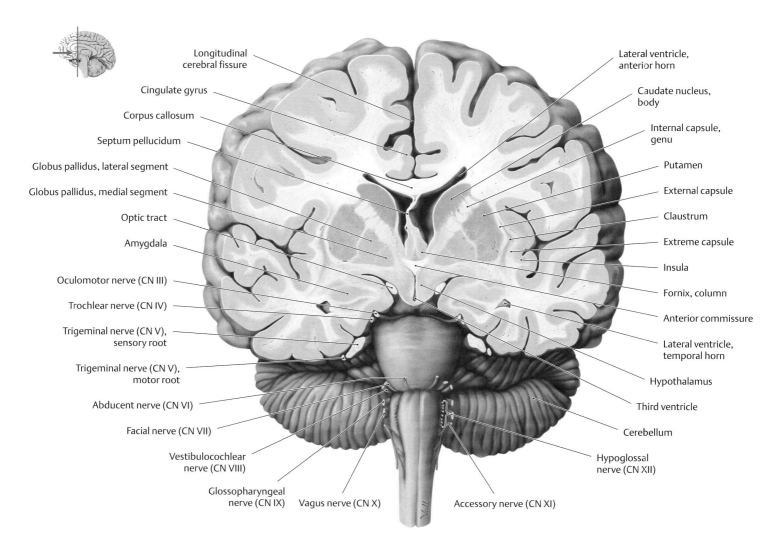

Longitudinal cerebral fissure

Cingulate gyrus

Corpus callosum

Septum pellucidum

Globus pallidus, lateral segment

Globus pallidus, medial segment

Optic tract

Amygdala

Oculomotor nerve (CN III)

Trochlear nerve (CN IV)

Trigeminal nerve (CN V), sensory root

Trigeminal nerve (CN V), motor root

Abducent nerve (CN VI)

Facial nerve (CN VII)

Vestibulocochlear nerve (CN VIII)

Glossopharyngeal nerve (CN IX)   Vagus nerve (CN X)

Lateral ventricle, anterior horn

Caudate nucleus, body

Internal capsule, genu

Putamen

External capsule

Claustrum

Extreme capsule

Insula

Fornix, column

Anterior commissure

Lateral ventricle, temporal horn

Hypothalamus

Third ventricle

Cerebellum

Hypoglossal nerve (CN XII)

Accessory nerve (CN XI)

A   Coronal section III
The inferior (temporal) horn of the lateral ventricle appears somewhat larger in the plane of this section. In the ventricular system, we can now see the floor of the *third ventricle* (see **B**) and the surrounding hypothalamus. The thalamus cannot yet be seen, as it lies slightly above and behind the hypothalamus. The *anterior commissure* appears in this plane as does the *globus pallidus*, which consists of a medial and a lateral segment. The large descending pathway, the *corticospinal tract*, passes through the *internal capsule*, which has a somatotopic organization. The genu of the internal capsule transmits axons for the pharynx, larynx, and jaw. The course of these axons is shown schematically in **C** (the fornix appears in **D**).

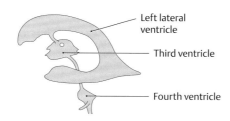

Left lateral ventricle

Third ventricle

Fourth ventricle

B   Ventricular system
Left lateral view.

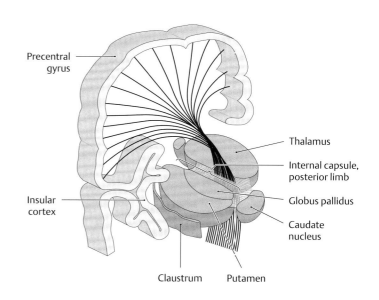

Precentral gyrus

Thalamus

Internal capsule, posterior limb

Insular cortex

Globus pallidus

Caudate nucleus

Claustrum   Putamen

C   Course of the pyramidal tract in the internal capsule
Left anterior view.

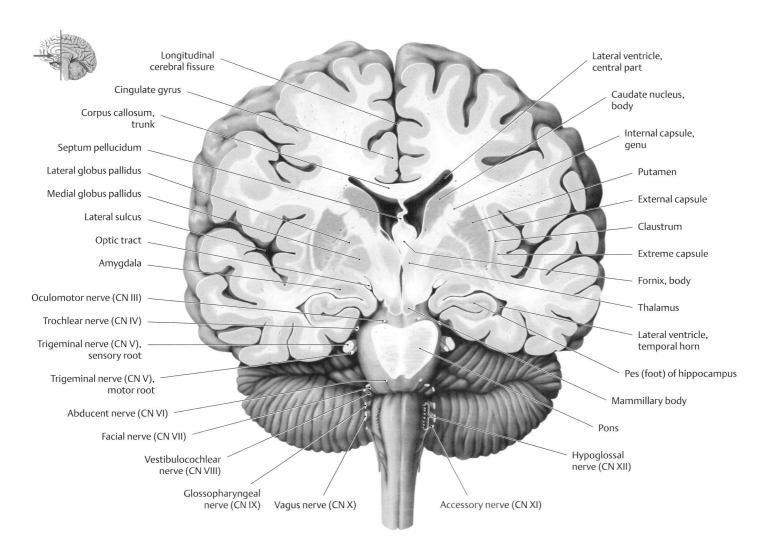

D Coronal section IV

The division of the globus pallidus into medial and lateral segments can now be seen clearly. This section displays the full width of both the inferior horn of the lateral ventricle and the *claustrum* (believed to be important in the regulation of sexual behavior). While the plane in **A** passed through the anterior commissure, this more occipital plane slices the mammillary bodies (see **E**). Pathological changes in the mammillary bodies can be found during autopsy of chronic alcoholics. The mammillary bodies are flanked on each side by the *foot of the hippocampus*. An important part of the limbic system, the mammillary bodies are con-

nected to the hippocampus by the *fornix* (see **F**). Due to the anatomical curvature of the fornix, its *column* is visible in more frontal sections (see **A**), while its *crura* appear as widely separated structures in more occipital sections (see **C**, p. 299). The *septum pellucidum* stretches between the fornix and corpus callosum, forming the medial boundary of the lateral ventricles (see **A** and **D**).

The first structure of the brainstem, the *pons,* can also be identified in this section.

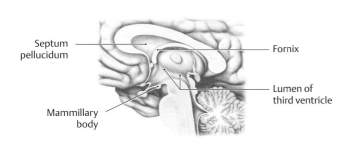

E Midsagittal section through the diencephalon and brainstem
Lateral view.

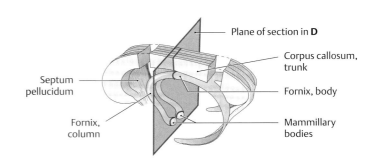

F Mammillary bodies and fornix

295

10.3 Coronal Sections: V and VI

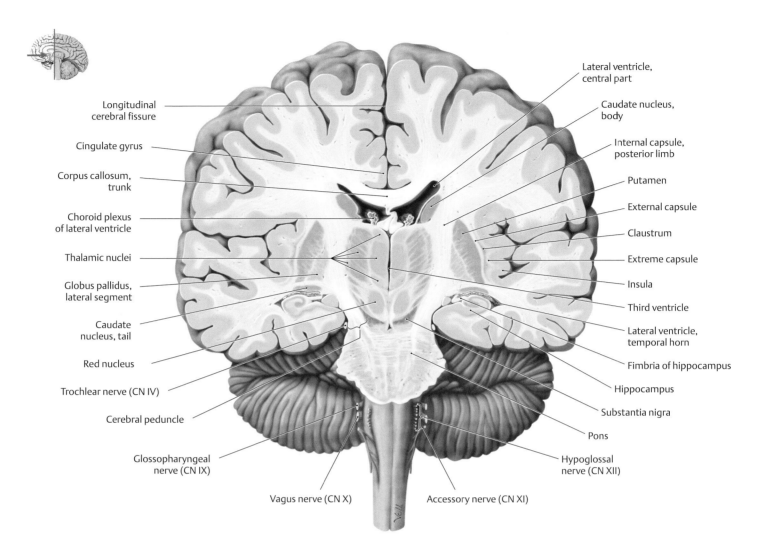

Longitudinal cerebral fissure

Cingulate gyrus

Corpus callosum, trunk

Choroid plexus of lateral ventricle

Thalamic nuclei

Globus pallidus, lateral segment

Caudate nucleus, tail

Red nucleus

Trochlear nerve (CN IV)

Cerebral peduncle

Glossopharyngeal nerve (CN IX)

Vagus nerve (CN X)

Lateral ventricle, central part

Caudate nucleus, body

Internal capsule, posterior limb

Putamen

External capsule

Claustrum

Extreme capsule

Insula

Third ventricle

Lateral ventricle, temporal horn

Fimbria of hippocampus

Hippocampus

Substantia nigra

Pons

Hypoglossal nerve (CN XII)

Accessory nerve (CN XI)

A Coronal section V

The appearance of the central nuclear region has changed markedly. The *caudate nucleus* is cut twice by the plane of this section. Its body borders the central part of the lateral ventricle, and a small portion of its tail borders the inferior horn of the ventricle (see **C** and **E**). Because the head and body of the caudate nucleus rim the lateral aspect of the anterior (frontal) horn and the central part of the lateral ventricle, the caudate nucleus has a curved shape similar to that of the ventricular system (see **C**). Thus, the tail of the caudate nucleus is ventral and lateral in relation to its head and body. Panel **E** shows that a coronal section through the tail of the caudate nucleus cuts the occipital portions of the *putamen*. A section in a slightly more occipital plane may not contain any part of the basal ganglia at all (see **B**). The central part of the lateral horn has

become much narrower due to the presence of the *thalamus*, visible here along with the thalamic nuclei. This is the first plane that displays the *choroid plexus*, which can be seen within the lateral ventricles. The choroid plexus extends from the interventricular foramen (not visible here) into the inferior horn. Because the foramen lies anterior to the thalamus, the plexus can be seen only in coronal sections that also pass through thalamic structures. Basal to the thalamus are the *red nucleus* and *substantia nigra*; these are important midbrain structures that bulge into the diencephalon and extend almost to the level of the globus pallidus (not visible here; see **B**). The *hippocampus* indents the floor of the temporal horn, and its fimbria can be seen. This section also shows how the fibers of the corticospinal tract pass through the *posterior limb* of the internal capsule and continue into the cerebral peduncles and pons.

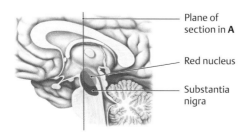

Plane of section in **A**

Red nucleus

Substantia nigra

B Red nucleus and substantia nigra
Midsagittal section.

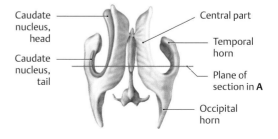

Caudate nucleus, head

Caudate nucleus, tail

Central part

Temporal horn

Plane of section in **A**

Occipital horn

C Ventricular system
Superior view.

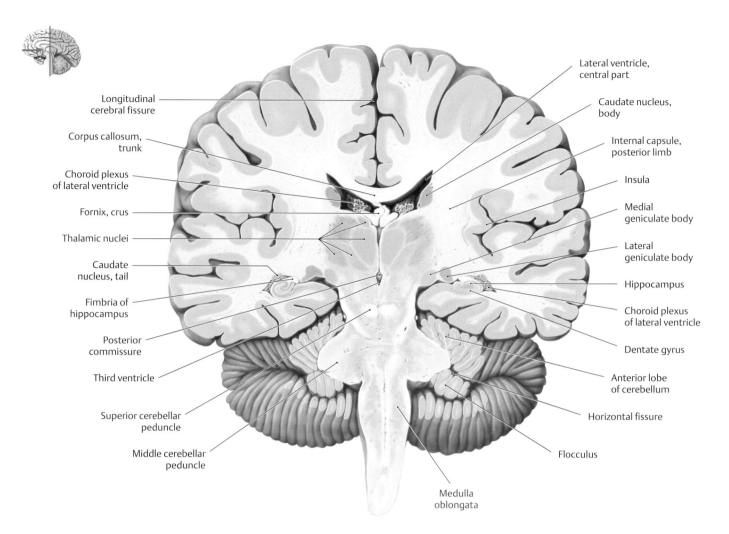

Longitudinal cerebral fissure

Corpus callosum, trunk

Choroid plexus of lateral ventricle

Fornix, crus

Thalamic nuclei

Caudate nucleus, tail

Fimbria of hippocampus

Posterior commissure

Third ventricle

Superior cerebellar peduncle

Middle cerebellar peduncle

Lateral ventricle, central part

Caudate nucleus, body

Internal capsule, posterior limb

Insula

Medial geniculate body

Lateral geniculate body

Hippocampus

Choroid plexus of lateral ventricle

Dentate gyrus

Anterior lobe of cerebellum

Horizontal fissure

Flocculus

Medulla oblongata

D Coronal section VI

The caudal thalamic nuclei are well displayed in this section, bordering the lateral ventricles from below and the third ventricle from the sides. The putamen lies at a more oral level and is no longer visible in this plane (see the transverse section on p. 306). This section passes through the *posterior limb* of the internal capsule (see also **C**, p. 294) and the anterior part of the *posterior commissure* (see **D**, p. 299). The *medial* and *lateral geniculate bodies*, which are components of the auditory and visual pathways, appear as two darker nuclei that flank the thalamus on the right and left sides at the same level as the commissure (see **F**). The crura of the fornix can be seen between the thalamus and corpus callosum. This is the first section that passes through part of the *cerebellum*. Here the *middle cerebellar peduncle* passes laterally toward the cerebellar hemispheres.

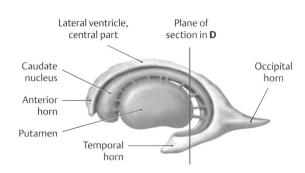

Lateral ventricle, central part

Plane of section in **D**

Caudate nucleus

Occipital horn

Anterior horn

Putamen

Temporal horn

E Topographical relationship between the caudate nucleus and ventricular system

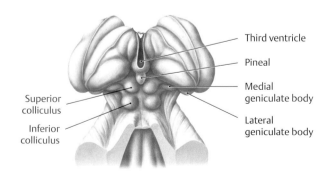

Third ventricle

Pineal

Medial geniculate body

Lateral geniculate body

Superior colliculus

Inferior colliculus

F The diencephalon (with geniculate bodies) and brainstem
Posterior view.

297

10.4 Coronal Sections: VII and VIII

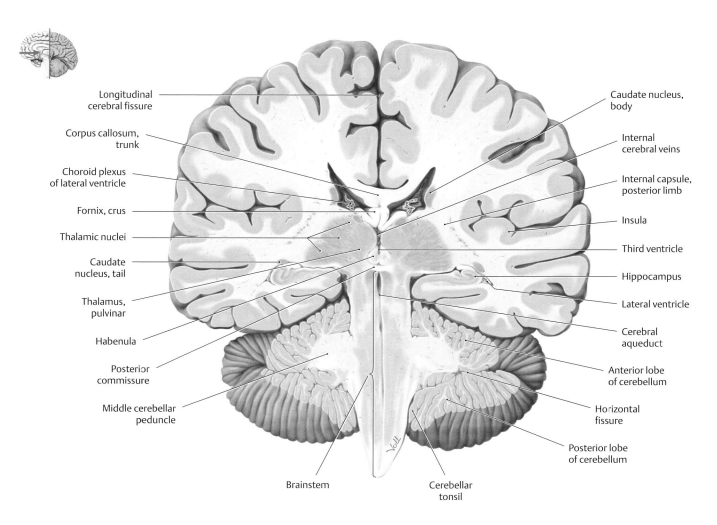

Longitudinal cerebral fissure

Corpus callosum, trunk

Choroid plexus of lateral ventricle

Fornix, crus

Thalamic nuclei

Caudate nucleus, tail

Thalamus, pulvinar

Habenula

Posterior commissure

Middle cerebellar peduncle

Brainstem

Caudate nucleus, body

Internal cerebral veins

Internal capsule, posterior limb

Insula

Third ventricle

Hippocampus

Lateral ventricle

Cerebral aqueduct

Anterior lobe of cerebellum

Horizontal fissure

Posterior lobe of cerebellum

Cerebellar tonsil

A Coronal section VII

Among the diencephalic and telencephalic nuclei, we can still identify the thalamus and occipital portions of the caudate nucleus, which become progressively smaller in the following sections until they finally disappear (see **C** and p. 300). The occipital part of the *hippocampus* can be seen below the medial wall of the lateral ventricle. This section cuts the brainstem along the *cerebral aqueduct* (see **C**). The cerebellum is connected to the brainstem by three white-matter stalks: the *superior cerebellar peduncle* (mainly efferent), *middle cerebellar peduncle* (afferent), and *inferior cerebellar peduncle* (afferent and efferent). Because the *middle*

cerebellar peduncle extends further anterior y than the other two peduncles (note its relationship to the brainstem axis), it is the first peduncle to appear in this frontal-to-occipital series of sections (see also **A**, p. 296, and **D**, p. 297). The *superior* cerebellar peduncle begins on the posterior side of the pons and thus appears in a later section (see **B** and p. 300). There are no natural anatomical boundaries between the middle and inferior cerebellar peduncles, and therefore the latter is not separately labeled in the sections. The superficial veins were removed from the brain when this section was prepared, and only the internal cerebral veins appear in this and the following section.

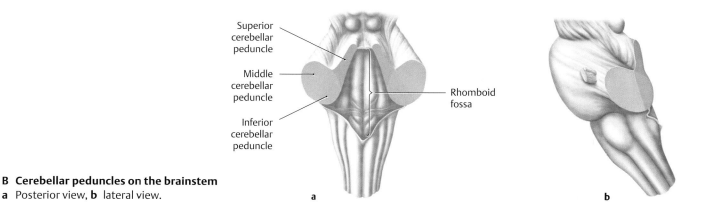

Superior cerebellar peduncle

Middle cerebellar peduncle

Inferior cerebellar peduncle

Rhomboid fossa

B Cerebellar peduncles on the brainstem

a Posterior view, **b** lateral view.

a

b

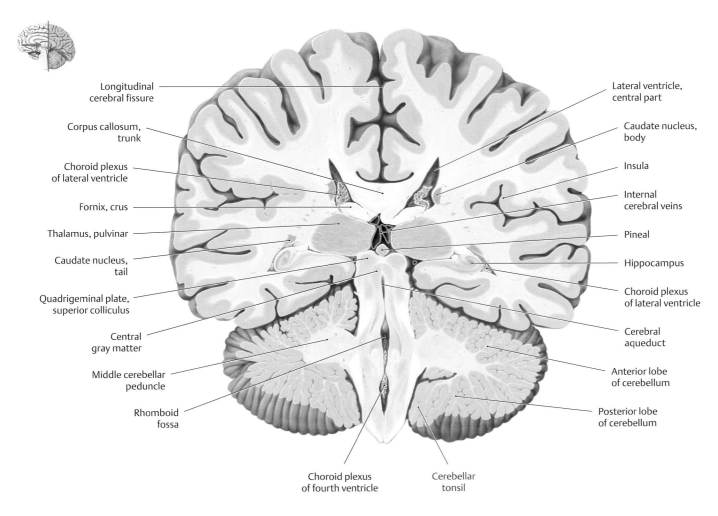

Longitudinal cerebral fissure

Corpus callosum, trunk

Choroid plexus of lateral ventricle

Fornix, crus

Thalamus, pulvinar

Caudate nucleus, tail

Quadrigeminal plate, superior colliculus

Central gray matter

Middle cerebellar peduncle

Rhomboid fossa

Choroid plexus of fourth ventricle

Cerebellar tonsil

Lateral ventricle, central part

Caudate nucleus, body

Insula

Internal cerebral veins

Pineal

Hippocampus

Choroid plexus of lateral ventricle

Cerebral aqueduct

Anterior lobe of cerebellum

Posterior lobe of cerebellum

C Coronal section VIII

The thalamic nuclei appear smaller than in previous sections, and more of the cerebellar cortex is seen. This plane passes through part of the cerebral aqueduct. The *rhomboid fossa*, which forms the floor of the fourth ventricle, is clearly visible in the dorsal part of the brainstem (see **D** and **Ba**). The quadrigeminal plate (lamina tecti) is also visible. Its smaller *superior* colliculi are particularly well displayed in this section, while the *inferior* colliculi are more prominent in the next section (see **A**, p. 300). The pineal is only partially visible because of its somewhat more occipi-

tal location (see **D**); a full cross-section can be seen in **A**, p. 300. The present section shows the division of the paired fornix tract into its two *crura* (see also **D**, p. 295). The hippocampus here borders on the inferior horn of the lateral ventricle on each side, bulging into its floor from the medial side (see also the previous sections and **E**). The hippocampus is an important component of the limbic system and is one of the first structures to undergo detectable morphological changes in Alzheimer's disease.

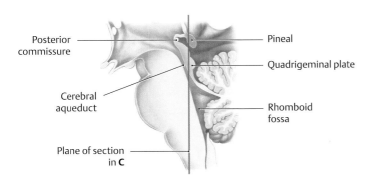

Posterior commissure

Cerebral aqueduct

Plane of section in **C**

Pineal

Quadrigeminal plate

Rhomboid fossa

D Midsagittal section through the rhombencephalon, mesencephalon, and diencephalon

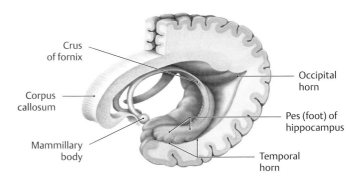

Crus of fornix

Corpus callosum

Mammillary body

Occipital horn

Pes (foot) of hippocampus

Temporal horn

E Hippocampal formation
Left lateral view.

10.5 Coronal Sections: IX and X

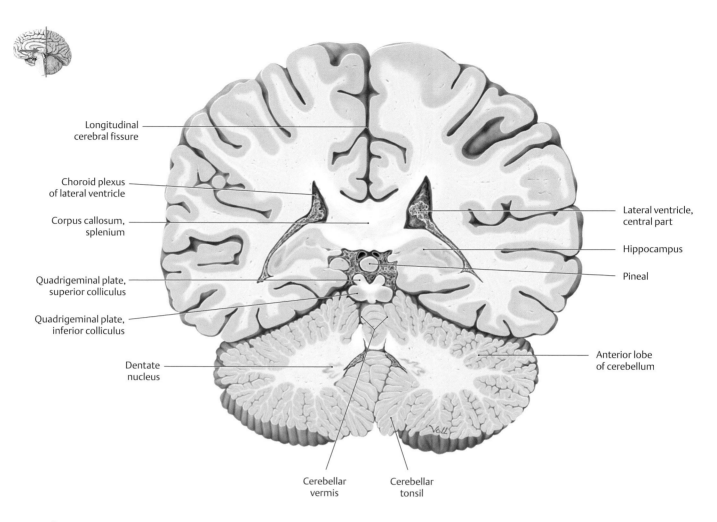

Longitudinal cerebral fissure

Choroid plexus of lateral ventricle

Corpus callosum, splenium

Quadrigeminal plate, superior colliculus

Quadrigeminal plate, inferior colliculus

Dentate nucleus

Lateral ventricle, central part

Hippocampus

Pineal

Anterior lobe of cerebellum

Cerebellar vermis

Cerebellar tonsil

A Coronal section IX
The pineal gland, a control center for circadian rhythms, is here displayed in full cross-section (contrast with the previous section; see also **D**, p. 299). Below it lies the quadrigeminal plate, the dorsal part of the midbrain (note its relationship to the brainstem axis). The larger *inferior* colliculi of the quadrigeminal plate are more prominent here than in the previous section (the inclination of the brainstem gives them a more posterior location). The *inferior* colliculi are part of the auditory pathway, while the *superior* colliculi (more clearly seen in the previous section) are part of the visual pathway. At the level of the cerebellum, the *vermis* can be identified as an unpaired midline structure. The only cerebellar nucleus visible at this level is the *dentate nucleus,* which is surrounded by the cerebellar white matter. The deep cerebral nuclei are no longer visible in the plane of this section.

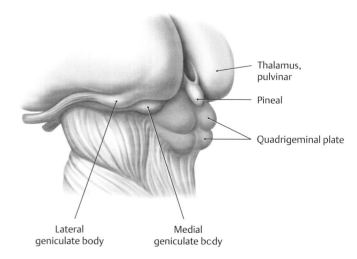

Thalamus, pulvinar

Pineal

Quadrigeminal plate

Lateral geniculate body

Medial geniculate body

B Quadrigeminal plate (lamina tecti)
Left posterior oblique view.

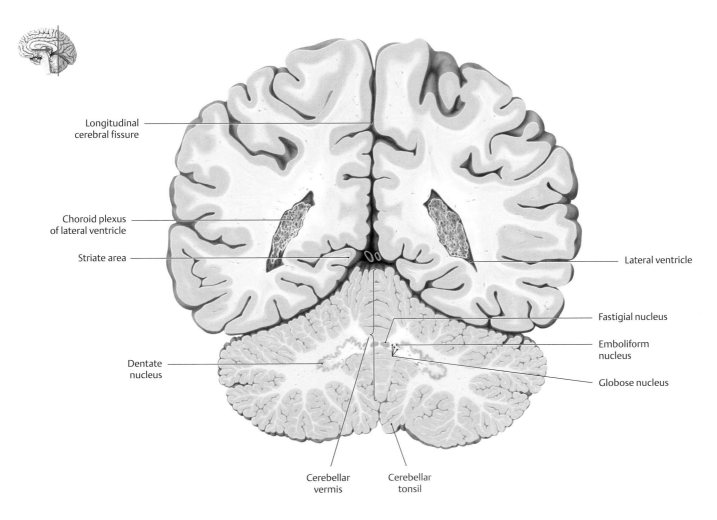

Longitudinal cerebral fissure

Choroid plexus of lateral ventricle

Striate area

Dentate nucleus

Lateral ventricle

Fastigial nucleus

Emboliform nucleus

Globose nucleus

Cerebellar vermis

Cerebellar tonsil

C Coronal section X

This plane presents the four *cerebellar nuclei:*

- Dentate nucleus (lateral cerebellar nucleus)
- Emboliform nucleus (anterior interpositus nucleus)
- Globose nucleus (posterior interpositus nucleus)
- Fastigial nucleus (medial cerebellar nucleus)

The longitudinally cut *cerebellar vermis* presents a larger area here than in the previous section. The fourth ventricle is no longer visible in the plane of this section.

10.6 Coronal Sections: XI and XII (Occipital)

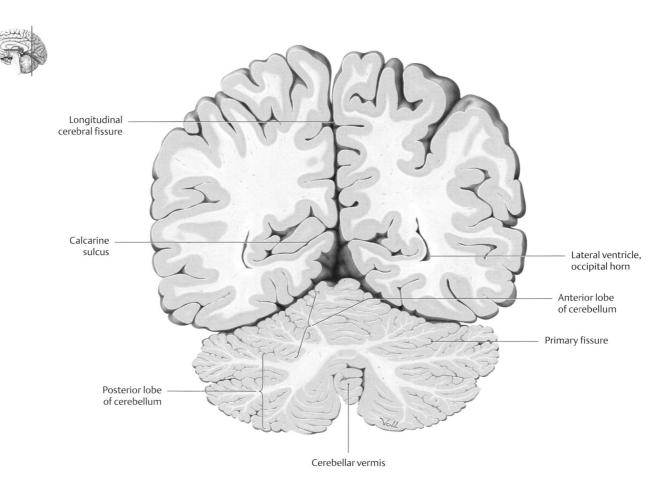

Longitudinal cerebral fissure

Calcarine sulcus

Lateral ventricle, occipital horn

Anterior lobe of cerebellum

Primary fissure

Posterior lobe of cerebellum

Cerebellar vermis

A Coronal section XI

The plane of this section clearly shows the posterior (occipital) horns of the lateral ventricles; these appear only as narrow slits in the next section (see **D**). The section also illustrates once again how the posterior horn is a prolongation of the inferior (temporal) horn (see **B**). Between the cerebellum and the occipital lobe of the cerebrum lies the *tentorium cerebelli* (see **C**). The tentorium contains the straight sinus, which passes to the confluence of the sinuses. It is one of the dural venous sinuses that drain blood from the brain, beginning at the confluence of the great cerebral vein and the inferior sagittal sinus (removed during preparation of the falx cerebri). Because the dura is removed from the brain in the preparation of most tissue sections, the sinuses enclosed by the dura mater also tend to be removed.

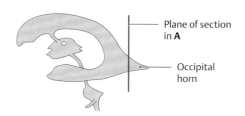

Plane of section in **A**

Occipital horn

B Ventricular system viewed from the left side

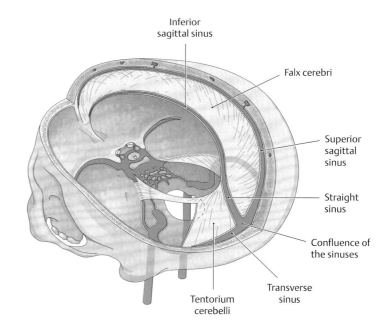

Inferior sagittal sinus

Falx cerebri

Superior sagittal sinus

Straight sinus

Confluence of the sinuses

Transverse sinus

Tentorium cerebelli

C The dural sinuses
Viewed from upper left.

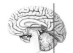

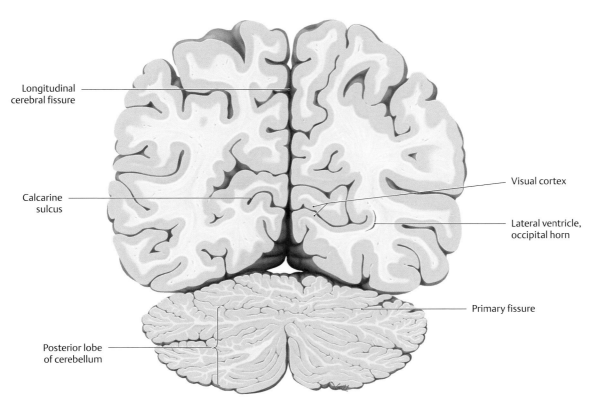

Longitudinal cerebral fissure

Calcarine sulcus

Visual cortex

Lateral ventricle, occipital horn

Primary fissure

Posterior lobe of cerebellum

D Coronal section XII

In the plane of this section, the posterior (occipital) horn of the lateral ventricle has dwindled to a narrow slit. The relatively long *calcarine sulcus* is visible in the occipital lobe of the cerebrum, and also appears in several of the proceeding sections. It is surrounded by the *striate area* (primary visual cortex, also called area 17 in the Brodmann brain map, p. 202), the size of which is best appreciated on the medial surface of the brain (see **E**). More occipital sections are not presented in this chapter, as they would show nothing but cortex and white matter.

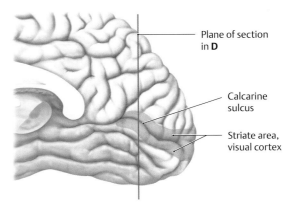

Plane of section in **D**

Calcarine sulcus

Striate area, visual cortex

E Right striate area (visual cortex)
Medial surface of the right hemisphere, viewed from the left side.

10.7 Transverse Sections: I and II (Cranial)

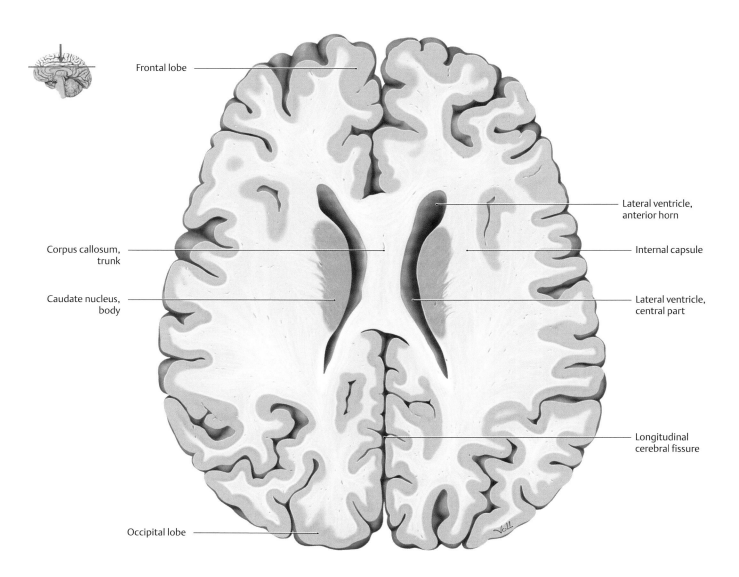

Frontal lobe

Lateral ventricle, anterior horn

Corpus callosum, trunk

Internal capsule

Caudate nucleus, body

Lateral ventricle, central part

Longitudinal cerebral fissure

Occipital lobe

General remarks on transverse brain sections

The sections in this series are viewed from above and behind the head; i.e., the observer is looking at the surface of the slice as it would typically appear in a brain autopsy or during a neurosurgical operation. Thus, the left side of the brain appears on the left side of the drawing. This contrasts with the image orientation in CT and MRI, where brain slices are always viewed from below; i.e., the left side of the brain appears on the right side of the image.

A Transverse section I

This highest of the transverse brain sections passes through frontal, parietal, and occipital structures of the telencephalon. Each of the two *lateral ventricles* is bordered laterally by the body of the caudate nucleus, and medially by the *trunk of the corpus callosum*. The corpus callosum transmits fiber tracts which interconnect areas in both hemispheres that serve the same function (*commissural tracts*). When viewed in cross section, the corpus callosum appears to be interrupted by the ventricles and caudate nucleus, when, in fact, it arches over these structures, forming the roof of the lateral ventricles. The course of the tracts that pass through the corpus callosum can be appreciated by looking at a coronal section (see **B**).

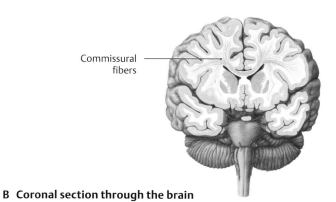

Commissural fibers

B Coronal section through the brain

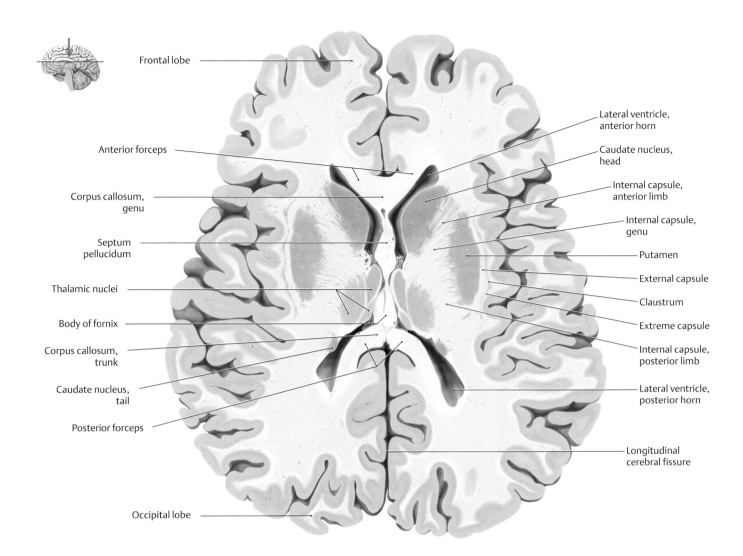

Frontal lobe

Anterior forceps

Corpus callosum, genu

Septum pellucidum

Thalamic nuclei

Body of fornix

Corpus callosum, trunk

Caudate nucleus, tail

Posterior forceps

Occipital lobe

Lateral ventricle, anterior horn

Caudate nucleus, head

Internal capsule, anterior limb

Internal capsule, genu

Putamen

External capsule

Claustrum

Extreme capsule

Internal capsule, posterior limb

Lateral ventricle, posterior horn

Longitudinal cerebral fissure

C Transverse section II

In this section, unlike the previous one, the *lateral ventricle* appears divided in two. Because this section is at a lower level, it cuts the anterior and posterior horns of the lateral ventricle separately, missing the central part of the ventricle (see **D**). It also cuts a broad swath of the *internal capsule* with its genu and anterior and posterior limbs. The optic radiation, which runs in the white matter of the occipital lobe, is not labeled here because it has no grossly visible anatomical boundaries. The *corpus callosum* also appears divided into two parts: the genu anteriorly and the trunk more posteriorly. This apparent division results from a second curvature of the corpus callosum at its genu ("knee"), where

it is anteriorly convex. The diagram in **E** demonstrates why this section passes successively through the genu of the corpus callosum, the septum pellucidum, the body of the fornix, and finally the trunk of the corpus callosum. The septum pellucidum forms the anteromedial wall of both lateral ventricles. The septum itself contains small nuclei. Sections of the thalamic nuclei (ventral lateral, lateral dorsal and anterior nuclei) are also visible along with the putamen and caudate nucleus. The head and tail of the caudate nucleus appear separately in the section (see also p. 306). The putamen, caudate nucleus, and intervening fibers of the internal capsule are collectively called the corpus striatum.

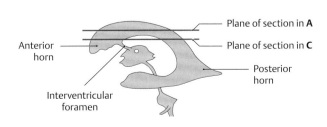

Anterior horn

Interventricular foramen

Plane of section in A

Plane of section in C

Posterior horn

D Lateral view of the ventricular system

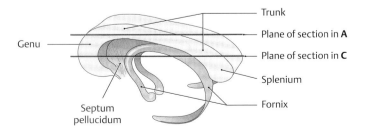

Genu

Trunk

Plane of section in A

Plane of section in C

Splenium

Fornix

Septum pellucidum

E Corpus callosum and fornix

10.8 Transverse Sections: III and IV

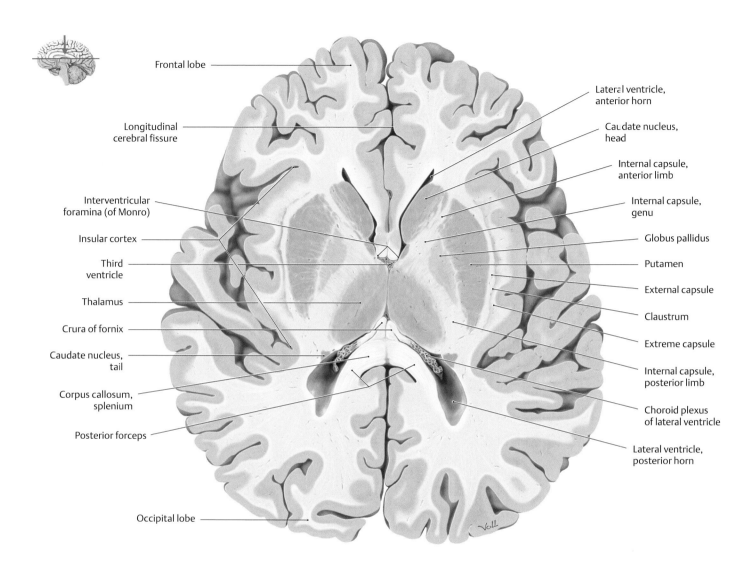

Frontal lobe

Longitudinal cerebral fissure

Interventricular foramina (of Monro)

Insular cortex

Third ventricle

Thalamus

Crura of fornix

Caudate nucleus, tail

Corpus callosum, splenium

Posterior forceps

Occipital lobe

Lateral ventricle, anterior horn

Caudate nucleus, head

Internal capsule, anterior limb

Internal capsule, genu

Globus pallidus

Putamen

External capsule

Claustrum

Extreme capsule

Internal capsule, posterior limb

Choroid plexus of lateral ventricle

Lateral ventricle, posterior horn

A Transverse section III

The lateral ventricles communicate with the third ventricle through the *interventricular foramina* (of Monro). They are located directly anterior to the thalamus (see **D**, p. 305, and **A**, p. 296). The nuclei of the telencephalon make up the deep gray matter of the cerebrum. The spatial relationship between the caudate nucleus and thalamus is illustrated in **B**. The caudate nucleus is larger frontally, and the thalamus larger occipitally. While the caudate nucleus and putamen of the motor system belong to the telencephalon, the thalamus of the sensory system belongs to the diencephalon. This transverse section passes through the caudate nucleus twice due to the anatomical curvature of the nucleus. This is the first transverse section that displays the globus pallidus, part of the motor system. The insular cortex is seen with the *claustrum* medial to it. The *crura of the fornix* are seen as posterior to the thalamus (see also **E**, p. 305). They unite at a slightly higher level to form the *body of the fornix,* which lies just below the corpus callosum and was visible in the previous section (see **C**, p. 305). The course of the internal capsule is visible in both this section and the last.

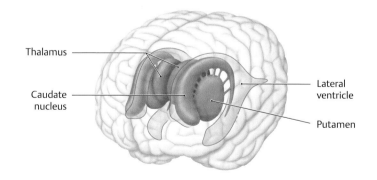

Thalamus

Caudate nucleus

Lateral ventricle

Putamen

B Spatial relationships of the caudate nucleus, putamen, thalamus, and lateral ventricles
Left anterior oblique view.

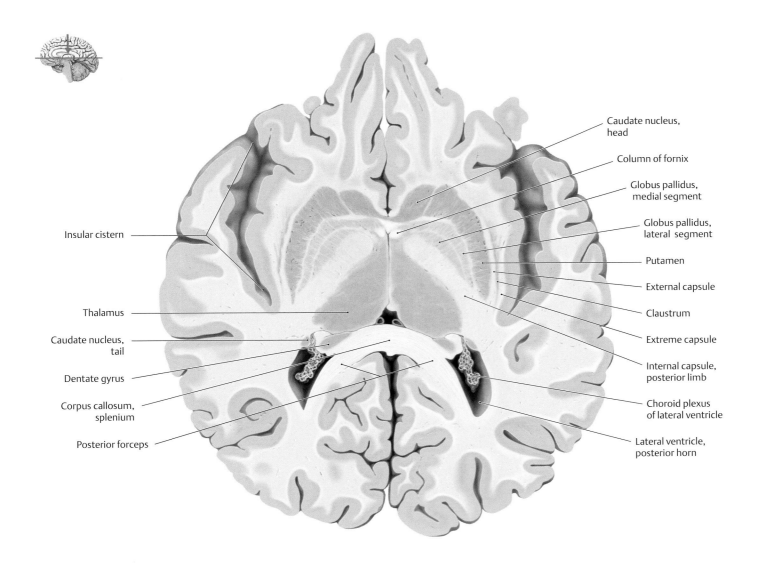

Caudate nucleus, head

Column of fornix

Globus pallidus, medial segment

Globus pallidus, lateral segment

Putamen

External capsule

Claustrum

Extreme capsule

Internal capsule, posterior limb

Choroid plexus of lateral ventricle

Lateral ventricle, posterior horn

Insular cistern

Thalamus

Caudate nucleus, tail

Dentate gyrus

Corpus callosum, splenium

Posterior forceps

C Transverse section IV
The nuclei shown in the previous section here appear as a roughly circular mass at the center of the brain, surrounded by the gray matter of the cerebral cortex, also called the *pallium* ("cloak") for obvious reasons. The choroid plexus is here visible in both lateral ventricles. This section cuts the occipital part of the corpus callosum, the *splenium,* as well as the basal portion of the *insular cortex.* The insula is a cortical region that lies below the surface and is covered by the opercula. The insular cistern should be used as a reference point, e.g., when comparing this section to **A** and **D**.

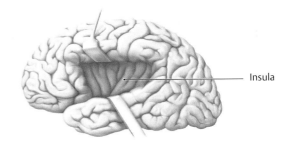

Insula

D Left insular region
Lateral view.

10.9 Transverse Sections: V and VI (Caudal)

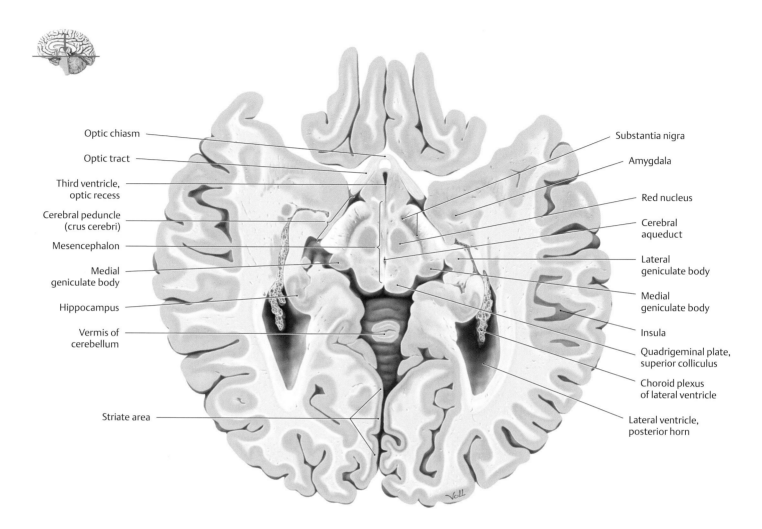

Optic chiasm

Optic tract

Third ventricle, optic recess

Cerebral peduncle (crus cerebri)

Mesencephalon

Medial geniculate body

Hippocampus

Vermis of cerebellum

Striate area

Substantia nigra

Amygdala

Red nucleus

Cerebral aqueduct

Lateral geniculate body

Medial geniculate body

Insula

Quadrigeminal plate, superior colliculus

Choroid plexus of lateral ventricle

Lateral ventricle, posterior horn

A Transverse section V
Structures visible in this section include the cerebral aqueduct, the basal part of the third ventricle (see also **B**, p. 294), and the *optic recess*. While the third ventricle is slitlike at this level, the section cuts a very large area of the ventricular system where it opens into the two posterior horns. This is the first transverse section that displays the midbrain (*mesencephalon*), passing through its oral portion (*note:* terms of location and direction refer to the brainstem axis, see p. 198). The cerebral peduncles (*crura cerebri*), the *substantia nigra*, and the *superior colliculi* of the quadrigeminal plate can also be seen. Visible structures of the *diencephalon* in this plane include the *medial* and *lateral geniculate bodies* (appearing only on the right side, see **B**) and the *optic tract*, which is an extension of the diencephalon.

Note: closely adjacent structures in the brain may belong to different ontogenetic regions. For example, the medial and lateral geniculate bodies are part of the diencephalon, while the superior and inferior colliculi (the latter is not visible), which make up the quadrigeminal plate, are part of the mesencephalon. It should be recalled, however, that the lateral geniculate body and superior colliculus are part of the visual pathway while the medial geniculate body and inferior colliculus are part of the auditory pathway.

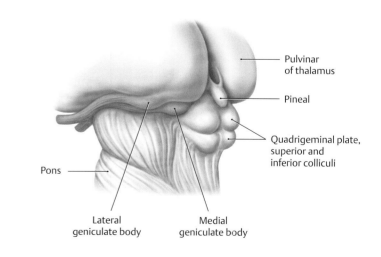

Pulvinar of thalamus

Pineal

Quadrigeminal plate, superior and inferior colliculi

Pons

Lateral geniculate body

Medial geniculate body

B Pons, midbrain, and adjacent diencephalon
Left posterior oblique view.

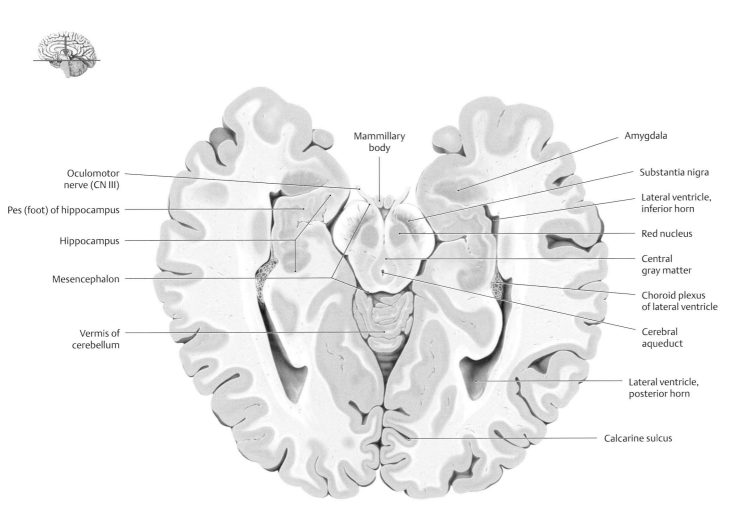

Mammillary body

Amygdala

Oculomotor nerve (CN III)

Substantia nigra

Pes (foot) of hippocampus

Lateral ventricle, inferior horn

Hippocampus

Red nucleus

Mesencephalon

Central gray matter

Choroid plexus of lateral ventricle

Vermis of cerebellum

Cerebral aqueduct

Lateral ventricle, posterior horn

Calcarine sulcus

C Transverse section VI

The structures that occupy the largest area at this level are the telencephalon, the medial portions of the mesencephalon, and the cerebellum. The nuclei located on the median aspect of each frontal lobe of the telencephalon are the *amygdalae*. The lower part of the section cuts the *calcarine sulcus* with the surrounding visual cortex. This section also passes through the choroid plexus of the lateral ventricles, whose *posterior* and *inferior horns* are displayed. Important structures of the *mesencephalon* are the substantia nigra and red nucleus, both of which are part of the motor system. The mammillary bodies are part of the *diencephalon* and are connected by the fornix (not visible in this section) to the hippocampus, which is part of the *telencephalon*. The mammillary bodies lie in the same horizontal plane as the hyppocampus and the same coronal plane as its pes (foot). These relationships result from the curved shape of the fornix (see **D**). More transverse sections at lower levels would supply little additional information on the cerebrum, and so our series of transverse sections ends here. The brainstem structures lying below the mesencephalon are displayed in a separate group of sections (see p. 234, 235).

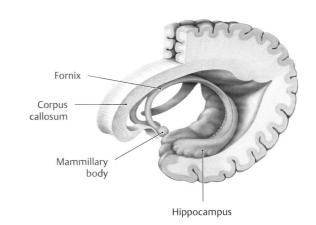

Fornix

Corpus callosum

Mammillary body

Hippocampus

D Fornix
Left anterior oblique view.

10.10 Sagittal Sections: I–III (Lateral)

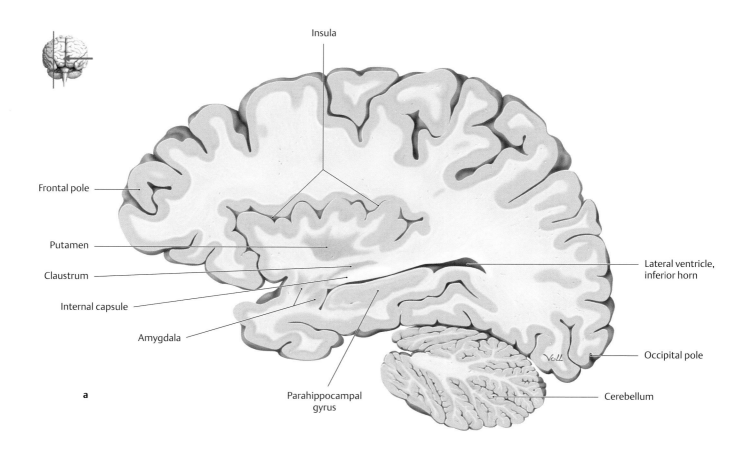

Insula

Frontal pole

Putamen

Claustrum

Internal capsule

Amygdala

Lateral ventricle, inferior horn

Occipital pole

Cerebellum

a

Parahippocampal gyrus

A Sagittal sections I–III
Left lateral view. The plane of section **a** passes through the *inferior (temporal) horn* of the lateral ventricle; the more medially situated *posterior (occipital) horn* is seen in **b** and **c** (see **C**, p. 296 for relative position of both horns). The *amygdala,* which is directly anterior to the inferior horn, lies in the same sagittal plane as the parahippocampal gyrus (**a–c**; see also **C**, p. 309). The internal capsule can also be seen in sections **a–c**; the long ascending and descending tracts pass through this structure. The most lateral section (**a**) offers the only view of the *insular cortex,* a part of the cerebral cortex that has sunk below the surface of the hemisphere (compare with the coronal sections on p. 293 and the following pages). The *putamen,* the most laterally situated among the basal ganglia of the telencephalon (see also **A**, p. 296) is also found in **a**, but appears larger in the more medial sections (**b, c**). A portion of the *claustrum* can be seen

ventral to the putamen (**a**), although most of the claustrum is lateral to the putamen (see **A**, p. 297) and outside the plane of the section. Section **b** just cuts the tail of the *caudate nucleus,* which is situated more laterally than its head and body (see also **D**, p. 279). The most medial section in this series (**c**) cuts the *calcarine sulcus* (see p. 312) and the *lateral geniculate body* which lies at the edge of the thalamus. The lateral segment of the globus pallidus can also be seen (**c**): the segments of the *globus pallidus* are actually medial to the putamen (see **D**, p. 295), but can be visualized here due to their concentric arrangement.

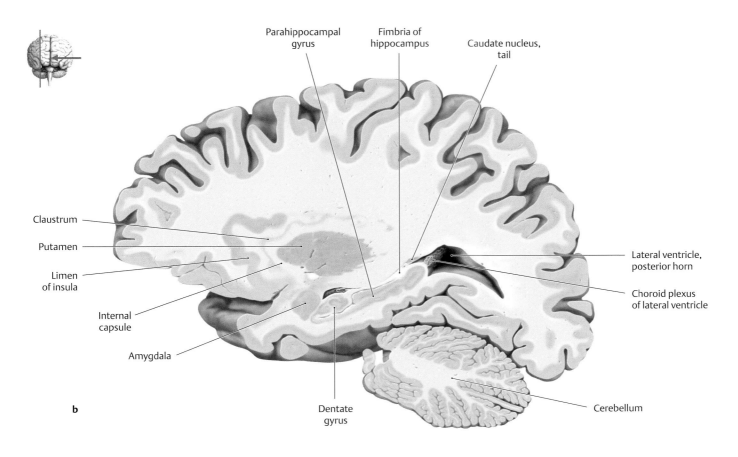

Parahippocampal gyrus

Fimbria of hippocampus

Caudate nucleus, tail

Claustrum

Putamen

Limen of insula

Internal capsule

Amygdala

Lateral ventricle, posterior horn

Choroid plexus of lateral ventricle

Cerebellum

Dentate gyrus

b

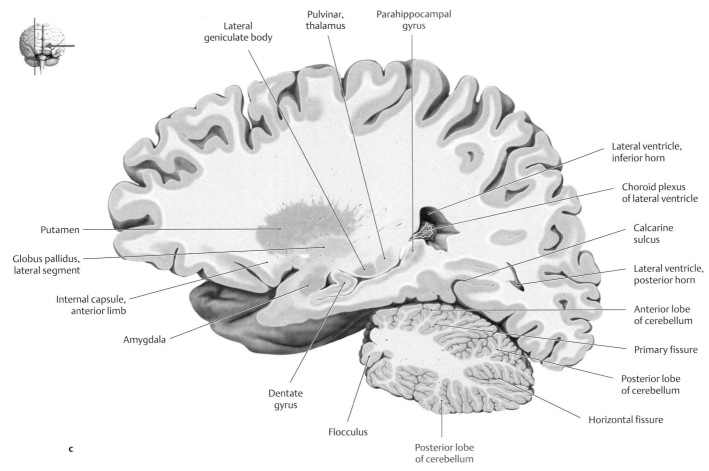

Lateral geniculate body

Pulvinar, thalamus

Parahippocampal gyrus

Putamen

Globus pallidus, lateral segment

Internal capsule, anterior limb

Amygdala

Dentate gyrus

Flocculus

Posterior lobe of cerebellum

Lateral ventricle, inferior horn

Choroid plexus of lateral ventricle

Calcarine sulcus

Lateral ventricle, posterior horn

Anterior lobe of cerebellum

Primary fissure

Posterior lobe of cerebellum

Horizontal fissure

c

311

10.11 Sagittal Sections: IV–VI

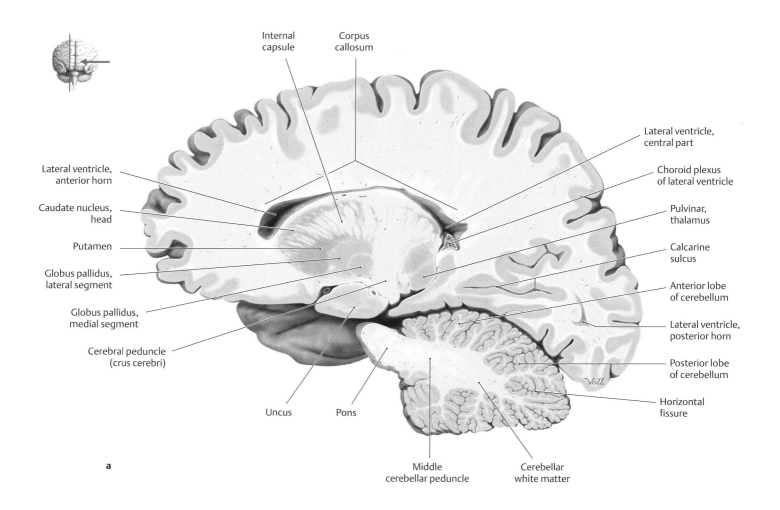

Internal capsule

Corpus callosum

Lateral ventricle, central part

Choroid plexus of lateral ventricle

Lateral ventricle, anterior horn

Pulvinar, thalamus

Caudate nucleus, head

Calcarine sulcus

Putamen

Globus pallidus, lateral segment

Anterior lobe of cerebellum

Globus pallidus, medial segment

Lateral ventricle, posterior horn

Cerebral peduncle (crus cerebri)

Posterior lobe of cerebellum

Horizontal fissure

Uncus

Pons

a

Middle cerebellar peduncle

Cerebellar white matter

A Sagittal sections IV–VI

Left lateral view. The dominant ventricular structures in all three of these sections are the anterior horn and central part of the *lateral ventricle* (the junction with the laterally situated posterior horn appears only in **a**). The *corpus callosum,* which connects functionally related areas of the two cerebral hemispheres (commissural tract), can be identified in the cerebral white matter although it is not sharply delineated (**a–c**). As the sections move closer to the cerebral midline, the putamen grows smaller while the caudate nucleus becomes increasingly prominent (**a–c**). These two bodies are known collectively as the *corpus striatum,* and their characteristic striations are seen particularly well in **a** (the white matter that separates the gray-matter streaks of the corpus striatum is the *internal capsule*). The previous sagittal sections showed only the lateral segment of the *globus pallidus* (see p. 310), but its medial segment is displayed in both **a** and **b**. As the globus pallidus disappears and

the putamen becomes less prominent, the nuclei of the medially situated thalamus become visible below the lateral ventricle (**c**; the subthalamic nuclei include the anterior, posterior, and lateral ventral nuclei of the diencephalon). The location of the thalamus explains why it is sometimes referred to as the *dorsal thalamus.* Section **c** also shows the *substantia nigra* in the mesencephalon (below the diencephalon), the inferior olivary nucleus in the underlying medulla oblongata, and the *dentate nucleus* of the cerebellum. The ascending and descending tracts previously visible only in the internal capsule can now be seen in the pons, part of the brainstem (**c**, corticospinal tract). The only visible portion of the fourth ventricle, barely sectioned in **c**, is its lateral recess.

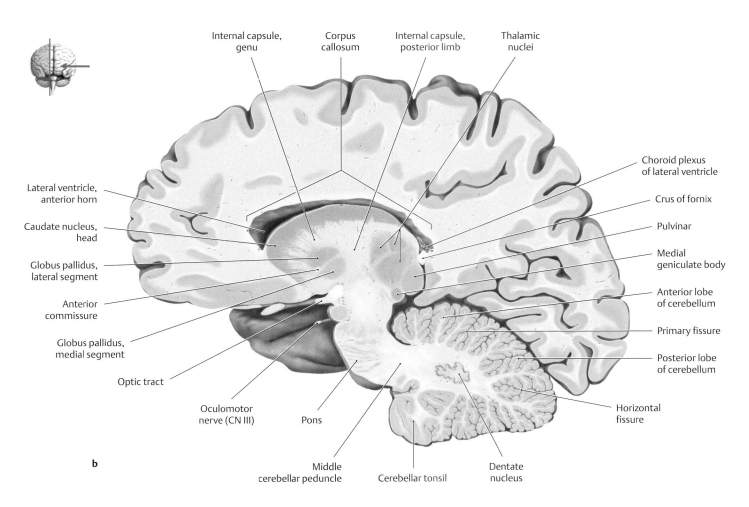

Internal capsule, genu

Corpus callosum

Internal capsule, posterior limb

Thalamic nuclei

Choroid plexus of lateral ventricle

Crus of fornix

Pulvinar

Medial geniculate body

Anterior lobe of cerebellum

Primary fissure

Posterior lobe of cerebellum

Horizontal fissure

Lateral ventricle, anterior horn

Caudate nucleus, head

Globus pallidus, lateral segment

Anterior commissure

Globus pallidus, medial segment

Optic tract

Oculomotor nerve (CN III)

Pons

Middle cerebellar peduncle

Cerebellar tonsil

Dentate nucleus

b

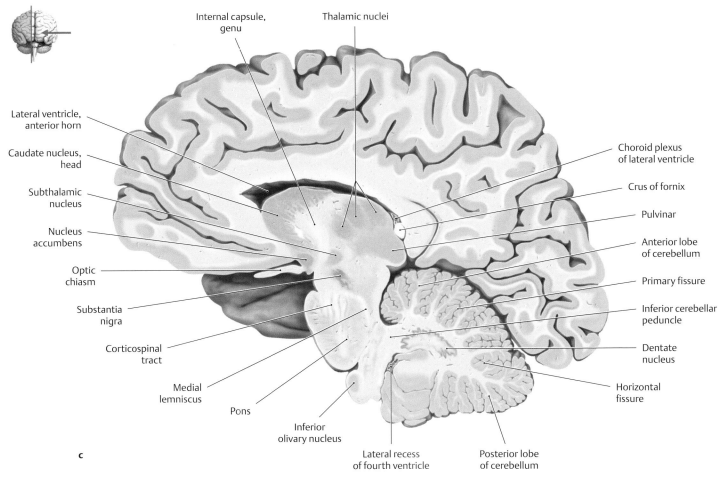

Internal capsule, genu

Thalamic nuclei

Choroid plexus of lateral ventricle

Crus of fornix

Pulvinar

Anterior lobe of cerebellum

Primary fissure

Inferior cerebellar peduncle

Dentate nucleus

Horizontal fissure

Posterior lobe of cerebellum

Lateral recess of fourth ventricle

Inferior olivary nucleus

Pons

Medial lemniscus

Corticospinal tract

Substantia nigra

Optic chiasm

Nucleus accumbens

Subthalamic nucleus

Caudate nucleus, head

Lateral ventricle, anterior horn

c

10.12 Sagittal Sections: VII and VIII (Medial)

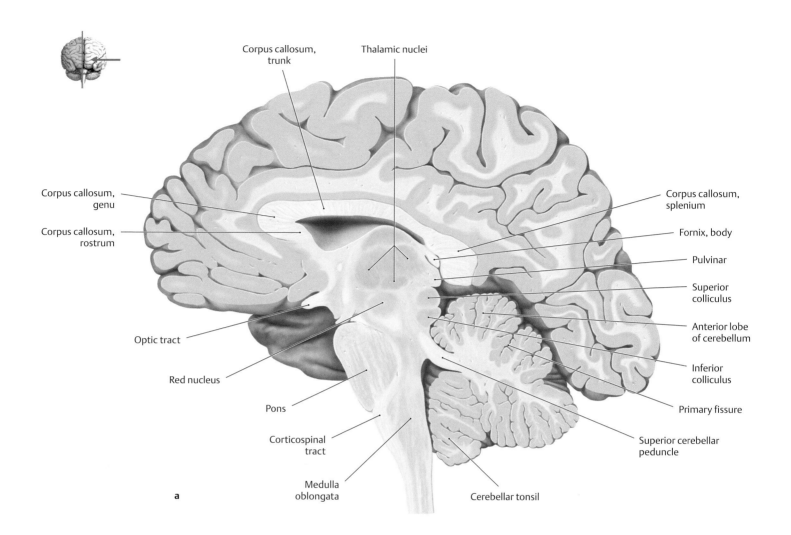

Corpus callosum, trunk

Thalamic nuclei

Corpus callosum, genu

Corpus callosum, rostrum

Optic tract

Red nucleus

Pons

Corticospinal tract

Medulla oblongata

Corpus callosum, splenium

Fornix, body

Pulvinar

Superior colliculus

Anterior lobe of cerebellum

Inferior colliculus

Primary fissure

Superior cerebellar peduncle

Cerebellar tonsil

a

A Sagittal sections VII and VIII
Left lateral view. This section (**a**) is so close to the midline that it passes through the principal paramedian structures: the substantia nigra, the red nucleus, and one each of the paired superior and inferior colliculi. The pyramidal tract (corticospinal tract) runs in front of the inferior olive in the medulla oblongata. A complete sagittal section of the corpus callosum is displayed, and most of the fornix tract is displayed in lon-

gitudinal section (**b**). The cerebellum has reached its maximum extent and forms the roof of the fourth ventricle (**b**). A portion of the *septum pellucidum*, which stretches between the fornix and corpus callosum, is also displayed.
When the brain is removed, the pituitary gland, which appears in **b**, remains in the sella turcica; i.e., it is always torn from the brain at its stalk when the brain is removed.

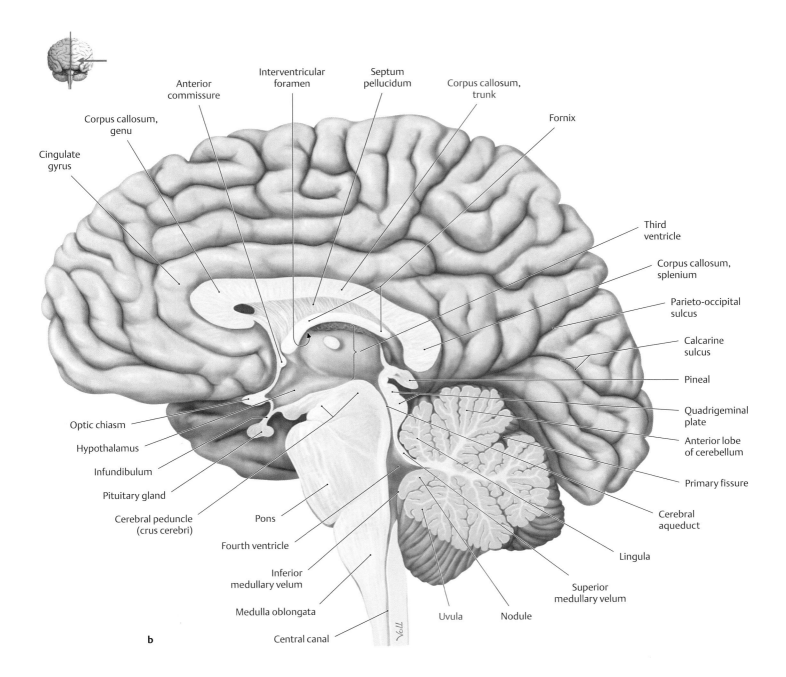

Anterior commissure

Interventricular foramen

Septum pellucidum

Corpus callosum, trunk

Corpus callosum, genu

Fornix

Cingulate gyrus

Third ventricle

Corpus callosum, splenium

Parieto-occipital sulcus

Calcarine sulcus

Pineal

Quadrigeminal plate

Optic chiasm

Anterior lobe of cerebellum

Hypothalamus

Primary fissure

Infundibulum

Pituitary gland

Cerebral aqueduct

Cerebral peduncle (crus cerebri)

Pons

Lingula

Fourth ventricle

Inferior medullary velum

Superior medullary velum

Medulla oblongata

Uvula

Nodule

b

Central canal

B Principal structures in the serial sections
The major structures seen in the serial sections are here assigned to their corresponding brain regions. Within each region, the structures are listed from most rostral to most caudal.

Telencephalon (endbrain)
- External capsule
- Extreme capsule
- Internal capsule
- Claustrum
- Anterior commissure
- Amygdala
- Corpus callosum
- Fornix
- Globus pallidus
- Cingulate gyrus
- Hippocampus
- Caudate nucleus
- Putamen
- Septum pellucidum

Diencephalon (interbrain)
- Lateral geniculate body
- Medial geniculate body
- Pineal gland
- Pulvinar of thalamus
- Thalamus
- Optic tract
- Mammillary body

Mesencephalon (midbrain)
- Cerebral aqueduct
- Quadrigeminal plate (lamina tecti)
  - Superior colliculus
  - Inferior colliculus
- Red nucleus
- Substantia nigra
- Cerebral peduncle (crus cerebri)

11.1 Sympathetic and Parasympathetic Nervous Systems, Organization

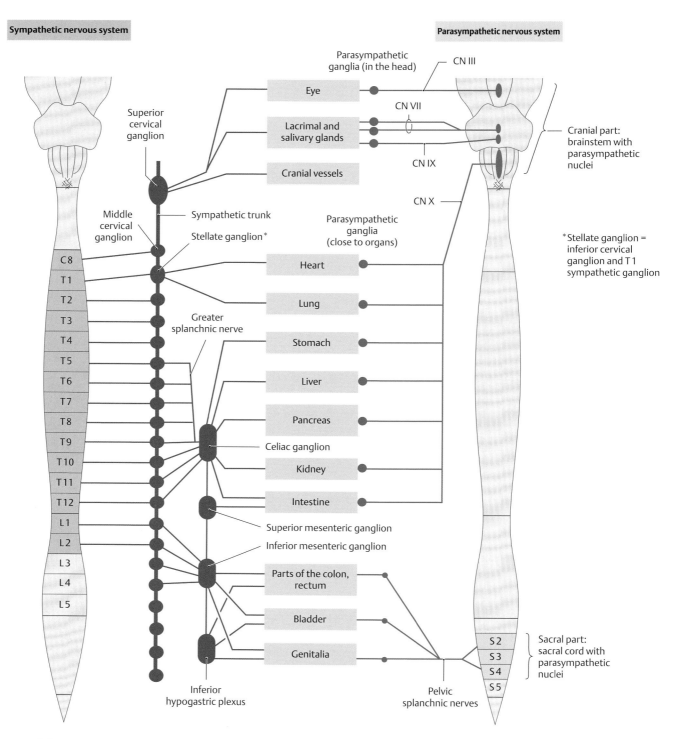

Sympathetic nervous system

Parasympathetic nervous system

Parasympathetic ganglia (in the head)

Eye

CN III

Superior cervical ganglion

Lacrimal and salivary glands

CN VII

Cranial vessels

CN IX

Cranial part: brainstem with parasympathetic nuclei

Middle cervical ganglion

Sympathetic trunk

Stellate ganglion*

CN X

Parasympathetic ganglia (close to organs)

*Stellate ganglion = inferior cervical ganglion and T 1 sympathetic ganglion

C 8

T 1

Heart

T 2

Lung

T 3

Greater splanchnic nerve

T 4

Stomach

T 5

T 6

Liver

T 7

T 8

Pancreas

T 9

Celiac ganglion

T 10

Kidney

T 11

T 12

Intestine

L 1

Superior mesenteric ganglion

L 2

Inferior mesenteric ganglion

L 3

Parts of the colon, rectum

L 4

L 5

Bladder

Genitalia

S 2

S 3

Sacral part: sacral cord with parasympathetic nuclei

S 4

S 5

Inferior hypogastric plexus

Pelvic splanchnic nerves

A Structure of the autonomic nervous system

The portion of the nervous system which innervates smooth muscle, cardiac muscle, and glands is called the *autonomic nervous system*. This is further subdivided into the *sympathetic* (red) and *parasympathetic* (blue) *systems,* each of which has a two-neuron sequence between the CNS and its target, consisting of a *presynaptic* neuron in the CNS, and a *postsynaptic* neuron in a ganglion (PNS) close to the target organ:

• **Sympathetic system:** presynaptic neurons located in the lateral horns of the cervical, thoracic, and lumbar spinal cords. Their axons exit the CNS via the ventral roots and synapse with postsynaptic neurons in sympathetic ganglia.

• **Parasympathetic system:** presynaptic neurons located in the brainstem and sacral spinal cord. Their axons exit the CNS via cranial nerves and pelvic splanchnic nerves to synapse with postsynaptic parasympathetic neurons, typically within the target organ.

The sympathetic and parasympathetic systems regulate blood flow, secretions and organ function, often acting in antagonistic ways on the same target (see **C**). In the abdomen, small clusters of neurons embedded in target organs form a network that can be considered a third autonomic division: the *enteric nervous system* (see p. 324). Although this network receives some presynaptic parasympathetic innervation via the vagus nerve (CN X), it typically functions independently, responding to local reflexes.

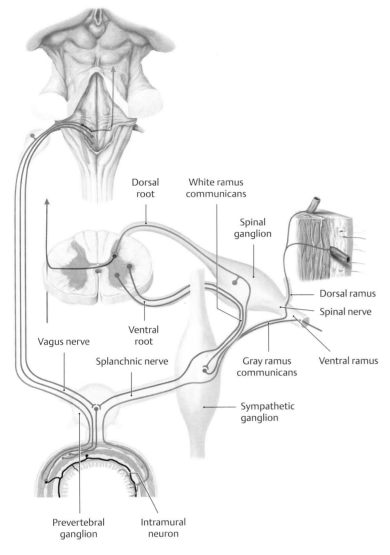

Dorsal root
White ramus communicans
Spinal ganglion
Dorsal ramus
Spinal nerve
Ventral root
Vagus nerve
Splanchnic nerve
Gray ramus communicans
Ventral ramus
Sympathetic ganglion
Prevertebral ganglion
Intramural neuron

B Synaptic organization of the autonomic nervous system

The sympathetic and parasympathetic portions of the nervous systems innervate many of the same targets, but use different transmitters, often with antagonistic effects (see **C**). These antagonistic systems also have differing patterns of organization, including unique paths to their targets and connections to the CNS. The cell bodies of the presynaptic motor neurons of the **sympathetic system** are located in the lateral horn of spinal cord segments T1 to L2 (sometimes C8 and L3). Their axons leave the spinal cord through thoracolumbar ventral roots, briefly travel in spinal nerves, and enter the paravertebral sympathetic trunk via white rami communicantes (white = myelinated). These axons terminate in synapses with postsynaptic neurons at three different levels:

1. Sympathetic ganglia along the paravertebral chain: The postsynaptic neurons send their axons back into the spinal nerves via gray rami communicantes (gray = unmyelinated). These axons travel in the spinal nerves to innervate local blood vessels, sweat glands, etc.
2. Prevertebral sympathetic ganglia: These ganglion cells send their axons along arterial plexuses to the bowel, kidneys, etc., providing innervation to both the organs and their vasculature.
3. Adrenal medulla (not shown): Adrenal medullary (endocrine) cells are developmentally related to sympathetic ganglion cells, and receive direct innervation from presynaptic sympathetic axons.

In contrast, the presynaptic neurons of the **parasympathetic system** are located in the CNS in the brainstem (cranial nerves III, VIII, IX, and X) and sacral spinal cord (S2–S4). The presynaptic axons leave the CNS via the cranial nerves noted above (the vagus nerve [CN X] is the example shown here), and pelvic splanchnic nerves. These presynaptic axons synapse with postsynaptic neurons in discrete cranial ganglia (ciliary, pterygopalatine, submandibular, and otic), which in turn send their axons in other cranial nerves to the target organ. Some presynaptic axons, particularly the vagus nerve, innervate scattered postsynaptic neurons that are embedded in the target organs themselves. Afferent fibers (shown in green), originating from pseudounipolar neurons in spinal (dorsal root) and cranial sensory ganglia, travel with autonomic motor axons. These sensory fibers carry information from visceral nociceptors (pain) and stretch receptors into the CNS. Efferent fibers are shown in purple, the ascending pain pathway in gray. For detailed description of the autonomic innervation of the viscera, see *Volume II, Neck and Internal Organs*.

C Synopsis of the sympathetic and parasympathetic nervous systems

This table summarizes the effects of the sympathetic and parasympathetic nervous systems on specific organs.

- The *sympathetic* nervous system is the excitatory part of the autonomic nervous system (fight or flight).
- The *parasympathetic* nervous system coordinates rest and digestive processes (rest and digest).
- Although the two systems have separate nuclei, they establish close anatomical and functional connections in the periphery.
- The transmitter at the target organ is *acetylcholine* in the parasympathetic and *norepinephrine* in the sympathetic nervous system (except for the adrenal medulla).
- Stimulation of the sympathetic or parasympathetic nervous system produces the following effects in specific organs (see table):

Organ	Sympathetic nervous system	Parasympathetic nervous system
Eye	Pupillary dilation	Pupillary constriction and increased curvature of the lens
Salivary glands	Decreased salivation (scant, viscous)	Increased salivation (copious, watery)
Heart	Rise in heart rate	Fall in heart rate
Lungs	Decreased bronchial secretions and bronchodilation	Increased bronchial secretions and bronchoconstriction
Gastrointestinal tract	Decrease in secretions and motility	Increase in secretions and motility
Pancreas	Decreased exocrine secretions	Increased exocrine secretions
Male sex organs	Ejaculation	Erection
Skin	Vasoconstriction, sweating, piloerection	No effect

11.2 Autonomic Nervous System, Actions and Regulation

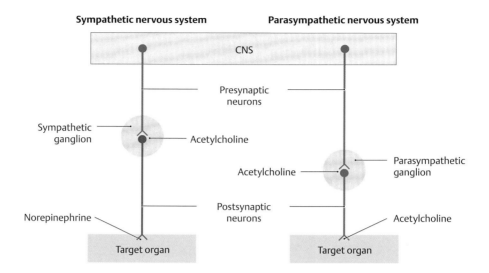

A Circuit diagram of the autonomic nervous system
The central first (presynaptic) neuron uses acetylcholine as a transmitter in both the sympathetic and parasympathetic nervous systems (cholinergic neuron, shown in blue). Acetylcholine is also used as a neurotransmitter by the second (postsynaptic) neuron in the parasympathetic nervous system. In the sympathetic nervous system, norepinephrine is used by the noradrenergic neuron (shown in red). *Note:* the target cell membrane contains different types of receptors (= transmitter sensors) for acetylcholine and norepinephrine. Each transmitters can produce entirely different effects, depending on the type of receptor.

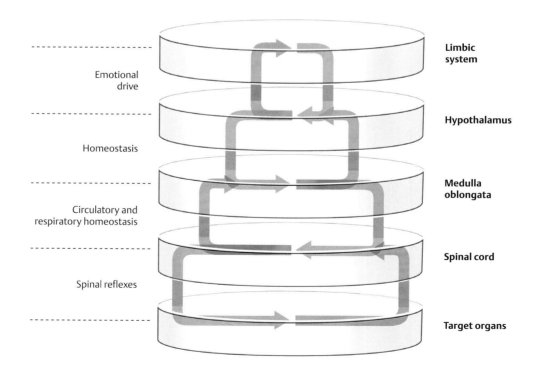

B Control of the peripheral autonomic nervous system (after Klinke and Silbernagl)
The peripheral actions of the autonomic nervous system are subject to control at various levels, the highest being the limbic system, whose efferent fibers act on the peripheral target organs (e.g., heart, lung, bowel; also affects sympathetic tone and cutaneous blood flow) through centers in the hypothalamus, medulla oblongata, and spinal cord. The higher the control center, the more subtle and complex its effect on the target organ. The limbic system receives signals from its target organs via afferent feedback mechanisms.

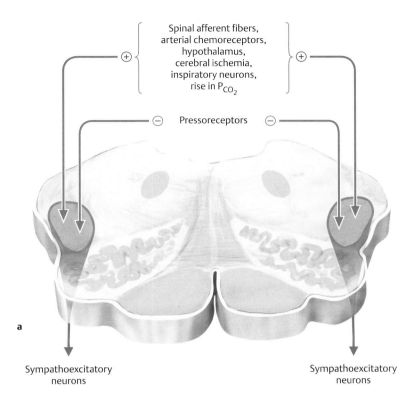

Spinal afferent fibers, arterial chemoreceptors, hypothalamus, cerebral ischemia, inspiratory neurons, rise in P_{CO_2}

⊕

⊖ Pressoreceptors ⊖

a

Sympathoexcitatory neurons

Sympathoexcitatory neurons

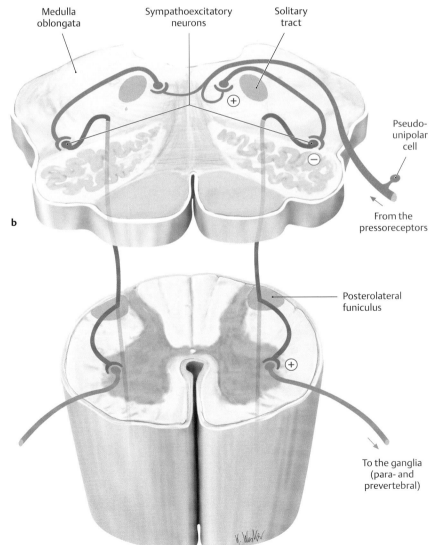

Medulla oblongata

Sympathoexcitatory neurons

Solitary tract

Pseudo-unipolar cell

b

From the pressoreceptors

Posterolateral funiculus

To the ganglia (para- and prevertebral)

C Excitatory and inhibitory effects on sympathoexcitatory neurons in the medulla oblongata

a Cross-section through the brainstem at the level of the medulla oblongata. To generate a baseline level of sympathetic outflow, the presynaptic visceral efferent sympathetic neurons in the spinal cord (intermediolateral and intermediomedial nuclei, see p. 271) must be stimulated by sympathoexcitatory neurons in the anterolateral part of the medulla oblongata. Numerous factors can inhibit or enhance the activity of these neurons which play a critical role in the regulation of blood pressure. If the blood pressure is too high, for example, afferent impulses from the pressoreceptors will inhibit sympathetic outflow.

b Afferent impulses from the factors listed in **a** are relayed in the medial nuclei of the solitary tract nucleus to secondary neurons, whose axons project back to the sympathoexcitatory neurons. When these neurons are inhibited, the peripheral resistance vessels relax and the blood pressure falls. The axons from these sympathoexcitatory neurons pass ipsilaterally through the posterolateral funiculus to presynaptic sympathetic neurons in the lateral horn of the spinal cord. Sensory neurons are shown in orange, motor neurons in green.

11.3 Parasympathetic Nervous System, Overview and Connections

A Overview: parasympathetic nervous system (cranial part)

There are four parasympathetic nuclei in the brainstem. The visceral efferent fibers of these nuclei travel along particular cranial nerves, listed below.

- Visceral oculomotor (Edinger–Westphal) nucleus: oculomotor nerve (CN III)
- Superior salivatory nucleus: facial nerve (CN VII)
- Inferior salivatory nucleus: glossopharyngeal nerve (CN IX)
- Dorsal vagal nucleus: vagus nerve (CN X)

The presynaptic parasympathetic fibers often travel with multiple cranial nerves to reach their target organs (for details see p. 81 and **E**, p. 85). The vagus nerve supplies all of the thoracic and abdominal organs as far as a point near the left colic flexure.
Note: The sympathetic fibers to the head travel along the arteries to their target organs.

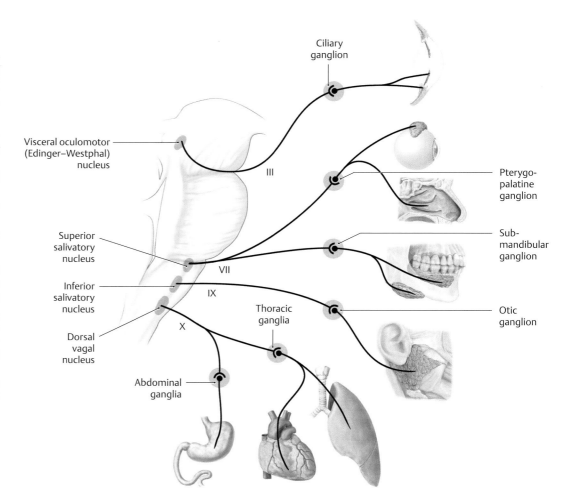

B Parasympathetic ganglia in the head

Nucleus	Path of presynaptic fibers	Ganglion	Postsynaptic fibers	Target organs
• Visceral oculomotor (Edinger-Westphal) nucleus	• Oculomotor nerve	• Ciliary ganglion	• Short ciliary nerves	• Ciliary muscle (accommodation) • Pupillary sphincter (miosis)
• Superior salivatory nucleus	• Nervus intermedius (facial nerve root) divides into:		• Maxillary nerve → zygomatic nerve → anastomosis → lacrimal nerve	• Lacrimal gland
	• Greater petrosal nerve → nerve of pterygoid canal	• Pterygopalatine ganglion	• Orbital branches • Lateral posterior nasal branches • Nasopalatine nerve • Palatine nerves	• Glands on: – posterior ethmoid cells – nasal conchae – anterior palate – hard and soft palate
	• Chorda tympani → lingual nerve	• Submandibular ganglion	• Glandular branches	• Submandibular gland • Sublingual gland
• Inferior salivatory nucleus	• Glossopharyngeal nerve → tympanic nerve → lesser petrosal nerve	• Otic ganglion	• Auriculotemporal nerve (CN V_3)	• Parotid gland
• Dorsal vagal nucleus	• Vagus nerve	• Ganglia near organs	• Fine fibers in organs, not individually named	• Thoracic and abdominal viscera

→ = is continuous with

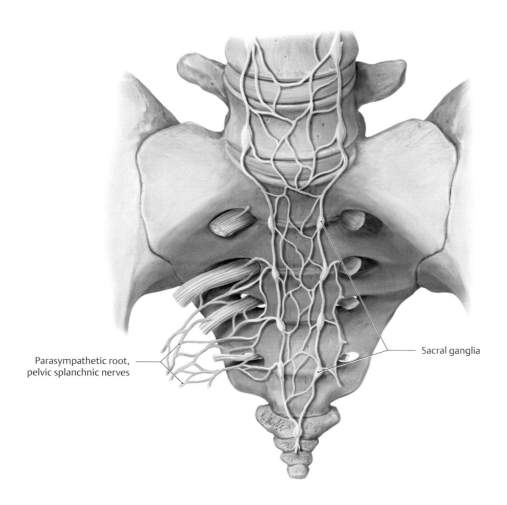

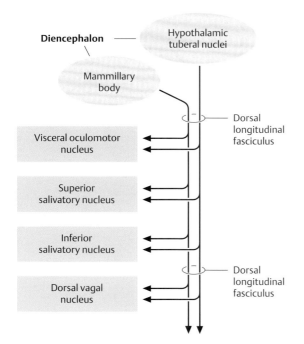

C Overview: parasympathetic nervous system (lumbrosacral part)
The portions of the bowel near the left colic flexure and the pelvic viscera are supplied by the sacral part of the parasympathetic nervous system. Efferent fibers emerge from the anterior sacral foramina in the ventral roots of segments S 2–S 4. The fibers are collected into bundles to form the pelvic splanchnic nerves. They blend with the sympathetic fibers and synapse in the ganglia in or near the organs.

D Connections of the dorsal longitudinal fasciculus
Increased salivation during eating results from stimulation of the salivary glands by the parasympathetic nervous system. To produce the coordinated stimulation of various glands, the cranial parasympathetic nuclei require excitatory impulses from higher centers (tuberal nuclei, mammillary bodies). The parasympathetic nuclei are then stimulated to increase the flow of saliva. The dorsal longitudinal fasciculus establishes the necessary connections with the higher centers. Besides the fibers that coordinate the parasympathetic nuclei, the fasciculus contains other fiber systems that are not shown in the diagram.

321

11.4 Autonomic Nervous System: Pain Conduction

A Pain afferents conducted from the viscera by the sympathetic and parasympathetic nervous systems
(after Jänig)

a Sympathetic pain fibers, **b** parasympathetic pain fibers.

It was originally thought that the sympathetic and parasympathetic nervous systems conveyed only efferent fibers to the viscera. More recent research has shown, however, that both systems also carry afferent nociceptive (pain) fibers (shown in green), many running parallel to visceral efferent fibers (shown in purple). It is likely that many of these fibers (which make up only 5% of all the afferent pain fibers in the body) are inactive during normal processes and may become active in response to organ lesions, for example.

a The pain-conducting (nociceptive) axons from the viscera course in the splanchnic nerves to the sympathetic ganglia and reach the spinal nerve by way of the white ramus communicans. The cell bodies of these neurons are located in the spinal ganglion. From the spinal nerve, the neurons pass through the dorsal roots to the posterior horn of the spinal cord. There they are relayed to establish a connection with the ascending pain pathway. Alternatively, a reflex arc may be established through interneurons (see **B**).
Note: unlike the efferent system, the afferent nociceptive fibers of the sympathetic and parasympathetic systems are not relayed in the peripheral ganglia.

b The cell bodies of the pain-conducting pseudounipolar neurons in the *cranial* parasympathetic system are located in the inferior or superior ganglion of the vagus nerve (CN X). Those of the *sacral* parasympathetic system are located in the sacral spinal ganglia of S2–S4. Their fibers run parallel to the efferent vagal fibers and establish a central connection with the pain-processing systems.

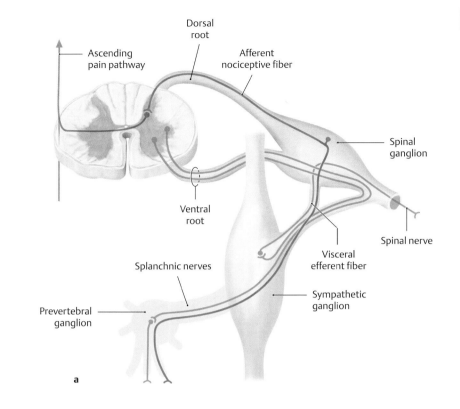

Ascending pain pathway

Dorsal root

Afferent nociceptive fiber

Spinal ganglion

Spinal nerve

Ventral root

Visceral efferent fiber

Splanchnic nerves

Sympathetic ganglion

Prevertebral ganglion

a

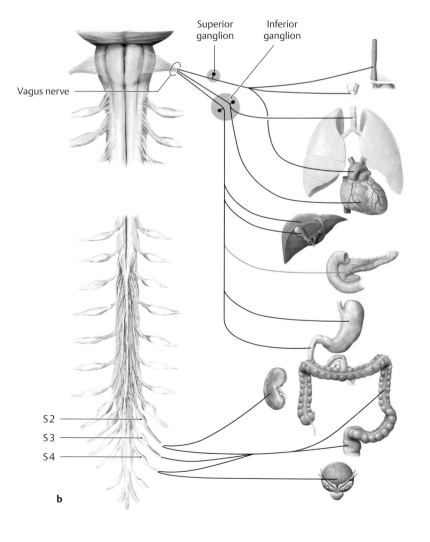

Vagus nerve

Superior ganglion

Inferior ganglion

S2

S3

S4

b

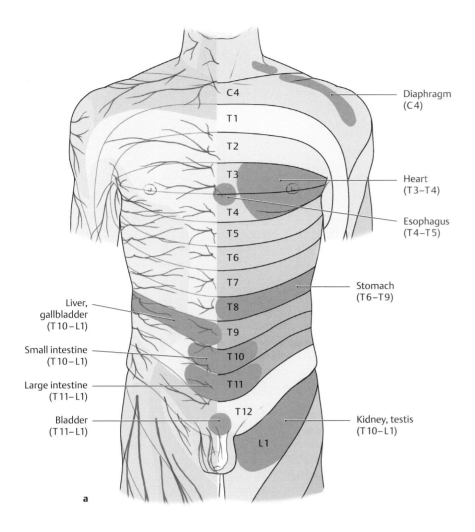

Diaphragm (C4)

Heart (T3–T4)

Esophagus (T4–T5)

Stomach (T6–T9)

Liver, gallbladder (T10–L1)

Small intestine (T10–L1)

Large intestine (T11–L1)

Bladder (T11–L1)

Kidney, testis (T10–L1)

a

B Referred pain

It is believed that nociceptive afferent fibers from dermatomes (somatic pain) and internal organs (visceral pain) terminate on the same relay neurons in the posterior horn of the spinal cord. The convergence of somatic and visceral afferent fibers (see **b**) confuses the relationship between the perceived and actual sites of pain, a phenomenon known as *referred pain*. The pain is typically perceived at the somatic site, as somatic pain is well-localized while visceral pain is not. Pain impulses from a particular internal organ are consistently projected to the same well-defined skin area (**a**); the pattern of pain projection is very helpful in determining the affected organ.

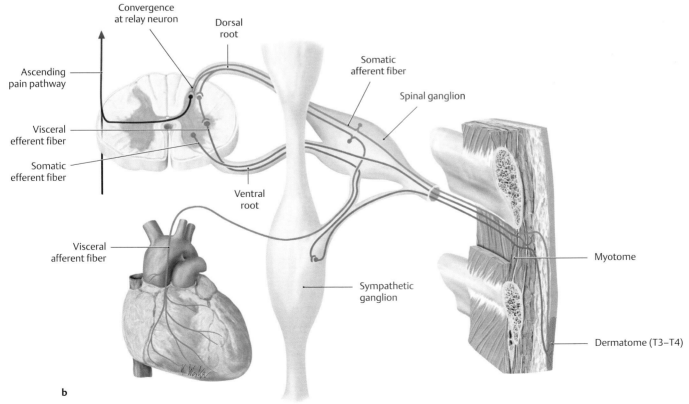

Convergence at relay neuron

Dorsal root

Ascending pain pathway

Somatic afferent fiber

Spinal ganglion

Visceral efferent fiber

Somatic efferent fiber

Ventral root

Visceral afferent fiber

Myotome

Sympathetic ganglion

Dermatome (T3–T4)

b

11.5 Enteric Nervous System

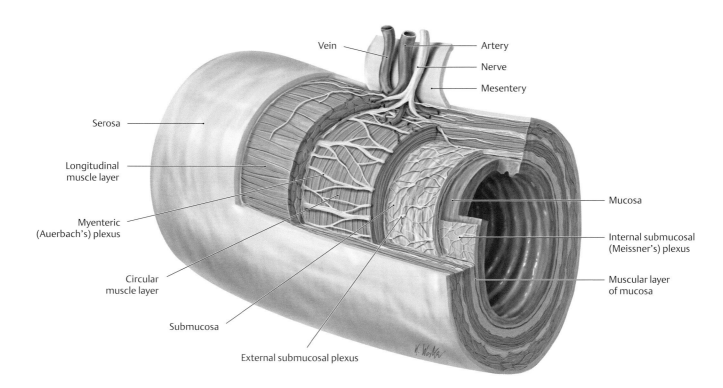

A Enteric nervous system in the small intestine

The enteric nervous system is the intrinsic nervous system of the bowel, consisting of small groups of neurons that form interconnected, microscopically visible ganglia in the wall of the digestive tube. Its two main divisions are the *myenteric* (Auerbach) *plexus* (located between the longitudinal and circular muscle fibers) and the *submucosal plexus* (located in the submucosa), which is subdivided into an *external* (Schabadasch) and *internal* (Meissner) *submucosal plexuses*. (Details on the fine lamina-

tion of the enteric nervous system can be found in textbooks of histology.) These networks of neurons are the foundation for autonomic reflex pathways. In principle they can function without external innervation, but their activity is intensely modulated by the sympathetic and parasympathetic nervous systems. Activities influenced by the enteric nervous system include enteric motility, secretion into the digestive tube, and local intestinal blood flow.

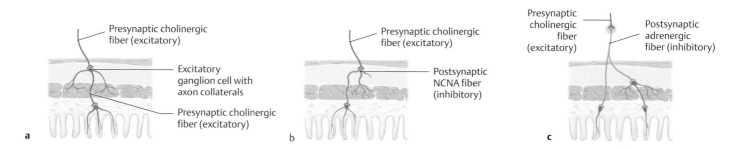

B Modulation of intestinal innervation by the autonomic nervous system

Although the parasympathetic nervous system ("rest and digest") generally promotes the activities of the digestive tube (secretion, motility), it may also produce inhibitory effects.

a Excitatory presynaptic cholinergic parasympathetic fibers terminate on excitatory cholinergic neurons that promote intestinal motility (mixing of the bowel contents to facilitate absorption).

b An inhibitory parasympathetic fiber synapses with an inhibitory ganglion cell that uses noncholinergic, nonadrenergic (NCNA) transmitters. These NCNA transmitters are usually neuropeptides that inhibit intestinal motility.

c Sympathetic fibers are not abundant in the muscular layers of the bowel wall. Postsynaptic adrenergic fibers inhibit the motor and secretory neurons in the plexuses.

The clinical importance of autonomic bowel innervation is illustrated below:

- During shock, the vessels in the bowel are constricted and the intestinal mucosa is accordingly deprived of oxygen. This results in disruption of the epithelial barrier, which may then be penetrated by microorganisms from the bowel lumen. This is an important mechanism contributing to multisystem failure in shock.
- There may be a cessation of intestinal motility (atonic bowel) after intestinal operations involving surgical manipulation of the digestive tube.
- Medications (especially opiates) may suppress the motility of the enteric nervous system, causing constipation.

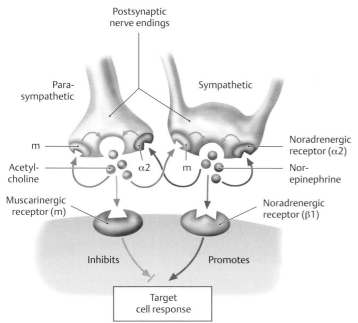

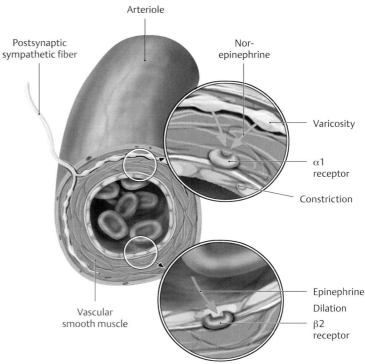

C Functional interactions of the sympathetic and parasympathetic nervous systems at the target organ

The transmitters of the sympathetic and parasympathetic nervous systems (norepinephrine and acetylcholine, respectively) act upon both the target organ and the (para)sympathetic nerve endings at the synapse. Noradrenergic receptors on the target tissue (β1, shown in blue) and nerve endings themselves (α2, shown in pink) modulate target cell responses on two levels: norepinephrine binding to the β1 receptor directly promotes a cellular response in heart tissue, while similar binding to the α2 receptors on the postsynaptic nerve endings allows for regulation of subsequent neurotransmitter release, through positive and negative feedback loops. The muscarinergic receptors (m, shown in green) mediate a similar process upon binding of acetylcholine. The neurotransmitters of the autonomic nervous system can therefore self- and cross-regulate in a multifaceted control mechanism.

D Sympathetic effects on arteries

An important function of the sympathetic nervous system is to regulate the caliber of the arterioles (blood pressure regulation). When sympathetic fibers release norepinephrine into the media of the arterioles, the α1 receptor mediates contraction of the vascular smooth muscle, and the blood pressure rises. Meanwhile, epinephrine from the blood acts on the β2 receptors in the sarcolemma of the same vascular smooth muscle cells, inducing vasodilation and a corresponding drop in blood pressure.

Note: Parasympathetic fibers do not terminate on blood vessels.

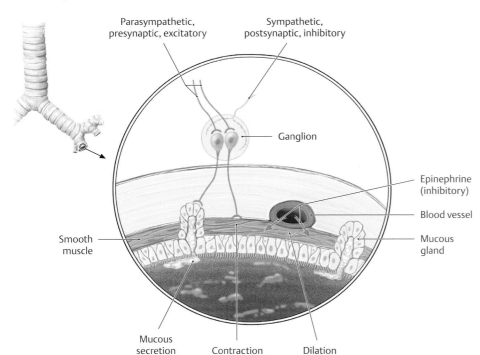

E Autonomic innervation of the trachea and bronchi

Parasympathetic stimulation of the local ganglia promotes secretion by the bronchial glands and narrowing of the bronchial passages. For this reason, the preparations for bronchoscopy include the administration of a drug (atropine) which blocks parasympathetic innervation, ensuring that mucous secretions will not obscure the bronchial mucosa. A similar reduction in bronchial secretions can be achieved through *sympathetic* stimulation. Epinephrine from the bloodstream acts on adrenergic β2 receptors to induce bronchodilation. This effect is applied therapeutically in the treatment of severe asthma attacks.

12.1 Sensory System, Overview

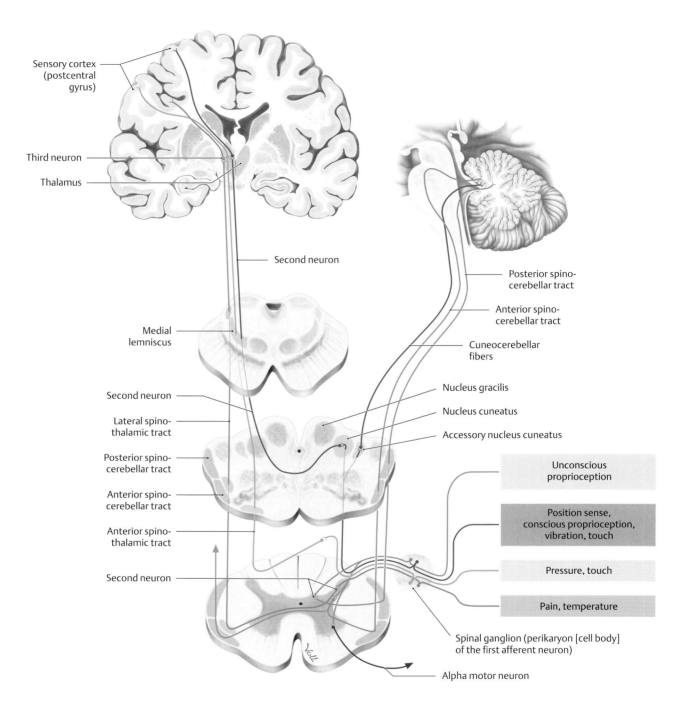

Sensory cortex (postcentral gyrus)

Third neuron

Thalamus

Second neuron

Posterior spino-cerebellar tract

Anterior spino-cerebellar tract

Medial lemniscus

Cuneocerebellar fibers

Second neuron

Nucleus gracilis

Lateral spino-thalamic tract

Nucleus cuneatus

Posterior spino-cerebellar tract

Accessory nucleus cuneatus

Anterior spino-cerebellar tract

Unconscious proprioception

Position sense, conscious proprioception, vibration, touch

Anterior spino-thalamic tract

Pressure, touch

Second neuron

Pain, temperature

Spinal ganglion (perikaryon [cell body] of the first afferent neuron)

Alpha motor neuron

A Simplified diagram of the sensory pathways of the spinal cord
Stimuli generate impulses in various receptors in the periphery of the body (see **C**, p. 179) which are transmitted to the cerebrum and cerebellum along the sensory (afferent) pathways or tracts shown here (see **B** for details). While most of the sensory qualities listed in **B** are intuitively clear (e.g. pain and temperature sensation), the concept of proprioception is more difficult to convey and will be explained in more detail. Proprioception is concerned with the position of the limbs in space (= position sense). The types of *information* involved in proprioception are complex: position sense (the position of the limbs in relation to one another) is distinguished from motion sense (speed and direction of joint movements) and force sense (the muscular force associated with joint movements). Accordingly, the receptors for proprioception (proprioceptors) consist mainly of muscle and tendon spindles and joint receptors

(see p. 328). We also distinguish between conscious and unconscious proprioception. Information on **conscious proprioception** travels in the posterior funiculus of the spinal cord (fasciculus gracilis and fasciculus cuneatus) and is relayed through its nuclei (nucleus gracilis and nucleus cuneatus) to the *thalamus.* From there it is conveyed to the *sensory cortex* (postcentral gyrus), where the information presumably rises to consciousness ("I know that my left hand is making a fist, even though my eyes are closed"). **Unconscious proprioception,** which enables us to ride a bicycle and climb stairs without thinking about it, is conveyed by the spinocerebellar tracts to the *cerebellum,* where it remains at the unconscious level. Sensory information from the head is mediated by the trigeminal nerve and is not depicted here (see p. 330).

B Synopsis of sensory pathways

The various stimuli generate impulses in different receptors which are transmitted in peripheral nerves to the spinal cord. The perikarya of the first afferent neuron (to which the receptors are connected) for all pathways are located in the spinal ganglion. The axons from the ganglion pass along various tracts in the spinal cord to the second neuron. Its axons either pass directly to the cerebellum or are relayed by a third neuron to the cerebrum.

Name of pathway	Sensory quality	Receptor	Course in the spinal cord	Central course (above the spinal cord)
Spinothalamic tracts				
Anterior spinothalamic tract	• Crude touch	• Hair follicles • Various skin receptors	The perikaryon of the second neuron is located in the posterior horn and may be up to 15 segments above or 2 segments below the entry of the first neuron. Its axons cross in the anterior commissure (see p. 274)	The axons of the second neuron (spinal lemniscus) terminate in the ventral posterolateral nucleus of the thalamus (see **D**, p. 219). There they synapse onto the third neuron, whose axons project to the postcentral gyrus
Lateral spinothalamic tract	• Pain and temperature	• Mostly free nerve endings	The perikaryon of the second neuron is in the substantia gelatinosa. Its axon crosses at the same level in the anterior commissure (see p. 274)	The axons of the second neuron (spinal lemniscus) terminate in the ventral posterolateral nucleus of the thalamus. There they synapse onto the third neuron, whose axons project to the postcentral gyrus
Tracts of the posterior funiculus				
Fasciculus gracilis	• Fine touch • Conscious proprioception of *lower* limb	• Vater-Pacini corpuscles • Muscle and tendon receptors	The axons of the first neuron pass to the nucleus gracilis in the lower medulla oblongata (second neuron) (see p. 276 and **B**, p. 233)	The axons of the second neuron cross in the brainstem and traverse the medial lemniscus (see **B**, p. 233) to the ventral posterolateral nucleus of the thalamus. There they synapse onto the third neuron, whose axons project to the postcentral gyrus
Fasciculus cuneatus	• Fine touch • Conscious proprioception of *upper* limb	• Vater-Pacini corpuscles • Muscle and tendon receptors	The axons of the first neuron pass to the nucleus cuneatus in the lower medulla oblongata (second neuron) (see p. 276 and **B**, p. 233)	The axons of the second neuron cross in the brainstem and traverse the medial lemniscus (see **B**, p. 233) to the ventral posterolateral nucleus of the thalamus. There they synapse onto the third neuron, whose axons project to the postcentral gyrus
Spinocerebellar tracts				
Anterior spinocerebellar tract (of Gowers)	• Unconscious crossed and uncrossed extero- and proprioception to the cerebellum	• Muscle spindles • Tendon receptors • Joint receptors • Skin receptors	The second neuron is located in the dorsal column in the central part of the gray matter. The axons of the second neuron run directly to the cerebellum, both crossed and uncrossed, without synapsing with a third neuron (see p. 278)	The axons of the second neuron pass through the superior cerebellar peduncle to the vermian part of the spinocerebellum (no third neuron) (see also p. 243)
Posterior spinocerebellar tract (of Flechsig)	• Unconscious uncrossed extero- and proprioception to the cerebellum	• Muscle spindles • Tendon receptors • Joint receptors • Skin receptors	The second neuron is located in the thoracic nucleus (Clarke column, Stilling nucleus) in the gray matter at the base of the posterior horn. The axons of the second neuron run directly to the cerebellum without crossing (see p. 278)	The axons of the second neuron pass through the inferior cerebellar peduncle to the vermian part of the spinocerebellum (no third neuron) (see also p. 243)

12.2 Sensory System: Stimulus Processing

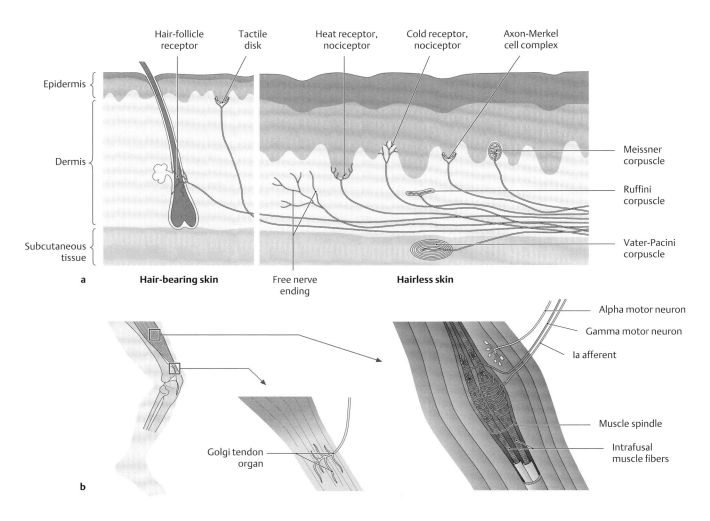

A Receptors of the somatosensory system

a Skin receptors: Various types of stimuli generate impulses in different receptors in the periphery of the body (illustrated here in sections through hair-bearing and hairless skin). These impulses are transmitted through peripheral nerves to the spinal cord, from which they are relayed and carried by specific tracts to the sensory cortex (see previous unit). Sensory qualities cannot always be uniquely assigned to specific receptors. The figure does not indicate the prevalence of the different receptor types. Nociceptors (= pain receptors), like heat and cold receptors, consist of free nerve endings. Nociceptors make up approximately 50 % of all receptors.

b Joint receptors: Proprioception encompasses position sense, motion sense, and force sense. Proprioceptors include muscle spindles, tendon sensors, and joint sensors (not shown).

B Receptive field sizes of cortical modules in the upper limb of a primate

Sensory information is processed in cortical "modules" (see **C**, p. 201). This drawing shows the size of the receptive fields supplied by modules. In areas where high resolution of sensory information is not required (e.g., the forearm), one module supplies a large receptive field. In areas that require finer tactile sensation (e.g., the fingers), one module supplies a much smaller receptive field. The size of these fields determines the overall proportions of the sensory homunculus (see **C**). Because one skin area may be innervated by several neurons, many of the receptive fields overlap. Information is transmitted from the receptive field to the cortex by a chain of neurons and their axons. These neurons and axons are located at specific sites in the CNS (topographical principle).

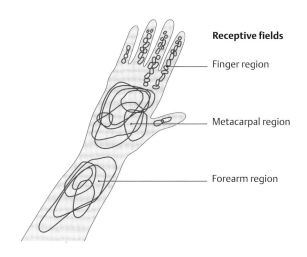

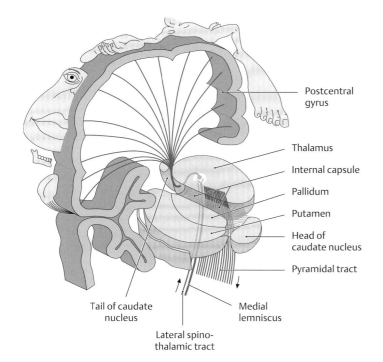

Postcentral gyrus

Thalamus

Internal capsule

Pallidum

Putamen

Head of caudate nucleus

Pyramidal tract

Tail of caudate nucleus

Medial lemniscus

Lateral spino-thalamic tract

C Arrangement of sensory pathways in the cerebrum

Anterior view of the right postcentral gyrus. The perikarya of the third neurons of the sensory pathways are located in the thalamus. Their axons project to the postcentral gyrus, where the primary somatosensory cortex is located. The postcentral gyrus has a somatotopic organization, meaning that each body region is represented in a particular cortical area. The body regions in the cortex are not represented in proportion to their actual size, but in proportion to the density of their sensory innervation. The fingers and head have abundant sensory receptors, and so their cortical representation is correspondingly large (see **B**). Conversely, the less dense sensory innervation of the buttocks and legs results in smaller areas of representation. Based on these varying numbers of peripheral receptors, we can construct a "sensory homunculus" whose parts correspond to the cortical areas concerned with their perception.

Note: The head of the homunculus is upright while the trunk is upside down.

The axons of the sensory neurons ascending from the thalamus travel side by side with the axons forming the pyramidal tract (red) in the dorsal part of the internal capsule. Because of this arrangement, a large cerebral hemorrhage involving the internal capsule produces sensory as well as motor deficits (see Kell et al.).

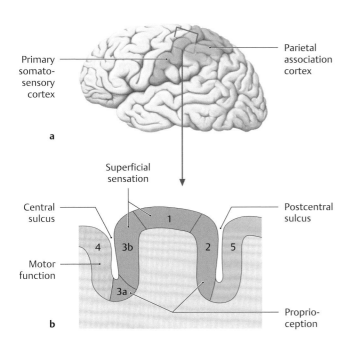

Primary somato-sensory cortex

Parietal association cortex

a

Superficial sensation

Central sulcus

Postcentral sulcus

Motor function

Proprioception

b

4 3b 1 2 5

3a

D Primary somatosensory cortex and parietal association cortex

a Left lateral view. The Brodmann areas are numbered in the sectional view (**b**). The contralateral body half is represented in the primary somatosensory cortex (except the perioral region, which is represented bilaterally: speech). This area of the cortex is concerned with somatosensory perception. The parietal association cortex receives information from both sides of the body. Thus, the processing of stimuli becomes increasingly complex in these cortical areas.

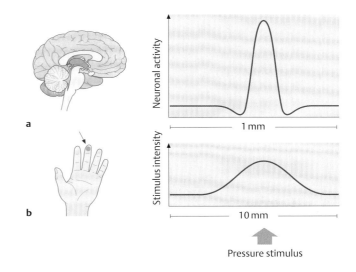

Neuronal activity

1 mm

a

Stimulus intensity

10 mm

b

Pressure stimulus

E Activity of cortical cell columns in the primary somatosensory cortex

a Amplitude of the neuronal response in the primary somatosensory cortex to a peripheral pressure stimulus. The intensity of the stimulus is shown in **b**. The diagrams illustrate the principle of sensory information processing in the cortex. When approximately 100 intensity detectors in the fingertip are stimulated by pressure, approximately 10,000 neurons in the corresponding cell column in the primary somatosensory cortex (see columnar organization of the cortex, p. 201) respond to the stimulus. Because the intensity of the peripheral pressure stimulus is maximal at the center and fades toward the edges, it is processed in the cortex accordingly. Cortical processing amplifies the contrast between the greater and lesser stimulus intensities, resulting in a sharper peak (**a**). While the stimulated area on the fingertip measures approximately 100 mm², the information is processed in only a 1-mm² area of the primary somatosensory cortex.

12.3 Sensory System: Lesions

A Sites of occurrence of lesions in the sensory pathways
  (after Bähr and Frotscher)
The central portions of the sensory pathways may be damaged at various sites from the spinal root to the somatosensory cortex as a result of trauma, tumor mass effect, hemorrhage, or infarction. The signs and symptoms are helpful in determining the location of the lesion. This unit deals strictly with lesions in conscious pathways. The innervation of the trunk and limbs is mediated by the spinal nerves. The innervation of the head is mediated by the trigeminal nerve, which has its own nuclei (see below).

Cortical or subcortical lesion (1, 2): A lesion at this level is manifested by paresthesia (tingling) and numbness in the corresponding regions of the trunk and limbs on the *opposite* side of the body. The symptoms may be most pronounced distally because of the large receptive fields on the fingers and the relatively small receptive fields on the trunk (see previous unit). The motor and sensory cortex are closely interlinked because fibers in the sensory tracts from the thalamus also terminate in the motor cortex, and because the cortical areas are adjacent (pre- and post-central gyrus).

Subthalamic lesion (3): All sensation is abolished in the *contralateral* half of the body (thalamus = "gateway to consciousness"). A partial lesion that spares the pain and temperature pathways (**4**) is characterized by hypesthesia (decreased tactile sensation) on the *contralateral* face and body. Pain and temperature sensation are unaffected.

Lesion of the trigeminal lemniscus and lateral spinothalamic tract (5): Damage to these pathways in the brainstem causes a loss of pain and temperature sensation in the *contralateral* half of the face and body. Other sensory qualities are unaffected.

Lesion of the medial lemniscus and anterior spinothalamic tract (6):
All sensory qualities on the *opposite* side of the body are abolished except for pain and temperature.
The medial lemniscus transmits the axons of the second neurons of the anterior spinothalamic tract and both tracts of the posterior funiculus.

Lesion of the trigeminal nucleus, spinal tract of the trigeminal nerve, and lateral spinothalamic tract (7): Pain and temperature sensation are abolished on the *ipsilateral* side of the face (uncrossed axons of the first neuron in the trigeminal ganglion) and on the *contralateral* side of the body (axons of the crossed second neuron in the lateral spinothalamic tract).

Lesion of the posterior funiculi (8): This lesion causes an *ipsilateral* loss of position sense, vibration sense, and two-point discrimination. Because coordinated motor function relies on sensory input that operates in a feedback loop, the lack of sensory input leads to ipsilateral sensory ataxia.

Posterior horn lesion (9): A circumscribed lesion involving one or a few segments causes an *ipsilateral* loss of pain and temperature sensation in the affected segment(s), because pain and temperature sensation are relayed to the second neuron within the posterior horn. Other sensory qualities including crude touch are transmitted in the posterior funiculus and relayed in the dorsal column nuclei; hence they are unaffected. The effects of a posterior horn lesion are called a "dissociated sensory deficit."

Dorsal root lesion (10): This lesion causes *ipsilateral*, radicular sensory disturbances that may range from pain in the corresponding dermatome to a complete loss of sensation. Concomitant involvement of the ventral root leads to segmental weakness. This clinical situation may be caused by a herniated intervertebral disk (see p. 345).

Lesions of *unconscious* cerebellar tracts that lead to sensorimotor deficits are not considered here. The volume on *General Anatomy and Musculoskeletal System* may be consulted for information on peripheral sensory nerve lesions.

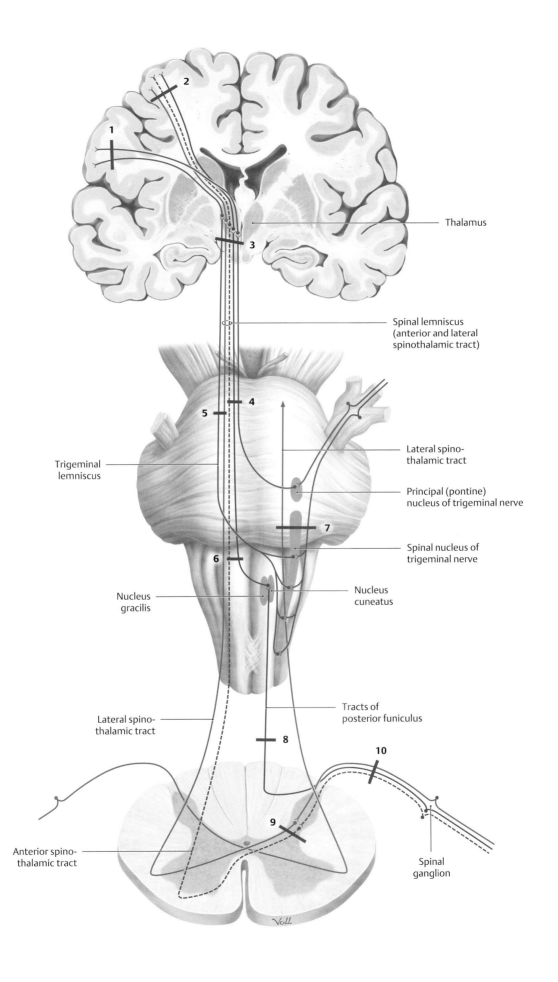

Thalamus

Spinal lemniscus
(anterior and lateral
spinothalamic tract)

Lateral spino-
thalamic tract

Principal (pontine)
nucleus of trigeminal nerve

Spinal nucleus of
trigeminal nerve

Nucleus
cuneatus

Trigeminal
lemniscus

Nucleus
gracilis

Tracts of
posterior funiculus

Lateral spino-
thalamic tract

Spinal
ganglion

Anterior spino-
thalamic tract

12.4 Sensory System: Pain Conduction

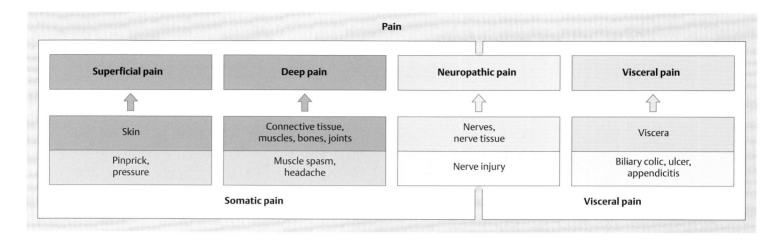

A Synopsis of pain modalities

The International Association for the Study of Pain defines pain as "an unpleasant sensory and emotional experience associated with actual or potential tissue damage, or described in terms of such damage." Pain is classified by its site of origin as *somatic* or *visceral*. Somatic pain generally originates in the trunk, limbs, or head, while visceral pain originates in the internal organs. *Neuropathic* pain is caused by damage to the nerves themselves. It may involve nerves of the somatic and/or autonomic nervous system. The somatic pain fibers described below travel with the spinal or cranial nerves, while the visceral pain fibers travel with the autonomic nerves (see p. 322).

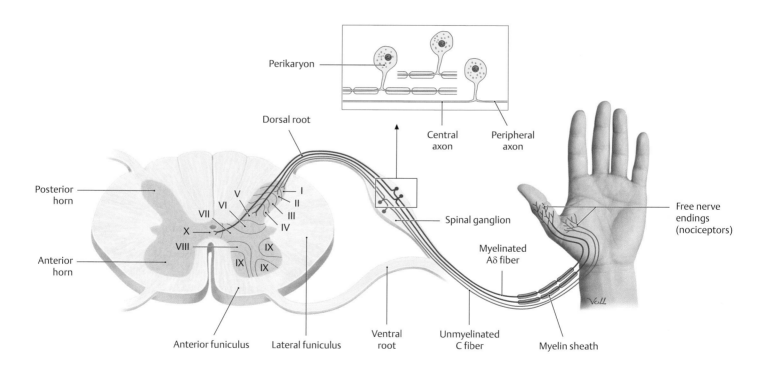

B Peripheral somatic pain conduction (after Lorke)

Somatic pain impulses from the trunk and limbs are conducted by myelinated Aδ fibers (temperature, pain, position) and unmyelinated C fibers (temperature, pain). The perikarya (cell bodies) for these afferent nerve fibers are located in the spinal ganglion (pseudounipolar neurons). Their axons terminate in the posterior horn of the spinal cord, chiefly in the Rexed laminae I, II, and IV—VI. The nociceptors, afferent fibers ascend after synapsing in the posterior horn (see **C**).
Note: Most somatosensory pain fibers are myelinated, while the viscerosensory fibers are unmyelinated.

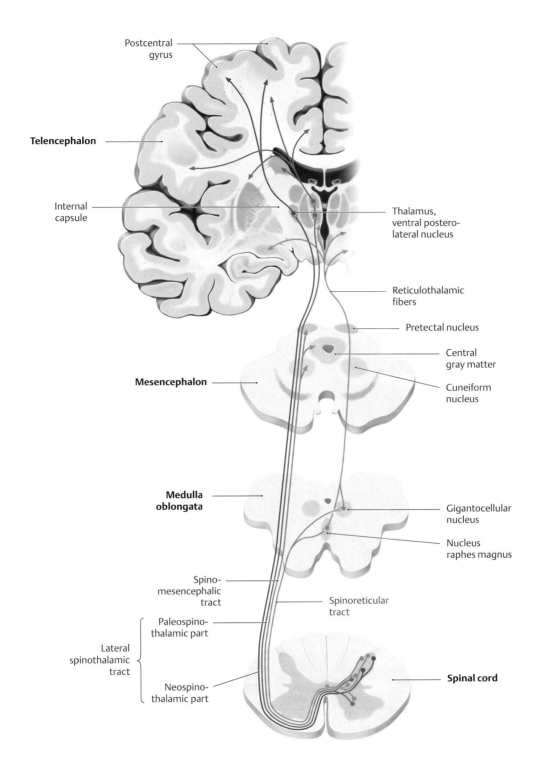

Postcentral gyrus

Telencephalon

Internal capsule

Thalamus, ventral postero-lateral nucleus

Reticulothalamic fibers

Pretectal nucleus

Central gray matter

Mesencephalon

Cuneiform nucleus

Medulla oblongata

Gigantocellular nucleus

Nucleus raphes magnus

Spino-mesencephalic tract

Spinoreticular tract

Paleospino-thalamic part

Lateral spinothalamic tract

Neospino-thalamic part

Spinal cord

C Ascending pain pathways from the trunk and limbs

The axons of the primary afferent neurons for pain sensation in the trunk and limbs terminate on the projection neurons (shown above) located in the posterior horn of the spinal-cord gray matter. The lateral spino-thalamic tract is subdivided into a neo- and paleospinothalamic part. The second neuron of the *neospinothalamic part* of the pain pathway (red) terminates in the ventral posterolateral nucleus of the thalamus. The third neuron projects from there to the primary somatosensory cortex (postcentral gyrus) of the brain. The second neuron of the *paleospino-thalamic tract* (blue) terminates in the intralaminar and medial nuclei of the thalamus, whose third neurons then project to a variety of brain regions. This pain pathway is mainly responsible for the emotional component of pain. In addition to these pain pathways that end in the cor-

tex, there are also pain pathways that end in *subcortical* regions—the spinomesencephalic tract and spinoreticular tract. The second neuron of the *spinomesencephalic tract* (green) terminates mainly in the central gray matter, which surrounds the aqueduct. Other axons terminate in the cuneiform nucleus or anterior pretectal nucleus. The second neuron of the *spinoreticular tract* (orange) ends in the reticular formation, represented here by the nucleus raphes magnus and the gigantocellular nucleus. Reticulothalamic fibers transmit the pain impulses onward to the medial thalamus, hypothalamus, and limbic system.

12.5 Sensory System: Pain Pathways in the Head and the Central Analgesic System

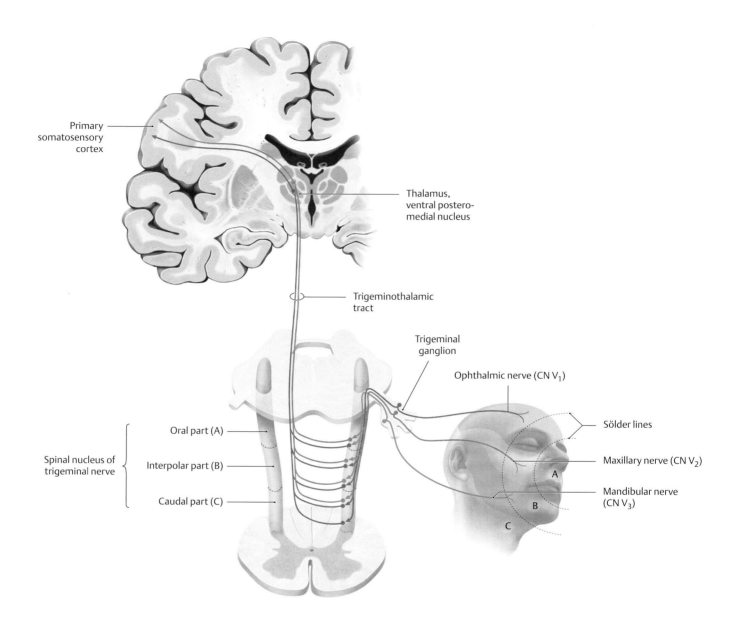

A Pain pathways in the head (after Lorke)

The pain fibers in the head accompany the principal divisions of the trigeminal nerve (CN V₁–V₃). The perikarya of these primary afferent neurons of the pain pathway are located in the trigeminal ganglion. Their axons terminate in the spinal nucleus of the trigeminal nerve.

Note the somatotopic organization of this nuclear region: The perioral region (**a**) is cranial and the occipital regions (**c**) are caudal. Because of this arrangement, central lesions lead to deficits that are distributed along the Sölder lines (see **D**, p. 75).

The axons of the second neurons cross the midline and travel in the trigeminothalamic tract to the ventral posteromedial nucleus and to the intralaminar thalamic nuclei on the opposite side, where they terminate. The third (thalamic) neuron of the pain pathway ends in the primary somatosensory cortex. Only the pain fibers of the trigeminal nerve are pictured in the diagram. In the trigeminal nerve itself, the other sensory fibers run parallel to the pain fibers but terminate in various trigeminal nuclei (see p. 74).

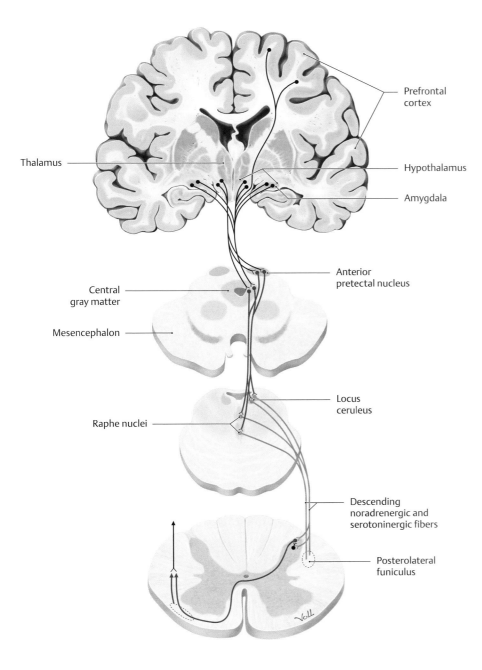

Prefrontal cortex

Thalamus

Hypothalamus

Amygdala

Anterior pretectal nucleus

Central gray matter

Mesencephalon

Locus ceruleus

Raphe nuclei

Descending noradrenergic and serotoninergic fibers

Posterolateral funiculus

B Pathways of the central descending analgesic system
(after Lorke)

Besides the ascending pathways that carry pain sensation to the primary somatosensory cortex, there are also descending pathways that have the ability to suppress pain impulses. The central relay station for the descending analgesic (pain-relieving) system is the central gray matter of the mesencephalon. It is activated by afferent input from the hypothalamus, the prefrontal cortex, and the amygdaloid bodies (part of the limbic system, not shown). It also receives afferent input from the spinal cord (see p. 333). The axons from the excitatory glutaminergic neurons (red) of the central gray matter terminate on serotoninergic neurons in the raphe nuclei and on noradrenergic neurons in the locus ceruleus (both shown in blue). The axons from both types of neuron descend in the posterolateral funiculus. They terminate directly or indirectly (via inhibitory neurons) on the analgesic projection neurons (second afferent neuron of the pain pathway), thereby inhibiting the further conduction of pain impulses.

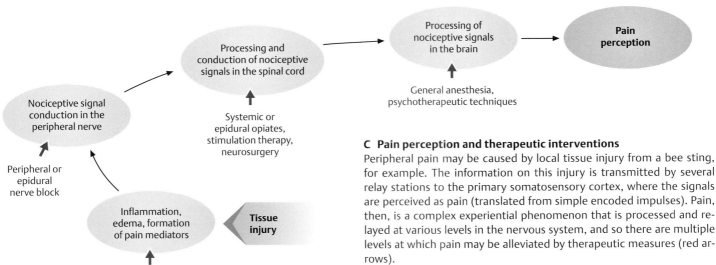

Processing of nociceptive signals in the brain

Pain perception

Processing and conduction of nociceptive signals in the spinal cord

General anesthesia, psychotherapeutic techniques

Nociceptive signal conduction in the peripheral nerve

Systemic or epidural opiates, stimulation therapy, neurosurgery

Peripheral or epidural nerve block

Inflammation, edema, formation of pain mediators

Tissue injury

Immobilization, cooling, analgesic medication, anti-inflammatory medication

C Pain perception and therapeutic interventions

Peripheral pain may be caused by local tissue injury from a bee sting, for example. The information on this injury is transmitted by several relay stations to the primary somatosensory cortex, where the signals are perceived as pain (translated from simple encoded impulses). Pain, then, is a complex experiential phenomenon that is processed and relayed at various levels in the nervous system, and so there are multiple levels at which pain may be alleviated by therapeutic measures (red arrows).

12.6 Motor System, Overview

A Simplified representation of the anatomical structures involved in a voluntary movement (pyramidal motor system)
(after Klinke and Silbernagl)

The first step in performing a voluntary movement is to plan the movement in the association cortex of the cerebrum (e.g., goal: "I want to pick up my coffee cup"). The cerebellar hemispheres and basal ganglia work in parallel to program the movement and inform the premotor cortex of the result of this planning. The premotor cortex passes the information to the primary motor cortex (M1), which relays the information through the *pyramidal tract* to the alpha motor neuron *(pyramidal motor system)*. The alpha motor neuron then initiates the process whereby the skeletal muscle transforms the program into a specific voluntary movement. Sensorimotor functions supply important feedback during this process (How far has the movement progressed? How strong is my grip on the cup handle?—different from gripping an eggshell, for example). Although some of the later figures portray the primary motor cortex as the starting point for a voluntary movement, this diagram shows that many motor centers are involved in the execution of a voluntary movement (including the *extrapyramidal motor system*, see **C** and **D**; cerebellum). For practical reasons, however, the discussion commonly begins at the primary motor cortex (M1).

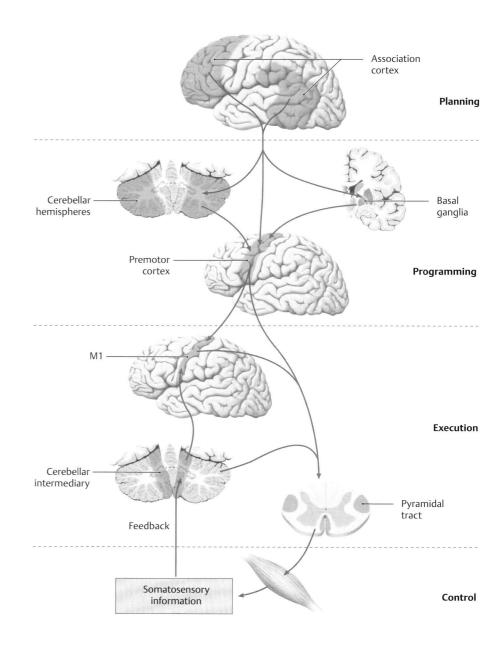

B Cortical areas with motor function: initiating a movement

Lateral view of the left hemisphere. The initiation of a voluntary movement (reaching for a coffee cup) results from the interaction of various cortical areas. The *primary motor cortex* (M1, Brodmann area 4) is located in the precentral gyrus (execution of a movement). The rostrally adjacent area 6 consists of the lateral premotor cortex and medial supplementary motor cortex (initiation of a movement). Association fibers (see p. 376) establish close functional connections with sensory areas 1, 2, and 3 (postcentral gyrus with primary somatosensory cortex, S1) and with areas 5 and 7 (= posterior parietal cortex), which have an associative motor function. These areas provide the cortical representation of space, which is important in precision grasping movements and eye movements.

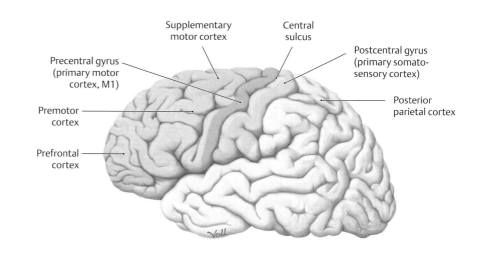

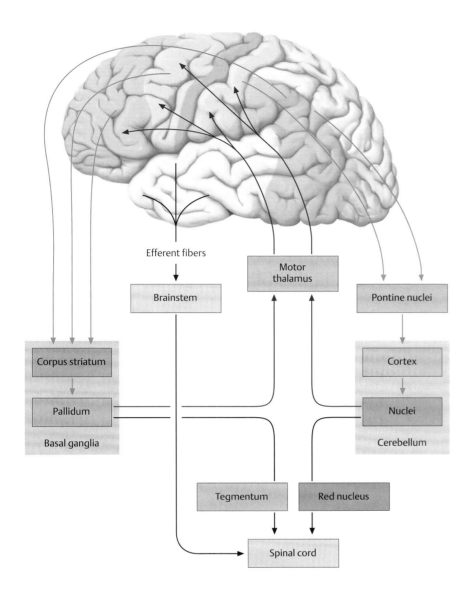

C Connections of the cortex with the basal ganglia and cerebellum: programming complex movements

The pyramidal motor system (the primary motor cortex and the pyramidal tract arising from it) is assisted by the basal ganglia and cerebellum in the planning and programming of complex movements. While afferent fibers of the motor nuclei (green) project directly to the basal ganglia (left) without synapsing, the cerebellum is indirectly controlled via pontine nuclei (right; see **C**, p. 233). The motor thalamus provides a feedback loop for both structures (see p. 341). The efferent fibers of the basal nuclei and cerebellum are distributed to lower structures including the spinal cord. The importance of the basal ganglia and cerebellum in voluntary movements can be appreciated by noting the effects of lesions in these structures. While diseases of the basal ganglia impair the initiation and execution of movements (e.g., in Parkinson's disease), cerebellar lesions are characterized by uncoordinated writhing movements (e.g., the reeling movements of inebriation, caused by a temporary toxic insult to the cerebellum).

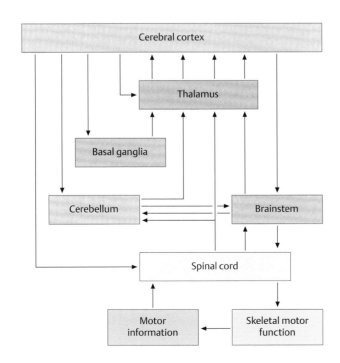

D Simplified block diagram of the sensorimotor system in movement control

Voluntary movements require constant feedback from the periphery (muscle spindles, tendon organs) in order to remain within the desired limits. Because the motor and sensory systems are so closely interrelated functionally, they are often described jointly as the sensorimotor system. The spinal cord, brainstem, cerebellum, and cerebral cortex are the three control levels of the sensorimotor system. All information from periphery, cerebellum, and the basal ganglia passes through the thalamus on its way to the cerebral cortex. The clinical importance of the sensory system in movement is illustrated by the sensory ataxia that may occur when sensory function is lost (see **D**, p. 353). The oculomotor component of the sensorimotor system is not shown.

12.7 Motor System: Pyramidal (Corticospinal) Tract

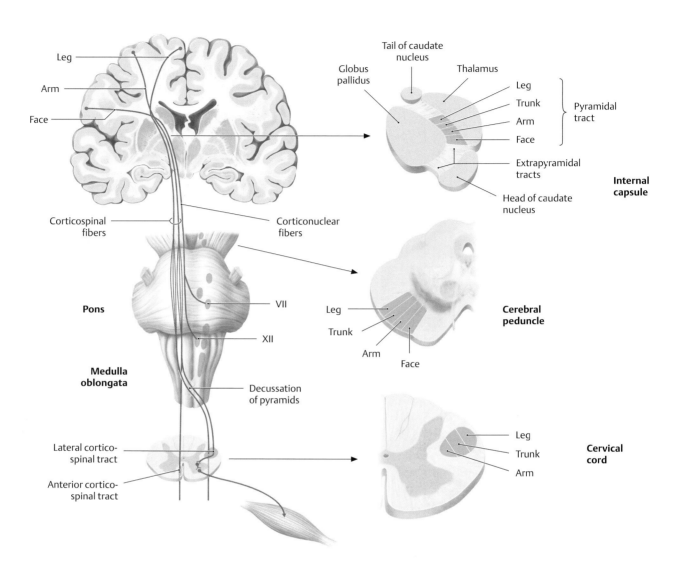

A Course of the pyramidal (corticospinal) tract

The pyramidal tract consists of three fiber systems: corticospinal fibers, corticonuclear fibers, and corticoreticular fibers (the latter are not shown here; they pass to the gigantocellular nucleus of the reticular formation in the brainstem and will not be discussed further). These groups of fibers constitute the descending motor pathways from the primary motor cortex. The corticospinal fibers pass to the motor anterior horn cells in the spinal cord, while the corticonuclear fibers pass to the motor nuclei of the cranial nerves.

Corticospinal fibers: Only a small percentage of the axons of the corticospinal fibers originate from the large pyramidal neurons in lamina V of the precentral gyrus (the laminar structure of the motor cortex is shown in **D**). Most of the axons arise from small pyramidal cells and other neurons in laminae V and VI. Other axons originate from adjacent brain regions. All of them descend through the internal capsule. Eighty percent of the fibers *cross the midline* at the level of the medulla oblongata (decussation of the pyramids) and descend in the spinal cord as the *lateral corticospinal (pyramidal) tract.* The *uncrossed* fibers descend in the cord as the *anterior corticospinal (pyramidal) tract* and cross later at the segmental level. Most of the axons terminate on intercalated cells whose synapses end on motor neurons.

Note: the basic pattern of somatotopic organization described earlier at the spinal cord level is found at all levels of the pyramidal tract. This facilitates localization of the lesion in the pyramidal tract.

Corticonuclear fibers: The motor nuclei and motor segments of the cranial nerves receive their axons from pyramidal cells in the facial region of the premotor cortex. These corticonuclear fibers terminate in the contralateral motor nuclei of cranial nerves III–VII and IX–XII in the brainstem (the fibers to other brainstem nuclei are shown in **C**). Besides this contralateral supply, axons also pass to several cranial nerve nuclei on the same (ipsilateral) side, resulting in a bilateral innervation pattern (not shown here). This dual supply is clinically important in lesions of the frontal branch of the facial nerve, for example (see **D**, p. 79).

Notes on the "pyramidal tract": Some authors interpret this term as applying strictly to the portion of the tract below the decussation of the pyramids, while other authors apply the term to the entire tract. Most publications, including this atlas, use "pyramidal tract" as a collective term for all of the fiber tracts described here. Some authors derive the term not from the decussation of the pyramids but from the giant pyramidal cells (Betz cells) in the cerebral cortex (see **D** and p. 281).

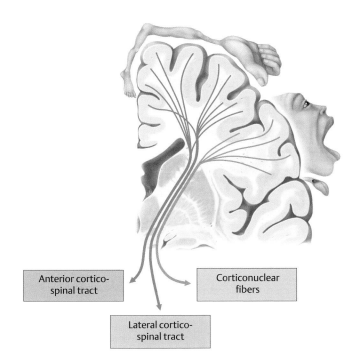

B Somatotopic representation of the skeletal muscle in the precentral gyrus (motor homunculus)

Anterior view. Regions in which the muscles are very densely innervated (e.g., the hand) must be supplied by many neurons in the precentral gyrus. As a result, they require a larger representation area in the cortex than regions supplied by fewer neurons (e.g., the trunk). This cortical representation is analogous to that in sensory innervation, where areas of varying size are also represented in the cortex (postcentral gyrus; compare with the sensory homunculus in **C**, p. 329). One cortical area is devoted to the trunk and limbs and another to the head. The axons for the head area are the corticonuclear fibers, and the axons for the trunk and limbs are the corticospinal fibers. The latter fibers split into two groups below the telencephalon, forming the lateral and anterior corticospinal tracts.

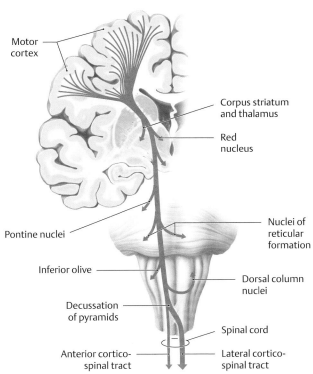

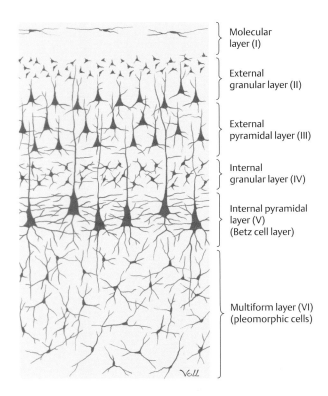

C Variety of cortical efferent fibers

Anterior view. Besides the corticospinal and corticonuclear fibers described above, a variety of axons descends from the cortex to various subcortical regions and into the spinal cord. The following subcortical regions also receive cortical efferent fibers: the corpus striatum, thalamus, red nucleus, pontine nuclei, reticular formation, inferior olive, dorsal column nuclei (these nuclear regions are described on p. 342), and spinal cord. The supraspinal efferent fibers listed above consist partially of axon collaterals from pyramidal tract neurons and partially of separate axons.

D Laminar structure of the motor cortex (= area 4 in the precentral gyrus)

The axons from giant pyramidal cells (Betz cells) in lamina V account for only a small percentage (< 4%) of the axons that make up the corticospinal tract. Small pyramidal cells and other neurons from laminae V and VI contribute the rest. In all, however, only about 40% of the axons of the pyramidal tract originate in area 4. The remaining 60% come from neurons in the supplementary motor fields (see p. 336).

339

12.8 Motor System: Motor Nuclei

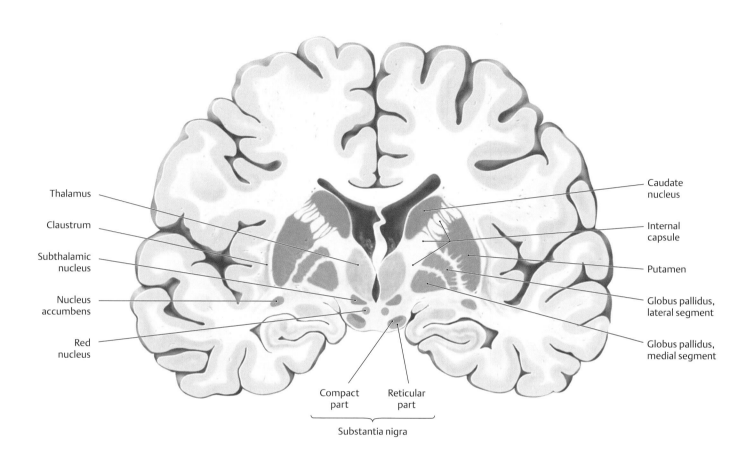

Thalamus

Claustrum

Subthalamic nucleus

Nucleus accumbens

Red nucleus

Caudate nucleus

Internal capsule

Putamen

Globus pallidus, lateral segment

Globus pallidus, medial segment

Compact part · Reticular part

Substantia nigra

A Motor nuclei

Coronal section. The basal ganglia are subcortical nuclei of the telencephalon that have a role in the planning and execution of movements. They are the central relay station of the extrapyramidal motor system and make up almost all the central gray matter of the cerebrum. The only other central gray-matter structure is the thalamus, which is primarily sensory ("gateway to consciousness") and is involved only secondarily, through feedback mechanisms, in motor sequences. The three largest motor nuclei are:

- Caudate nucleus,
- Putamen, and
- Globus pallidus (developmentally, part of the diencephalon).

These three nuclei are sometimes known by varying collective designations:

- The *lentiform nucleus* is formed by the putamen, globus pallidus, and intervening fiber tracts.

- The *corpus striatum consists* of the putamen, caudate nucleus, and intervening streaks of gray matter. In addition to these three nuclei, there are other nuclei that are considered functional components of the motor system (also shown here).

In a strictly anatomical sense, only the telencephalic structures listed above are constituents of the basal ganglia. Some textbooks mistakenly include the *subthalamic nucleus* of the diencephalon (see p. 224) and the *substantia nigra* of the mesencephalon (see p. 228) among the basal ganglia because of their close functional relationship to nuclei. Functional disturbances of the basal nuclei are characterized by movement disorders (e.g., Parkinson's disease).

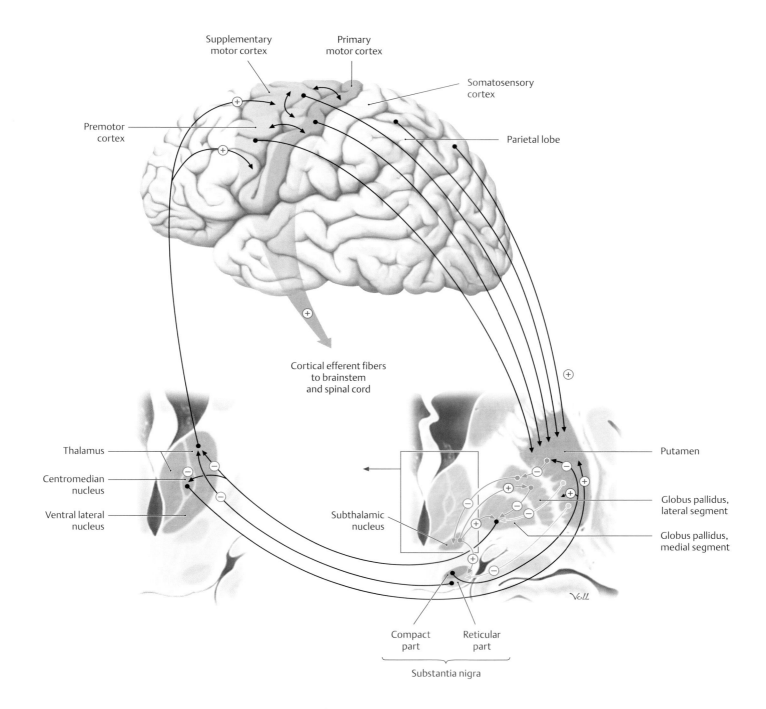

Supplementary motor cortex

Primary motor cortex

Somatosensory cortex

Premotor cortex

Parietal lobe

Cortical efferent fibers to brainstem and spinal cord

Thalamus

Centromedian nucleus

Ventral lateral nucleus

Subthalamic nucleus

Putamen

Globus pallidus, lateral segment

Globus pallidus, medial segment

Compact part

Reticular part

Substantia nigra

B Flow of information between motor cortical areas and basal ganglia: motor loop

The basal ganglia are concerned with the controlled, purposeful execution of fine voluntary movements (e.g., picking up an egg without breaking it). They integrate information from the cortex and subcortical regions, which they process in parallel and then return to motor cortical areas via the thalamus (feedback). Neurons from the premotor, primary motor, supplementary motor, and somatosensory cortex and from the parietal lobe send their axons to the putamen (see p. 209). Initially there is a direct (yellow) and indirect (green) pathway for relaying the information out of the putamen. Both pathways ultimately lead to the motor cortex by way of the thalamus. In the *direct* pathway (yellow), the neurons of the putamen project to the medial globus pallidus and to the reticular part of the substantia nigra. Both nuclei then return feedback signals to the motor thalamus, which projects back to motor areas of the cortex. The *indirect* pathway (green) leads from the putamen

through the lateral globus pallidus and subthalamic nucleus back to the medial globus pallidus, which then projects to the thalamus. An alternate indirect route leads from the subthalamic nucleus to the reticular part of the substantia nigra, which in turn projects to the thalamus. When inhibitory dopaminergic neurons in the compact part of the substantia nigra cease to function, the indirect pathway is suppressed and the direct pathway is no longer facilitated. Both effects lead to the increased inhibition of thalamocortical neurons, resulting in decreased movements (= *hypokinetic disorder*, e.g., in Parkinson's disease). Conversely, reduced activation of the internal part of the globus pallidus and the reticular part of the substantia nigra leads to increased activation of the thalamocortical neurons, resulting in abnormal spontaneous movements (= *hyperkinetic disorder*, e.g., Huntington's disease).

The diagram at lower left shows a close-up view of the boxed area (thalamus).

12.9 Motor System: Extrapyramidal Motor System and Lesions

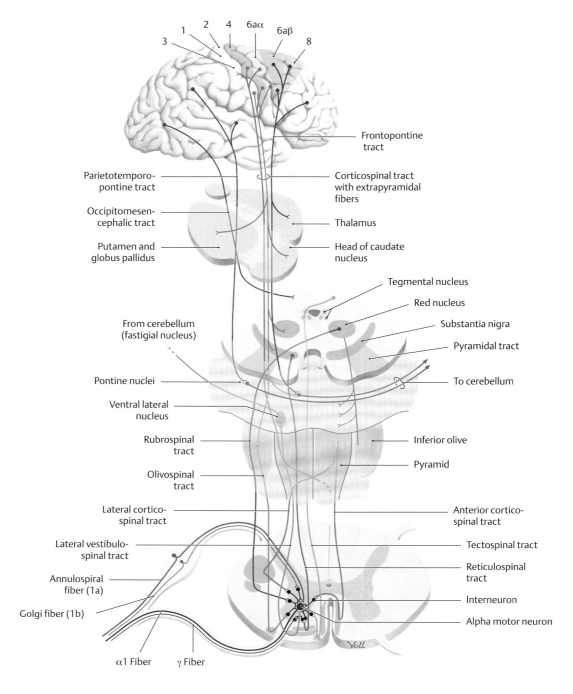

Labels on figure:

2 4 6aα 6aβ
1 8
3

Frontopontine tract

Parietotemporo-pontine tract

Corticospinal tract with extrapyramidal fibers

Occipitomesen-cephalic tract

Thalamus

Putamen and globus pallidus

Head of caudate nucleus

Tegmental nucleus

Red nucleus

From cerebellum (fastigial nucleus)

Substantia nigra

Pyramidal tract

Pontine nuclei

To cerebellum

Ventral lateral nucleus

Rubrospinal tract

Inferior olive

Pyramid

Olivospinal tract

Lateral cortico-spinal tract

Anterior cortico-spinal tract

Lateral vestibulo-spinal tract

Tectospinal tract

Reticulospinal tract

Annulospiral fiber (1a)

Interneuron

Golgi fiber (1b)

Alpha motor neuron

α1 Fiber   γ Fiber

A Descending tracts of the extrapyramidal motor system

The neurons of origin of the descending tracts of the extrapyramidal motor system* arise from a heterogeneous group of nuclei that includes the basal ganglia (putamen, globus pallidus, and caudate nucleus), the red nucleus, the substantia nigra, and even motor cortical areas (e.g., area 6). The following descending tracts are part of the extrapyramidal motor system:

- Rubrospinal tract
- Olivospinal tract
- Vestibulospinal tract
- Reticulospinal tract
- Tectospinal tract

These long descending tracts terminate on interneurons which then form synapses onto alpha and gamma motor neurons, which they con-

trol. Besides these long descending motor tracts, the motor neurons additionally receive sensory input (blue). All impulses in these pathways are integrated by the alpha motor neuron and modulate its activity, thereby affecting muscular contractions. The functional integrity of the alpha motor neuron is tested clinically by reflex testing.

* The term "extrapyramidal motor system" has been criticized because its functional and anatomical components are so closely linked to the pyramidal motor system that the distinction seems arbitrary in an anatomical sense—particularly since the system does not include cerebellar tracts that are also involved in the control of motor function.

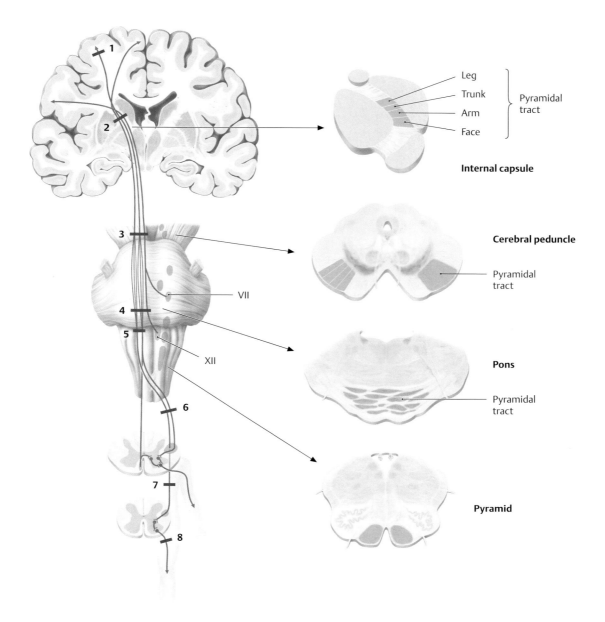

Leg
Trunk
Arm
Face

Pyramidal tract

Internal capsule

Cerebral peduncle

Pyramidal tract

VII

XII

Pons

Pyramidal tract

Pyramid

B Lesions of the central motor pathways and their effects

Lesion near the cortex (1): paralysis of the muscles innervated by the damaged cortical area. Because the face and hand are represented by particularly large areas in the motor cortex (see **B**, p. 339), paralysis often affects primarily the arm and face ("brachiofacial" paralysis). The paralysis invariably affects the side opposite the lesion (decussation of the pyramids) and is flaccid and partial *(paresis)* rather than complete because the extrapyramidal fibers are not damaged. If the extrapyramidal fibers were also damaged, the result would be *complete spastic paralysis* (see below).

Lesion at the level of the internal capsule (2): This leads to chronic, contralateral, spastic hemi*plegia* (= complete paralysis) because the lesion affects both the pyramidal tract and the extrapyramidal motor pathways,* which mix with pyramidal tract fibers in front of the internal capsule. Stroke is a frequent cause of lesions at this level.

Lesion at the level of the cerebral peduncles (crura cerebri) (3): contralateral spastic hemi*paresis*.

Lesion at the level of the pons (4): contralateral hemiparesis or bilateral paresis, depending on the size of the lesion. Because the fibers of the pyramidal tract occupy a larger cross-sectional area in the pons than in the internal capsule, not all of the fibers are damaged in many cases. For example, the fibers for the facial nerve and hypoglossal nerve are usually unaffected because of their dorsal location. Damage to the ab-

ducent nucleus may cause ipsilateral damage to the trigeminal nucleus (not shown).

Lesion at the level of the pyramid (5): Flaccid contralateral paresis occurs because the fibers of the extrapyramidal motor pathways (e.g., the rubrospinal and tectospinal tract) are more dorsal than the pyramidal tract fibers and are therefore unaffected by an isolated lesion of the pyramid.

Lesion at the level of the spinal cord (6, 7): A lesion at the level of the cervical cord (6) leads to ipsilateral spastic hemiplegia because the fibers of the pyramidal and extrapyramidal system are closely interwoven at this level and have already crossed to the opposite side. A lesion at the level of the thoracic cord (7) leads to spastic paralysis of the ipsilateral leg.

Lesion at the level of the peripheral nerve (8): This lesion damages the axon of the alpha motor neuron, resulting in flaccid paralysis.

---

* Thus, spastic paralysis is actually a sign of extrapyramidal motor damage. This fact was unknown when pyramidal tract lesions were first described, however, and it was assumed that a *pyramidal tract lesion* led to spastic paralysis. Because this fact has few practical implications, spasticity is still described in some textbooks as the classic sign of a pyramidal tract lesion. It would be better simply to regard spastic paralysis as a form of central paralysis.

12.10 Radicular Lesions: Sensory Deficits

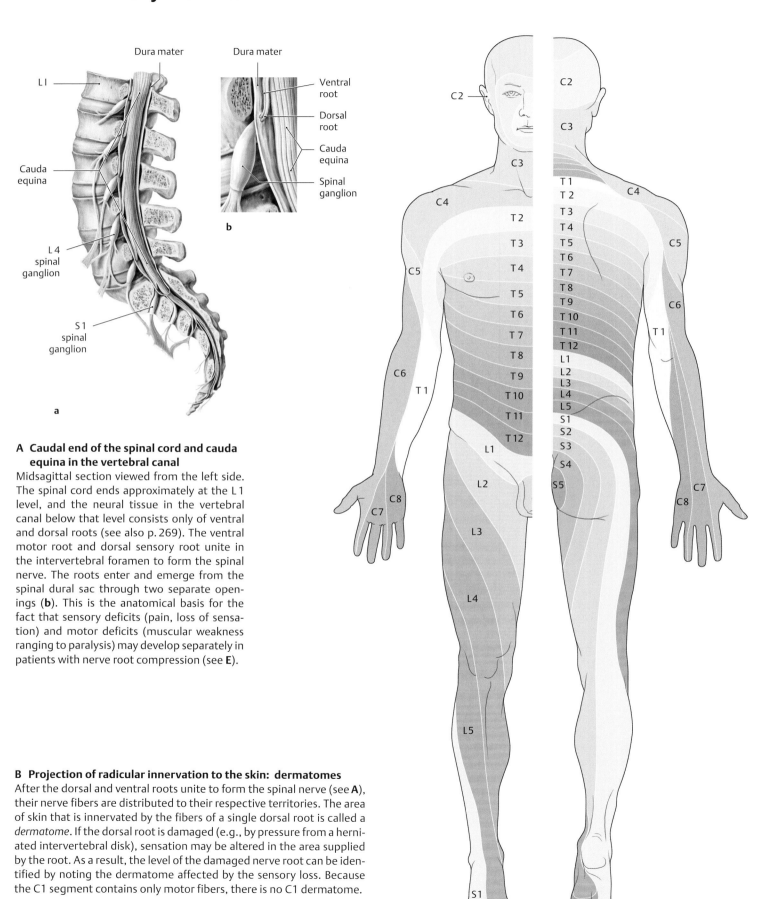

Dura mater

L I

Cauda equina

L 4 spinal ganglion

S 1 spinal ganglion

a

Dura mater

Ventral root

Dorsal root

Cauda equina

Spinal ganglion

b

A Caudal end of the spinal cord and cauda equina in the vertebral canal

Midsagittal section viewed from the left side. The spinal cord ends approximately at the L 1 level, and the neural tissue in the vertebral canal below that level consists only of ventral and dorsal roots (see also p. 269). The ventral motor root and dorsal sensory root unite in the intervertebral foramen to form the spinal nerve. The roots enter and emerge from the spinal dural sac through two separate openings (**b**). This is the anatomical basis for the fact that sensory deficits (pain, loss of sensation) and motor deficits (muscular weakness ranging to paralysis) may develop separately in patients with nerve root compression (see **E**).

B Projection of radicular innervation to the skin: dermatomes

After the dorsal and ventral roots unite to form the spinal nerve (see **A**), their nerve fibers are distributed to their respective territories. The area of skin that is innervated by the fibers of a single dorsal root is called a *dermatome*. If the dorsal root is damaged (e.g., by pressure from a herniated intervertebral disk), sensation may be altered in the area supplied by the root. As a result, the level of the damaged nerve root can be identified by noting the dermatome affected by the sensory loss. Because the C1 segment contains only motor fibers, there is no C1 dermatome.

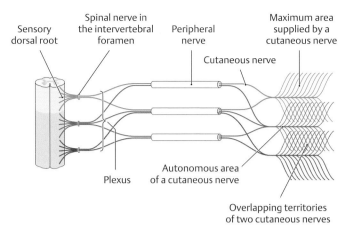

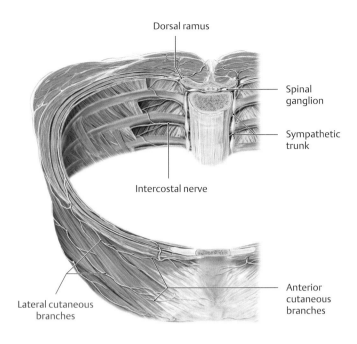

C Location of a radicular lesion

A radicular lesion is located on the ventral motor root or dorsal sensory root between its site of emergence from the spinal cord and the union of both roots to form a peripheral nerve. Accordingly, a lesion of the ventral root leads to motor deficits (see p. 346) while a dorsal root lesion leads to sensory disturbances in the corresponding dermatome. The dermatomes on the limbs are shifted because of migratory processes during embryonic development, but the dermatomes on the trunk retain their segmental pattern of innervation (see **B** and **D**). Due to the overlap between adjacent dermatomes, the sensory loss that results from damage to a dermatome may be smaller than the size of the dermatome as it appears in the diagram. The brain does not "know" the location of the lesion; it processes information as if the lesion were located in the area supplied by the nerve, i.e., in the dermatone.

D Radicular innervation of the trunk

The segmental arrangement of the musculature is preserved in the trunk, and so the trunk retains a segmental (radicular) innervation pattern. Because the nerves in the trunk do not form plexuses, the radicular innervation pattern continues into the peripheral territory of a cutaneous nerve (T 2 – T 12; see **B**). It can be seen that afferent fibers from the sympathetic trunk reach the peripheral nerves distal to the roots. This explains why radicular lesions are usually not associated with autonomic deficits in the affected dermatomes.

E Pressure on spinal nerve roots from a herniated lumbar disk of L 4/5

A herniated intervertebral disk may exert pressure on the spinal nerve root or cauda equina. The disk consists of a central gelatinous core (nucleus pulposus) and a peripheral ring of fibrocartilage (anulus fibrosus). When the anulus fibrosus is damaged, material from the gelatinous core may be extruded through the ring defect and impinge upon the root at its entry into the intervertebral foramen. This is a frequent cause of radicular symptoms, which have two grades of severity:

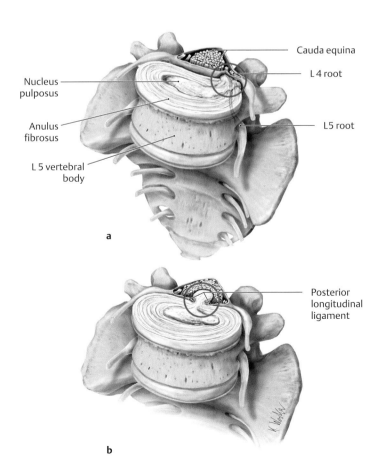

- Irritation of the nerve root in the region of the intervertebral foramen. This leads to pain in the low back (lumbago), potentially accompanied by pain radiating into the lower limb in the dermatone of the affected root (sciatica).
- A large disk herniation may compress the dorsal and/or ventral spinal nerve root, causing severe pain in addition to sensory deficits and (if the ventral root is affected) motor deficits.

- a **Posterolateral disk herniation** at the L 4/5 level. This damages the L 5 root passing behind the herniated disk but not the descending L 4 root, which has already entered the intervertebral foramen at that level. As a result, the sensory deficits are manifested in the L 5 dermatome (see **B**). Only a far lateral disk herniation will damage the root that exits at the same level as the affected disk.
- b **Posteromedial disk herniation** at the L 4/5 level. The material herniates through the posterior longitudinal ligament and impinges on the cauda equina. *Cauda equina syndrome* may develop if a lesion in this region compresses multiple roots. The locations of the deficits associated with specific root lesions are described in the next unit.

12.11 Radicular Lesions: Motor Deficits

A Indicator muscles of radicular lesions—limb muscles and diaphragm (after Kunze)

While a lesion of the sensory dorsal roots leads to sensory disturbances in specific dermatomes (see p. 344 and **C**, p. 345), a lesion of the *motor ventral roots* will cause weakness to develop in specific muscles. Just as the affected dermatome indicates the site of the sensory root lesion, the affected muscle indicates the level of the damaged spinal cord segment or its root. The muscles that are predominantly supplied by a particular spinal cord segment are called its *indicator muscles* (analogous to the dermatomes for the dorsal roots). Because indicator muscles are supplied predominantly but, as a rule, not exclusively by a single segment, a lesion in one segment or spinal nerve root usually causes weakness (paresis) of the affected muscle rather than complete paralysis (plegia). Slight weakness may also be noted in muscles that receive some innervation from the affected segment but are not principally supplied by it. The indicator muscles in the upper and lower limbs are listed in the tables below. Whereas sensory (dorsal) root lesions may occur in isolation, motor (ventral) root lesions usually occur in association with dorsal root lesions, and therefore the dermatomes are also listed in the tables.

Note: Because these nerves of the trunk are derived directly from the spinal nerve roots without any intervening plexuses, the pattern of segmental innervation in the trunk is identical to the pattern of peripheral innervation.

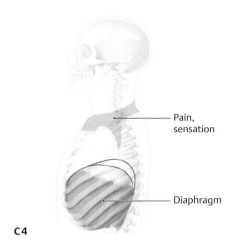

Pain, sensation

Diaphragm

C4

Location of pain or sensory disturbance	Shoulder
Indicator muscle	Diaphragm
Reflexes abolished by a segmental lesion	None

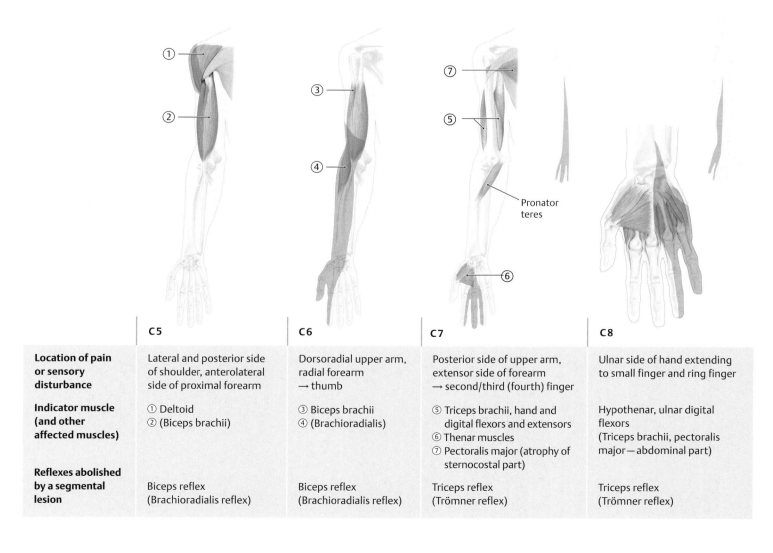

	C5	C6	C7	C8
Location of pain or sensory disturbance	Lateral and posterior side of shoulder, anterolateral side of proximal forearm	Dorsoradial upper arm, radial forearm → thumb	Posterior side of upper arm, extensor side of forearm → second/third (fourth) finger	Ulnar side of hand extending to small finger and ring finger
Indicator muscle (and other affected muscles)	① Deltoid ② (Biceps brachii)	③ Biceps brachii ④ (Brachioradialis)	⑤ Triceps brachii, hand and digital flexors and extensors ⑥ Thenar muscles ⑦ Pectoralis major (atrophy of sternocostal part)	Hypothenar, ulnar digital flexors (Triceps brachii, pectoralis major—abdominal part)
Reflexes abolished by a segmental lesion	Biceps reflex (Brachioradialis reflex)	Biceps reflex (Brachioradialis reflex)	Triceps reflex (Trömner reflex)	Triceps reflex (Trömner reflex)

Pronator teres

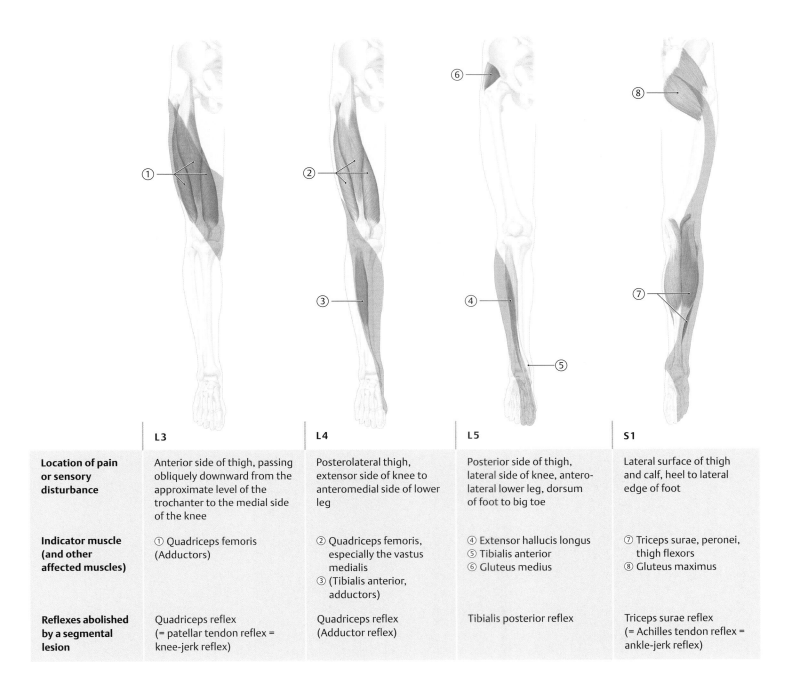

	L3	L4	L5	S1
Location of pain or sensory disturbance	Anterior side of thigh, passing obliquely downward from the approximate level of the trochanter to the medial side of the knee	Posterolateral thigh, extensor side of knee to anteromedial side of lower leg	Posterior side of thigh, lateral side of knee, antero-lateral lower leg, dorsum of foot to big toe	Lateral surface of thigh and calf, heel to lateral edge of foot
Indicator muscle (and other affected muscles)	① Quadriceps femoris (Adductors)	② Quadriceps femoris, especially the vastus medialis ③ (Tibialis anterior, adductors)	④ Extensor hallucis longus ⑤ Tibialis anterior ⑥ Gluteus medius	⑦ Triceps surae, peronei, thigh flexors ⑧ Gluteus maximus
Reflexes abolished by a segmental lesion	Quadriceps reflex (= patellar tendon reflex = knee-jerk reflex)	Quadriceps reflex (Adductor reflex)	Tibialis posterior reflex	Triceps surae reflex (= Achilles tendon reflex = ankle-jerk reflex)

B Principal indicator muscles of the spinal cord segments
The table lists the typical indicator muscles for each cord segment.

Cord segment	Indicator muscle
C4	Diaphragm
C5	Deltoid
C6	Biceps brachii
C7	Triceps brachii
C8	Hypothenar muscles, long digital flexors on ulnar side
L3	Quadriceps femoris
L4	Quadriceps femoris, vastus medialis
L5	Extensor hallucis longus, tibialis anterior
S1	Triceps surae, peronei, gluteus maximus

C Clinical manifestations of nerve root irritation

- Pain in the affected dermatome
- Sensory losses in the affected dermatome
- Increased pain during coughing, sneezing, or straining
- Pain fibers more severely affected than other sensory fibers
- Motor deficits in the indicator muscles of the segment
- Reflexes associated with the affected segment are absent or diminished.

12.12 Lesions of the Brachial Plexus

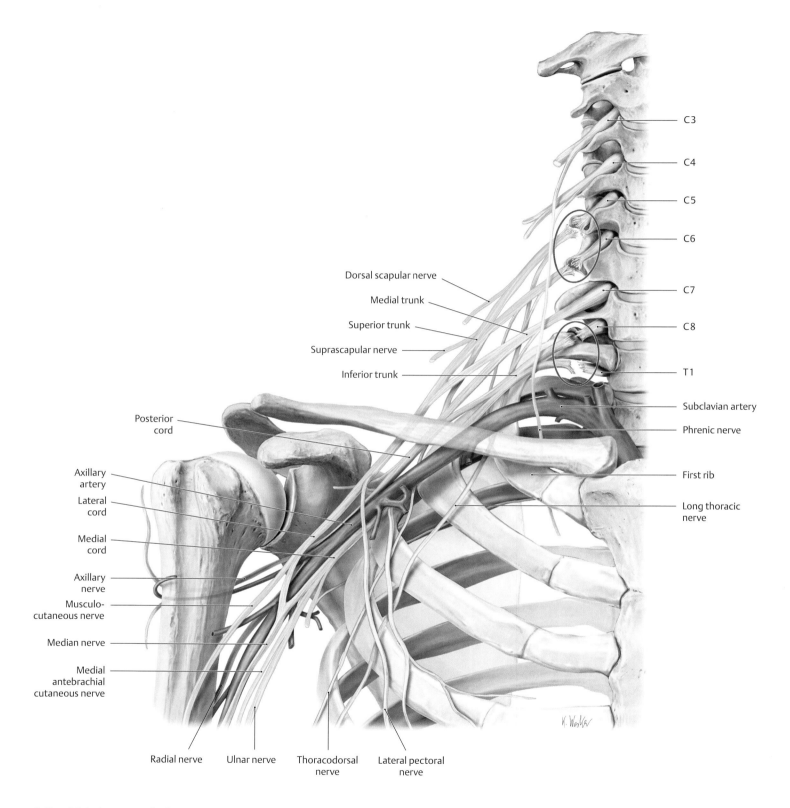

Labels on the figure:
- C3
- C4
- C5
- C6
- Dorsal scapular nerve
- Medial trunk
- Superior trunk
- Suprascapular nerve
- Inferior trunk
- C7
- C8
- T1
- Subclavian artery
- Phrenic nerve
- First rib
- Long thoracic nerve
- Posterior cord
- Axillary artery
- Lateral cord
- Medial cord
- Axillary nerve
- Musculo-cutaneous nerve
- Median nerve
- Medial antebrachial cutaneous nerve
- Radial nerve
- Ulnar nerve
- Thoracodorsal nerve
- Lateral pectoral nerve

A Brachial plexus paralysis

Anterior view of the right side. Lesions are circled. By definition, two forms of brachial plexus paralysis are distinguished: *upper brachial plexus paralysis*, which is caused by a lesion of the C5 and C6 ventral rami (see **C**), and *lower brachial plexus paralysis*, which is caused by a lesion of the C8 and T1 ventral rami (see **D**). C7 forms a "watershed" between the two forms of paralysis and is typically unaffected by either form. A complete lesion of the brachial plexus may also occur in severe trauma.

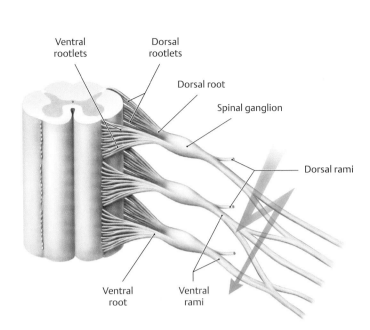

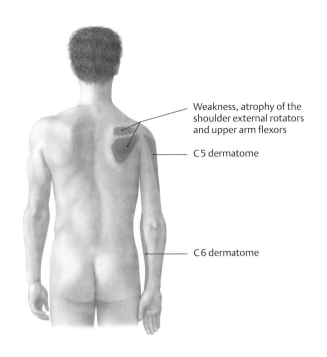

B Site of lesion in brachial plexus paralysis

A brachial plexus lesion affects the ventral rami of several spinal nerves, which transmit afferent signals to the plexus. Because the ventral rami carry both motor and sensory fibers, a brachial plexus lesion always causes a combination of motor and sensory deficits. The resulting paralysis (see **C**) is always of the flaccid type because of its peripheral nature (= lesion of the second motor neuron).

C Example: upper brachial plexus paralysis (Erb's palsy)

This condition results from a lesion of the ventral rami of the C5 and C6 spinal nerves, causing paralysis of the abductors and external rotators of the shoulder joint and of the upper arm flexors and supinator. The arm hangs limply at the side (loss of the upper arm flexors), and the palm faces backward (loss of the supinator with dominance of the pronators). There may also be partial paralysis of the extensor muscles of the elbow joint and hand. Typical cases present with sensory disturbances on the lateral surface of the upper arm and forearm, but these signs may be absent. A frequent cause of upper brachial plexus paralysis is obstetric trauma.

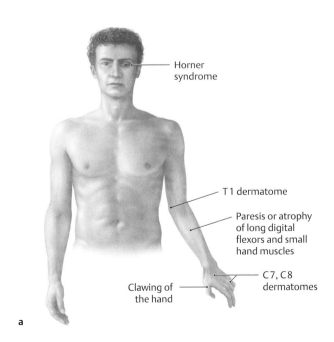

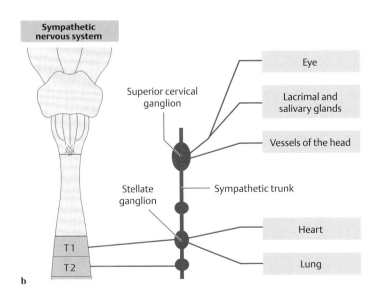

D Example: lower brachial plexus paralysis (Dejerine–Klumpke palsy)

This paralysis results from a lesion of the ventral rami of the C8 and T1 spinal nerves (see **A**). It affects the hand muscles, the long digital flexors, and the flexor muscles in the wrist (claw hand with atrophy of the small hand muscles, **a**). Sensory disturbances affect the ulnar surfaces of the forearm and hand. Because the sympathetic fibers for the head leave the spinal cord at T1 (**b**), the sympathetic innervation of the head is also lost. This is manifested by a *unilateral Horner syndrome*, characterized by miosis (contracted pupil due to paralysis of the dilator pupillae) and narrowing of the palpebral fissure (not ptosis) due to a loss of sympathetic innervation to the superior and inferior tarsal muscles. The narrowed palpebral fissure mimics enophthalmos (sinking of the eyeball into the orbit).

349

12.13 Lesions of the Lumbosacral Plexus

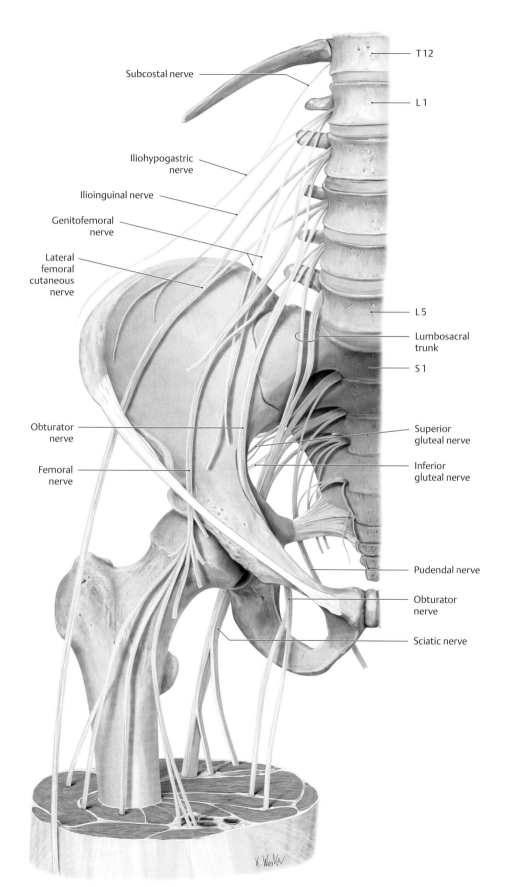

Subcostal nerve

Iliohypogastric nerve

Ilioinguinal nerve

Genitofemoral nerve

Lateral femoral cutaneous nerve

Obturator nerve

Femoral nerve

T 12

L 1

L 5

Lumbosacral trunk

S 1

Superior gluteal nerve

Inferior gluteal nerve

Pudendal nerve

Obturator nerve

Sciatic nerve

A Lumbosacral plexus

Anterior view. The lumbosacral plexus is divided into a lumbar plexus (T 12–L 4) and sacral plexus (L 5–S 4).

Note: The nerves of the lumbar part (yellow) pass anteriorly while those of the sacral part (green) pass posteriorly. The connection between the two parts of the plexus is the lumbosacral trunk.

Because the lumbosacral plexus is in a protected location deep within the pelvis, it is less commonly affected by lesions than the brachial plexus, which is much more superficial. The lumbosacral plexus may be injured by pelvic ring fractures, a sacral bone fracture, or hip fractures, or as a complication of hip replacement.

Weakness and atrophy of the hip flexors, knee extensors, and external rotators and adductors of the thigh

Intact sweating

Anhidrosis

Left foot

Right foot

a

b

B Lesion of the left lumbar plexus (T 12–L 4)

The dominant feature of this condition is femoral nerve paralysis affecting the hip flexors, knee extensors, and the external rotators and adductors of the thigh (**a**). A sensory deficit is found on the anteromedial aspect of the thigh and calf. The lesion also disrupts the sympathetic fibers for the leg, which arise from the lumbar cord and pass through the lumbar plexus. The clinical manifestations (**b**) include: increased warmth of the foot (loss of sympathetic vasoconstriction) and anhidrosis on the sole of the foot (sweating is absent because of loss of sympathetic innervation to the sweat glands). When sweating is intact, the ninhydrin test is positive (footprint on a sheet of paper stains purple with 1 % ninhydrin solution).

Note: Manifestations in the limbs are recognized by comparison with the unaffected side.

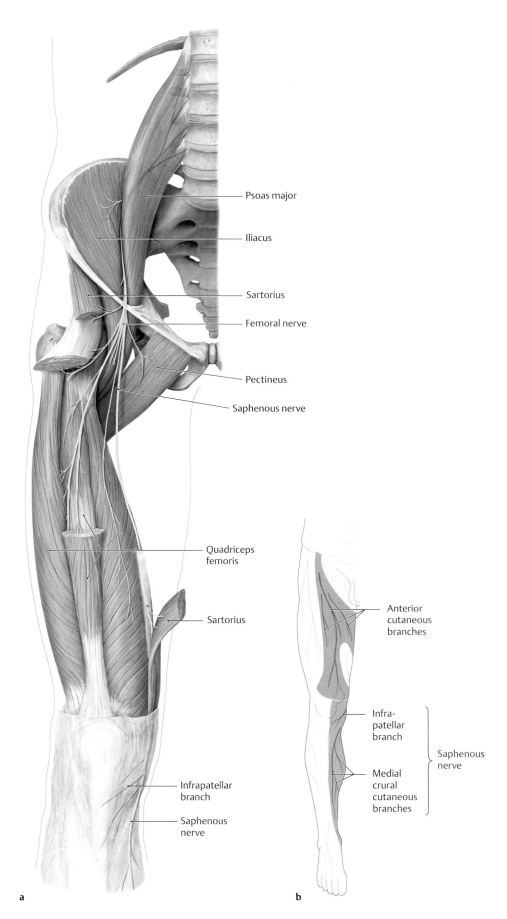

Psoas major

Iliacus

Sartorius

Femoral nerve

Pectineus

Saphenous nerve

Quadriceps femoris

Sartorius

Infrapatellar branch

Saphenous nerve

a

Anterior cutaneous branches

Infra-patellar branch

Saphenous nerve

Medial crural cutaneous branches

b

C Muscular and cutaneous distribution of the femoral nerve (L1–L4)
Anterior view.

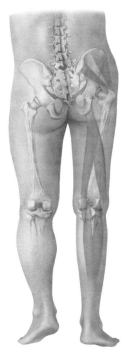

D Lesion of the right sacral plexus (L5–S4)
This lesion presents clinically with *paralysis of the sciatic nerve* and its two main branches, the tibial and common fibular nerves, which are jointly affected. The results are loss of plantar flexion (tibial nerve paralysis, inability to walk on the toes) and paralysis of the foot and toe extensors (common fibular nerve, steppage gait: the patient must raise the knee abnormally high while walking to avoid dragging the toes on the ground). Sensory disturbances are noted on the posterior surfaces of the thigh, lower leg, and foot. Because the *superior gluteal nerve* is involved, the gluteus medius and minimus are also paralyzed. These two muscles stabilize the pelvis of the stationary side during gait. When they are paralyzed, the pelvis tilts toward the swinging leg, producing a "waddling" gait (known also as a positive Trendelenburg sign). The superior gluteal nerve also innervates the tensor fasciae latae, which normally acts in the same manners as the two gluteal muscles. Specific categories of peripheral nerve lesions are described in the volume on *General Anatomy and Musculoskeletal System*.

12.14 Lesions of the Spinal Cord and Peripheral Nerves: Sensory Deficits

Overview of the next three units (after Bähr and Frotscher)
Two questions should be addressed in the diagnostic evaluation of spinal cord lesions:

1. What structure(s) within the *cross-section* of the spinal cord is (are) affected? This is determined systematically by proceeding from the periphery of the cord toward the center.
2. At what level of the spinal cord (in longitudinal section) is the lesion located?

In these units we will first correlate various deficit patterns (syndromes) with the structures in the cross-section of the spinal cord. We will then discuss the level of the lesion in the longitudinal or craniocaudal dimension. Since these syndromes present with deficits that result from damage to specific anatomical structures, they can be explained in anatomical terms. Based on the lesions and syndromes described here, the reader can test his or her ability to relate what has already been learned to the locations and effects of spinal cord lesions.

A Spinal ganglion syndrome illustrated for an isolated lesion of T 6
As part of the dorsal roots, the spinal ganglia are concerned with the transmission of sensory information. (Recall that the ganglia contain the perikarya of the first sensory neuron.) When only a single spinal ganglion is affected (e.g., by a viral infection such as herpes zoster), the resulting pain and paresthesia are limited to the sensory distribution (dermatome) of the ganglion. Because the dermatomes show considerable overlap, adjacent dermatomes can assume the function of the affected dermatome. As a result, the area that shows absolute sensory loss, called the "autonomous area" of the dermatome, may be quite small.

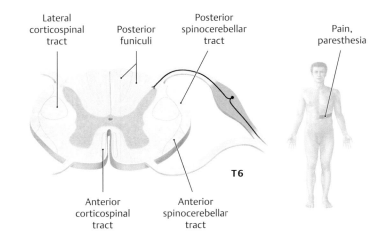

Lateral corticospinal tract — Posterior funiculi — Posterior spinocerebellar tract — Pain, paresthesia

Anterior corticospinal tract — Anterior spinocerebellar tract

T 6

B Dorsal root syndrome illustrated for a lesion at the C 4 – T 6 level
When a lesion (trauma, degenerative spinal changes, tumor) affects multiple successive dorsal roots as in this example, complete sensory loss occurs in the affected dermatomes. When this sensory loss affects the afferent limb of a reflex, that reflex will be absent or diminished. If the sensory dorsal roots are irritated but not disrupted, as in the case of a herniated intervertebral disk, severe pain may sometimes be perceived in the affected dermatome. Because pain fibers do not overlap as much as other sensory fibers, the examiner should have no difficulty in identifying the affected dermatome, and thus the corresponding spinal cord segment, from the location of the pain.

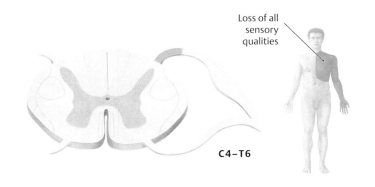

Loss of all sensory qualities

C 4–T 6

C Posterior horn syndrome illustrated for a lesion at the C 5 – C 8 level
This lesion, like a dorsal *root* lesion of the spinal nerves, is characterized by a segmental pattern of sensory disturbance. But with a posterior *horn* lesion of the spinal cord, unlike a dorsal *root* lesion, the resulting sensory deficit is incomplete. Pain and temperature sensation are abolished in the dermatomes on the ipsilateral side because the first peripheral/afferent neuron of the lateral spinothalamic tract is relayed in the posterior horn, which is within the damaged area. Position sense and vibration sense are unaffected because the fibers for these sensory qualities are both conveyed in the posterior funiculus. Bypassing the posterior horn, these fibers pass directly via the posterior funiculi to their synapses in the nucleus gracilis or nucleus cuneatus (see p. 276). A lesion of the anterior spinothalamic tract does not produce striking clinical signs. The deficit (loss of pain and temperature sensation with preservation of position and vibration sense) is called a *dissociated sensory loss*. Pain and temperature sensation are preserved below the lesion because the tracts in the white matter (lateral spinothalamic tract) are undamaged. This type of dissociated sensory loss occurs in syringomyelia, a congenital or acquired condition in which threre is an expanded cavity in or near the central canal of the spinal cord. (According to the strictest terminology, expansion of the central canal itself = hydromyelia).

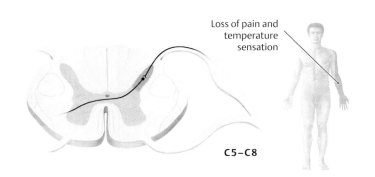

Loss of pain and temperature sensation

C 5–C 8

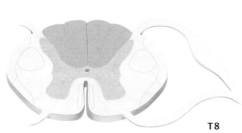

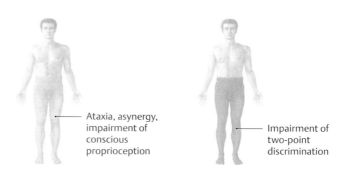

D Lesion of the posterior funiculi at the T 8 level

A lesion of the posterior funiculi (see also p. 276) is characterized by a loss of:

- Position sense,
- Vibration sense, and
- Two-point discrimination.

These deficits occur distal to the lesion, hence they involve the legs and lower trunk when the lesion is at the T 8 level. When the legs are affected, as in the present example, the loss of position sense (mediated by proprioception, see p. 179) leads to an unsteady gait (ataxia). When

the arm is affected (not shown here), the only clinical finding is sensory impairment. The lack of feedback to the motor system also prevents the precise interaction of different muscle groups during fine movements (asynergy). Ataxia results from the fact that information on body position is essential for carrying out movements. Vision can (partly) compensate for this loss of information when the eyes are open, and so the ataxia worsens when the eyes are closed (Romberg's sign). This *sensory ataxia* differs from *cerebellar ataxia* in that the latter cannot be compensated by visual control.

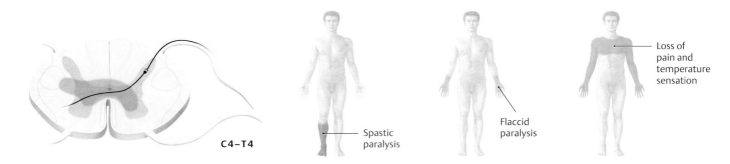

E Gray matter syndrome illustrated for a lesion at the C 4 – T 4 level

This syndrome results from a pathological process (e.g., a tumor) in and around the central canal. All tracts that cross through the gray matter are damaged, i.e., the anterior and lateral spinothalamic tracts. The result is a dissociated sensory loss (loss of pain and temperature sensation with preservation of position, vibration, and touch), in this case involving the arms and upper chest (compare with **C**). A relatively large

lesion may additionally affect the anterior horns, which contain the alpha motor neuron, causing a flaccid paralysis in the distal portions of the upper limb. An even larger lesion may concomitantly affect the pyramidal tract, causing spastic paralysis of the distal muscles (here in the legs). This syndrome may result from syringomyelia (see **C**) or tumors located near the central canal.

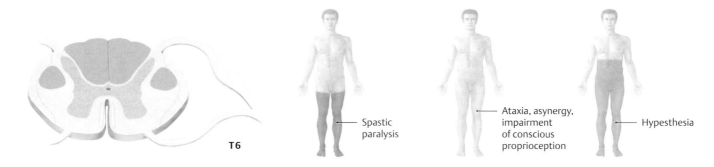

F Combined disease of the posterior funiculi and pyramidal tract illustrated for a lesion at the T 6 level

A *lesion of the posterior funiculi* leads to loss of position and vibration sense. A concomitant *pyramidal tract lesion* additionally leads to spastic paralysis of the legs and abdominal muscles below the affected dermatome, i.e., below T 6 in the example. This predominantly cervico-

thoracic lesion typically occurs in funicular myelosis (vitamin B$_{12}$ deficiency), in which the posterior funiculi are affected initially, followed by the pyramidal tract. This disease is characterized by degeneration of the myelin sheaths.

353

12.15 Lesions of the Spinal Cord and Peripheral Nerves: Motor Deficits

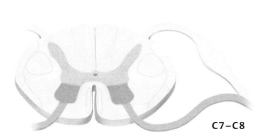

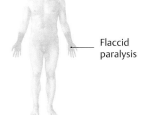

A Anterior horn syndrome illustrated for a lesion at the C 7 – C 8 level

Damage to the motor anterior horn cells leads to ipsilateral paralysis, in this case involving the hands and forearm muscles because the lesion is at C 7 – C 8 and these segments innervate the muscles in this region. The paralysis is flaccid because the alpha motor neuron that supplies the muscles (lower motor neuron = second motor neuron, see p. 181) has ceased to function. Because larger muscles are supplied by motor neurons from more than one segment (see **A**, p. 270), damage to a single segment may lead only to muscular weakness (paresis) rather than complete paralysis of the affected muscle group. When the lateral horns are additionally involved, decreased sweating and vasomotor function will also be noted because the lateral horns contain the cell bodies of the sympathetic neurons that subserve these functions. This type of lesion may occur in poliomyelitis or in spinal muscular atrophy, for example. These relatively rare diseases are relentlessly progressive.

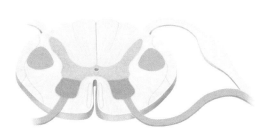

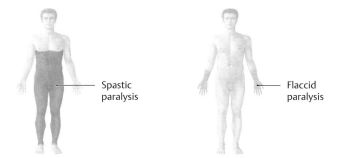

B Combined lesions of the anterior horn and lateral corticospinal tract

These lesions produce a combination of flaccid and spastic paralysis. Damage to the motor anterior horns or "lower" motor neuron (= second motor neuron) causes flaccid paralysis, while a lesion of the lateral corticospinal tract or "upper" motor neuron (= first motor neuron) causes spastic paralysis. The degree of injury to both types of neuron may be highly variable. In the example shown, an anterior horn lesion at the C 7 – C 8 level has caused flaccid paralysis of the forearm and hand. By contrast, a lesion of the lateral corticospinal tract at the T 5 level would cause spastic paralysis of the abdominal and leg muscles.

Note: When the second motor neuron in the anterior horn is already damaged (flaccid paralysis), an additional lesion of the lateral corticospinal tract at the level of the same segment will not produce any noticeable effects.

This lesion pattern occurs in amyotrophic lateral sclerosis, in which the first cortical motor neuron (pyramidal tract lesion) and second spinal motor neuron (anterior horn lesion) both undergo progressive degeneration (etiology unclear). The end stage is marked by additional involvement of the motor cranial nerve nuclei, with swallowing and speaking difficulties (bulbar paralysis).

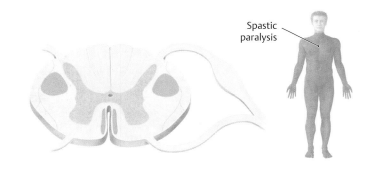

C Corticospinal tract syndrome

Progressive spastic spinal paralysis (Erb-Charcot disease) is characterized by a progressive degeneration of the cortical neurons in the motor cortex with increasing failure of the corticospinal pathways (axonal degeneration of the first motor neuron). The course of the disease is marked by a progressive spastic paralysis of the limbs that begins in the legs and eventually reaches the arms.

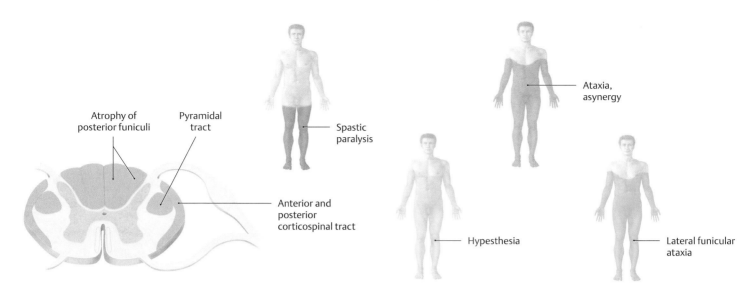

D Combined lesions of the posterior funiculus, spinocerebellar tracts, and pyramidal tract

This syndrome begins with destruction of the neurons in the spinal ganglia, which transmit information on conscious position sense (loss: ataxia, asynergy), vibration sense, and two-point discrimination. This neuronal destruction leads to atrophy of the posterior funiculi. There is little or no impairment of pain and temperature sensation, which are still transmitted to higher centers in the unaffected lateral spinothalamic tract. The loss of conscious proprioception alone is sufficient to cause

sensory ataxia (lack of feedback to the motor system, see **D**, p. 353). But the lesions additionally affect the spinocerebellar tracts (unconscious proprioception), injury to which suffices to cause ataxia, and so this dual injury causes a particularly severe loss of conscious and unconscious proprioception. This is the main clinical feature of the disease. Spastic paralysis also develops as a result of pyramidal tract dysfunction. The prototype of this disease is hereditary Friedreich ataxia, which has several variants. The gene has been localized to chromosome 19.

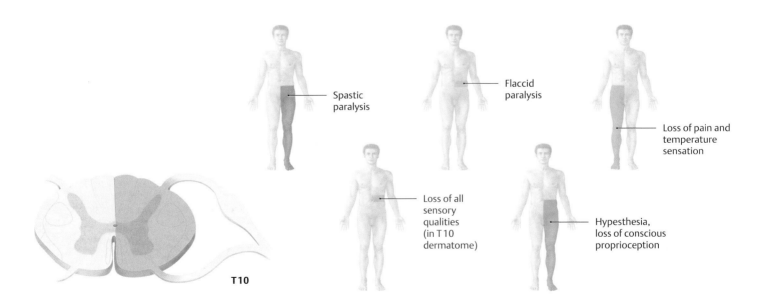

E Spinal hemiplegia syndrome (Brown–Séquard syndrome) illustrated for a lesion at the T 10 level on the left side

Hemisection of the spinal cord, though uncommon (e.g., in stab injuries), is an excellent model for testing our understanding of the function and course of the nerve tracts in the spinal cord. Spastic paralysis due to interruption of the pyramidal tract (see footnote on p. 343) occurs on the side of the lesion (and below the level of the lesion). The interruption of the posterior funiculi (pathways for conscious proprioception) causes a loss of position and vibration sense and two-point discrimination on the side of the lesion. After spinal shock has subsided, spastic paralysis develops below the level of the lesion (here affecting the left leg). Of course, this paralysis does not produce an ataxia like that described

following interruption of the posterior funiculi. Destruction of the alpha motor neurons in the locally damaged segment (in this case T 10) leads to ipsilateral flaccid paralysis associated with this segment. Because the axons of the lateral spinothalamic tract have already crossed to the unaffected side below the lesion, pain and temperature sensation are preserved on the *ipsilateral* side below the lesion. These two types of sensation are lost on the *contralateral* side, however, because the crossed axons on the opposite side have been interrupted at the level of the lesion. If spinal root irritation occurs at the level of the lesion, radicular pain may occur because of the descending course of the sensory (and motor) roots in the segment above the lesion (see **E**, p. 345).

12.16 Lesions of the Spinal Cord, Assessment

A Deficits caused by complete cord lesions at various levels

Having explored the manifestations of lesions at different sites in the cross-section of the spinal cord, we will now consider the effects of lesions at various levels of the cord. An example is the paralysis caused by a *complete spinal cord lesion,* which occurs acutely after a severe injury and is considerably more common than the incomplete lesions described earlier (see **E**, p. 355). A complete cord lesion following acute trauma is initially manifested by *spinal shock,* the pathophysiology of which is not yet fully understood. This condition is marked by complete flaccid paralysis below the site of the lesion, with a loss of all sensory qualities from the level of the lesion downward. Loss of bladder and rectal function and impotence are also present. Because the lesion also interrupts the sympathetic fibers, sweating and thermoregulation are impaired. The gray matter of the spinal cord recovers over a period ranging from a few days to eight weeks. The spinal reflexes return, and the flaccid paralysis changes to a spastic paralysis. There is a recovery of bladder and rectal function, but only at a reflex level since voluntary control has been permanently lost. Impotence is permanent. **Lesions of the cervical cord** above C 3 are swiftly fatal because they disrupt the efferent supply of the phrenic nerve (main root at C 4), which innervates the diaphragm and maintains abdominal respiration, while innervation to the intercostal muscles is also lost, causing a failure of thoracic respiration. A complete lesion of the lower cervical cord causes paralysis of all four limbs (quadriplegia), and respiration is precarious because of paralysis of the intercostal muscles. **Lesions of the upper thoracic cord** (T 2 downward) spare the arms but respiration is compromised because of paralysis of the abdominal muscles. A lesion of the **lower thoracic cord** (the exact site is unimportant) has little or no effect on the abdominal muscles, and respiration is not impaired. If the sympathetic splanchnic nerves are also damaged, there may be compromise of visceral motor function ranging to paralytic ileus (see p. 324). With

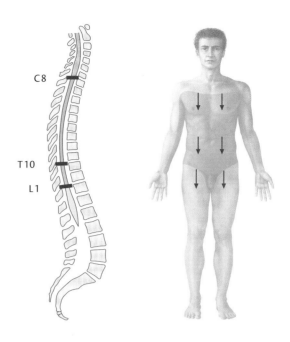

lesions of the lumbar cord, a distinction is drawn between epiconus syndrome (L 4 – S 2) and conus syndrome (S 3 downward). *Epiconus syndrome* is characterized by a flaccid paralysis of the legs (only the roots are affected, causing peripheral paralysis), and reflex but not conscious emptying of the bladder and rectum is preserved. Sexual potency is lost. In *conus syndrome,* the legs are not paralyzed and only the foregoing autonomic disturbances are present. The motor deficits described here are also associated with sensory deficits (see **B**).

B Deficits associated with complete spinal cord lesions at various levels (after Rohkamm)

Level of lesion	Motor deficits	Sensory deficits	Autonomic deficits
C 1 – C 3 (high cervical cord lesion)	• Quadriplegia • Paralysis of nuchal muscles • Spasticity • Respiratory paralysis (immediate death if not artificially ventilated)	• Sensory loss from occiput or mandibular border downward • Pain in occipital region, back of neck, and shoulder region	• Reflex visceral functions (bladder, bowel) with no voluntary control • Horner syndrome
C 4 – C 5	• Quadriplegia • Diaphragmatic respiration only	• Sensory loss from clavicle or shoulder downward	• See above
C 6 – C 8 (lower cervical cord lesion)	• Quadriplegia • Diaphragmatic respiration • Spasticity	• Sensory loss from upper chest wall and back downward, and on the arms (sparing the shoulders)	• See above
T 1 – T 5	• Paraplegia • Decreased respiratory volume	• Sensory loss from inside of forearm, upper chest wall and back	• Reflex function of bladder and rectum • Erection without voluntary control
T 5 – T 10	• Paraplegia, spasticity	• Sensory loss from affected level in chest wall and back	• See above
T 11 – L 3	• Paraplegia	• Sensory loss from groin region or front of thigh, depending on site of lesion	• See above
L 4 – S 2 (epiconus, spinal nerve roots paralyzed)	• Distal paraplegia	• Sensory loss from front of thigh, dorsum of foot, sole of foot, or back of thigh, depending on site of lesion	• Flaccid paralysis of bladder and rectum • Impotence
S 3 – S 5 (conus)	• No deficit	• Sensory loss in perianal region and inside of thigh	• See above

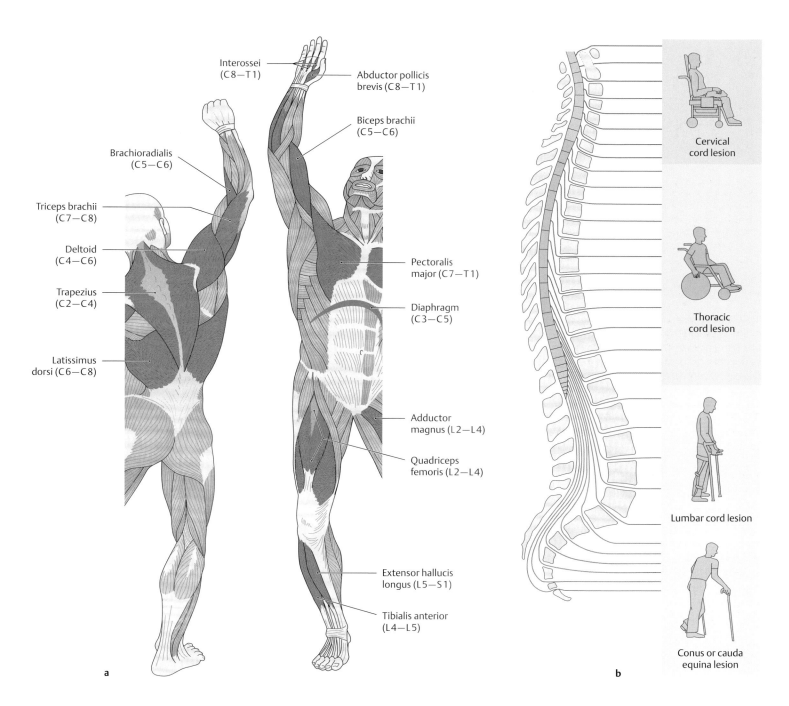

Interossei (C8–T1)

Abductor pollicis brevis (C8–T1)

Biceps brachii (C5–C6)

Brachioradialis (C5–C6)

Triceps brachii (C7–C8)

Deltoid (C4–C6)

Trapezius (C2–C4)

Latissimus dorsi (C6–C8)

Pectoralis major (C7–T1)

Diaphragm (C3–C5)

Adductor magnus (L2–L4)

Quadriceps femoris (L2–L4)

Extensor hallucis longus (L5–S1)

Tibialis anterior (L4–L5)

a

Cervical cord lesion

Thoracic cord lesion

Lumbar cord lesion

Conus or cauda equina lesion

b

C Determining the level of spinal cord lesions

a Muscles and the spinal cord segments that innervate them. Most muscles are multisegmental, i.e., they receive innervation from several spinal cord segments. Thus, for example, a lesion at the C7 level will not necessarily cause complete paralysis of the latissimus dorsi, because that muscle is also innervated by C6. This is not the case with the "indicator muscles," which are supplied almost exclusively by a single segment (see **B**, p. 347). A lesion at the L3 level, for example, will cause almost complete paralysis of the quadriceps femoris because that muscle is innervated almost entirely by L3.

b The degree of disability varies, depending on the level of the complete cord lesion.

357

12.17 Visual System, Overview and Geniculate Part

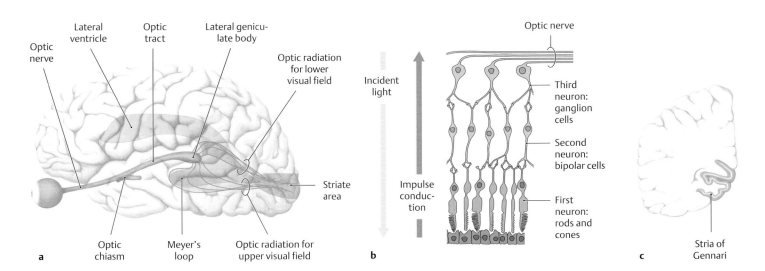

a — Optic nerve, Lateral ventricle, Optic tract, Lateral geniculate body, Optic radiation for lower visual field, Optic chiasm, Meyer's loop, Optic radiation for upper visual field, Striate area, Incident light, Impulse conduction

b — Optic nerve, Third neuron: ganglion cells, Second neuron: bipolar cells, First neuron: rods and cones

c — Stria of Gennari

A Overview of the visual pathway

Left lateral view. The visual pathway extends from the eye, an anterior prolongation of the diencephalon, back to the occipital pole. Thus it encompasses almost the entire longitudinal axis of the brain. The principal stations are as follows:

Retina. The retina contains the first three neurons of the visual pathway (**b**):

- First neuron: photoreceptor rods and cones, located on the deep retinal surface opposite to the direction of the incoming light ("inversion of the retina").
- Second neuron: bipolar cells.
- Third neuron: ganglion cells whose axons are collected to form the optic nerve.

Optic nerve, optic chiasm, and **optic tract:** This neural portion of the visual pathway is part of the central nervous system (optic nerve = cranial nerve II) and is surrounded by meninges. Thus, the optic nerve is actually a tract rather than a true nerve. The optic nerves join below the base of the diencephalon to form the optic chiasm, which then divides into the two optic tracts. Each of these tracts divides in turn into a lateral and medial root.

Lateral geniculate body: Ninety percent of the axons of the third neuron (= 90% of the optic nerve fibers) terminate in the lateral geniculate body on neurons that project to the striate area (visual cortex, see below). This is the *geniculate part of the visual pathway* (discussed here). It is concerned with *conscious* visual perception and is conveyed by the lateral root of the optic tract. The remaining 10% of the third-neuron axons in the visual pathway do not terminate in the lateral geniculate body. This is the *nongeniculate part of the visual pathway* (medial root, see **B**, p. 361), and its signals are not consciously perceived.

Optic radiation and **visual cortex** (striate area): The optic radiation begins in the lateral geniculate body, forms a band that winds around the inferior and posterior horns of the lateral ventricles, and terminates in the visual cortex or striate area (= Brodmann area 17). Located in the occipital lobe, the visual cortex can be grossly identified by a prominent stripe of white matter in the otherwise gray cerebral cortex (the stria of Gennari, see **c**). This white stripe runs parallel to the brain surface and is shown in the inset, where the gray matter of the visual cortex is shaded light red.

☐ Left half of visual field

▨ Right half of visual field

B Representation of each visual field in the contralateral visual cortex

Superior view. The light rays in the *nasal* part of each visual field are projected to the *temporal* half of the retina, while those from the temporal part are projected to the retinal half. Because of this arrangement, the left half of the visual field projects to the visual cortex of the right occipital pole, and the right half projects to the visual cortex of the left occipital pole. For clarity, each visual field in the diagram is divided into two halves, and the reader should understand this basic division before we explore how the visual fields are divided into four quadrants (**C**).

Note: The axonal fibers from the nasal half of each retina cross to the opposite side at the optic chiasm and then travel with the uncrossed fibers from the temporal half of each retina.

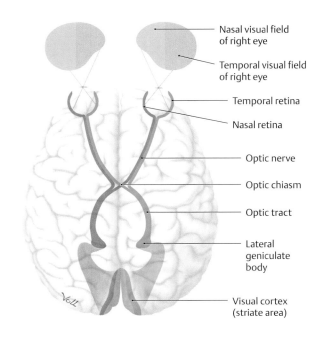

Nasal visual field of right eye
Temporal visual field of right eye
Temporal retina
Nasal retina
Optic nerve
Optic chiasm
Optic tract
Lateral geniculate body
Visual cortex (striate area)

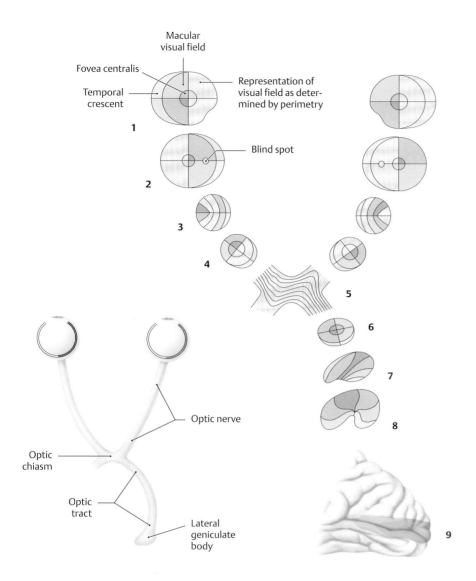

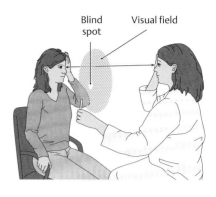

D Informal visual field examination with the confrontation test

The visual field examination is an essential step in the examination of lesions of the visual pathway (see **A**, p. 360). The **confrontation test** is an *informal* test in which the examiner (with an intact visual field) and the patient sit face-to-face, cover one eye, and each fixes their gaze on the other's open eye, creating identical visual axes. The examiner then moves his or her index finger from the outer edge of the visual field toward the center until the patient signals that he or she can see the finger. With this test the examiner can make a gross assessment as to the presence and approximate location of a possible visual field defect. The *precise* location and extent of a visual field defect can be determined by **perimetry**, in which points of light replace the examiner's finger. The results of the test are entered in charts that resemble the small diagrams in **C**.

C Topographic organization of the geniculate part of the visual pathway

The fovea centralis, the point of maximum visual acuity on the retina, has a high receptor density. Accordingly, a great many axons pass centrally from its receptors, and so the fovea centralis is represented by an exceptionally large area in the visual cortex. Other, more peripheral portions of the retina contain fewer receptors and therefore fewer axons, resulting in a smaller representational area in the visual cortex.

Note: Only the left half of the complete visual field is shown. It is subdivided into four quadrants (clockwise from top left in 1): upper temporal, upper nasal, lower nasal, and lower temporal. The representation of this subdivision is continued into the visual cortex.

1 The three zones that make up a particular **visual hemifield** (left, in this case) are each indicated by color shading of decreasing intensity:

- The smallest and darkest zone is at the center of the fovea centralis; it corresponds to the central visual field.
- The largest zone is the macular visual field, which also contains the "blind spot" (= optic disk, see **2**).
- The "temporal crescent" represents the temporal, monocular part of the visual field.
- Note that the lower nasal quadrant of each visual field is indented by the nose (small medial depression).

2 Because all light that reaches the retina must first pass through the narrow pupil (which is like the aperture of a camera), up/down and temporal/nasal are exactly reversed when the image is projected onto the **retina**.

3, 4 In the initial part of the optic nerve, the fibers that represent the macular visual field first occupy a lateral position (**3**) and then move increasingly toward the center of the nerve (**4**).

5 In traversing the **optic chiasm**, the nasal fibers of the optic nerve cross the midline to the opposite side.

6 At the **start of the optic tract**, the fibers from the corresponding halves of the retinae unite — the right halves of the retinae in the right tract, the left halves in the left tract. The impulses from the right visual field finally terminate in the left striate area. Initially the macular fibers continue to occupy a central position in the optic tract.

7 At the **end of the optic tract**, just before it enters the lateral geniculate body, the fibers are collected to form a wedge.

8 In the **lateral geniculate body**, the wedge shape is preserved, the macular fibers occupying almost half the wedge. After the fibers are relayed to the fourth neuron, they project to the posterior end of the occipital pole (= visual cortex).

9 This figure shows that the central part of the visual field is represented by the largest area in the **visual cortex** compared with other portions of the field. This is due to the large number of axons that run to the optic nerve from the fovea centralis. This large proportion of axons is continued into the visual cortex, establishing a point-to-point (retinotopic) correlation between the fovea centralis and the visual cortex. The other parts of the visual field also show a point-to-point correlation but have fewer axons. The central lower half of the visual field is represented by a large area on the occipital pole above the calcarine sulcus, while the central upper half of the visual field is represented below the sulcus. The region of central vision also occupies the largest area within the lateral geniculate body (see **8**).

12.18 Visual System, Lesions and Nongeniculate Part

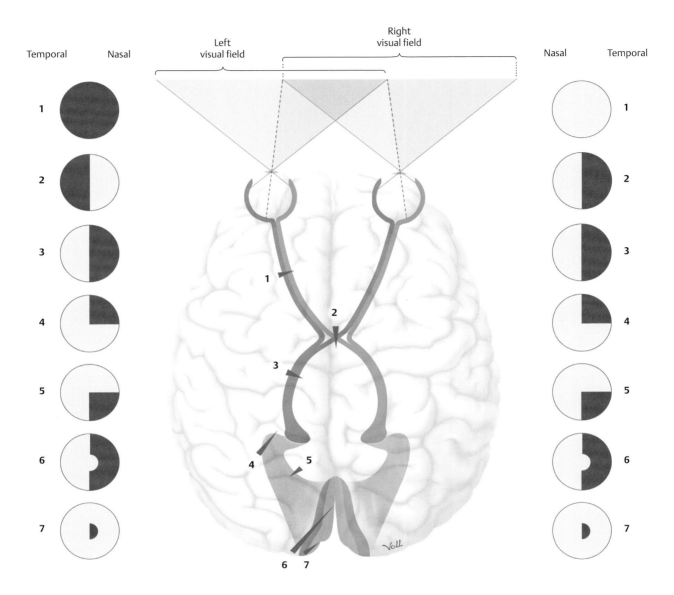

A Visual field defects (scotomata) and their location along the visual pathway

Visual field defects and lesion sites are illustrated here for the left visual pathway. Lesions of the visual pathway may result from a large number of neurological diseases. The patient perceives the lesion as a visual disturbance. Because the nature of the visual field defect often points to the location of the lesion, it is clinically important to know the patterns of defects that may be encountered. Division of the visual field into four quadrants is helpful in determining the location of a lesion. The quadrants are designated as upper and lower temporal, and upper and lower nasal (see also p. 359).

1 A unilateral optic nerve lesion produces blindness (amaurosis) in the affected eye only.
2 A lesion of the optic chiasm causes bitemporal hemianopia (as in a horse wearing blinders) because it interrupts the fibers from the nasal portions of the retina (the only ones that cross in the optic chiasm), which represent the temporal visual fields
3 A unilateral lesion of the optic tract causes contralateral homonymous hemianopia because it interrupts fibers from the *temporal* portions of the retina on the ipsilateral side and the *nasal* portions on the opposite side. Thus the right or left half of the visual field is affected in each eye.

Note: All homonymous visual field defects are caused by a retrochiasmal lesion.

4 A unilateral lesion of the optic radiation in the anterior temporal lobe (Meyer's loop) leads to contralateral upper quadrantanopia (a "pie-in-the sky"deficit). This occurs because the affected fibers wind around the inferior horn of the lateral ventricle in the temporal lobe and are separated from the fibers that come from the lower half of the visual field (see p. 358).
5 A unilateral lesion in the medial part of the optic radiation in the parietal lobe leads to contralateral lower quadrantanopia. This occurs because the fibers course superior to those for the upper quadrant in Meyer's loop (see p. 358).
6 A lesion of the occipital lobe leads to homonymous hemianopia. Because the optic radiation fans out widely before entering the visual cortex, lesions of the occipital lobe have been described that spare foveal vision. These lesions are most commonly due to intracerebral hemorrhage. The visual field defects may vary considerably because of the variable size of the hemorrhage.
7 A lesion confined to the cortical areas of the occipital pole, which represent the macula, is characterized by a homonymous hemianopic central scotoma.

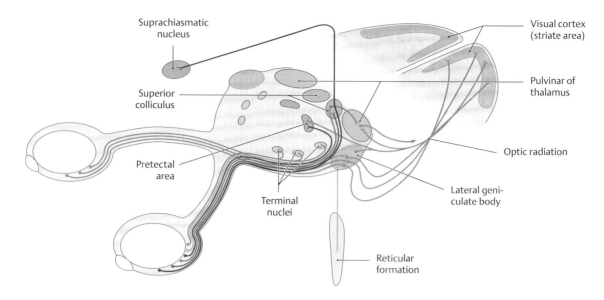

B Nongeniculate part of the visual pathway

Approximately 10% of the axons of the optic nerve do not terminate on neurons in the lateral geniculate body for projection to the visual cortex. They continue along the medial root of the optic tract, forming the *nongeniculate part* of the visual pathway. The information from these fibers is not processed at a conscious level but plays an important role in the unconscious regulation of various vision-related processes and in visually mediated reflexes (e.g., the afferent limb of the pupillary light reflex). Axons from the nongeniculate part of the visual pathway terminate in the following regions:

- Axons to the superior colliculus: transmit kinetic information that is necessary for tracking moving objects by unconscious eye and head movements (retinotectal system).

- Axons to the pretectal area: afferents for pupillary responses and accommodation reflexes (retinopretectal system). Subdivision into

specific nuclei has not yet been accomplished in humans, and so the term "area" is used.

- Axons to the suprachiasmatic nucleus of the hypothalamus: influence circadian rhythms.
- Axons to the thalamic nuclei (optic tract) in the tegmentum of the mesencephalon and to the vestibular nuclei: afferent fibers for optokinetic nystagmus (= jerky, physiological eye movements during the tracking of fast-moving objects). This has also been called the "accessory visual system."
- Axons to the pulvinar of the thalamus: visual association cortex for oculomotor function (neurons are relayed in the superior colliculus).
- Axons to the parvocellular nucleus of the reticular formation: arousal function.

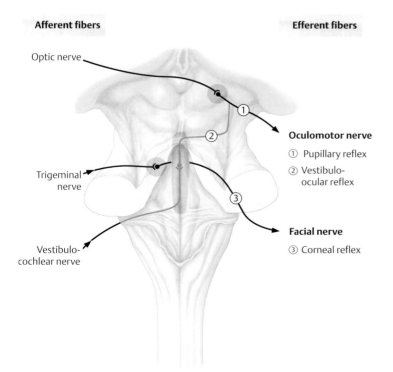

C Brainstem reflexes: clinical importance of the nongeniculate part of the visual pathway

Brainstem reflexes are important in the examination of comatose patients. Loss of all brainstem reflexes is considered evidence of brain death. Three of these reflexes are described below:

Pupillary reflex: The pupillary reflex relies on the nongeniculate parts of the visual pathway (see p. 363). The afferent fibers for this reflex come from the optic nerve, which is an extension of the diencephalon (since the diencephalon is not part of the brainstem, "brainstem reflex" is a somewhat unfortunate term). The efferents for the pupillary reflex come from the accessory nucleus of the oculomotor nerve (CN III), which is located in the brainstem. Loss of the pupillary reflex may signify a lesion of the diencephalon (interbrain) or mesencephalon (midbrain).

Vestibulo-ocular reflex: Irrigating the ear canal with cold water in a normal individual evokes nystagmus that beats toward the opposite side (afferent fibers are conveyed in the vestibulocochlear nerve = CN VIII, efferent fibers in the oculomotor nerve = CN III). When the vestibulo-ocular reflex is absent in a comatose patient, it is considered a poor sign because this reflex is the most reliable clinical test of brainstem function.

Corneal reflex: This reflex is not mediated by the visual pathway. The afferent fibers for the reflex (elicited by stimulation of the cornea, as by touching it with a sterile cotton wisp) are conveyed in the trigeminal nerve and the efferent fibers (contraction of the orbicularis oculi in response to corneal irritation) in the facial nerve. The relay center for the corneal reflex is located in the pontine region of the brainstem.

361

12.19 Visual System: Reflexes

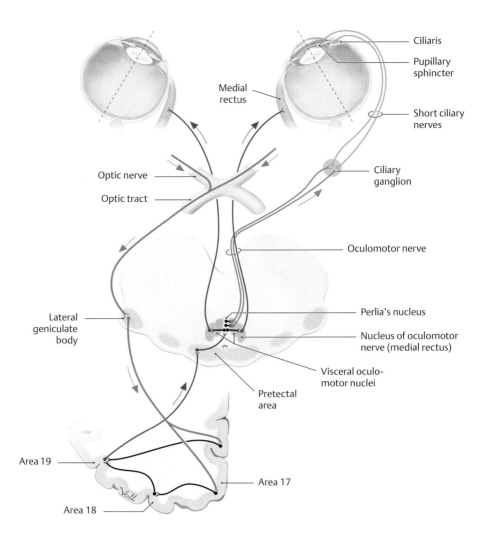

Ciliaris

Pupillary sphincter

Medial rectus

Short ciliary nerves

Optic nerve

Optic tract

Ciliary ganglion

Oculomotor nerve

Lateral geniculate body

Perlia's nucleus

Nucleus of oculomotor nerve (medial rectus)

Visceral oculo-motor nuclei

Pretectal area

Area 19

Area 17

Area 18

A Pathways for convergence and accommodation

When the head moves closer to an object, the visual axes of the eyes must move closer together (convergence) and *simultaneously* the lenses must adjust their focal length (accommodation). Both processes are necessary for a sharp, three-dimensional visual impression. Three sub-processes can be identified in convergence and accommodation:

1. In **convergence**, the two medial rectus muscles move the ocular axis inward to keep the image of the approaching object on the fovea centralis.
2. In **accommodation**, the curvature of the lens is increased to keep the image of the object sharply focused on the retina. The lens is flattened by contraction of the lenticular fibers, which are attached to the cili-ary muscle. When the ciliary muscle contracts during accommoda-tion, it relaxes the tension on the lenticular fibers, and the intrinsic pressure of the lens causes it to assume a more rounded shape.
3. The pupil is constricted by the sphincter pupillae to increase visual acuity.

Convergence and accommodation may be conscious (fixing the gaze on a near object) or unconscious (fixing the gaze on an approaching au-tomobile). Most of the axons of the third neuron in the visual pathway course in the optic nerve to the lateral geniculate body. There they are relayed to the fourth neuron, whose axons project to the primary visual cortex (area 17). Axons from the secondary visual area (19) finally reach

the pretectal area by way of synaptic relays and interneurons. Another relay occurs at that level, and the axons from these neurons terminate in Perlia's nucleus, which is located between the two Edinger-Westphal nuclei (= visceral oculomotor nuclei). Two functionally distinct groups of neurons are located in Perlia's nucleus:

- For accommodation, one group of neurons relays impulses to the *somatomotor* oculomotor nucleus, whose axons pass directly to the medial rectus muscle.
- The other group relays the neurons responsible for accommoda-tion and pupillary constriction to the *visceromotor* (parasympathetic) accessory nuclei of the oculomotor nerve (parasympathetic inner-vation is illustrated here for one side only).

After synapsing in this nuclear region, the preganglionic parasympa-thetic axons pass to the ciliary ganglion, where the central neuron synapses with the peripheral parasympathetic neuron. Again, two groups of neurons are distinguished: one passes to the ciliary muscle (accommodation) and the other to the pupillary sphincter (pupillary constriction). The pupillary sphincter light response is abolished in ter-tiary syphilis, while accommodation (ciliary muscle) and convergence are preserved. This phenomenon, called an Argyll Robertson pupil, sug-gests that the connections to the ciliary and pupillary sphincter muscles are mediated by different tracts, although the anatomy of these tracts is not yet fully understood.

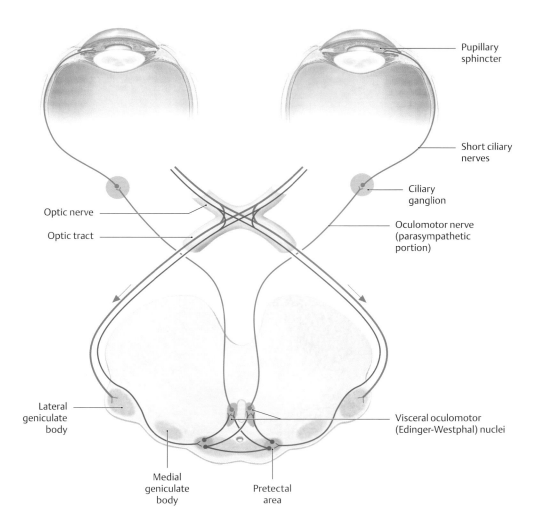

Pupillary sphincter

Short ciliary nerves

Ciliary ganglion

Oculomotor nerve (parasympathetic portion)

Optic nerve

Optic tract

Lateral geniculate body

Visceral oculomotor (Edinger-Westphal) nuclei

Medial geniculate body

Pretectal area

B Regulation of pupillary size—the light reflex

The pupillary light reflex enables the eye to adapt to varying levels of brightness. When a large amount of light enters the eye, like the beam of a flashlight, the pupil constricts (to protect the photoreceptors in the retina); when the light fades, the pupil dilates. As the term "reflex" implies, this adaptation takes place without conscious input (*nongeniculate* part of the visual pathway).

Afferent limb of the light reflex: The first three neurons (first neurons: rods and cones; second neurons: bipolar cells; third neurons: ganglion cells) in the *afferent* limb of the light reflex are located in the retina. The axons from the ganglion cells form the optic nerve. The axons responsible for the light reflex (light blue) pass to the pretectal area (nongeniculate part of the visual pathway) in the medial root of the optic tract. The other axons pass to the lateral geniculate body (dark blue). After synapsing in the pretectal nucleus, the axons from the fourth neurons pass to the parasympathetic nuclei (accessory nuclei of the oculomotor nerve = Edinger-Westphal nuclei) of the oculomotor nerve. Because both sides are innervated, a *consensual light response* can occur (see below).

Efferent limb of the light reflex: The fifth neurons located in the Edinger-Westphal nucleus (*central* parasympathetic neurons) distribute their axons to the ciliary ganglion. There they are relayed to the sixth neurons (*peripheral* parasympathetic neurons), whose axons then pass to the pupillary sphincter.

The *direct* pupillary light response is distinguished from the *indirect* response:

The **direct light response** is tested by covering both eyes of the conscious, cooperative patient and then uncovering one eye. After a short latency period, the pupil of the light-exposed eye will contract.

To test the **indirect light response**, the examiner places his hand on the bridge of the patient's nose, shading one eye from the beam of a flashlight while shining it into the other eye. The object is to test whether shining the light into one eye will cause the pupil of the shaded eye to contract as well (*consensual light response*).

Loss of the light response due to certain lesions: With a unilateral optic nerve lesion, shining a light into the *affected* side will induce no direct light response on the affected side. The consensual light response on the opposite side will also be lost because of impairment of the afferent limb of the light response on the affected side. Illumination of the *unaffected* side will, of course, elicit pupillary contraction on that side (direct light response). A consensual light response is also present because the afferent signals for this reflex are mediated by the unaffected side while the efferent signals are not mediated by the optic nerve. With a lesion of the parasympathetic oculomotor nucleus or ciliary ganglion, the efferent limb of the reflex is lost. In either case the patient has no direct or indirect pupillary light response on the affected side. A lesion of the optic radiation or visual cortex (*geniculate* part of the visual pathway) does not abolish this reflex, as it will affect only the geniculate part of the visual pathway.

12.20 **Visual System:**
Coordination of Eye Movement

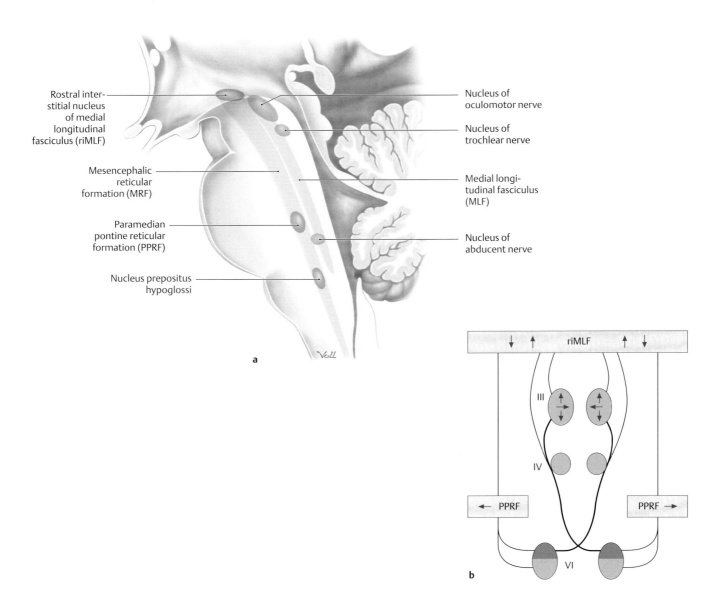

Rostral inter-
stitial nucleus
of medial
longitudinal
fasciculus (riMLF)

Mesencephalic
reticular
formation (MRF)

Paramedian
pontine reticular
formation (PPRF)

Nucleus prepositus
hypoglossi

Nucleus of
oculomotor nerve

Nucleus of
trochlear nerve

Medial longi-
tudinal fasciculus
(MLF)

Nucleus of
abducent nerve

a

riMLF

III

IV

PPRF   PPRF

VI

b

A Oculomotor nuclei and their higher connections in the brainstem

a Midsagittal section viewed from the left side. **b** Circuit diagram showing the supranuclear organization of eye movements.

When we shift our gaze to a new object, we swiftly move the axis of vision of our eyes toward the intended target. These rapid, precise, "ballistic" eye movements are called *saccades*. They are preprogrammed and, once initiated, cannot be altered until the end of the saccadic movement. The nuclei of all the nerves that supply the eye muscles (nuclei of cranial nerves III, IV, and VI, shaded red) are involved in carrying out these movements. They are interconnected for this purpose by the *medial longitudinal fasciculus* (shaded blue; see **B** for its location). Because these complex movements essentially involve all of the extraocular muscles and the nerves supplying them, the activity of the nuclei must be coordinated at a higher or *supranuclear* level. This means, for

example, that when we gaze to the right with the *right* eye, the right lateral rectus muscle (CN VI, abducent nucleus activated) must contract while the right medial rectus muscle (CN III, oculomotor nucleus inhibited) must relax. For the *left* eye, the left lateral rectus (CN VI) must relax while the left medial rectus (CN III) must contract. Movements of this kind that involve both eyes are called *conjugate eye movements*. These movements are coordinated by several centers (premotor nuclei, shaded purple). Horizontal gaze movements are programmed in the nuclear region of the paramedian pontine reticular formation (PPRF), while vertical gaze movements are programmed in the rostral interstitial nucleus of the medial longitudinal fasciculus (riMLF). Both gaze centers establish bilateral connections with the nuclei of cranial nerves III, IV, and VI. The tonic signals for maintaining the new eye position originate from the nucleus prepositus hypoglossi (see **a**).

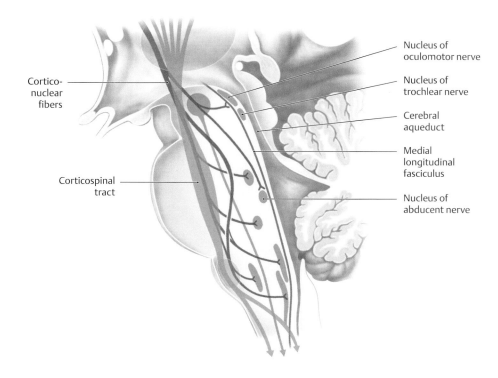

Cortico-nuclear fibers

Corticospinal tract

Nucleus of oculomotor nerve

Nucleus of trochlear nerve

Cerebral aqueduct

Medial longitudinal fasciculus

Nucleus of abducent nerve

B Course of the medial longitudinal fasciculus in the brainstem

Midsagittal section viewed from the left side. The medial longitudinal fasciculus runs anterior to the cerebral aqueduct on both sides and continues from the mesencephalon to the cervical spinal cord. It transmits fibers for the coordination of conjugate eye movements. A lesion of the MLF results in internuclear ophthalmoplegia (see **C**).

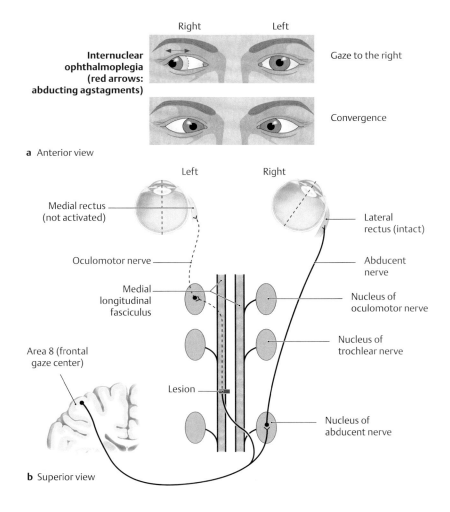

Right   Left

Internuclear ophthalmoplegia (red arrows: abducting agstagments)

Gaze to the right

Convergence

a Anterior view

Left   Right

Medial rectus (not activated)

Oculomotor nerve

Medial longitudinal fasciculus

Area 8 (frontal gaze center)

Lesion

Lateral rectus (intact)

Abducent nerve

Nucleus of oculomotor nerve

Nucleus of trochlear nerve

Nucleus of abducent nerve

b Superior view

C Lesion of the medial longitudinal fasciculus and internuclear ophthalmoplegia

The medial longitudinal fasciculus interconnects the oculomotor nuclei and also connects them with the opposite side (**b**). When this "information highway" is interrupted, internuclear ophthalmoplegia develops. This type of lesion most commonly occurs between the nucleus of the abducent nerve and the oculomotor nucleus. It may be unilateral or bilateral. Typical causes are multiple sclerosis and diminished blood flow. The lesion is manifested by the loss of conjugate eye movements (**a**). With a lesion of the left medial longitudinal fasciculus, as shown here, the left medial rectus muscle is no longer activated during gaze to the right. The eye cannot be moved *inward* on the side of the lesion (loss of the medial rectus), and the opposite eye goes into an abducting nystagmus (lateral rectus is intact and innervated by the abducent nerve). Reflex movements such as convergence are not impaired, as there is no peripheral or nuclear lesion and this reaction is not mediated by the medial longitudinal fasciculus.

365

12.21 Auditory Pathway

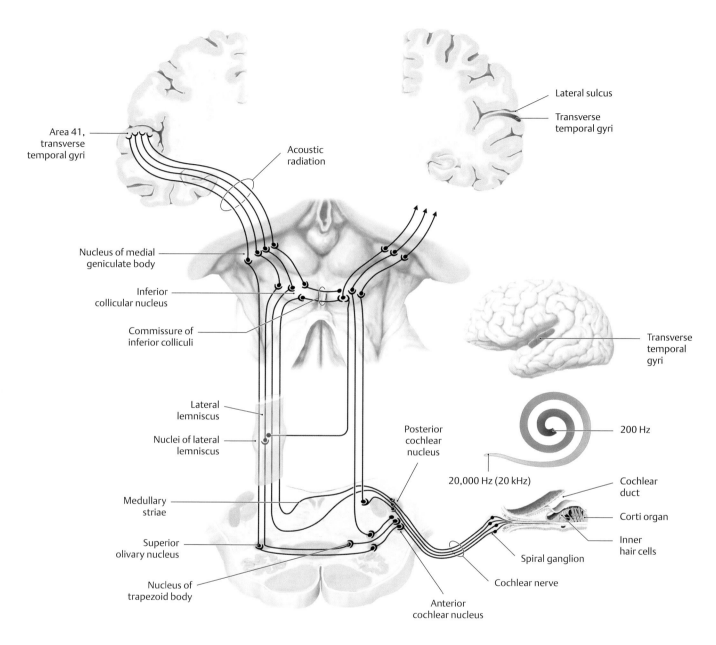

Area 41, transverse temporal gyri

Acoustic radiation

Lateral sulcus

Transverse temporal gyri

Nucleus of medial geniculate body

Inferior collicular nucleus

Commissure of inferior colliculi

Transverse temporal gyri

Lateral lemniscus

Nuclei of lateral lemniscus

Posterior cochlear nucleus

200 Hz

20,000 Hz (20 kHz)

Cochlear duct

Medullary striae

Corti organ

Inner hair cells

Superior olivary nucleus

Spiral ganglion

Nucleus of trapezoid body

Cochlear nerve

Anterior cochlear nucleus

A Afferent auditory pathway of the left ear

The receptors of the auditory pathway are the inner hair cells of the organ of Corti. Because they lack neural processes, they are called *secondary sensory cells*. They are located in the cochlear duct of the basilar membrane and are studded with stereocilia, which are exposed to shearing forces from the tectorial membrane in response to a traveling wave. This causes bowing of the stereocilia (see p. 151). These bowing movements act as a stimulus to evoke cascades of neural signals. Dendritic processes of the bipolar neurons in the spiral ganglion pick up the stimulus. The bipolar neurons then transmit impulses via their axons, which are collected to form the cochlear nerve, to the anterior and posterior cochlear nuclei. In these nuclei the signals are relayed to the second neuron of the auditory pathway. Information from the cochlear nuclei is then transmitted via 4–6 nuclei to the primary auditory cortex, where the auditory information is consciously perceived (analogous to the visual cortex). The primary auditory cortex is located in the transverse temporal gyri (Heschl gyri, Brodmann area 41). The auditory pathway thus contains the following key stations:

- Inner hair cells in the organ of Corti
- Spiral ganglion
- Anterior and posterior cochlear nuclei
- Nucleus of the trapezoid body and superior olivary nucleus
- Nucleus of the lateral lemniscus
- Inferior collicular nucleus
- Nucleus of medial geniculate body
- Primary auditory cortex in the temporal lobe (transverse temporal gyri = Heschl gyri or Brodmann area 41)

The individual parts of the cochlea are correlated with specific areas in the auditory cortex and its relay stations. This is known as the *tonotopic organization of the auditory pathway*. This organizational principle is similar to that in the visual pathway. Binaural processing of the auditory information (= stereo hearing) first occurs at the level of the superior olivary nucleus. At all further stages of the auditory pathway there are also interconnections between the right and left sides of the auditory pathway (for clarity, these are not shown here). A cochlea that has ceased to function can sometimes be replaced with a cochlear implant.

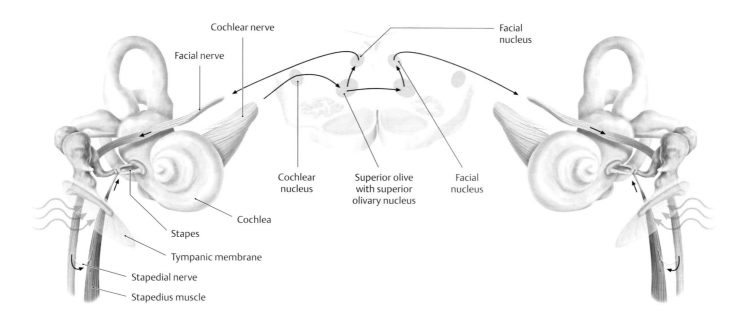

B The stapedius reflex

When the volume of an acoustic signal reaches a certain threshold, the stapedius reflex triggers a contraction of the stapedius muscle. This reflex can be utilized to test hearing without the patient's cooperation ("objective" auditory testing). The test is done by introducing a sonic probe into the ear canal and presenting a test noise to the tympanic membrane. When the noise volume reaches a certain threshold, it evo-

kes the stapedius reflex and the tympanic membrane stiffens. The change in the resistance of the tympanic membrane is then measured and recorded. The *afferent* limb of this reflex is in the cochlear nerve. Information is conveyed to the facial nucleus on each side by way of the superior olivary nucleus. The *efferent* limb of this reflex is formed by special visceromotor fibers of the facial nerve.

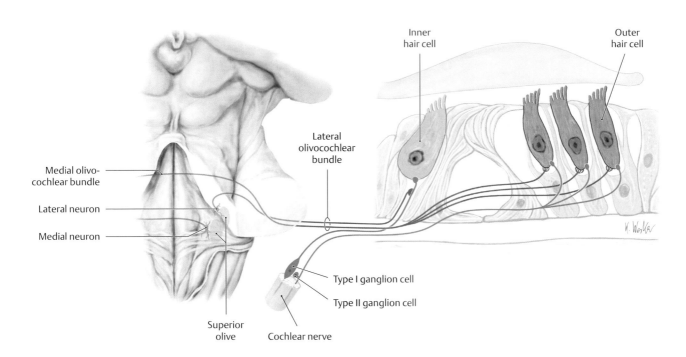

C Efferent fibers from the olive to the Corti organ

Besides the afferent fibers from the organ of Corti (see **A**, shown here in blue), which form the vestibulocochlear nerve, there are also efferent fibers (red) that pass to the organ of Corti in the inner ear and are concerned with the active preprocessing of sound ("cochlear amplifier") and acoustic protection. The efferent fibers arise from neurons that are located in either the lateral or medial part of the superior olive and project from there to the cochlea (lateral or medial olivocochlear bundle). The

fibers of the lateral neurons pass *uncrossed* to the dendrites of the *inner* hair cells, while the fibers of the medial neurons *cross* to the opposite side and terminate at the base of the *outer* hair cells, whose activity they influence. When stimulated, the outer hair cells can actively amplify the traveling wave. This increases the sensitivity of the inner hair cells (the actual receptor cells). The activity of the efferents from the olive can be recorded as otoacoustic emissions (OAE). This test can be used to screen for hearing abnormalities in newborns.

12.22 **Vestibular System**

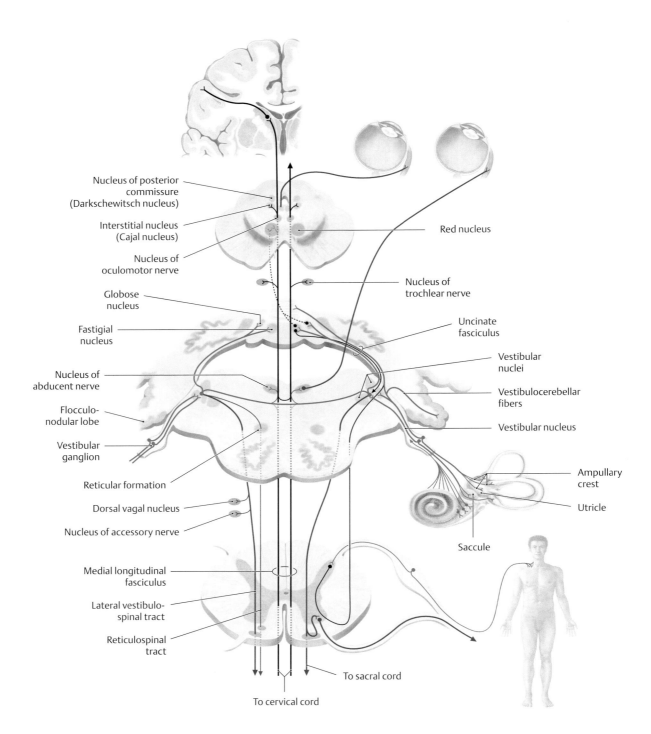

Nucleus of posterior commissure (Darkschewitsch nucleus)

Interstitial nucleus (Cajal nucleus)

Nucleus of oculomotor nerve

Globose nucleus

Fastigial nucleus

Nucleus of abducent nerve

Flocculo-nodular lobe

Vestibular ganglion

Reticular formation

Dorsal vagal nucleus

Nucleus of accessory nerve

Medial longitudinal fasciculus

Lateral vestibulo-spinal tract

Reticulospinal tract

Red nucleus

Nucleus of trochlear nerve

Uncinate fasciculus

Vestibular nuclei

Vestibulocerebellar fibers

Vestibular nucleus

Ampullary crest

Utricle

Saccule

To sacral cord

To cervical cord

A **Central connections of the vestibular nerve**

Three systems are involved in the regulation of human balance:

- Vestibular system
- Proprioceptive system
- Visual system

The latter two systems have already been described. The peripheral receptors of the *vestibular system* are located in the membranous labyrinth (see petrous bone, pp. 140, 152), which consists of ythe utricle and saccule and the ampullae of the three semicircular ducts. The maculae of the utricle and saccule respond to linear acceleration, while the semicircular duct organs in the ampullary crests respond to angular (rotational) acceleration. Like the hair cells of the inner ear, the receptors of the vestibular system are *secondary* sensory cells. The basal portions of

the secondary sensory cells are surrounded by dendritic processes of bipolar neurons. Their perikarya are located in the vestibular ganglion. The axons from these neurons form the vestibular nerve and terminate in the four vestibular nuclei (see **C**). Besides input from the vestibular apparatus, these nuclei also receive sensory input (see **B**). The vestibular nuclei show a topographical organization (see **C**) and distribute their efferent fibers to three targets:

- Motor neurons in the spinal cord via the lateral vestibulospinal tract . These motor neurons help to maintain upright stance, mainly by increasing the tone of extensor muscles.
- Flocculonodular lobe of the cerebellum (archicerebellum) via vestibulocerebellar fibers .
- Ipsilateral and contralateral oculomotor nuclei via the ascending part of the medial longitudinal fasciculus.

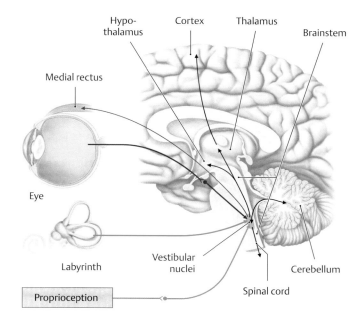

B Central role of the vestibular nuclei in the maintenance of balance

The afferent fibers that pass to the vestibular nuclei and the efferent fibers that emerge from them demonstrate the central role of these nuclei in maintaining balance. The vestibular nuclei receive afferent input from the vestibular system, proprioceptive system (position sense, muscles, and joints), and visual system. They then distribute efferent fibers to nuclei that control the motor systems important for balance. These nuclei are located in the:

- Spinal cord (motor support),
- Cerebellum (fine control of motor function), and
- Brainstem (oculomotor nuclei for oculomotor function).

Efferents from the vestibular nuclei are also distributed to the following regions:

- Thalamus and cortex (spatial sense)
- Hypothalamus (autonomic regulation: vomiting in response to vertigo)

Note: Acute failure of the vestibular system is manifested by rotary vertigo.

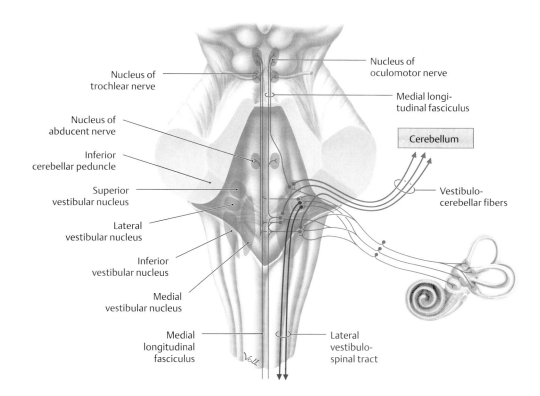

C Vestibular nuclei: topographic organization and central connections

Four nuclei are distinguished:

- Superior vestibular nucleus (of Bechterew)
- Lateral vestibular nucleus (of Deiters)
- Medial vestibular nucleus (of Schwalbe)
- Inferior vestibular nucleus (of Roller)

The vestibular system has a topographic organization:

- The afferent fibers of the saccular macula terminate in the inferior vestibular nucleus and lateral vestibular nucleus.
- The afferent fibers of the utricular macula terminate in the medial part of the inferior vestibular nucleus, the lateral part of the medial vestibular nucleus, and the lateral vestibular nucleus.

- The afferent fibers from the ampullary crests of the semicircular canals terminate in the superior vestibular nucleus, the upper part of the inferior vestibular nucleus, and the lateral vestibular nucleus.

The efferent fibers from the lateral vestibular nucleus pass to the lateral vestibulospinal tract. This tract extends to the sacral part of the spinal cord, its axons terminating on motor neurons. Functionally it is concerned with keeping the body upright, chiefly by increasing the tone of the extensor muscles. The vestibulocerebellar fibers from the other three nuclei act through the cerebellum to modulate muscular tone. All four vestibular nuclei distribute ipsilateral and contralateral axons via the medial longitudinal fasciculus to the three motor nuclei of the nerves to the extraocular muscles (i.e., the nuclei of the abducent, trochlear, and oculomotor nerves).

369

12.23 **Gustatory System (Taste)**

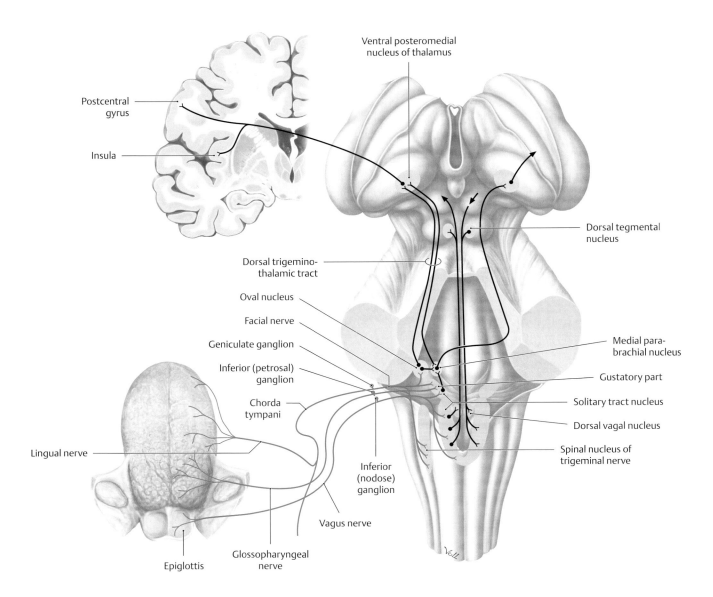

A Gustatory pathway

The receptors for the sense of taste are the taste buds of the tongue (see **B**). Unlike other receptor cells, the receptor cells of the taste buds are specialized epithelial cells (secondary sensory cells, as they do not have an axon). When these epithelial cells are chemically stimulated, the base of the cells releases glutamate, which stimulates the peripheral processes of afferent cranial nerves. These different cranial nerves serve different areas of the tongue. It is rare, therefore, for a complete loss of taste (ageusia) to occur.

- The *anterior two-thirds* of the tongue are supplied by the facial nerve (CN VII), the afferent fibers first passing in the lingual nerve (branch of the trigeminal nerve) and then in the chorda tympani to the geniculate ganglion of the facial nerve.
- The *posterior third of the tongue* and the *vallate papillae* are supplied by the glossopharyngeal nerve (CN IX).
- The *epiglottis* is supplied by the vagus nerve (CN X).

Peripheral processes from pseudounipolar ganglion cells (which correspond to pseudounipolar spinal ganglion cells) terminate on the taste buds. The central portions of these processes convey taste information to the gustatory part of the nucleus of the solitary tract. Thus, they function as the first afferent neuron of the gustatory pathway. Their

perikarya are located in the geniculate ganglion for the facial nerve, in the inferior (petrosal) ganglion for the glossopharyngeal nerve, and in the inferior (nodose) ganglion for the vagus nerve. After synapsing in the gustatory part of the nucleus of the solitary tract, the axons from the second neuron are believed to terminate in the medial parabrachial nucleus, where they are relayed to the third neuron. Most of the axons from the third neuron cross to the opposite side and pass in the dorsal trigeminothalamic tract to the contralateral ventral posteromedial nucleus of the thalamus. Some of the axons travel uncrossed in the same structures. The fourth neurons of the gustatory pathway, located in the thalamus, project to the postcentral gyrus and insular cortex, where the fifth neuron is located. Collaterals from the first and second neurons of the gustatory afferent pathway are distributed to the superior and inferior salivatory nuclei. Afferex impulses in these fibers induce the secretion of saliva during eating ("salivary reflex"). The parasympathetic preganglionic fibers exit the brainstem via cranial nerves VII and IX (see the descriptions of these cranial nerves for details). Besides this purely gustatory pathway, spicy foods may also stimulate trigeminal fibers (not shown), which contribute to the sensation of taste. Finally, olfaction (the sense of smell), too, is a major component of the sense of taste as it is subjectively perceived: patients who cannot smell (anosmosia) report that their food tastes abnormally bland.

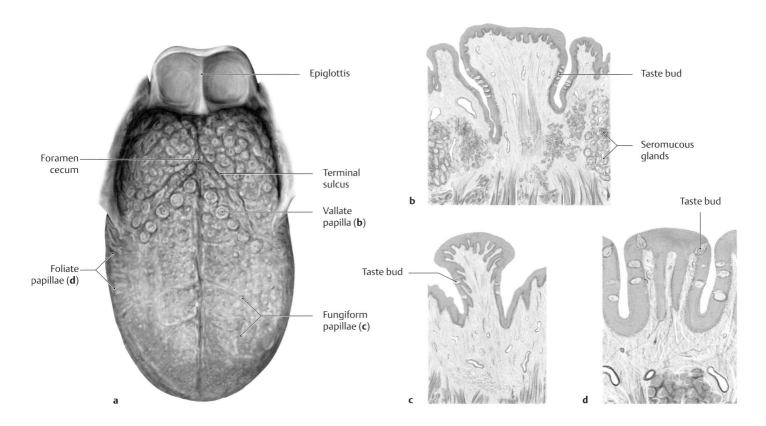

Epiglottis

Foramen cecum

Terminal sulcus

Vallate papilla (**b**)

Foliate papillae (**d**)

Fungiform papillae (**c**)

Taste bud

Seromucous glands

b

Taste bud

Taste bud

a

c

d

B Organization of the taste receptors in the tongue

The human tongue contains approximately 4600 taste buds in which the secondary sensory cells for taste perception are collected. The taste buds (see **C**) are embedded in the epithelium of the lingual mucosa and are located on the surface expansions of the lingual mucosa—the vallate papillae (principal site, **b**), the fungiform papillae (**c**), and the foliate papillae (**d**). Additionally, isolated taste buds are located in the mucous membranes of the soft palate and pharynx. The surrounding serous glands of the tongue (Ebner glands), which are most closely associated with the vallate papillae, constantly wash the taste buds clean to allow for new tasting. Humans can perceive five basic taste qualities: sweet, sour, salty, bitter, and a fifth "savory" quality, called umami, which is activated by glutamate (a taste enhancer).

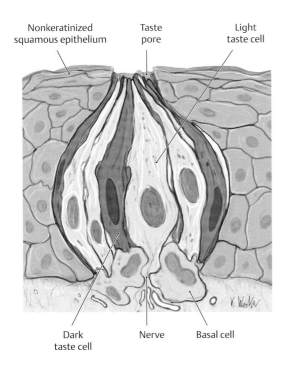

Nonkeratinized squamous epithelium

Taste pore

Light taste cell

Dark taste cell

Nerve

Basal cell

C Microscopic structure of a taste bud

Nerves induce the formation of taste buds in the oral mucosa. Axons of cranial nerves VII, IX, and X grow into the oral mucosa from the basal side and induce the epithelium to differentiate into the light and dark taste cells (= modified epithelial cells). Both types of taste cell have microvilli that extend to the gustatory pore. For sweet and salty, the taste cell is stimulated by hydrogen ions and other cations. The other taste qualities are mediated by receptor proteins to which the low-molecular-weight flavored substances bind (details may be found in textbooks of physiology). When the low-molecular-weight flavored substances bind to the receptor proteins, they induce signal transduction that causes the release of glutamate, which excites the peripheral processes of the pseudounipolar neurons of the three cranial nerve ganglia. The taste cells have a life span of approximately 12 days and regenerate from cells at the base of the taste buds, which differentiate into new taste cells.

Note: The old notion that particular areas of the tongue are sensitive to specific taste qualities has been found to be false.

12.24 **Olfactory System (Smell)**

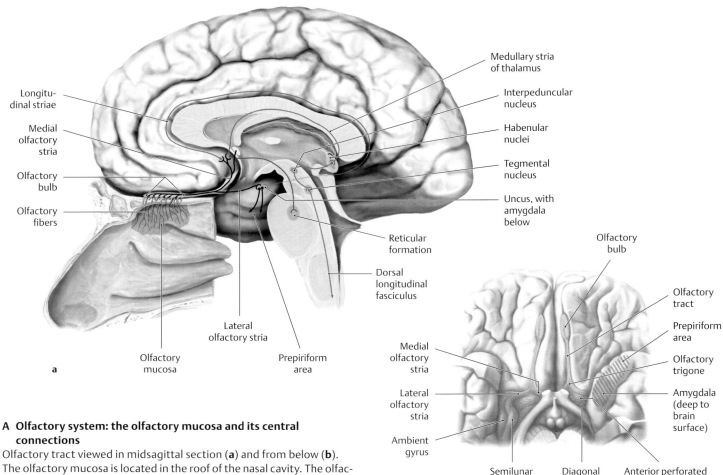

A Olfactory system: the olfactory mucosa and its central connections

Olfactory tract viewed in midsagittal section (**a**) and from below (**b**). The olfactory mucosa is located in the roof of the nasal cavity. The olfactory cells (= primary sensory cells) are bipolar neurons. Their peripheral receptor-bearing processes terminate in the epithelium of the nasal mucosa, while their central processes pass to the olfactory bulb (see **B** for details). The olfactory bulb, where the second neurons of the olfactory pathway (mitral and tufted cells) are located, is considered an extension of the telencephalon. The axons of these second neurons pass centrally as the *olfactory tract*. In front of the anterior perforated substance, the olfactory tract widens to form the olfactory trigone and splits into the lateral and medial olfactory striae.

- Some of the axons of the olfactory tract run in the **lateral olfactory stria** to the olfactory centers: the amygdala, semilunar gyrus, and ambient gyrus. The prepiriform area (Brodmann area 28) is considered to be the primary olfactory cortex in the strict sense. It contains the third neurons of the olfactory pathway.
  Note: The prepiriform area is shaded in **b**, lying at the junction of the basal side of the frontal lobe and the medial side of the temporal lobe.
- Other axons of the olfactory tract run in the **medial olfactory stria** to nuclei in the septal (subcallosal) area, which is part of the limbic system (see p. 374), and to the olfactory tubercle, a small elevation in the anterior perforated substance.
- Yet other axons of the olfactory tract terminate in the **anterior olfactory nucleus**, where the fibers that cross to the opposite side branch off and are relayed. This nucleus is located in the olfactory trigone, which lies between the two olfactory striae and in front of the anterior perforated substance.

Note: None of these three tracts are routed through the thalamus. Thus, the olfactory system is the only sensory system that is not relayed in the thalamus before reaching the cortex. There is, however, an indirect route from the primary olfactory cortex to the neocortex passing throug the thalamus and terminating in the basal forebrain. The olfactory signals are further analyzed in these basal portions of the forebrain (not shown).

The olfactory system is linked to other brain areas well beyond the primary olfactory cortical areas, with the result that olfactory stimuli can evoke complex emotional and behavioral responses. Noxious smells may induce nausea, while appetizing smells evoke watering of the mouth. Presumably these sensations are processed by the hypothalamus, thalamus, and limbic system (see next unit) via connections established mainly by the medial forebrain bundle and the medullary striae of the thalamus. The medial forebrain bundle distributes axons to the following structures:

- Hypothalamic nuclei
- Reticular formation
- Salivatory nuclei
- Dorsal vagal nucleus

The axons that run in the medullary striae of the thalamus terminate in the habenular nuclei. This tract also continues to the brainstem, where it stimulates salivation in response to smell.

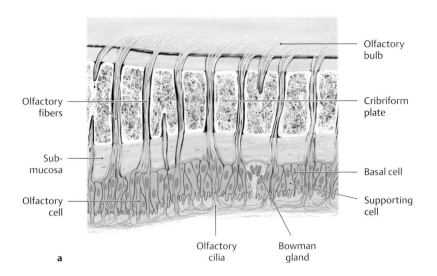

Olfactory fibers
Sub-mucosa
Olfactory cell
Olfactory bulb
Cribriform plate
Basal cell
Supporting cell
Olfactory cilia
Bowman gland

a

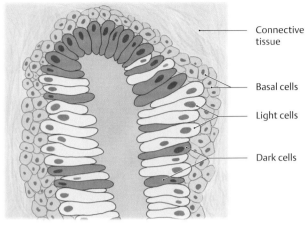

Connective tissue
Basal cells
Light cells
Dark cells

c

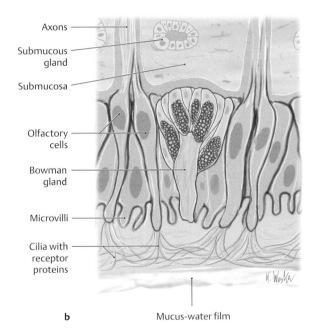

Axons
Submucous gland
Submucosa
Olfactory cells
Bowman gland
Microvilli
Cilia with receptor proteins
Mucus-water film

b

B Olfactory mucosa and vomeronasal organ (VNO)

The **olfactory mucosa** occupies an area of approximately 2 cm² on the roof of each nasal cavity, and 10^7 primary sensory cells are concentrated in each of these areas (**a**). At the molecular level, the olfactory receptor proteins are located in the cilia of the sensory cells (**b**). Each sensory cell has only one specialized receptor protein that mediates signal transduction when an odorant molecule binds to it. Although humans are microsmatic, having a sense of smell that is feeble compared with other mammals, the olfactory receptor proteins still make up 2 % of the human genome. This underscores the importance of olfaction in humans. The primary olfactory sensory cells have a life span of approximately 60 days and regenerate from the basal cells (life-long division of neurons). The bundled central processes (axons) from hundreds of olfactory cells form olfactory fibers (**a**) that pass through the cribriform plate of the ethmoid bone and terminate in the *olfactory bulb* (see **C**), which lies above the cribriform plate. The vomeronasal organ (**c**) is located on both sides of the anterior nasal septum. Its central connections in humans are unknown. It responds to steroids and evokes unconscious reactions in subjects (possibly influences the choice of a mate). Mate selection in many animal species is known to be mediated by olfactory impulses that are perceived in the vomeronasal organ.

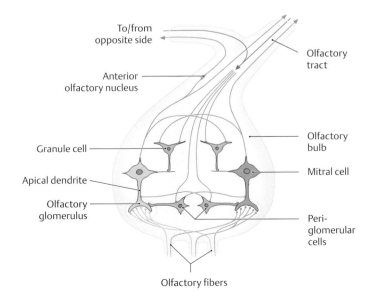

To/from opposite side
Anterior olfactory nucleus
Granule cell
Apical dendrite
Olfactory glomerulus
Olfactory fibers
Olfactory tract
Olfactory bulb
Mitral cell
Peri-glomerular cells

C Synaptic patterns in an olfactory bulb

Specialized neurons in the olfactory bulb, called mitral cells, form apical dendrites that receive synaptic contact from the axons of thousands of primary sensory cells. The dendrite plus the synapses make up the *olfactory glomeruli*. Axons from sensory cells with the same receptor protein form glomeruli with only one or a small number of mitral cells. The basal axons of the mitral cells form the olfactory tract. The axons that run in the olfactory tract project primarily to the olfactory cortex but are also distributed to other nuclei in the CNS. The axon collaterals of the mitral cells pass to granule cells: both granule cells and periglomerular cells inhibit the activity of the mitral cells, causing less sensory information to reach higher centers. These inhibitory processes are believed to heighten olfactory contrast, which aids in the more accurate perception of smells. The tufted cells, which also project to the primary olfactory cortex, are not shown.

373

12.25 **Limbic System**

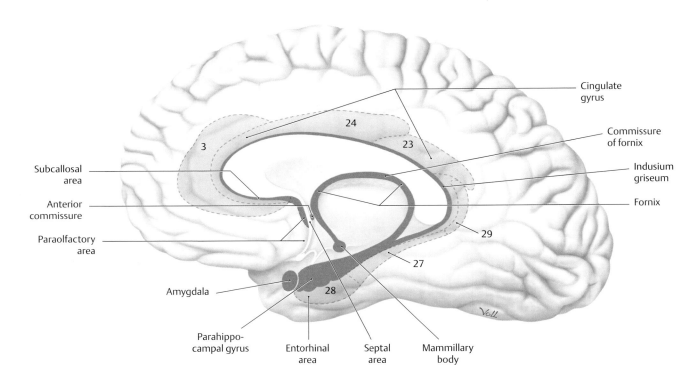

Cingulate gyrus

Commissure of fornix

Indusium griseum

Fornix

Subcallosal area

Anterior commissure

Paraolfactory area

Amygdala

Parahippo-campal gyrus

Entorhinal area

Septal area

Mammillary body

A Limbic system viewed through the partially transparent cortex
Medial view of the right hemisphere. The term "limbic system" (Latin *limbus* = "border" or "fringe") was first used by Broca in 1878, who collectively described the gyri surrounding the corpus callosum, diencephalon, and basal ganglia as the *grand lobe limbique*. The limbic system encompasses neo-, archi- and paleocortical regions as well as subcortical nuclei. The anatomical extent of the limbic system is such that it can exchange and integrate information between the telencephalon (cerebral cortex), diencephalon, and mesencephalon. Viewed from the medial aspect of the cerebral hemispheres, the limbic system is seen to consist of an inner arc and an outer arc. The outer arc is formed by:

- Parahippocampal gyrus,
- Cingulate gyrus (also called the limbic gyrus),
- Subcallosal area (paraolfactory area), and
- Indusium griseum.

The inner arc is formed by:

- Hippocampal formation,
- Fornix,
- Septal area (also known simply as the septum),
- Diagonal band of Broca (not visible in this view), and
- Paraterminal gyrus.

The limbic system also includes the amygdalae and mammillary bodies. The following nuclei are also considered part of the limbic system but are not shown: the anterior thalamic nucleus, habenular nucleus, dorsal tegmental nucleus, and interpeduncular nucleus.
The limbic system is concerned with the regulation of drive and affective behavior and plays a crucial role in memory and learning. The numbers in the diagram indicate the Brodmann areas.

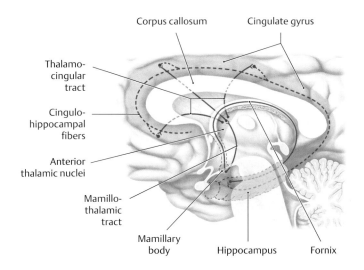

Corpus callosum

Cingulate gyrus

Thalamo-cingular tract

Cingulo-hippocampal fibers

Anterior thalamic nuclei

Mamillo-thalamic tract

Mamillary body

Hippocampus

Fornix

B Neuronal circuit (Papez circuit)
View of the medial surface of the right hemisphere. Several nuclei of the limbic system are interconnected by a *neuronal circuit* (see below) called the Papez circuit after the anatomist who first described it. The sequence below indicates the nuclei (normal print) and tracts (*italic print*) that are the successive stations of this neuronal circuit:

Hippocampus → *fornix* → mammillary body → *mammillothalamic tract* (Vicq d'Azyr bundle) → anterior thalamic nuclei → *thalamocingular tract (radiation)* → cingulate gyrus → *cingulohippocampal fibers* → hippocampus.

This neuronal circuit interconnects ontogenically distinct parts of the limbic system. It establishes a connection between information stored in the unconscious and conscious behavior.

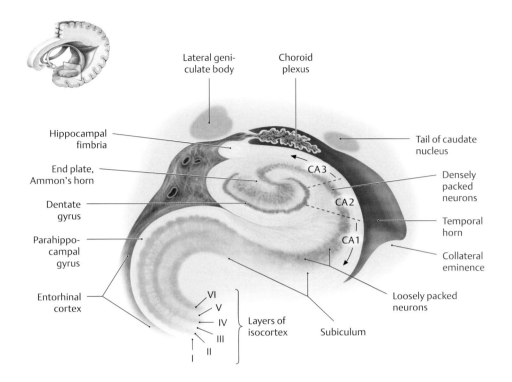

Lateral geni-culate body

Choroid plexus

Hippocampal fimbria

End plate, Ammon's horn

Dentate gyrus

Parahippo-campal gyrus

Entorhinal cortex

Tail of caudate nucleus

CA3

CA2

Densely packed neurons

CA1

Temporal horn

Collateral eminence

Loosely packed neurons

VI
V
IV
III
II
I

Layers of isocortex

Subiculum

C Cytoarchitecture of the hippocampal formation (after Bähr and Frotscher)

View from anterior left.

Note: The hippocampal formation has a three-layered allocortex instead of a six-layered iso-cortex (lower left in diagram). It is a phylogenet-ically older structure than the isocortex. At the center of the allocortex is a band of neurons that forms the neuronal layer of the hippocampus (= hippocampus proper = Ammon's horn). The neurons in this layer are mainly pyramidal cells. Three regions, designated CA1–CA3, can be distinguished based on differences in the density of the pyramidal cells. *Region CA 1,* called also the "Sommer sector," is important in neuropathology, as the death of neurons in this sector is the first morphologically de-tectable sign of cerebral hypoxia. Besides the hippocampus proper, we can also identify the cellular sheet of the dentate gyrus (dentate fascia), which consists mainly of granule cells.

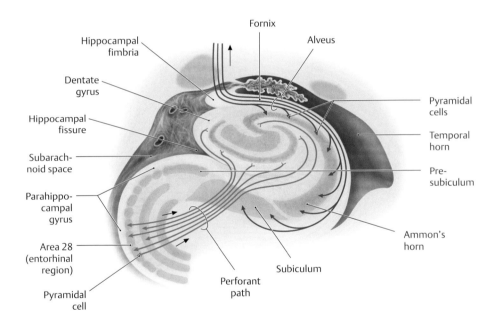

Fornix

Alveus

Hippocampal fimbria

Dentate gyrus

Hippocampal fissure

Subarach-noid space

Parahippo-campal gyrus

Area 28 (entorhinal region)

Pyramidal cell

Perforant path

Subiculum

Pyramidal cells

Temporal horn

Pre-subiculum

Ammon's horn

D Connections of the hippocampus

Left anterior view. The most important affer-ent pathway to the hippocampus is the *perforant path* (blue), which extends from the entorhinal region (triangular pyramidal cells of Brodmann area 28) to the hippo-campus (where it ends in a synapse). The neu-rons that project from area 28 into the hippo-campus receive afferent input from many brain regions. Thus, the entorhinal region is consid-ered the gateway to the hippocampus. The pyramidal cells of Ammon's horn (triangles) send their axons into the fornix, and the axons transmitted via the fornix continue to the mammillary body (Papez neuronal circuit) or to the septal nuclei.

E Important definitions pertaining to the limbic system

Archicortex

Phylogenetically old structures of the cerebral cortex; does not have a six-layered architecture

Hippocampus (retrocommissural)

Ammon's horn (hippocampus proper), dentate gyrus (dentate fascia), subiculum (some authors consider it part of the hippocampal formation rather than the hippocampus itself)

Hippocampal formation

Hippocampus plus the entorhinal area of the parahippocampal gyrus

Limbic system

Important coordinating system for memory and emotions. Includes the following *telencephalic* structures: cingulate gyrus, parahippocampal gyrus, hippocampal formation, septal nuclei, and amygdala. Its *diencephalic* components include the anterior thalamic nucleus, mammillary bodies, nucleus accumbens, and habenular nucleus. Its *brainstem* components are the raphe nuclei. The medial forebrain bundle and the dorsal longitudinal fasciculus contribute to the fiber tracts of the limbic system.

Periarchicortex

A broad transitional zone around the hippocampus, consisting of the cingulate gyrus, the isthmus of the cingulate gyrus, and the parahippo-campal gyrus

12.26 **Brain: Fiber Tracts**

A Fiber tracts

Fiber tracts are the "information highways" of the white matter of the brain and spinal cord. The most important terms pertaining to CNS fiber tracts are listed in the table.

Projection fibers	Connect the cerebral cortex to subcortical centers, either ascending or descending
• **Ascending fibers**	Connect subcortical centers to the cerebral cortex
• **Descending fibers**	Connect the cerebral cortex to deeper centers
Association fibers	Connect different cortical areas within one hemisphere
Commissural fibers	Connect like cortical areas in both hemispheres (= interhemispheric association fibers)
Fornix	Special projection tract of the limbic system

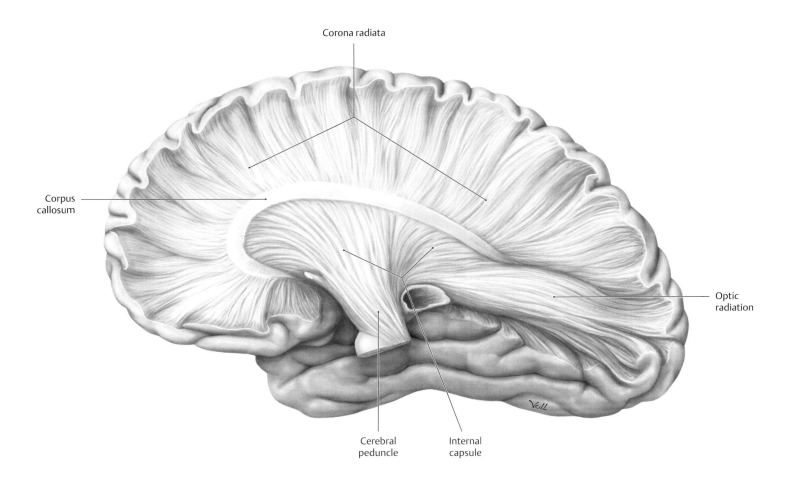

Corona radiata

Corpus callosum

Optic radiation

Cerebral peduncle

Internal capsule

B Brain specimen prepared to show the structure of the projection fibers

Medial view of the right hemisphere. This type of specimen is prepared by fixing the brain in formaldehyde and then freezing it. The gray matter, which has a high water content, is destroyed by ice-crystal formation, while the lipid-containing white matter remains relatively intact. The frozen brain is then thawed, and the tissue is dissected and teased with a spatula to bring out the fiber architecture of the white matter. The fibers represent bundled axons that pass collectively from their site of origination to their destination. Because the brain has a topographic organization, many equidirectional axons pass through the white matter as fasciculi (for the designations of different fiber types, see **A**, above). The projection fibers shown here connect the cerebral cortex to subcortical structures (e.g., basal ganglia, spinal cord). A distinction is drawn between ascending and descending fibers and their systems. In descending systems, the cell bodies of the neurons are located in the cerebral cortex and their axons terminate in subcortical structures (e.g., the corticospinal tract). In ascending systems, the neurons from subcortical structures terminate in the cerebral cortex (e.g., sensory tracts from the spinal cord).

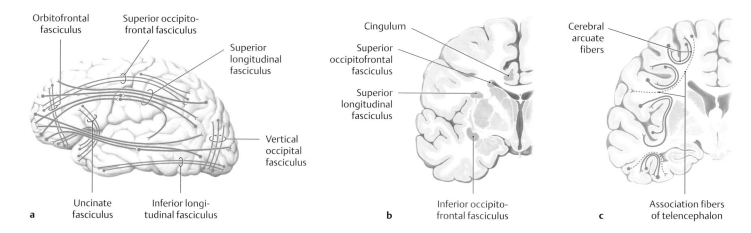

a

Orbitofrontal fasciculus
Superior occipito-frontal fasciculus
Superior longitudinal fasciculus
Vertical occipital fasciculus
Uncinate fasciculus
Inferior longitudinal fasciculus

b

Cingulum
Superior occipitofrontal fasciculus
Superior longitudinal fasciculus
Inferior occipito-frontal fasciculus

c

Cerebral arcuate fibers
Association fibers of telencephalon

C Association fibers

a Lateral view of the left hemisphere. **b** Anterior view of the right hemisphere. **c** Anterior view of short association fibers.

Long association fibers interconnect different brain areas that are located in different lobes, whereas short association fibers interconnect cortical areas within the same lobe. Adjacent cortical areas are interconnected by short, U-shaped arcuate fibers, which run just below the cortex.

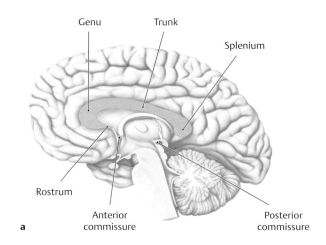

Genu
Trunk
Splenium
Rostrum
Anterior commissure
Posterior commissure

a

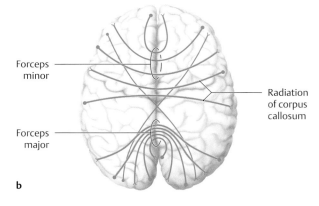

Forceps minor
Forceps major
Radiation of corpus callosum

b

D Commissural fibers

a Medial view of the right hemisphere. **b** Superior view of the transparent brain.

Commissural fibers interconnect the two hemispheres of the brain. The most important connecting structure between the hemispheres is the corpus callosum. If the corpus callosum is intentionally divided, as in a neurosurgical procedure, the two halves of the brain can no longer communicate with each other ("split-brain" patient, see p. 380). There are other, smaller commissural tracts besides the corpus callosum (anterior commissure, fornical commissure).

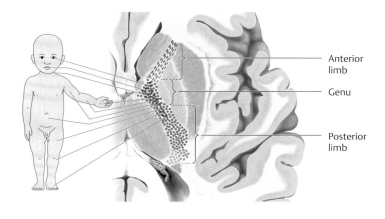

Anterior limb
Genu
Posterior limb

E Somatotopic organization of the internal capsule

Transverse section. Both ascending and descending projection fibers pass through the internal capsule. If blood flow to the internal capsule is interrupted, as by a stroke, these ascending and descending tracts undergo irreversible damage. The figure of the child shows how the sites where the pyramidal tract fibers pass through the internal capsule can be assigned to peripheral areas of the human body. Thus, we see that smaller lesions of the internal capsule may cause a loss of central innervation (= spastic paralysis) in certain areas of the body. This accounts for the great clinical importance of this structure. The internal capsule is bounded medially by the thalamus and the head of the caudate nucleus, and laterally by the globus pallidus and putamen. The internal capsule consists of an anterior limb, a genu, and a posterior limb, which are traversed by specific tracts:

Anterior limb	• Frontopontine tracts (red dashes) • Anterior thalamic peduncle (blue dashes)
Genu of internal capsule	• Corticonuclear fibers (red dots)
Posterior limb	• Corticospinal fibers (red dots) • Posterior thalamic peduncle (blue dots) • Temporopontine tract (orange dots) • Posterior thalamic peduncle (light blue dots)

377

12.27 Brain: Functional Organization

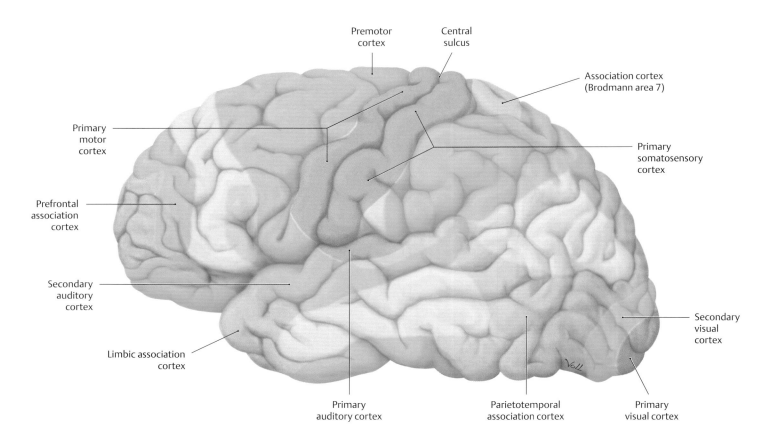

Premotor cortex

Central sulcus

Association cortex (Brodmann area 7)

Primary motor cortex

Primary somatosensory cortex

Prefrontal association cortex

Secondary auditory cortex

Secondary visual cortex

Limbic association cortex

Primary auditory cortex

Parietotemporal association cortex

Primary visual cortex

A Functional organization of the neocortex

Left lateral view. The primary sensory and motor areas are shown in red, and the areas of the association cortex are shown in different shades of green. Projection tracts begin or end, respectively, in the primary motor or sensory areas. More than 80% of the cortical surface area is association cortex, which is secondarily connected to the primary sensory or primary motor areas. The neuronal processing of differentiated behavior and intellectual performance takes place in the association cortex,

which has increased greatly in size over the course of human evolution. The functional organization pattern shown here, such as the localization of the primary motor cortex in the precentral gyrms, can be demonstrated in living subjects with modern imaging techniques. The results of such studies are illustrated in the figures below. Interestingly, the correlations described in these studies correspond reasonably well with the cortical areas defined by Brodmann.

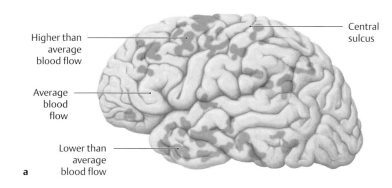

Higher than average blood flow

Central sulcus

Average blood flow

Lower than average blood flow

a

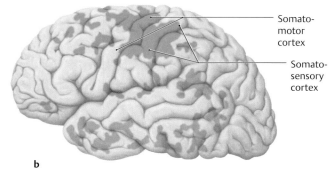

Somato-motor cortex

Somato-sensory cortex

b

B Analysis of brain function based on studies of regional cerebral blood flow

Left lateral view of the brain. When neurons are activated they consume more glucose and oxygen, which must be delivered to them via the bloodstream. This may produce a detectable increase in regional blood flow. These brain maps illustrate the local patterns of cerebral blood flow at rest (**a**) and during movement of the right hand (**b**). When the

right hand is moved, increased blood flow is recorded in the left precental gyrus, which contains the motor representation of the right hand (see motor homunculus in **B** on p. 339). Simultaneous activation is noted in the sensory cortex of the postcentral region, showing that the sensory cortex is also active during motor function (feedback loop).

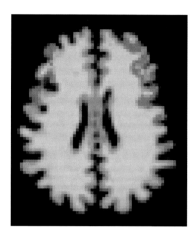

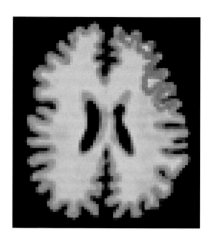

Female

Male

C Sex differences in neuronal processing
(after Stoppe, Hentschel, and Munz)
Patterns of brain activity can also be demonstrated by functional magnetic resonance imaging (fMRI). This provides a noninvasive method for investigating the metabolic activity of the brain. Because no human brain is identical to any other, a comparison of several brains will show slight variations in the distribution of specific functions. By superimposing the results of examinations in different brains, we can produce a generalized map that shows the approximate distribution of brain functions. Compare the summation map for female brains on the left with a map for male brains on the right. Both groups of subjects were given phonological tasks based on recognizing differences in the meaning of spoken sounds. While the female subjects activated both sides of their brain when solving the tasks, the male subjects activated only the left side (the sectional images are viewed from below).

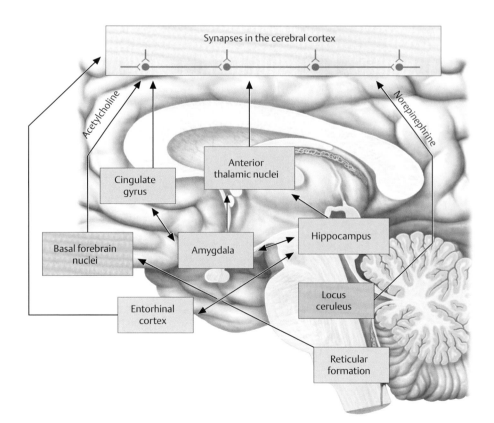

D Modulating subcortical centers
The cerebral cortex, the seat of our conscious thoughts and actions, is influenced by various subcortical centers. The parts of the limbic system that are crucial for learning and memory are indicated in light red.

12.28 Brain: Hemispheric Dominance

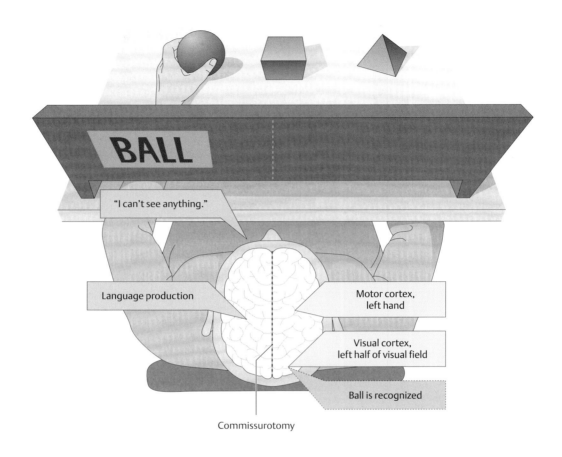

A Demonstration of hemispheric dominance for language in split-brain patients (after Klinke, Pape, and Silbernagl)

The corpus callosum is by far the most important commissural tract, interconnecting areas of like function in both hemispheres of the brain. Because lesions of the corpus callosum were once considered to have no clinical effects, surgical division of the corpus callosum was commonly performed at one time in epileptic patients to keep epileptic seizures from spreading across the brain. This operation interrupts the connections in the *upper telencephalon* while leaving intact the more deeply situated *diencephalon,* which contains the optic tract. Patients who have undergone this operation are called "split-brain patients." They have no obvious clinical abnormalities, but special neuropsychological tests reveal deficits, the study of which has improved our understanding of brain function. In one test the patient sits in front of a screen on which words are projected. Meanwhile, the patient can grasp objects behind the screen without being able to see them. When the word "Ball" is flashed briefly on the left side of the screen, the patient perceives it in the visual cortex on the right side (the optic tract has not been cut). Because language production resides in the *left* hemisphere in 97% of the population, the patient cannot verbalize the projected word out loud because communication between the hemispheres has been interrupted at the level of the telencephalon (seat of speech production). But the patient is still able to feel the ball manually and pick it out from other objects. The function of the corpus callosum is to enable both hemispheres (which can function independently to a degree) to communicate with each other when the need arises. Because of the phenomenon of hemispheric dominance, the corpus callosum in humans is more elaborately developed than in other animal species.

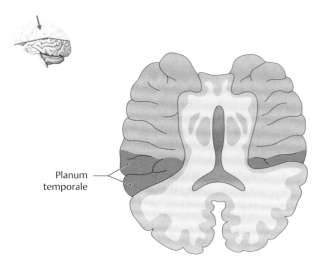

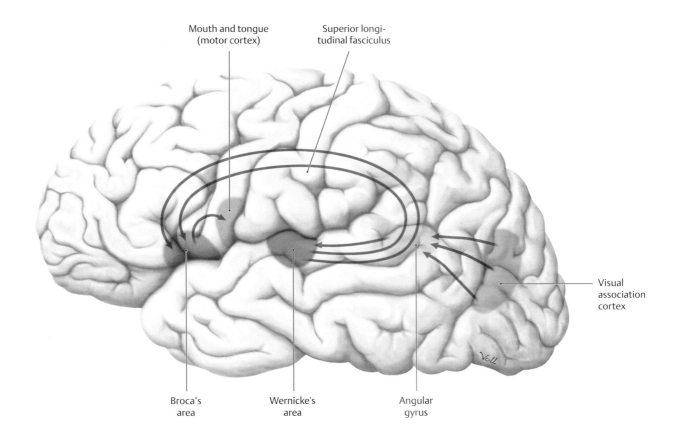

B Hemispheric asymmetry (after Klinke and Silbernagl)
Superior view of the temporal lobe of a brain that has been taken apart (i.e., the frontal lobes have been removed) along the lateral fissure. The *planum temporale,* located on the posterior and superior surface of the temporal lobe, has different contours on the two sides of the brain, being more pronounced on the left side than on the right in two-thirds of individuals. The functional significance of this asymmetry is uncertain. We cannot explain it simply by noting that Wernicke's speech area is located in that part of the temporal lobe, because while temporal asymmetry is present in only 67% of the population, the speech area is located on the left side in 97%.

C Language areas in the normally dominant left hemisphere
Lateral view. The brain contains several language areas whose loss is associated with typical clinical symptoms. *Wernicke's area* (the posterior part of area 22) is necessary for language comprehension, while *Broca's area* (area 44) is concerned with language production. The two areas are interconnected by the superior longitudinal (arcuate) fasciculus. Broca's area activates the mouth and tongue region of the motor cortex for the articulation of speech. The angular gyrus coordinates the inputs from the visual, acoustic, and somatosensory cortices and relays them onward to Wernicke's area.

12.29 Brain: Clinical Findings

The figures in this unit illustrate the correlations that have been discovered between specific brain areas and clinical findings. Studies of this kind have enabled us to link particular patterns of behavior, some abnormal, and particular clinical symptoms to specific areas in the brain.

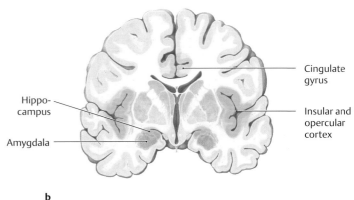

Cingulate gyrus

Hippo-campus

Insular and opercular cortex

Amygdala

b

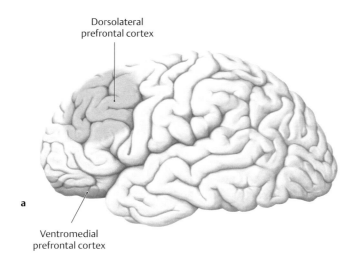

Dorsolateral prefrontal cortex

a

Ventromedial prefrontal cortex

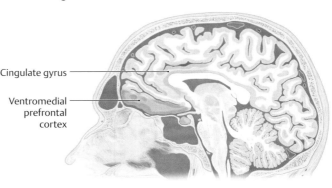

Cingulate gyrus

Ventromedial prefrontal cortex

c

A Neuroanatomy of emotions (after Braus)
a Lateral view of the left hemisphere. **b** Anterior view of a coronal section through the amygdala. **c** Midsagittal section of the right hemisphere, medial aspect.
Emotion is linked to specific regions of the brain. The ventromedial prefrontal cortex is connected primarily to the amygdaloid bodies and is believed to modulate emotion, while the dorsolateral prefrontal cortex is connected primarily to the hippocampus. This is the area of the cortex in which memories are stored along with their emotional valence. Abnormalities of this network are believed to play a role in depression.

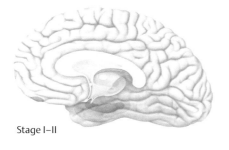

Stage I–II

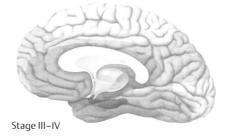

Stage III–IV

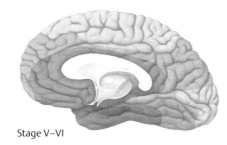

Stage V–VI

B Spread of Alzheimer's disease through the brain
(after Braak and Braak)
Medial view of the right hemisphere. Alzheimer's disease is a relentlessly progressive disease of the cerebral cortex that causes memory loss and, eventually, profound dementia. The progression of the disease can be demonstrated with special staining methods and can be divided into stages using the classification of Braak and Braak:

- Stages I–II: the appearance of the nerve cells is altered in the periphery of the entorhinal cortex (= transentorhinal region), which is considered part of the allocortex (see p. 204). These stages are still asymptomatic.

- Stages III–IV: the lesions have spread to involve the limbic system (also part of the allocortex), and initial clinical symptoms appear. These stages may be detectable by imaging studies in some cases.
- Stages V–VI: the entire isocortex is involved, and the clinical manifestations are fully developed.

Thus, the allocortex is important in brain pathophysiology as the site of origin of Alzheimer's dementia, even though it makes up only 5% of the cerebral cortex.

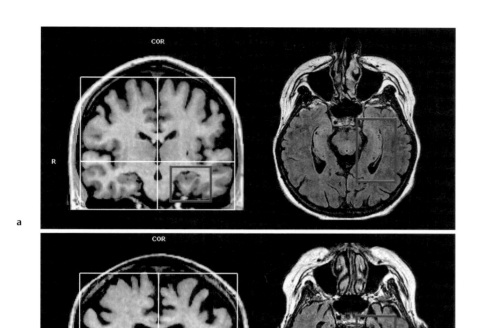

C MRI changes in the hippocampus in a patient with Alzheimer's dementia
Comparing the brain of a healthy subject (**a**) with that of a patient with Alzheimer's dementia (**b**), we notice that the latter shows atrophy of the hippocampus, a brain region that is part of the allocortex. We notice, too, that the lateral ventricles are enlarged in the patient with Alzheimer dementia (from D. F. Braus: *Ein Blick ins Gehirn.* Thieme, Stuttgart 2004).

Enlarged lateral ventricle

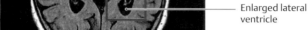

Atrophy of the hippocampus

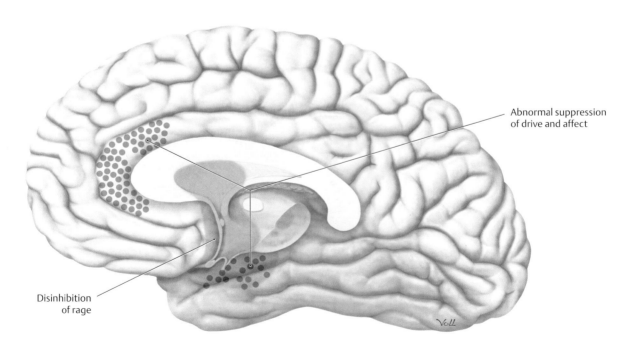

Abnormal suppression of drive and affect

Disinhibition of rage

D Lesions of certain brain areas and associated behavioral changes
(after Poeck and Hartje)
Medial view of the right hemisphere. Bilateral lesions of the medial temporal lobe and the frontal part of the cingulate gyrus (blue dots) lead to a suppression of drive and affect. This structural abnormality in the limbic system produces clinical changes that include apathy, a blank facial expression, monotone speech, and a dull, nonspontaneous mode of behavior. The condition may be caused by tumors, decreased blood flow, or trauma. On the other hand, tumors involving the septum pellucidum and hypothalamus (pink-shaded area) and certain forms of epilepsy may cause a disinhibition of anger, and the patient may respond to seemingly trivial events with attacks of "hypothalamic rage" accompanied by screaming and biting. This outburst is not directed against any particular person or object and persists for some time.

Appendix

List of References

Barr, M. L., J. A. Kiernan: The Human Nervous System, 5th ed. J. B. Lippincott, Philadelphia 1988

Bähr, M., M. Frotscher: Duus' Neurologisch-topische Diagnostik, 8. Aufl. Thieme, Stuttgart 2003

Bear, M. F., B. W. Connors, M. A. Paradiso: Neuroscience. Exploring the Brain. 2. Aufl. Williams u. Wilkins, Baltimore 2000

Braak, H., E. Braak: Neuroanatomie. In: Demenzen (hrsg. von K. Beyreuther, K. M. Einhäupl, H. Förstl und A. Kurz) Thieme, Stuttgart 2002, 118–129

Braus, D. F.: EinBlick ins Gehirn, Thieme, Stuttgart 2004

Calabria, G., M. Rolando: Strutture e funzioni del film lacrimale. Proceedings of the 6th Symposium of the Italian Ophthalmological Society (S.O.I.), Genua 1984, 9–35

Delank, H. W., W. Gehlen: Neurologie, 10. Aufl. Thieme, Stuttgart 2003

Duus, P.: Neurologisch-topische Diagnostik, 7. Aufl. Thieme, Stuttgart 2001

Faller, A., M. Schünke: Der Körper des Menschen, 14. Aufl. Thieme, Stuttgart 2004

Feneis, H., W. Dauber: Anatomisches Bildwörterbuch, 9. Aufl. Thieme, Stuttgart 2005

Frick, H., H. Leonhardt, D. Starck: Allgemeine und spezielle Anatomie. Taschenlehrbuch der gesamten Anatomie, Bd. 1 und 2, 4. Aufl. Thieme, Stuttgart 1992

Hempelmann, G., C. Krier, J. Schulte am Esch (Hrsg.): Gesamtreihe ains. 4 Bände, Thieme, Stuttgart 2001

Herrick, J. C.: Brains of Rats and Men. University of Chicago Press, Chicago 1926

Ingvar, D. H.: Functional landscapes of the dominant hemisphere. Brain Res. 107 (1976), 181–197

Jänig, W.: Visceral afferent neurones: Neuroanatomy and functions, organ regulations and sensations. In: Vaitl, D., R. Schandry (eds.): From the heart to the brain. Peter Lang, Frankfurt am Main 1995, 5–34

Kahle, W., M. Frotscher: Taschenatlas der Anatomie, Bd. 3, 9. Aufl. Thieme, Stuttgart 2005

Kell, Ch. A., K. von Kriegstein, A. Rösler, A. Kleinschmidt, H. Laufs: The Sensory Cortical Representation of the Human Penis: Revisiting Somatotopy in the Male Homunculus. J. Neurosci., Jun 2005; 25: 5984–5987

Klinke, R., S. Silbernagl: Lehrbuch der Physiologie, 3. Aufl. Thieme, Stuttgart 2001

Klinke, R., H. C. Pape, S. Silbernagl: Physiologie, 5. Aufl. Thieme, Stuttgart 2005

Kunze, K.: Lehrbuch der Neurologie. Thieme, Stuttgart 1992

Lang, G.: Augenheilkunde, 3. Aufl. Thieme, Stuttgart 2004

Lorke, D.: Schmerzrelevante Neuroanatomie. In: ains, Bd. 4, Schmerztherapie (hrsg. von H. Beck, E. Martin, J. Motsch, J. Schulte am Esch), Thieme, Stuttgart 2001, 13–28

Masuhr, K. F., M. Neumann: Neurologie, 5. Aufl. Thieme, Stuttgart 2004

Maurer, J.: Neurootologie. Thieme, Stuttgart 1999

Meyer, W: Die Zahn-Mund- und Kiefer-Heilkunde, Bd. 1, Urban & Schwarzenberg, München 1958

Mumenthaler, M., M. Stöhr, H. Müller-Vahl: Läsion peripherer Nerven und radikuläre Syndrome, 8. Aufl. Thieme, Stuttgart 2003

Nieuwenhuys, R., J. Voogd, Chr. van Huijzen: Das Zentralnervensystem des Menschen, 2. Aufl. Springer, Berlin 1991

Platzer, W.: Atlas der topografischen Anatomie. Thieme, Stuttgart 1982

Poeck, K., W. Hartje: Störungen von Antrieb und Affektivität. In: Klinische Neuropsychologie (hrsg. von W. Hartje und K. Poeck), 5. Aufl. Thieme, Stuttgart 2002, 412–422

Probst, R., G. Grevers, H. Iro: Hals-Nasen-Ohren-Heilkunde, 2. Aufl. Thieme, Stuttgart 2004

Rauber/Kopsch: Anatomie des Menschen, Bd. 1–4, Thieme, Stuttgart. Bd. 1., 2. Aufl.: 1997, Bd. 2 und 3: 1987, Bd. 4: 1988

Rohkamm. R.: Taschenatlas Neurologie, 2. Aufl. Thieme, Stuttgart 2003

Scheibel, M. E., A. B. Scheibel: Activity cycles in neurons of the reticular formation. Recent Adv Biol Psychiatry. 1965; 8: 283–93

Schmidt, F.: Zur Innervation der Articulatio temporomandibularis. Gegenbaurs morphol. Jb. 1967; 110: 554–573

Schumacher, G. H., G. Aumüller: Topographische Anatomie des Menschen, 6. Aufl. G. Fischer, 1994

Siegenthaler, W.: Klinische Pathophysiologie, 8. Aufl. Thieme, Stuttgart 2000

Stoppe, G., F. Hentschel, D. L. Munz: Bildgebende Verfahren in der Psychiatrie. Thieme, Stuttgart 2000

Tillmann, B.: Farbatlas der Anatomie Zahnmedizin-Humanmedizin. Thieme, Stuttgart 1997

von Lanz, T., W. Wachsmuth: Praktische Anatomie, Bd. 1/1B Kopf. Gehirn- und Augenschädel. Springer, Berlin 2004

Subject Index

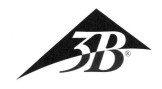

CONTACT DETAILS 3B SCIENTIFIC GROUP OF COMPANIES

HEADQUARTER
3B Scientific Hamburg
Rudorffweg 8
21031 Hamburg - Germany
Phone: +49-(0)40-739 66 0
Fax: +49-(0)40-739 66 100
E-Mail: 3b@3bscientific.com
Internet: www.3bscientific.com

UNITED KINGDOM
UK 3B Scientific
8, Beaconsfield Road
Weston-super-Mare, Somerset, BS23 1YE
Tel.: +44-(0)1934-425 333
Fax: +44-(0)1934-425 334
E-Mail: uk3bs@3bscientific.com
Internet: www.3bscientific.co.uk

USA
American 3B Scientific
2189 Flintstone Drive, Unit O, Tucker
Georgia 30084
Phone: +1-770.492.91.11
Fax: +1-770.492.01.11
E-Mail: info@a3bs.com
Internet: www.a3bs.com

ITALY
Italia 3B Scientific
Via Progresso 46
40064 Ozzano dell'Emilia (BO)
Tel.: +39-051-790 505
Fax: +39-051-469 5098
E-Mail: i3bs@3bscientific.com
Internet: www.3bscientific.it

GERMANY
3B Scientific Dresden
Heidelberger Straße 26
01189 Dresden
Tel.: +49-(0)351-403 90 0
Fax: +49-(0)351-403 90 90
E-Mail: vertrieb@3bscientific.com
Internet: www.3bscientific.de

HUNGARY
Biocalderoni
Kozma u. 9-11
1108 Budapest
Tel.: +36 1 431 09 17
Fax: +36 1 262 33 93
E-Mail: biocalderoni@biocalderoni.hu
Internet: www.biocalderoni.hu

FRANCE
France 3B Scientific
8 Rue Jean Monnet, Z.I. Parc 3
68870 Bartenheim
Téléphone : +33-(0)3 89 70 75 20
Fax : +33-(0)3 89 70 75 21
E-Mail : f3bs@3bscientific.com
Internet : www.3bscientific.fr

JAPAN
Nihon 3B Scientific
2-5-18 Sonoki
Niigata-shi, 950-1135
Tel.: +81-025-282 3228
Fax: +81-025-282 3229
E-Mail: 3b@3bs.jp
Internet: www.3bs.jp

SPAIN
España 3B Scientific
Calle Cofrentes 9
46183 Valencia
Téléphone: +34-96-2725-237
Fax: +34-96-2725-238
E-Mail: marco.polidori@3bscientific.com
Internet: www.3bscientific.es

CHINA
Suzhou 3B Scientific
45 HuoJu Road, Suzhou New District
Suzhou New District S&T Industrial Park
215009 Suzhou, Jiangsu
Phone: +86 512 6808 1123
Fax: +86 512 6825 8957
E-Mail: c3bs@3bscientific.cn
Internet: www. 3bscientific.cn

3B SCIENTIFIC —
ANATOMY
IN
3
DIMENSIONS

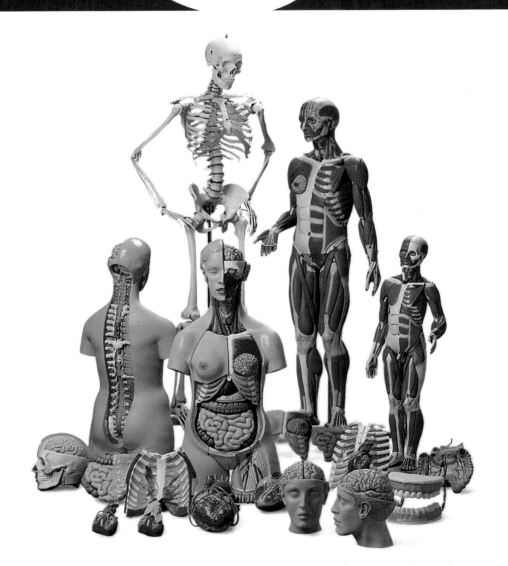